Pre-Invasive Disease: Pathogenesis and Clinical Management

Rebecca C. Fitzgerald
Editor

Pre-Invasive Disease: Pathogenesis and Clinical Management

Springer

Editor
Rebecca C. Fitzgerald
Programme Leader, MRC Cancer Cell Unit
Hutchison-MRC Research Centre
Hills Road
Cambridge CB2 0XZ
UK
rcf@hutchison-mrc.cam.ac.uk

ISBN 978-1-4419-6693-3 e-ISBN 978-1-4419-6694-0
DOI 10.1007/978-1-4419-6694-0
Springer New York Dordrecht Heidelberg London

Library of Congress Control Number: 2010936286

Cover illustration: Biopsy of Barrett's oesophagus (metaplastic oesophageal epithelium which predisposes to adenocarcinoma) stained with Alexa 555-labelled lectin called wheat germ agglutinin (WGA). Non-dysplastic areas within the biopsy demonstrate strong WGA staining of both the apical epithelial membrane and the superficial epithelial mucous globules. The superficial epithelial mucous globule staining is lost in areas of low grade dysplasia and in high grade dysplasia, this as well as the apical membrane staining is almost entirely lost. (Picture provided by Dr. Elizabeth Bird-Lieberman)

Printed on acid-free paper

Springer is part of Springer Science+Business Media (www.springer.com)

Preface

On a weekly basis, as we discuss new oesophago-gastric cancer cases within a multidisciplinary team, I am reminded of how dismal cancer is for the majority of patients. The lucky ones in whom we can achieve a cure are, generally speaking, those who present with early-stage disease.

It has been recognized for almost two centuries that pre-cancerous conditions exist, and indeed it is now known that most cancers develop over a period of years through a series of pre-invasive stages. This being the case there should be ample opportunity to intervene early in the natural history of cancer in order to improve outcomes. To do this effectively requires an understanding of the molecular and cellular basis for the disease.

Whilst the concept of early detection and prevention of cancer is an attractive one there are many questions which remain unanswered. For example, what are the causes of pre-invasive lesions, are they as a result of inherited genetic susceptibility or environmental factors, and how then can we use this information to minimize risk? At a population level, one could intervene through promotion of a healthier diet or smoking cessation programmes; at an individual level, one could implement screening programmes to identify individuals at increased risk due to pre-invasive lesions. Screening is already widely adopted for colon, cervix, and breast cancers but remains a controversial subject. It is hotly debated whether the magnitude of the risk justifies screening interventions which incur individual and societal costs, both fiscal and psychological. Once pre-invasive lesions are identified the clinician is faced with complex management decisions which might entail monitoring (surveillance), chemoprevention, or removal through endoscopic or surgical means.

There are currently exciting opportunities to revolutionise our approach to pre-invasive disease with an explosion of technological advances for understanding the cancer genome at an increasing level of detail. Clinical modalities have also progressed rapidly with the advent of new imaging and therapeutic options which incorporate knowledge of the molecular characteristics of the disease. Surgery is becoming less and less invasive and minimally invasive approaches using endoscopy and laparoscopy are ideally placed to treat small, early lesions.

Whilst cancer is widely studied and written about, pre-invasive disease has lagged behind. In addition, discourse on basic biology and clinical approaches to pre-invasive disease are seldom brought together. The purpose of this monograph is to bring together expert knowledge on this area in one volume. It has been a pleasure to bring this book to fruition, and I hope that it will be a valuable resource for all those interested in this fascinating area of research and clinical practice. Most of all I hope that it spurs us all on, as there are many unanswered questions still to be addressed.

Cambridge, UK Rebecca Fitzgerald

Foreword

Questions in the Study of Epithelial Preneoplasia

Bruce Ponder

The practical interest in preneoplasia is because it offers the possibility of diagnosis of cancer at an early, pre-invasive stage, and of successful intervention by local (endoscopy, surgery, irradiation) or systemic therapies. The preneoplastic lesion can potentially be the means to recognition of the developing cancer, to insights into mechanism and hence strategies for treatment and prevention, and to early read-out of response.

This however raises several questions, many of them still awaiting a complete answer.

The yield: what proportion of cancers with lethal potential at different sites evolve through an identifiable pre-invasive stage and so in principle could be detected and dealt with early?

The answer must be defined in terms of the methods at hand. Estimates are hard to find even though they would presumably be part of the public health decisions that underlie screening policy. For colorectal cancer, it seems that 90% or more of potentially lethal cancers are detectable at a curable stage by endoscopy; for breast cancer and mammography maybe 25% of deaths are prevented; for prostate cancer and PSA screening possibly 50%; for adenocarcinoma of the oesophagus by detection and follow-up of the Barrett's lesion, maybe 50% or fewer [1]. This is with current detection methods: can we make any estimate of which cancers have the best potential for improvement, if methods could be improved?

More sensitive detection raises a second question, the reverse side of the coin:

The trade-off: what is the potential cost of early detection in terms of over-diagnosis and over-treatment?

The prevalence, in all of us, of multiple lesions in different tissues that have morphological features of early cancer but which have very low or uncertain probability of progression to clinically significant disease, has been recognised for many years. In the context of PSA screening for early diagnosis of prostate cancer, it has been estimated that 48 men must undergo radical treatment to save one prostate cancer death [2]. CT scan-based screening for lung cancer detects many peripheral lung nodules with the morphological appearances of cancer; but the screening studies show no shift in the stage distribution of lung cancers away from the more advanced stages [3]. It was shown in the 1970s that 30% of moderate or severe dysplasia detected in cervical cancer screening regressed without treatment [4]; more recent studies show that even in patients with recognised pre-invasive lesions such as dysplasia of the bronchial epithelium or Barrett's oesophagus, the annual probability of invasive cancer is of the order of 1 in 100 or less. This implies prolonged surveillance of large groups of individuals and possibly quite significant interventions, for small yield and the possibility of inadvertent harm.

There is thus a balance to be struck between the potential costs and benefits of programmes of early detection and surveillance, which demands attention. To resolve this balance in each case requires better information about risk and to predict behaviour of each lesion. Will the new technologies of genetic analysis, applied to either lesion or normal tissue of the host, allow us to achieve this? For discussion this question can be split into three overlapping parts. The first relates to predicting the behaviour of a specific lesion, the second to the risks and behaviour of future lesions and thus to issues of intervention and surveillance, and the third to overall estimates of individual risk and thus to stratification of the population into groups at different risk and hence different potential to benefit from programmes of early detection.

Predicting the behaviour of a specific lesion and the need for intervention.

If we knew which screen-detected lesions were of clinical significance, we could match the treatment appropriately and avoid over-treatment – as for example in PSA-detected prostate cancer, described above. Pathologists have for many years used morphological criteria on tissue sections to do this: but the examples of localised breast cancer, PSA-detected prostate cancer and of Barrett's oesophagus show that, as detection methods become more sensitive and the prevalence of pre-invasive and early invasive lesions increases, these criteria are no longer sufficient. Gene expression profiling of the primary lesion has the potential to do better, as for example in breast cancer, where the subset of apparently localised cancers that have metastasised can be identified with useful sensitivity and specificity by gene expression profiling of the primary tumour. This provides optimism that molecular analysis can predict the behaviour of a single lesion. The next question is whether it can also be predictive for other lesions in the same tissue:

Can analysis of a single lesion predict the risks and behaviour of subsequent lesions within the same epithelium?

If this were so, the prediction would be useful for the design of programmes of surveillance, and of possible tissue-wide efforts at prevention. The underlying question is one of biology. The development of a cancer is thought of as the accumulation of successive stochastic genetic or epigenetic events. Are these events truly independent in multiple cancers within a single tissue, or are they to some extent determined or constrained by host factors – genetic background or exposure? If the latter, then depending upon the strength of the constraints, different lesions within an individual will tend to be similar, and the characteristics of one lesion will to some degree be predictive for others.

Evidence that such constraints exist comes from studies of inherited susceptibility. In familial breast cancer, the gene expression profiles (and estrogen receptor (ER) status) of tumours from women who carry a mutation in BRCA1, in BRCA2, or in neither gene, are different [5]. BRCA mutations are strongly predisposing, so this might be discounted as an extreme case: but characteristic molecular subtypes and ER status are also seen in the associations between common, weakly predisposing gene variants such as FGFR2 and breast cancer [6]. Specific exposures may also drive characteristic patterns of altered gene expression: for example the changes in the airway epithelium in response to cigarette smoke [7].

In principle, then, multiple lesions within a single epithelium are likely to be more similar, because of host factors, than lesions from different individuals. This similarity may be even greater if the lesions have arisen from within the same extended mutant clone, and so share some of the initial events. Whether and in what circumstances these effects are strong enough to provide clinically useful predictors is for empirical test. Formal data are hand to find, but current clinical practice suggests that these circumstances are few.

If such constraints exist, they will presumably be mediated through, or reflected in, the molecular and cellular phenotype of the cognate normal epithelium – the "soil" in which the malignancies arise. This leads to the final question:

Can analysis of the apparently normal tissue from which the cancer will arise provide a prediction of future cancer risk (and possibly behaviour)?

If this were so the prediction would have important applications in stratification of the population in terms of risk, and thus in terms of the cost/benefit balance of entry into programmes of early detection. If the prediction were not just of risk of cancer, but of risk of clinically significant cancer, the application would be even greater.

The factors that will differ between individuals and which can be expected to influence risks of cancer and cancer type are, broadly, individual genetic make-up and exposure. What is the potential size of these effects and how can they be measured?

The majority of strongly predisposing genes for cancer have been identified, but these account for under 5% of overall cancer incidence. For most of the common cancers (e.g. breast, prostate, lung) some 70% of the estimated inherited cancer risk is still unexplained. This 70% is thought to be made up of probably hundreds of common and rare genetic variants, each of small effect, but in combination these may be potentially very significant in terms of distribution of risk in the population, and hence in terms of application to the stratification of risk. Imagine these normal genetic variants dealt out at conception like a hand of cards: it has been estimated that for breast cancer the 20% of women with the "worst" hand will have on average a 30–40-fold greater risk than the 20% with the "best" hand [8]. This means that half of all breast cancers will occur in the 12% of women at greatest [genetic] risk. As noted above, some of these variants increase the risk of different molecular subtypes of breast cancer more than others; and it is possible that they may also influence aggressiveness and outcome.

Most environmental exposures are difficult to quantify. Smoking is relatively easy because it is a well-defined behaviour that can be measured in pack-years of exposure reaching back many years, and so is UV damage resulting in sunburn; but accurate dietary history is notoriously difficult to obtain even in the present, let alone after the lapse of many years. Even if data on exposures and genetics were available, the multiple interactions between the hundreds of components would present a daunting problem.

An interesting possibility, so far not widely explored, is that the history of these genetic effects and exposure and their many interactions, in so far as it impinges on cancer risk and behaviour, should be written in an integrated form in the tissue from which the cancers will arise. (This is not to exclude direct effects on the emerging cancer: but many of these, for example differences in DNA repair, or immune or paracrine effects may also be written in the uninvolved tissue).

Following this idea, cancer – and other diseases such as diabetes – can be thought of as "an emergent property of a regulatory network" [9]: a gene regulatory network which can be perturbed by inherited or somatic mutation, normal genetic variation, or causes external to the tissue (for example hormones, or external exposures and the damage resulting from them). If this is correct, gene expression profiles of uninvolved tissue would be expected to differ between individuals, and it might be possible using the training set/validation set approach that has been extensively applied to cancer tissues to define subsets of those cancers, also to define patterns in the uninvolved tissue that are predictive of the risk of cancer. There are obvious pitfalls to be avoided, for example the possibility of sampling emergent altered clones that are not representative: but there are already several reports suggesting that this approach might work. They include a series of papers (e.g. 10) by Spira and colleagues on the patterns of gene expression in bronchial and upper airway epithelium, showing a similar signature of smoking, but different signatures in smokers with and without lung cancer; and publications reporting on a variety of phenotypic measures in colorectal mucosa and their association with the presence of polyps [11, 12]. Further prospective validation of these potential predictors is however required.

Schadt and others [13] have taken the analysis a step further to the definition of specific gene regulatory networks, and putative functional molecules within them. Others have defined gene expression profiles in terms of signatures of the activities of different signalling pathways [14]. Kopelovich [15] pointed out a decade ago the potential of using accessible tissues as surrogates for tissues difficult to access (for example, oral or nasal epithelium for bronchus), an important concept that also requires further validation.

Summary

Setting aside practical issues of access to certain tissues, the challenges that currently threaten to limit the use of preneoplasias as a route to cancer prevention, are about the balance of cost and benefit. The costs are in terms of resources and false positive diagnosis, when screening for preneoplasias at the population level; and in terms of over-treatment by interventions for lesions only a minority of which will progress to clinically significant disease. The commonly used multi-stage process of screening, combining sensitivity with increasing levels of specificity, recognises this. Careful phenotyping of the epithelium from which the lesions arise, as well as analysis of the lesions themselves, may allow us to refine and improve this process.

References

1. Reid BJ et al (2010) Barrett's oesophagus and oesophageal adenocarcinoma: time for a new synthesis. Nat Rev Cancer 10:87–101
2. Schroeder FH et al (2009) Screening and Prostate-Cancer Mortality in a Randomized European Study. New Engl J Med 360:1320–1328
3. Bach PB (2008) Is our natural history model of lung cancer wrong? Lancet Oncology 9:693–697
4. Spriggs AI (1971) Follow-up of untreated carcinoma-in-situ of cervix uteri. Lancet ii:599–600
5. Hedenfalk I et al (2001) Gene expression profiles in hereditary breast cancer. New Engl J Med 344:539–548
6. Garcia-Closas M et al (2008) Heterogeneity of breast cancer associations with five susceptibility loci by clinical and pathological characteristics. PLOS Genetics 4:e1000054
7. Sridhar S et al (2008) Smoking-induced gene expression changes in the bronchial airway are reflected in nasal and buccal epithelium. BMC Genomics 9:259–272
8. Pharoah PDP et al (2002) Polygenic susceptibility to breast cancer and implications for prevention. Nat Genet 31:33–36
9. Chen Y et al (2008) Variations in DNA elucidate molecular networks that cause disease. Nature 452:429–435
10. Spira A et al (2007) Airway epithelial gene expression in the diagnostic evaluation of smokers with suspect lung cancer. Nat Med 13:361–366
11. Roy HK et al (2009) Association between Rectal Optical Signatures and Colonic Neoplasia: Potential Applications for Screening. Cancer Res 69:4476–4483
12. Chen L-C et al (2004) Alteration of Gene Expression in Normal-Appearing Colon Mucosa of *APCmin* Mice and Human Cancer Patients. Cancer Res 64:3694–3700
13. Emilsson V et al (2008) Genetics of gene expression and its effect on disease. Nature 452:423–428
14. Bild AH et al (2006) Oncogenic pathway signatures in human cancers as a guide to targeted therapies. Nature 439:353–357
15. Kopelovich L et al (1999) Surrogate Anatomic/Functional Sites for Evaluating Cancer Risk: An Extension of the Field Effect. Clin Cancer Res 5:3899–3905

Contents

Contributors

Craig D. Allred
Department of Pathology and Immunology, Washington University
School of Medicine, 660 South Euclid Avenue, Campus Box 8118,
St. Louis, MO 63110, USA
dcallred@path.wustl.edu

Fran Balkwill
Centre for Cancer and Inflammation, Institute of Cancer, Barts and The London
School of Medicine and Dentistry, Queen Mary University of London,
Charterhouse Square, London EC1M 6BQ, UK
f.balkwill@qmul.ac.uk

Anindo K. Banerjee
Consultant Respiratory Physician, Southampton General Hospital,
Southampton, UK

Michael Baudis
Institute of Molecular Biology, University of Zurich, Switzerland

Ornella Belvedere
Leeds Institute of Molecular Medicine,
University of Leeds, St. James's University Hospital,
Bekett Street, LS9 7TF, Leeds, UK
ornella.belvedere@gmail.com

Maria Antonia Bianco
Gastroenterology Units, Hospital A. Maresca of Torre del Greco, Italy

Jane M. Blazeby
Department of Social Medicine, University of Bristol, Bristol, UK;
Division of Surgery, Head & Neck, University Hospitals Bristol NHS Foundation
Trust, Bristol, BS2 8HW, UK
J.M.Blazeby@bristol.ac.uk

Alexander D. Borowsky
Department of Pathology and Laboratory Medicine, Center for Comparative Pathology, University of California, School of Medicine, 95616, Davis, California, USA

Alex Boussioutas
Cancer Genomics and Predictive Medicine, Peter MacCallum Cancer Centre East Melbourne 3002, Australia
Department of Medicine RMH/WH, University of Melbourne, Western Hospital, Footscray 3011, Australia
alexb@unimelb.edu.au

Kevin M. Brindle
Cancer Research UK, Cambridge Research Institute, Li Ka Shing Centre, Robin way, Cambridge CB2 ORE, UK and Department of Biochemistry, University of Cambridge, Tennis Court Road, Cambridge CB2 1GA, UK
kmb 1001@cam.ac.uk

John P. Brown
Research Oncology, Division of Cancer Studies, King's College London, 3rd Floor, Bermondsey Wing, Guy's Hospital, Great Maze Pond SE1 9RT, London, UK

Federico Buffoli
Gastroenterology Units, Hospital of Cremona Cremona, Italy

Rita A. Busuttil
Cancer Genomics and Predictive Medicine, Peter MacCallum Cancer Centre, East Melbourne 3002, Australia

Robert D. Cardiff
Department of Pathology and Laboratory Medicine, Center for Comparative Pathology, University of California, Davis, School of Medicine, Davis, CA 95616, USA

Elisa Cattaneo
Institute of Molecular Cancer Research, University of Zurich, Switzerland

Wen-Chung Chen
Departments of Pathology, The Johns Hopkins Medical Institutions, Baltimore, MD 21231, USA

Stefan David
Department of Gastroenterology, Johns Hopkins School of Medicine, Baltimore, MD, USA
Sdavida@jhmi.edu

Mark Eveleigh
Department of Social Medicine, University of Bristol, Bristol, UK

Rebecca Fitzgerald
MRC Cancer Cell Unit, Hutchison-MRC Research Centre, Hills Road
CB22 0XZ, Cambridge, UK
rcf@hutchison-mrc.cam.ac.uk

Jean Marie Houghton
Department of Cancer Biology, University of Massachusetts Medical School,
LRB 2nd floor 209, 364 Plantation street, Worcester, MA 01635, USA
jeanmarie.houghton@umassmed.edu

Richard A. Hubner
Specialist Registrar, Department of Medicine,
Royal Marsden Hospital, London, UK
richard.hubner@icr.ac.uk

S. Y. Catherine Kang
Department of Cancer Control Research, British Columbia Cancer Agency
Research Centre, University of British Columbia, Vancouver BC, Canada and
Department of Biomedical Physiology and Kinesiology, Simon Fraser University,
Burnaby, BC, Canada

Kareem M. Shariff
Cancer Cell Unit, Hutchison-MRC Research Centre, CB22 OXZ,
Cambridge, UK

Evelyn Kurt-Jones
Department of Medicine, University of Massachusetts Medical School,
Worcester, MA 01635, USA

Alastair D. Lamb
CRUK Cambridge Research Institute, Addenbrooke's Hospital,
University Department of Uro-Oncology,
Cambridge CB2 0QQ, Cambridge, UK
alastair.lamb@cancer.org.uk

Scott K. Lyons
Cancer Research UK, Cambridge Research Institute,
Li Ka Shing Centre, Robinson way, Cambridge CB2 ORE, UK and
Department of Biochemistry, University of Cambridge, Tennis Court Road,
Cambridge CB2 1GA, UK

Barbara Ma
Department of Pathology, The Johns Hopkins School of Medicine,
Baltimore, MD
21231, USA

Calum E. MacAulay
Integrative Oncology, British Columbia Cancer Agency Research Centre, University of British Columbia, Vancouver, BC, Canada

Anirban Maitra
The Sol Goldman Pancreatic Cancer Research Center, Johns Hopkins University School of Medicine, 1550 Orleans Street, CRB-2, Suite 345, 21231, Baltimore, MD, USA
amaitra1@jhmi.edu

Carlo C. Maley
Molecular and Cellular Oncogenesis Program, The Wistar Institute, 3600 Spruce St., Philadelphia, PA 19104, USA
cmaley@alum.mit.edu

Chih-Ping Mao
Departments of Pathology, The Johns Hopkins School of Medicine, Baltimore, MD 21231, USA

Giancarlo Marra
Institute of Molecular Cancer Research, University of Zurich, Winterthurerstrasse 190, 8057 Zurich, Switzerland
marra@imcr.uzh.ch

Hanno Matthaei
The Sol Goldman Pancreatic Cancer Research Center, Johns Hopkins University School of Medicine, 1550 Orleans Street, CRB-2, Suite 345, 21231, Baltimore, MD, USA;

Stephen J. Meltzer
Department of Gastroenterology, Johns Hopkins School of Medicine, Baltimore, MD, USA;
The Sidney Kimmel Comprehensive Cancer Center, Baltimore, MD 21231, USA

David E. Neal
CRUK Cambridge Research Institute, Addenbrooke's Hospital, Cambridge, CB2 0QQ, UK
den22@cam.ac.uk

Paul D. P. Pharoah
Departments of Oncology and Public Health and Primary Care, University of Cambridge, Cambridge CB1 8RN, UK
paul.pharoah@srl.cam.ac.uk

Pierre Lao-Sirieix
Cancer Cell Unit, Hutchison-MRC Research Centre, Cambridge CB22 0XZ, UK
pss@hutchison-mrc.cam.ac.uk

Sarah E. Pinder
Professor of Breast Pathology, Research Oncology,
Division of Cancer Studies, King's College London, 3rd Floor,
Bermondsey Wing, Guy's Hospital, Great Maze Pond, SE1 9RT, London, UK
sarah.pinder@kcl.ac.uk

Catherine F. Poh
Integrative Oncology, British Columbia Cancer Agency Research Centre,
University of British Columbia, Vancouver, BC, Canada
Faculty of Dentistry, University of British Columbia, Vancouver, BC, Canada

John D. Potter
Division of Public Health Sciences,
Fred Hutchinson Cancer Research Center,
1100 Fairview Avenue North, PO Box 19024, Seattle, WA 98109-1024, USA
jpotter@fhcrc.org

Shelley Potter
Department of Social Medicine, University of Bristol, Bristol, UK;
Division of Surgery, Head & Neck, University Hospitals Bristol NHS
Foundation Trust, BS2 8HW, Bristol, UK

Pamela Rabbitts
Professor of Experimental Respiratory Research,
Leeds Institute of Molecular Medicine, University of Leeds, UK

Brian J. Reid
Divisions of Human Biology and Public Health Sciences, Fred Hutchinson
Cancer Research Center, P.O. Box 19024, Seattle, WA 98109, USA;
Departments of Medicine and Genome Sciences, University of Washington,
Seattle, WA 98195, USA

Miriam P. Rosin
BC Oral Cancer Prevention Program, British Columbia Cancer Agency
Research Centre, 675 West 10th Avenue, Vancouver BC, Canada
mrosin@bccrc.ca

Souzan Sanati
Department of Pathology and Immunology, Washington University School
of Medicine, 660 South Euclid Avenue, Campus Box 8118, St. Louis, MO 63110,
USA

Eva Szabo
Lung and Upper Aerodigestive Cancer Research Group, Division of Cancer
Prevention, National Cancer Institute, National Institutes of Health,
6130 Executive Blvd., Rm 2132, Bethesda, MD 20892, USA

Namasivayam Vikneswaran
Division of Gastroenterology and Hepotology, Mayo Clinic, 200 2nd SW
Rochester, MN, 55905, USA

Kenneth K. Wang
Division of Gastroenterology and Hepatology, Mayo Clinic,
200 2nd St SW, Rochester, MN 55905, USA
wang.kenneth@mayo.edu

Anne Y. Warren
Addenbrooke's Hospital, University Department of Pathology,
Cambridge, CB2 0QQ, UK
anne.warren@nhs.net

Robert N. Whistance
Department of Social Medicine, University of Bristol, Bristol, UK;
Division of Surgery, Head & Neck, University Hospitals Bristol NHS Foundation Trust, Bristol, BS2 8HW, UK

Nicholas A. Wright
Histopathology Lab, Cancer Research UK, 44, Lincoln's Inn Fields,
London WC2A 3PX, UK;
The Blizard Institute of Cell and Molecular Science, Barts and the London School of Medicine and Dentistry, Queen Mary University of London, Mile End Road, London, UK
warden@qmul.ac.uk

T-C Wu
Department of Pathology, The Johns Hopkins Medical Institutions,
Cancer Research Building II, Room 309, 1550 Orleans Street,
Baltimore, MD, USA; Department of Obstetrics and Gynecology, The Johns Hopkins Medical Institutions, Baltimore, MD, USA;
Department Molecular Microbiology and Immunology, The Johns Hopkins Medical Institutions, Orleans Street, Baltimore, MD, USA;
Department of Oncology, The Johns Hopkins Medical Institutions, Baltimore, MD, USA
wutc@jhmi.edu

Lewei Zhang
Faculty of Dentistry, University of British Columbia, Vancouver, BC, Canada

Fausto Zorzi
Department of Pathology, Poliambulanza Hospital, Brescia, Italy

Part I
Pathogenesis

Chapter 1
Stem Cells in Intraepithelial Neoplasia

Nicholas A. Wright

Abstract Tumours are thought to contain a subpopulation of self-renewing stem cells, the so-called *cancer stem cells*, which maintain the tumour. Moreover, tumours themselves are thought to arise from *organ-specific stem cells*. In epithelia, transformation of these cells leads to spread of a *mutated stem cell clone* through the epithelial sheet, leading to the development of a *pre-invasive lesion.* Barrett's oesophagus is used as an example of the role of stem cells in the development of such a pre-invasive lesion. This is an intriguing condition where the stratified squamous epithelium of the lower oesophagus is replaced with a metaplastic epithelium, which usually shows goblet cell-containing crypts. A similar metaplasia occurs in the stomach in chronic atrophic gastritis. In both cases these epithelial fields can becomes genetically unstable and develop a considerable mutation burden, including mutations in important tumour-suppressor genes, setting in motion the so-called metaplasia/dysplasia/carcinoma sequence. There has long been argument about the nature of this metaplasia, but in the stomach we have shown that it represents a clonal proliferation and arises through a process of *monoclonal conversion* from gastric stem cells to the intestinal phenotype in individual gastric glands. We have further shown clonal spread of the metaplastic process within the epithelium, mediated through the mechanism of crypt fission. In Barrett's mucosa however, we have shown that the mucosa is composed of numbers of discrete mutated clones, all of which may compete, providing a stimulus for clonal progression and thus malignant change. We also propose that the origin of these multiple clones is from stem cells in the ducts of the oesophageal glands found in the lower oesophagus.

N.A. Wright (✉)
Histopathology Lab, Cancer Research UK, 44, Lincoln's Inn Fields, London WC2A 3PX, UK
and
The Blizard Institute of Cell and Molecular Science, Barts and the London School of Medicine and Dentistry, Queen Mary University of London, Mile End Road, London, UK
e-mail: warden@qmul.ac.uk

R.C. Fitzgerald (ed.), *Pre-Invasive Disease: Pathogenesis and Clinical Management*,
DOI 10.1007/978-1-4419-6694-0_1,

Introduction

There is a now a growing appreciation that tumours contain a subpopulation of self-renewing stem cells, the so-called *cancer stem cells*, held to be responsible for maintaining the tumour and for the development of a hierarchy of proliferating and differentiating cells which are claimed – by their proponents – to be responsible for the well-recognised phenomenon of tumour heterogeneity (see for example [1]). At the same time it is now widely accepted that tumours arise as a result of a series of mutations occurring in an appropriate cell. In the colonic epithelium, for example, many of the mutations necessary for malignant progression have been identified. A shibboleth of modern tumour biology is that such a series of mutations accumulates in a *single cell*: this single cell, through mutation and selection, acquires properties which endow it with characteristics which ensure it's growth and survival as a *mutant clone*, which then undergoes a series of divisions which results in the development of a neoplasm. Similar series of molecular events is envisioned for the development of other epithelial tumours – for example the lung, the stomach and the skin [2]. This immediately raises the problem of the identification of these important cells. There is a growing school of thought, which proposes that such cells are the *organ-specific stem cells*.

Once established within the epithelium, a mechanism must exist for the growth and propagation of the mutant clone within the epithelium. This can occur by the accumulation of a discrete mass of such transformed cells within the epithelium, sometimes termed an *adenoma* in tissues such as the colon, stomach or skin. Perhaps more commonly there is diffuse spread of a mutated clone through the epithelium, often over considerable distances. This is usually often accompanied by morphological changes of malignancy, termed *dysplasia*, and accompanies conditions such as ulcerative colitis in the colon, squamous metaplasia in the bronchus, actinic keratosis in the skin, ductal carcinoma in situ (DCIS) in the breast, pancreatic intra-epithelial neoplasia (PIN) in the pancreas and is also thought to occur in Barrett's oesophagus. These are the pre-invasive lesions, and it is a general rule that all epithelial tumours go through such a stage before invading into the subjacent stroma and metastasising.

It is the purpose of this chapter to examine some of the recent evidence for this proposal that tumours arise from epithelial organ-specific stem cells, and to use the example of the phenomenon of intestinal metaplasia – widely accepted as the precursor lesion for dysplasia in the stomach and in Barrett's oesophagus – for an in-depth look at the role of stem cells in the development of the pre-invasive lesion which leads to Barrett's carcinoma.

The Stem Cell Origin of Cancer

It is an interesting proposal that all tumours arise from stem cells. This chapter will address this concept with special reference to pre-invasive disease, a common feature of most, if not all, epithelial cancers. So, why do we propose that all such tumours originate in a stem cell or stem cells? This is usually explained on two major counts: firstly they possess the self-renewal mechanisms required for the maintenance and expansion of stem cell numbers, and secondly particularly in renewing populations such as the gut and skin, stem cells are thought to be located in a *stem cell niche* in which they stay, maintaining their numbers by asymmetric cell division, which provides the requisite time for the acquisition of further mutations. Daughter cells are lost relatively quickly from the population, and might not be thought to linger long enough to accumulate the necessary mutation burden required for transformation.

An excellent example of this is seen in the intestine, where the pre-invasive lesion is the *adenoma*: it has been known for many years that most carcinomas in the intestine originate in the adenoma – the so-called *adenoma: carcinoma sequence* (see [3] for review). Thus, in mouse small intestine there is both a stem cell compartment at about 4–5 cell positions from the base, thought to be slowly cycling [4] together with a rapidly cycling stem cell compartment composed of slender cells – the crypt base columnar cells sited between the Paneth cells at the base of the crypt [5]. This is usually regarded as the intestinal stem cell niche, considered to be a privileged site where stem cells derive – from their daughter cells – all lineages within the tissue, maintaining their own numbers by asymmetric division. Genetic lineage tracking techniques show that at cell position 4–5 cells the cells express Bmi1, and knocking in a tamoxifen-inducible *Cre* into the *Bmi1* locus in Bmi1Cre-ER/+; Rosa26LacZ/+ mice gave clones containing all intestinal lineages – thus the cells are *multipotential*. The crypt base columnar cells express the *Wnt* target gene *Lgr5* but are also multipotential, shown by an inducible *Cre* knock-in allele in the *Lgr5* locus crossed with the Cre-activatable RosalacZ reporter [5]. That these cells are the origin to adenomas was shown by targeted deletion of *Apc* in the *Lrg5*-expressing crypt base columnar cells (using *Lgr5*-EGFP-creERT2/*Apc*flox/flox mice), which gives rapidly growing adenomas. However, and importantly, deletion of *Apc* in the dividing transit or amplifying cells found higher in the crypt (using Ah-cre/Rosa26R/ *Apc*flox/flox mice) produced no adenomas [6]. *Thus underlines the importance of having the mutation in the stem cell population.* In fact, Lgr5 expression in mice overlaps with prominin 1 (CD133) expression, and induction of Wnt signaling in these cells with a Cre-dependent mutant allele of β-catenin (Ctnnb1lox (ex3)) showed origin of the adenomas from prominin 1-positive cells [7]. In both these models established colonic and small intestinal adenomas contained about 6.5% of Lgr5-positive cells, and interestingly the frequency of prominin 1-positive cells in the adenomas at 7% was the same.

However, stem cells at positions 4–5 can also apparently initiate intestinal tumours: it is here that Wip1 phosphatase, an enzyme that inhibits the DNA damage response, is located in cells at this position. *ApcMin/+/Wip1*-null mice have a severely reduced adenoma burdens, mediated by p53-dependent apoptosis of stem cells [8]. Loss of CD44 will also reduce adenoma burden in *Apc/Min/+* mice, possibly through increased apoptosis of initiated cells, since CD44 is putatively expressed only by the crypt base columnar cells and early transit amplifying cells, and hence the cells that presumably start adenoma formation [9].

In the prostate, it was generally accepted that tumours arise from the androgen receptor-negative basal cells [10]. Inhibition of androgen actions does not reduce the clonogenicity in prostatic cancer cell lines but the size of the colonies was reduced, suggesting that androgen-independent self-renewal of cells with stem cell properties occurs, but that transit amplifying cells were androgen-dependent [11]. However, it has been reported that in human prostate cancer cell lines the CD133+ tumour propagating cells are positive for androgen receptor, indicating an origin from luminal cells [12] Returning to the mouse, after castration a very small (<1%) population of luminal cells, which are castration-resistant, express the Nkx3-1 homeodomain-containing transcription factor. The properties of these cells include self-renewal and bipotential differentiation capacity: when androgen is given to mice with targeted deletion of *Pten* in these cells, prostatic intraepithelial neoplasia is seen with microinvasion [13]. Consequently, the prostate may contain two distinct target cells for tumour initiation: since basal cells are absent from prostatic adenocarcinoma, a luminal origin would be consistent with these observations.

In the breast also, there may be more than one cell type from which cancer develops. Many breast cancers are believed to have their origins in undifferentiated oestrogen receptor (ER)-negative multipotential stem cells, but in basal-like breast cancers, gene expression profiling suggests that they originate from luminal progenitors. Moreover luminal progenitors are expanded in preneoplastic tissue from BRCA1 mutation carriers [14]. Furthermore, in the testis, pluripotent germ cell tumours (teratomas) are thought to arise from the maturation arrest of foetal germ cells or gonocytes – cells bearing a close resemblance to the likely probable precursor lesion, carcinoma in situ (CIS) of the testis [15].

The liver is thought to have two distinct (stem) cell populations, which can give rise to hepatocellular carcinoma. A derivation of this tumour from hepatocytes has been suggested in several animal models of hepatocellular carcinoma, since transgenes, which induce such tumours, can be conveniently driven by the albumin promoter. But hepatic progenitor cells (HPCs) originate from a so-called *facultative stem cell compartment*, thought to be derived from small biliary ductules, which proliferate in response to chronic liver damage such as cirrhosis. In most incidences, cirrhosis is itself the usual precursor lesion of hepatocellular carcinoma. This makes these cells probable carcinogen target cells [16]. Thus should tumours arise from HPCs, then there could be a block in stem cell differentiation, so-called 'stem cell maturation arrest'. In this respect it has been suggested that there are four subtypes of hepatocellular carcinoma, which corresponds to a hierarchy of liver cell lineages [17]. It is interesting to note that those patients with the poorest prognosis show a larger fraction of either EpCAM+/AFP+ cells (which show the features of embryonic hepatoblasts) or EpCAM–/AFP+ cells which are HPC-like: however, patients with EpCAM–/AFP– cells – resembling mature hepatocytes or EpCAM+/AFP– cells – cholangiocyte-like – had a more favourable outcome. Gene expression profiling has also revealed a subset of HCCs, which share a poor prognosis, which also have a profile suggesting an origin from HPCs [18]. When these tumours are divided into categories with high and low expression of the HPC marker CK19–, a group of patients can be recognised who experience a shorter time to recurrence [19].

There are several different histological types of lung cancer, in addition to which many show a mixed phenotype. This heterogeneity, often said to be related to their anatomical location within the lung, may reflect of region-specific variations in the stem cell composition of the tracheobronchial tree [20]. These stem cells may occupy a so-called *pro-oncogenic stem cell niche*: there are mouse models where global knock-down of a tumour suppressor gene such as p53 has been achieved – or indeed up-regulation of an oncogene regulated by a lung-specific promoter which is widely expressed in the lung. This produces a phenomenon called in humans *field cancerization*, where the same pro-oncogenic genetic change is found over large areas of the tracheobronchial epithelium. Such a situation was described by Franklin et al. [21], where the same p53 mutation was found throughout the tracheobronchial epithelium of a smoker. Nevertheless, although *k-ras* mutations are often seem in human non-small cell lung cancer [22], mouse models with widespread *k-ras* mutations give rise only to bronchioalveolar adenocarcinomas [23]. This is possibly due to the induction of self-renewing, multipotent bronchioalveolar stem cells (BASCs) which are found at the bronchioalveolar duct junction [24]. Human small cell lung cancers usually arise from mid-level bronchioles where the neuroendocrine precursors are found, but squamous cell carcinomas originate in the proximal major bronchi, possibly developing from CK14-positive basal cells located in the submucosal gland ducts or the inter-cartilaginous boundaries [25].

Stem Cells in the Development of Intestinal Metaplasia and Barrett's Oesophagus

I shall now explore in more detail the possible role of stem cells in the initiation and progression of a relatively common pre-invasive lesion – Barrett's oesophagus, widely-regarded as the precursor of oesophageal adenocarcinoma. Carcinoma of the oesophagus is one of the sixth leading causes of deaths from cancer in men in the Western World, and increasing in incidence. While squamous cell carcinoma arises from the stratified squamous oesophageal epithelium, it is the *adenocarcinoma*, which is known to arise in a fascinating lesion called *Barrett's esophagus*, which is responsible for the increase in interest in carcinoma of the oesophagus. The English surgeon Norman Barrett first brought this condition to prominence: Barrett's oesophagus is the replacement of the normal oesophageal stratified squamous epithelium with metaplastic glandular epithelium in response to inflammation and ulceration. It is probably provoked by duodeno-gastroesophageal reflux, with chronic exposure to acid and bile, which causes damage and inflammation in the oesophageal squamous epithelium.

The diagnosis of Barrett's depends on endoscopic examination with biopsy and the recognition of characteristic histological appearances is required. These usually include the appearance of a metaplastic epithelium very dissimilar from the stratified squamous epithelium of the native oesophagus, in which many as essential for the diagnosis regard the presence of mucin-secreting goblet cells. It is from this metaplastic epithelium which oesophageal adenocarcinoma can arise from progression through a *metaplasia–dysplasia–carcinoma* sequence. The presence of Barrett's oesophagus increases the risk of oesophageal adenocarcinoma by 30–40% [26].

Management of Barrett's oesophagus consists of treating the reflux, and controversially by surveillance for the early detection of carcinoma. Treatment consists of medications such as proton pump inhibitors, which reduce acid output, or by anti-reflux surgery.

In the prediction of malignancy, the histological grade of dysplasia is usually been used to assess the probability of progression towards malignancy. Lesions are graded variously as negative for dysplasia, indefinite for dysplasia, low-grade dysplasia, high-grade dysplasia or carcinoma. There is no degree of certainty in this process, since while some grades do indeed progress, others regress, and some lesions can remain stable for many years. Moreover, histological interpretation shows considerable inter- and intra-observer variation [27].

Aspects of Molecular Changes in Barrett's Oesophagus

Invaluable information has been derived from taking serial biopsies from cohorts of patients with Barrett's oesophagus and subjecting them to molecular analysis. In this way the evolution of mutations common tumour suppressor genes throughout the progression of the metaplasia/dysplasia/carcinoma sequence. Two of the most important genes are the cyclin-dependent kinase N2 (p16) and TP53 (p53) tumour suppressor genes: inactivation of these genes occurs early in the metaplasia/dysplasia/carcinoma sequence [28] – as many as 88% of Barrett's patient's without dysplasia show a p16 lesion [29]. Similar studies showed that clonal p16 and p53 lesions were seen throughout long segments of Barrett's oesophagus [28,30] has led to the proposal that there exists a precursor cell or cells that expands in a *clonal* manner, with the important prediction that there has to be *a founder mutation* which is maintained in all descendant cells. This is indeed a useful way of looking at the clonal expansion of cells with mutations: a basic premise of this idea is the concept that Barrett's – or a mutated cell in any other genetically unstable epithelial field progresses as a consequence of sequential tumour suppressor gene inactivation which causes a selective growth advantage. This leads to the establishment of the mutated cell and its direct descendants – a *mutant clone*. Consequent to this there is preferential expansion of this mutated clone. When the mutation has expanded throughout an entire field, extinguishing all competing clones, it is said to have 'gone to fixation' (see Fig. 1.1). The process by which this occurs is thought to be natural selection acting through the selective advantage possessed by the clone, driving a mutation to fixation and is

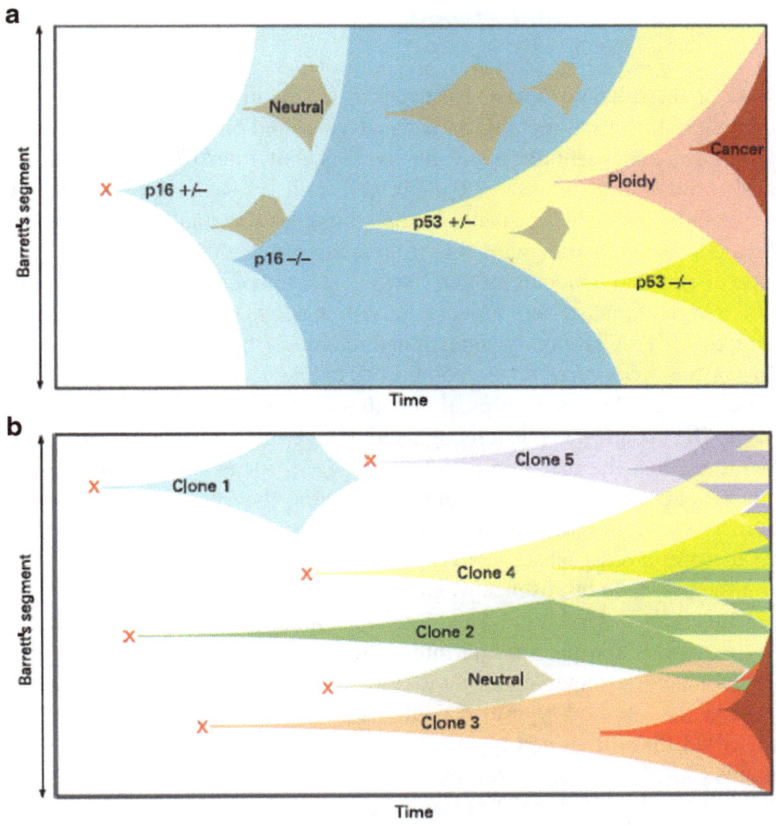

Fig. 1.1 Different models for clonal evolution models in Barrett's oesophagus and similar pre-invasive lesions. (**a**) The model of clonal evolution according to Carlo Maley and colleagues [31] A founder mutation (red cross) occurs in a single progenitor (stem cell) and giving that cell a growth advantage leading to a *selective sweep*. Then successive selective sweeps leads to progression along the metaplasia–dysplasia pathway. In this model clone bifurcation is responsible for clonal heterogeneity (**b**) The model according to Leedham et al. [32] based on the mutation of multiple progenitor or stem cells within the oesophageal gland squamous ducts (red crosses). Here multiple independent clones occur which evolve separately. The giving rise to a mosaic clonal pattern of the Barrett's segment shown by the striped areas (from [32] with permission)

sometimes called a selective sweep [33,34]. Thus loss of both p16 alleles is thought to cause a selective sweep: consequently p16 mutation fixation occurs early in the progression of Barrett's oesophagus [34]. There is good evidence that widespread clonal expansion with fixation of p16 mutations occurs in Barrett's oesophagus [29].

To understand what is happening in Barrett's we need to look closely at the nature of the morphological change in Barrett's mucosa – usually called *intestinal metaplasia*.

The Nature of Intestinal Metaplasia

Most work on intestinal metaplasia has been carried out in the context of its occurrence in the stomach. Intestinal metaplasia is usually defined on the basis of its histological appearance and particularly by the presence of intestinal-type cells such as goblet, absorptive and sometimes Paneth, cells and is usually found in the context of chronic and/or atrophic gastritis. In the stomach, intestinal metaplasia has long been regarded as a pre-malignant condition leading to the development of the intestinal type of gastric adenocarcinoma. Various attempts have been made to identify which histological features are associated with the development of malignancy (see for example [35]). Classically, intestinal metaplasia has been classified into the *complete* or the *incomplete* type – sometimes called Type I and Type II, dependent on the presence of absence of typical Paneth and absorptive cells. However, a Type IIb or Type III metaplasia is also recognised, where the mucus cells contain sulphomucins rather than the usual acid sialomucin (see, for example [36,37]). Though these classifications have been generally accepted, they have overemphasized the characteristics common to cells in the small intestine, while neglecting to take into account the preserved gastric phenotype. Others have proposed classifications are based on the presence or absence of gastric-type cells in intestinal metaplasia – for example that due to [38,39], where intestinal metaplasia is subdivided into two major types, (a) mixed gastric and intestinal type and (b) a solely intestinal type. Thus intestinal type metaplastic glands are composed entirely of intestinal type cells, whereas the mixed-type also contains gastric cells. However, these authors have observed that the mixed typed glands appear to gradually become intestinal type glands [38]. It is clear, therefore, that a conversion of glands formed of gastric type cells to wholly intestinal lineages is occurring though an intermediate stage where the gland contains both lineages: how does this occur?

The Stem Cell/Clonal Origins of Intestinal Metaplasia

There has been some dispute about whether gastric glands in both animals and man are clonally derived – i.e. derived originally from the progeny of a single stem cell. Using male: female chimaeric mice, Thompson et al. [40] showed that gastric glands in the mouse were indeed clonal populations. Nomura et al. [41] showed that, like intestinal crypts, stomach glands commence development as polyclonal units, but by adulthood (6 weeks), the majority had progressed to monoclonal units. However, this has not been the story in the human stomach: thus, using X-chromosome inactivation with the human androgen receptor gene (HUMARA), Nomura et al. [42] reported that sixty percent of single corpus glands were *homotypic* or clonally derived, but 40% were heterotypic – containing mixed cells of different allelic methylation: moreover, when the clonality of the upper parts and that of the lower parts were analyzed separately, eleven glands were heterotypic in either part and four glands were homotypic in the upper part and in the lower part. However, ninety-six percent of the single pyloric glands were homotypic and therefore clonal. This argues for complex stem cell architecture in normal human corpus gastric glands.

Studies using the same method on intestinal metaplastic glands showed that 48% were heterotypic while 52% were homotypic, although once again almost all the single pyloric glands were homotypic [43]. Importantly, 11 of 13 intestinal metaplastic mucosae that were 6 mm in diameter contained glands that had originated from different cells. In this respect, Mihara et al. [44], analysing methylation of multiple CpG islands in several genes in a single gland, showed that of those isolated from a gland with intestinal metaplasia, most were methylated. It was suggested that methylation occurred multifocally and that that methylation of multiple genes occurs independently in multiple glands, each possessing its own stem cell, Thus, on this view, intestinal metaplastic glands initially appear multifocally in the pyloric area – multiple gastric glands aberrantly differentiate into those with intestinal characteristics, and then gradually spread into the corpus area as an independent and polyclonal process. Mihara et al. [44] regarded the presence of a very variable pattern (eight patterns among eight methylated DNA molecules) of methylation in a non-cancerous gastric mucosae confirmed the polyclonal origins of intestinal metaplasia. But even in populations known to be clonal, methylation patterns soon diverge (Graham et al. in preparation).

Thus prevailing opinion states that intestinal metaplastic glands are polyclonal, and each gland arises independently of its neighbour by an altered pattern of differentiation in its stem cell(s). Thus intestinal metaplasia is regarded as quintessentially a polyclonal disorder of the stomach. On the other hand there is now good evidence that normal *colonic* and *small intestinal* crypts are clonal populations. Using the X-inactivation inactivation of a defective glucose-6-phosphate dehydrogenase (G6PD) gene in a population of Sardinian women, Novelli et al. [45] showed that human small intestinal crypts were clonal, staining for either the defective gene product or for the wild type protein – there were no mixed crypts. Similarly, in a very rare XO/XY patient with familial adenomatous polyposis (FAP) the crypts were either positive or negative for the Y chromosome and again never mixed [46], again indicating the clonal nature of human intestinal crypts. Taking advantage of naturally occurring mutations in the cytochrome c oxidase gene, a gene encoded by the mitochondrial genome, a technique introduced by Taylor et al. [47], we have used enzyme histochemistry for cytochrome c oxidase and succinate dehydrogenase in normal human duodenal crypts together with laser-capture, and the entire mitochondrial genome was amplified using a nested PCR protocol. Sequencing identified mutations and immunohistochemistry demonstrated specific cell lineages. We were able to show that all negative crypts contained the same clonal mutation and all differentiated epithelial lineages were present, indicating a common stem cell origin. Mixed crypts were also detected, confirming the existence of multiple stem cells. Thus normal human intestinal crypts are clonal and are maintained by multiple stem cells. We were able to show that patches of mutated crypts contained the same mutation, and that thus mutations spread in the small intestine [48] and that these mutations spread by crypt fission [49].

Similarly, there is now good evidence that corpus glands in the human also clonal populations: McDonald et al. [50] using the same technique of enzyme histochemistry for cytochrome c oxidase and succinate dehydrogenase coupled with laser microdissection and mtDNA sequencing, have observed gastric units that were partially mutated, evidence for the presence of multiple stem cells in such corpus gastric glands, since such units contain at least two different populations of stem cells, one expressing and one not expressing cytochrome c oxidase activity. But there are also entirely mutated gastric units in which a mutated stem cell has expanded to take over the entire stem cell population. Different regions of cytochrome c oxidase-deficient gastric units which have been laser-captured and the mitochondrial genome sequenced, showed that the foveolus, neck region, and base of the negative gastric unit possess the same mtDNA mutation whereas the neighbouring cytochrome c oxidase-positive glands were wild type. Its is clear that *monoclonal conversion* of the gastric unit has taken place where one cytochrome c oxidase-deficient stem cell has stochastically replaced all the cytochrome c oxidase-normal stem cells, resulting in a clonally deficient unit. Thus, contrary to findings using the HUMARA method, *corpus gastric glands are clonal populations, and all cell types are clonally derived* from the contained stem cells (Fig. 1.2).

Intestinal Metaplasia is a Clonal Proliferation

The understanding of the nature of metaplasia in Barrett's is really now dependent of our appreciation of the changes in the organ-specific stem cells which are thought to initiate the change. It is therefore worthwhile asking again whether intestinal metaplasia is really a clonal phenomenon and due to re-programming of stem cells – in the stomach these would be gastric stem cells, and in the oesophagus, presumably the stem cells of the oesophageal squamous epithelium.

We have discussed above results from X-inactivation and methylation studies, which suggest that the progression of intestinal metaplasia occurs in a polyclonal manner. However, we have been able to show that intestinal metaplastic crypts in the human stomach is clonal: we demonstrated the presence of entirely cytochrome c oxidase-deficient metaplastic crypts from a region of intestinal metaplasia and also show partially mutated crypts, suggesting that intestinal metaplastic crypts have multiple stem cells ([50]; Fig. 1.3). We were also able to show that all the differentiated intestinal-type epithelial cells are present within a cytochrome c oxidase-deficient crypt, and thus contain multipotential stem cells. Patches of multiple cytochrome c oxidase-deficient metaplastic crypts were also observed, and the same mutation was only in the cytochrome c oxidase-deficient crypts and not in the positive ones, showing that the patch is derived from a single founder crypt that has been expanded by fission (Fig. 1.3). We therefore conclude that intestinal metaplasia is a clonal proliferation, due to a change in stem cell determination, and that patches of intestinal metaplasia, and therefore mutations, expand by crypt or gland fission.

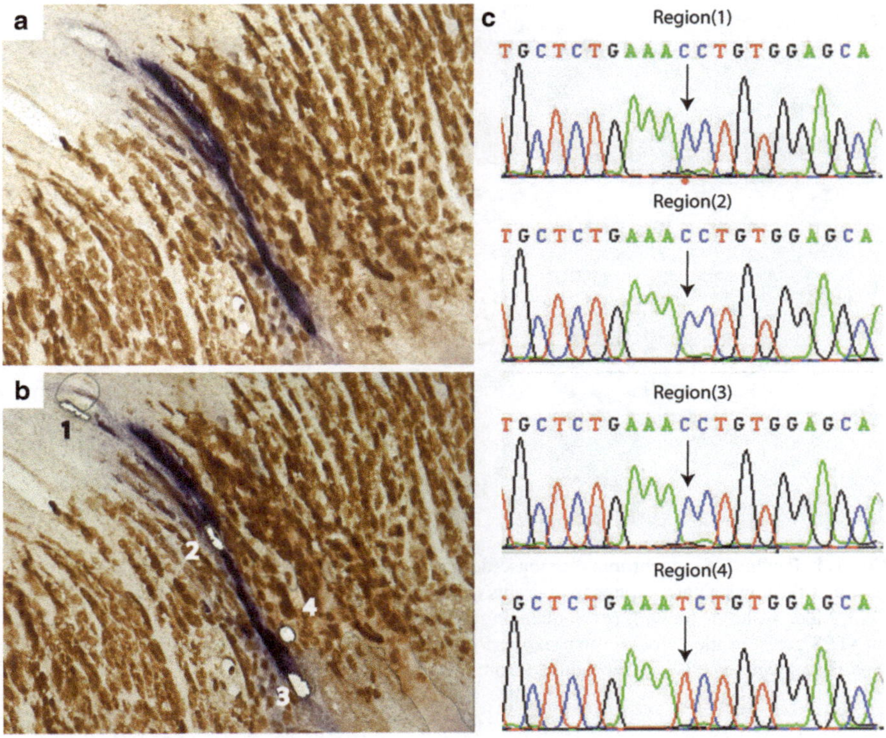

Fig. 1.2 Normal human gastric glands are shown to be clonal. (**a**) A cytochrome c oxidase-deficient gastric gland. (**b**) Negative cells have been dissected from the foveolus (1), from the neck region (2) and the base (3) of a negative-staining gland, and also from the base (4) of an adjacent positive gland. (**c**) MtDNA sequencing showed a T→C transition at position 8181 (reproduced from [50] with permission)

In work in preparation we have shown that other mutations, such as in p53 and APC, are also clonal in intestinal metaplastic crypts and expand clonally in the same manner. Thus there is good evidence that intestinal metaplasia is a clonal proliferation, initiated by a change in a single stem cell.

The Origin of Barrett's Metaplasia

It is becoming clear that, far from there being a singe clone source in Barrett's oesophagus, the epithelium contains multiple mutated clones (see [31,32], and Fig. 1.1). We should note at the outset that the reason for the clonal heterogeneity seen in both of these models is different: in the Maley model clone bifurcation is responsible, while in the Leedham model multiple independent clones then arise which evolve separately. The question then rises – what is the source of

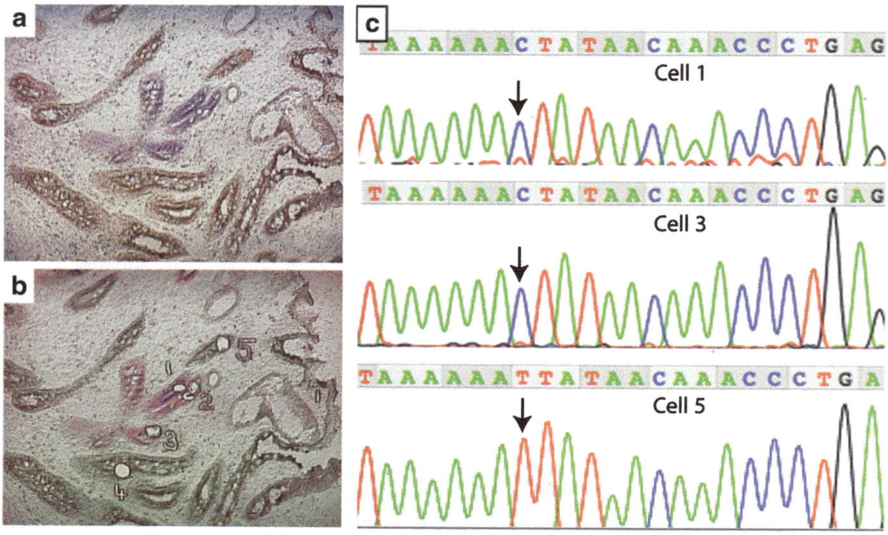

Fig. 1.3 Patches of cytochrome c oxidase-deficient metaplastic crypts are clonal and expand by fission. (**a**) Shows a patch of negative crypts (blue) crypts pre-laser capture. (**b**) Post-laser capture (1–3, blue; 4 and 5, brown). (**c**) Sequencing showed a T→C transition (at position 8503 in the mtATP8 gene) in the cytochrome c oxidase-deficient cells (1 and 3), but not in the cytochrome c oxidase-positive cells (5) (reproduced from [50] with permission)

these multiple clones? A clue to this can be found in the origin of the neo-squamous islands of epithelium that arise within Barrett's oesophagus, usually as a consequence of medical or surgical therapy, or after endoscopic ablation. Paulson et al. [51] isolated islands of the neo-squamous epithelium and the surrounding Barrett's epithelium looked for genetic alterations in the p16 or the TP53 genes. In nearly all the patients studied the neo-squamous islands were wild-type for p16 or TP53, indicating that it originates in cells different from those responsible for Barrett's epithelium.

We have suggested that non-mutated squamous ducts are likely to be the source of wild-type squamous islands [52]. When we analysed the genotype of neo-squamous islands, all but one of the dissected squamous islands were wild-type, even though they were surrounded by mutated Barrett's crypts. Wild-type squamous islands were also seen growing over mutated deeper Barrett's crypts. As we previously showed [52], squamous islands are almost always situated overlying deeper oesophageal glands or gland ducts, if traced in serial section. We were able to show a squamous island arising from an oesophageal gland duct, and while the surrounding Barrett's epithelium revealed a p53 non-sense point mutation, the underlying squamous island and oesophageal gland squamous duct were p53 wild-type, and thus of a different clonal origin to the surrounding Barrett's dysplastic mucosa [32]. Moreover, in another case the metaplastic epithelium revealed a silent point mutation in exon 2 of p16, also present in the duct (and in the underlying oesophageal gland). Although the mutation was non-coding it serves as a useful marker, suggesting a clonal origin of both epithelial lineages, and also that metaplastic epithelium arises from the duct. That the same mutation was found in the oesophageal gland acini suggests a bi-directional flow of cells perhaps from a stem cell niche in somewhere in the duct, as has been reported for Brunner's glands [53].

Together with the demonstration of multiple competing independent clones and a possible identification of the origin of Barrett's oesophagus from the oesophageal gland duct, structures which are present throughout the length of the oesophagus, suggests to us that reflux-induced ulceration and consequent inflammation induce tumour suppressor gene mutations in the stem cell populations in oesophageal gland ducts. These multiple clones then compete until the fittest clone outstrips the rest to progress to carcinoma. This introduces the concept of clonal competition.

The Nature of Clonal Competition

How does competition between clones increase the propensity for malignant change, and how do such clones expand at the expense of others? These are important questions for which there are as yet no convincing answers, but a good deal of interesting speculation, some of it based on experiment. Merlo et al. [54] have analysed the development of cancer as an evolutionary and ecological process: ecology usually entails analysing the dynamics of communities of species and their interactions and can be classified by the effects of the *fitness* of the individual – here a clone – on other individuals. In this context, fitness usually defined in terms of both survival and reproduction capability and thus its average contribution to future generations. There are several such interactions possible, of which competition is just one.

In a population of cells such as occurs in Barrett's oesophagus, competition can of course exist as compete for resources such as oxygen [54] but there is increasing evidence that mutated clones can directly influence the growth of their neighbours: thus two subpopulations of tumour cells isolated from the same colonic tumour in rats, when injected into opposite flanks of syngeneic rats, can inhibit the growth of the other [55]. But some of the best evidence for competition between clones has come from work on *Drosophila*, where several genetic methods can be used to make patches of mutant cells in a field of wild-type tissue – not dissimilar, it might be thought, from the situation in Barrett's mucosa [56,57]. When cells which have mutations in ribosomal genes (*Minutes*) were mixed with wild-type cells, *Minute* heterozygous cells proliferate less and are replaced by surrounding wild-type cells. Thus the loss of the slower growing clones was caused by the wild-type cells – cell *competition* Moreover, in the mouse, when wild-type cells were injected into heterozygous blastocysts wild-type cells contribute much more to several tissues.

Additionally, in *Drosophila*, clones mutant for *dMyc*, the homologue of *myc*, lose out to wild-type cells in the developing wing imaginal discs, and importantly, cells over-expressing *dMyc* can eliminate wild-type cells, so-called *super-competitors*, and take over the entire wing epithelia. Although the dMyc-over-expressing cells grow at a faster rate, this excess growth is accompanied by the death of wild-type cells so that cell numbers were not altered and no morphological malformations appear in the discs or in the wing structure. The Salvador–Warts–Hippo (SWH) pathway is thought to control organ size through the modulation of cell growth, proliferation and apoptosis, and in *Drosophila* marked increases in organ size occur when this pathway is dysregulated [58]. SWH pathway components are conserved from yeast to humans, and the pathway has been implicated in the development of human cancers. This pathway may also be involved in clonal competition [59]. Cells expressing such mutations show overgrowth in the presence of wild-type cells. The fact that both deregulation of *dMyc* and the *Hippo* pathway are associated with tumorigenesis points to a possible link between cell super competition and cancer.

These mechanisms may act through apoptosis: if apoptosis is prevented then both clones survive both groups coexist, even though the proliferation advantage remains. Thus it is the killing surrounding cells that allows the expansion of the dominant cell or clone [57]. There are therefore several steps in this process: after a mutation in *Minute* or *dMyc* the fitness of a clone is altered which appears to result in imbalances in morphogen and survival factor signalling. Cells appear able to monitor the signalling levels of adjacent clones and a secreted signal to kill the 'loser' clone, possibly via a secreted molecule. Finally, c-jun N-terminal kinase signalling and caspase activation in the loser clone induces an engulfment response in the dominant clone, which is removed from the epithelial layer [57].

Of course, in the context of Barrett's oesophagus, even in the presence of dysplasia, clones are disposed within crypts. There is little doubt that clonal expansion, at least in non-dysplastic crypts, occurs by the process of crypt fission [50], although when severe dysplasia occurs, there is evidence that the dysplastic epithelium can invade other crypt territories from the surface [60]. We do not presently know what molecular events enable clones of crypts to dominate through this fission process, but Leedham et al. [60] examined individual crypts from the non-cancerous mucosa of patients with colitis-associated neoplasia. APC, p53, K-RAS, and 17p LOH and mutation burden was established and in most lesions an oncogenic mutation could be identified in all crypts across the lesion independent of the morphological appearances, indicating origin from a single crypt. We have seen above that localised sweeps of clonal expansion among multiple independent clones occurs in Barrett's mucosa, and again it is probable that this occurs by crypt fission. Whether such dominant clones of crypts achieve clonal dominance in the manner suggested by the above experiments in *Drosophila* is an interesting possibility.

Conclusion

We have seen that there is good emerging evidence supporting the proposal that epithelial tumours arise from the lineage-labelling, organ-specific stem cells. We have used the example of Barrett's oesophagus – an interesting condition where the squamous epithelium of the lower oesophagus is replaced with an intestinalised epithelium composed of crypt systems. We have discussed the stem cell and thus clonal architecture of such intestinal metaplasia, and concluded that it is a clonal proliferation. The changes which occur in the mucosa during the development of dysplasia and carcinoma are complex, but appear to involve the evolution of multiple clones, which, through competition leads to the emergence of a dominant clone which evolves into dysplasia and hence to carcinoma. We need to find out much more about how mutant clones become dominant and spread, and how competition between clones promotes the development of cancer in humans.

Acknowledgements I thank Malcolm Alison, Stuart McDonald, Lydia Gutierrez-Gonzalez, Simon Leedham and Trevor Graham for much help with this work, and Cancer Research UK for funding.

References

1. Hermann PC, Huber SL, Herrler T, Aicher A, Ellwart JW, Guba M, Bruns CJ, Heeschen C (2007) Distinct populations of cancer stem cells determine tumor growth and metastatic activity in human pancreatic cancer. Cell Stem Cell 1:313–323
2. Garcia S, Park HS, Novelli M, Wright NA (1999) Field cancerization, clonality, and epithelial stem cells: the spread of mutated clones in epithelial sheets. J Pathol 187:61–81
3. Rosenberg DW, Giardina C, Tanaka T (2009) Mouse models for the study of colon carcinogenesis. Carcinogenesis 30(2):183–196
4. Sangiorgi E, Capecchi MR (2008) Bmi1 is expressed in vivo in intestinal stem cells. Nat Genet 40:915–920
5. Barker N, van Es JH, Kuipers J, Kujala P, van den Born M, Cozijnsen M, Haegebarth A, Korving J, Begthel H, Peters PJ, Clevers H (2007) Identification of stem cells in small intestine and colon by marker gene Lgr5. Nature 449:1003–1007
6. Barker N, Ridgway RA, van Es JH, van de Wetering M, Begthel H, van den Born M, Danenberg E, Clarke AR, Sansom OJ, Clevers H (2009) Crypt stem cells as the cells-of-origin of intestinal cancer. Nature 457:608–611
7. Zhu L, Gibson P, Currle DS, Tong Y, Richardson RJ, Bayazitov IT, Poppleton H, Zakharenko S, Ellison DW, Gilbertson RJ (2009) Prominin 1 marks intestinal stem cells that are susceptible to neoplastic transformation. Nature 457:603–607
8. Demidov ON, Timofeev O, Lwin HN, Kek C, Appella E, Bulavin DV (2007) Wip1 phosphatase regulates p53-dependent apoptosis of stem cells and tumorigenesis in the mouse intestine. Cell Stem Cell 1:180–190
9. Zeilstra J, Joosten SP, Dokter M, Verwiel E, Spaargaren M, Pals ST (2008) Deletion of the WNT target and cancer stem cell marker CD44 in Apc(Min/+) mice attenuates intestinal tumorigenesis. Cancer Res 68:3655–3661
10. Maitland NJ, Collins AT (2008) Inflammation as the primary aetiological agent of human prostate cancer: a stem cell connection? J Cell Biochem 105:931–939
11. Bisson I, Prowse DM (2009) WNT signaling regulates self-renewal and differentiation of prostate cancer cells with stem cell characteristics. Cell Res 19:683–697
12. Vander Griend DJ, Karthaus WL, Dalrymple S, Meeker A, DeMarzo AM, Isaacs JT (2008) The role of CD133 in normal human prostate stem cells and malignant cancer-initiating cells. Cancer Res 68:9703–9711
13. Wang X, Kruithof-de Julio M, Economides KD, Walker D, Yu H, Halili MV, Hu YP, Price SM, Abate-Shen C, Shen MM (2009) A luminal epithelial stem cell that is a cell of origin for prostate cancer. Nature 461:495–500

14. Lim E, Vaillant F, Wu D, Forrest NC, Pal B, Hart AH, Asselin-Labat ML, Gyorki DE, Ward T, Partanen A, Feleppa F, Huschtscha LI, Thorne HJ, kConFab, Fox SB, Yan M, French JD, Brown MA, Smyth GK, Visvader JE, Lindeman GJ (2009) Aberrant luminal progenitors as the candidate target population for basal tumor development in BRCA1 mutation carriers. Nat Med 15:907–913
15. Kristensen DM, Sonne SB, Ottesen AM, Perrett RM, Nielsen JE, Almstrup K, Skakkebaek NE, Leffers H, Meyts ER (2008) Origin of pluripotent germ cell tumours: the role of microenvironment during embryonic development. Mol Cell Endocrinol 288:111–118
16. Alison MR, Islam S (2009) Attributes of adult stem cells. J Pathol 217:144–160
17. Yamashita T, Forgues M, Wang W, Kim JW, Ye Q, Jia H, Budhu A, Zanetti KA, Chen Y, Qin LX, Tang ZY, Wang XW (2008) EpCAM and alpha-fetoprotein expression defines novel prognostic subtypes of hepatocellular carcinoma. Cancer Res 68:1451–1461
18. Lee JS, Heo J, Libbrecht L, Chu IS, Kaposi-Novak P, Calvisi DF, Mikaelyan A, Roberts LR, Demetris AJ, Sun Z, Nevens F, Roskams T, Thorgeirsson SS (2006) A novel prognostic subtype of human hepatocellular carcinoma derived from hepatic progenitor cells. Nat Med 12:410–416
19. Durnez A, Verslype C, Nevens F, Fevery J, Aerts R, Pirenne J, Lesaffre E, Libbrecht L, Desmet V, Roskams T (2006) The clinicopathological and prognostic relevance of cytokeratin 7 and 19 expression in hepatocellular carcinoma. A possible progenitor cell origin. Histopathology 49:138–151
20. Alison MR, Islam S, Lim S (2009) Stem cells in liver regeneration, fibrosis and cancer: the good, the bad and the ugly. J Pathol 217:282–298
21. Franklin WA, Gazdar AF, Haney J, Wictuba II, La Rossa FG, Kennedy T, Ricthey DM, Miller YE (1997) Widely dispersed p53 mutations in respiratory epithelium. J Clin Invest 100:2133–2137
22. Riely GJ, Marks J, Pao W (2009) KRAS mutations in non-small cell lung cancer. Proc Am Thorac Soc 6:201–205
23. Jackson EL, Willis N, Mercer K, Bronson RT, Crowley D, Montoya R, Jacks T, Tuveson DA (2001) Analysis of lung tumor initiation and progression using conditional expression of oncogenic K-ras. Genes Dev 15:3243–3248
24. Kim CF, Jackson EL, Woolfenden AE, Lawrence S, Babar I, Vogel S, Crowley D, Bronson RT, Jacks T (2005) Identification of bronchioalveolar stem cells in normal lung and lung cancer. Cell 121:823–835
25. Barth PJ, Koch S, Muller B, Unterstab F, von Wichert P, Moll R (2000) Proliferation and number of Clara cell 10-kDa protein (CC10)-reactive epithelial cells and basal cells in normal, hyperplastic and metaplastic bronchial mucosa. Virchows Arch 437:648–655
26. Jankowski JA, Wright NA, Meltzer SJ et al (1999) Molecular evolution of the metaplasia–dysplasia–adenocarcinoma sequence in the esophagus. Am J Pathol 154:965–973
27. Montgomery E, Bronner MP, Goldblum JR, Greenson JK, Haber MM, Hart J, Lamps LW, Lauwers GY, Lazenby AJ, Lewin DN et al (2001) Reproducibility of the diagnosis of dysplasia in Barrett esophagus: a reaffirmation. Hum Pathol 32:368–378
28. Barrett MT, Sanchez CA, Prevo LJ et al (1999) Evolution of neoplastic cell lineages in Barrett oesophagus. Nat Genet 22:106–109
29. Wong DJ, Paulson TG, Prevo LJ et al (2001) p16(INK4a) lesions are common, early abnormalities that undergo clonal expansion in Barrett's metaplastic epithelium. Cancer Res 61:8284–8289
30. Galipeau PC, Prevo LJ, Sanchez CA et al (1999) Clonal expansion and loss of heterozygosity at chromosomes 9p and 17p in premalignant esophageal (Barrett's) tissue. J Natl Cancer Inst 91:2087–2095
31. Maley CC, Galipeau PC, Finley JC et al (2006) Genetic clonal diversity predicts progression to esophageal adenocarcinoma. Nat Genet 38:468–473
32. Leedham SJ, Preston SL, McDonald SA, Elia G, Bhandari P, Poller D, Harrison R, Novelli MR, Jankowski JA, Wright NA (2008) Individual crypt genetic heterogeneity and the origin of metaplastic glandular epithelium in human Barrett's oesophagus. Gut 57(8):1041–1048
33. Maley CC, Galipeau PC, Li X et al (2004) Selectively advantageous mutations and hitchhikers in neoplasms: p16 lesions are selected in Barrett's esophagus. Cancer Res 64:3414–3427

34. Maley CC, Reid BJ (2005) Natural selection in neoplastic progression of Barrett's esophagus. Semin Cancer Biol 15:474–483
35. Jass JR, Filipe MI (1979) A variant of intestinal metaplasia associated with gastric carcinoma: a histochemical study. Histopathology 3:191–199
36. Filipe MI, Barbatis C, Sandey A, MA J (1988) Expression of intestinal mucin antigens in the gastric epithelium and its relationship with malignancy. Hum Pathol 19:19–26
37. Filipe MI, Potet F, Bogomoletz WV, Dawson PA, Fabiani B, Chauveinc P, Fenzy A, Gazzard B, Goldfain D, Zeegen R (1985) Incomplete sulphomucin-secreting intestinal metaplasia for gastric cancer. Preliminary data from a prospective study from three centres. Gut 26: 1319–1326
38. Inada K, Nakanishi H, Fujimitsu Y, Shimizu N, Ichinose M, Miki K, Nakamura S, Tatematsu M (1997) Gastric and intestinal mixed and solely intestinal types of intestinal metaplasia in the human stomach. Pathol Int 47:831–841
39. Inada K, Tanaka H, Nakanishi H, Tsukamoto T, Ikehara Y, Tatematsu K, Nakamura S, Porter EM, Tatematsu M (2001) Identification of Paneth cells in pyloric glands associated with gastric and intestinal mixed-type intestinal metaplasia. Virchows Arch 439:14–20
40. Thompson M, Fleming KA, Evans DJ, Fundele R, Surani MA, Wright NA (1990) Gastric endocrine cells share a clonal origin with other gut cell lineages. Development 110(2):477–481
41. Nomura S, Esumi H, Job C, Tan SS (1998) Lineage and clonal development of gastric glands. Clonal analysis of isolated intestinal metaplastic glands of stomach using X linked polymorphism. Dev Biol 204(1):124–135
42. Nomura S, Kaminishi M, Sugiyama K, Oohara T, Esumi H (1996) Clonal analysis of isolated single fundic and pyloric gland of stomach using X-linked polymorphism. Biochem Biophys Res Commun 226(2):385–390
43. Nomura S, Kaminishi M, Sugiyama K, Oohara T, Esumi H (1998) Clonal analysis of isolated intestinal metaplastic glands of stomach using X linked polymorphism. Gut 42(5):663–668
44. Mihara M, Yoshida Y, Tsukamoto T et al (2006) Methylation of multiple genes in gastric glands with intestinal metaplasia. A disorder with polyclonal origins. Am J Pathol 169:1643–1651
45. Novelli M, Cossu A, Oukrif D, Quaglia A, Lakhani S, Poulsom R et al (2003) X-inactivation patch size in human female tissue confounds the assessment of tumor clonality. Proc Natl Acad Sci U S A 100:3311–3314
46. Novelli MR, Williamson JA, Tomlinson IP, Elia G, Hodgson SV, Talbot IC et al (1996) Polyclonal origin of colonic adenomas in an XO/XY patient with FAP. Science 272:1187–1190
47. Taylor RW, Barron MJ, Borthwick GM, Gospel A, Chinnery PF, Samuels DC et al (2003) Mitochondrial DNA mutations in human colonic crypt stem cells. J Clin Invest 112:1351–1360
48. Gutierrez-Gonzalez L, Deheragoda M, Elia G, Leedham SJ, Shankar A, Imber C, Jankowski JA, Turnbull DM, Novelli M, Wright NA, McDonald SA (2009) Analysis of the clonal architecture of the human small intestinal epithelium establishes a common stem cell for all lineages and reveals a mechanism for the fixation and spread of mutations. J Pathol 217(4):489–496
49. Greaves LC, Preston SL, Tadrous PJ, Taylor RW, Barron MJ, Oukrif D et al (2006) Mitochondrial DNA mutations are established in human colonic stem cells, and mutated clones expand by crypt fission. Proc Natl Acad Sci U S A 103:714–719
50. McDonald SA, Greaves LC, Gutierrez-Gonzalez L, Rodriguez-Justo M, Deheragoda M, Leedham SJ et al (2008) Mechanisms of field cancerization in the human stomach: the expansion and spread of mutated gastric stem cells. Gastroenterology 134:500–510
51. Paulson TG, Xu L, Sanchez C et al (2006) Neosquamous epithelium does not typically arise from Barrett's epithelium. Clin Cancer Res 12:1701–1706
52. Coad RA, Woodman AC, Warner PJ et al (2005) On the histogenesis of Barrett's oesophagus and its associated squamous islands: a three-dimensional study of their morphological relationship with native oesophageal gland ducts. J Pathol 206:388–394
53. Ahnen DJ, Poulsom R, Stamp GW et al (1994) The ulceration-associated cell lineage (UACL) reiterates the Brunner's gland differentiation programme but acquires the proliferative organization of the gastric gland. J Pathol 173:317–326

54. Merlo LM, Pepper JW, Reid BJ, Maley CC (2006) Cancer as an evolutionary and ecological process. Nat Rev Cancer 6(12):924–935
55. Caignard A, Martin MS, Michel MF, Martin F (1985) Interaction between two cellular subpopulations of a rat colonic carcinoma when inoculated to the syngeneic host. Int J Cancer 36:273–279
56. Moreno E (2008) Is cell competition relevant to cancer? Nat Rev Cancer 8(2):141–147
57. Rhiner C, Moreno E (2009) Super competition as a possible mechanism to pioneer precancerous fields. Carcinogenesis 30(5):723–728
58. Harvey K, Tapon N (2007) The Salvador–Warts–Hippo pathway – an emerging tumour-suppressor network. Nat Rev Cancer 7:182–191
59. Tyler DM et al (2007) Genes affecting cell competition in Drosophila. Genetics 175:643–657
60. Leedham SJ, Graham TA, Oukrif D, McDonald SA, Rodriguez-Justo M, Harrison RF, Shepherd NA, Novelli MR, Jankowski JA, Wright NA (2009) Clonality, founder mutations, and field cancerization in human ulcerative colitis-associated neoplasia. Gastroenterology 136:542–550

Chapter 2
The Inflammatory Tissue Microenvironment and the Early Stages of Malignancy

Fran Balkwill

Abstract The microenvironment has a critical impact on the malignant potential and eventual outcome of a pre-invasive lesion. A tumour-promoting microenvironment contains many of the cells and mediators of chronic inflammation. The origins of this may be extrinsic i.e. inflammatory stimuli cause or exacerbate the evolution of cells with malignant potential, or intrinsic i.e. the oncogenic changes in the initiated cells induce inflammatory pathways.

Introduction

The microenvironment has a critical impact on the malignant potential and eventual outcome of a pre-invasive lesion. An initiated cell with malignant potential can be seen as a troublesome youth – put in a 'good' environment with schools, parks, youth clubs etc. their future will be positive; in a 'bad' environment with poor housing, drugs, gangs etc. their future will be uncertain.

In terms of pre-invasive cancers, the 'bad' microenvironment has many of the cells and mediators of chronic inflammation. The origins of this inflammatory microenvironment may be extrinsic i.e. inflammatory stimuli cause or exacerbate the evolution of cells with malignant potential, or intrinsic i.e. the oncogenic changes in the initiated cells induce inflammatory pathways [1]. These two pathways are not mutually exclusive and the outcomes are essentially the same. In pre-invasive lesions, cancer-related inflammation can exacerbate genetic damage in initiated/malignant cells, stimulate their survival and growth, inhibit useful anti-tumour immune responses, recruit tumor-promoting leukocytes and construct a

F. Balkwill (✉)
Centre for Cancer and Inflammation, Institute of Cancer, Barts and The London School of Medicine and Dentistry, Queen Mary University of London, Charterhouse Square, London EC1M 6BQ, UK
e-mail: f.balkwill@qmul.ac.uk

R.C. Fitzgerald (ed.), *Pre-Invasive Disease: Pathogenesis and Clinical Management*, DOI 10.1007/978-1-4419-6694-0_2,

tissue microenvironment where neo-vascularisation and tissue remodeling aid the growth and spread of the malignant cells. While these actions are the same in a variety of cancers, the effector cells and mediators seem to vary with different tissues and oncogenic changes [2].

An inflammatory pro-tumour microenvironment is involved every stage of malignancy but is particularly well defined in studies of experimental pre-invasive lesions.

Malignant Change Induces Inflammatory Pathways

The presence of an inflammatory component in the microenvironment of pre-invasive lesions that have no epidemiologic link to inflammatory disease, suggested that genetic events causing neoplasia could be responsible for the development of an inflammatory microenvironment. One of the first papers to provide evidence for this idea came from Mantovani and colleagues and concerned papillary thyroid carcinoma, PTC. Rearrangement of the RET tyrosine kinase (RET/PTC) represents a frequent, early, causative and sufficient genetic event in the pathogenesis of PTC. In primary human thyrocytes, RET/PTC activates an inflammatory program [3]. The transcriptome of RET/PTC-activated cells includes colony-stimulating factors, CSFs, which promote leukocyte recruitment and survival; interleukin-1, IL-1, a major inflammatory cytokine; cyclooxygenase 2, COX2, an inflammatory enzyme that is frequently over-expressed in cancer; chemokines attracting monocytes and dendritic cells CCL2, CCL20; angiogenic chemokines e.g. CXCL8. In addition RET/PTC activation induces the chemokine receptor CXCR4 on the initiated cells. Key elements of the RET/PTC-activated inflammatory programme were found in biopsy specimens and patients with lymph node metastasis showed higher levels of the inflammatory molecules in their primary tumours [3]; these results show that this early, causative and sufficient genetic event involved in the pathogenesis of a human tumour directly promotes an inflammatory microenvironment [3, 4].

Ras is the most frequently mutated dominant oncogene in human cancer and activated oncogenic components of the ras–raf signalling pathway also induce the production of tumor promoting inflammatory cytokines and chemokines [5, 6]. Myc is over-expressed in many human tumours – its activation initiates and maintains key aspects of the tumour phenotype. In addition to promoting cell autonomous proliferation, myc instructs remodelling of the extracellular microenvironment with inflammatory cells and mediators playing key roles. In a pancreatic islet tumour model, a first wave of myc-driven angiogenesis in early pre-invasive lesion was induced by the inflammatory cytokine IL-1 [7]. The myc-activated genetic programme also included chemokines recruiting mast cells that sustained new vessel formation and tumour growth [8].

Mutations in tumour suppressor genes can also regulate inflammatory pathways and two examples of this involve von Hippel Lindau, VHL, tumour suppressor gene and transforming growth factor β (TGF-β). The VHL is part of a molecular complex that targets degradation of hypoxia inducible factor (HIF-1α). VHL mutations increase HIF-1α protein in malignant cells and this increases the cell and tissue response to hypoxia, including angiogenesis. HIF-1α interfaces with NF-κB and increases protein levels of the inflammatory cytokine TNF-α[9] and the chemokine receptor CXCR4 in human renal cell carcinoma cells [10].

Similarly, genetic inactivation of the type II TGF-β receptor unleashes production of the chemokines CXCL5 and CXCL12 [11]. These chemokines attract immune suppressive myeloid derived suppressor cells (MDSC) that may inhibit a useful antitumor immune response and directly facilitate metastasis.

Thus, oncogenes representative of different molecular classes and modes of action (tyrosine kinases; ras-raf; nuclear oncogenes; tumour suppressors) are all able to orchestrate pro-inflammatory programs. These programs involve the major inflammatory cytokines known to be involved in cancer-related inflammation, TNF-α [12] IL-1β [13] and IL-6 [14], and/or certain chemokines [15]. In addition, induction of at least one chemokine receptor CXCR4 that is involved in survival and chemotactic migration of the malignant cells, has been linked to oncogenic mutations [16]. The oncogene-orchestrated inflammatory response also appears to share common elements e.g. a link to angiogenesis and recruitment of cells of myelomonocytic origin.

Recent experiments have implicated the inflammatory cytokine IL-6 in an even earlier event in carcinogenesis, the switch from an immortalised to a transformed cell. Interestingly, this key step in cancer progression involved an epigenetic switch in response to autocrine inflammatory stimuli, as opposed to a mutational change in a tumor suppressor gene or oncogene. When the Src oncoprotein was transiently activated in immortalised mammary epithelial cells, it caused a stable epigenetic switch to transformed cells that formed self-renewing mammospheres containing cancer stem cells and grew in nude mice [17]. The mechanism of this stable but epigenetic change involved activation of NF-κB and the microRNA suppressor Lin28 that led to a rapid reduction of let-7 microRNA levels. Let-7 inhibits IL-6 hence there was a rapid increase in IL-6 production in the Src transformed cells. IL-6 alone could transform the immortalized mammary cells and anti-IL-6 antibodies inhibited their growth in vitro and in vivo. There was a strong inverse correlation between let-7a and IL-6 expression levels in human breast, prostate and hepatocellular carcinoma tissues. Thus, the epigenetic switch that led to stable transformation of cells was caused by an inflammatory positive feedback loop, a transient inflammatory signal being converted to a chronic inflammatory state maintained by activated NF-κB.

Tumor-Promoting Inflammation and Pre-invasive Malignancies

One of the founding tenets of research into cancer-related inflammation is evidence that many inflammatory stimuli or chronic inflammatory conditions increase the incidence of malignancy [1, 18]. Whether the stimuli are due to infection, chemicals, irradiation or chronic inflammation of unknown cause, pre-invasive lesions that progress to invasive cancers are commonly found at sites of inflammation. Well-documented examples in humans include chronic *Helicobacter pylori* infection leading to gastric cancer and MALT lymphoma; hepatitis and hepatocellular carcinoma; schistosomiasis and bladder cancer; asbestosis and mesothelioma; prostatitis and prostate cancer; pancreatitis and pancreatic cancer, inflammatory bowel disease and colon cancers; Barrett's oesophagus and oesophageal carcinoma.

Mouse models have provided experimental evidence that many different inflammatory stimuli can induce pre-invasive cancers that progress to invasive lesions. Examples are chemically induced hepatitis [19, 20] and colitis [21, 22] and mouse models of *Helicobacter* gastritis [23]. Such models have again identified inflammatory cytokines such as TNF-α and IL-6 and the transcription factor complexes STAT3 and NF-κB as being key molecular mediators [24]. Myeloid cells have important tumor-promoting influences in many of the models, such as M2-like tumour associated macrophages or myeloid-derived suppressor cells and inflammatory signaling from both non-malignant leukocytes and the malignant cells is important in the evolution of these cancers.

Links Between the Intrinsic and Extrinsic Pathways of Cancer-Related Inflammation

The intrinsic and extrinsic pathways that lead to a tumour-promoting microenvironment in pre-invasive lesions are not mutually exclusive. For instance, the carcinogenic activity of *H. pylori* is genetically linked with the inflammatory cytokine TNF-α – members of the Tipα gene family in *H. pylori* are potent TNF inducers and in combination with Ras activation, can render gastric epithelial cells malignant [25].

Another example relates to pancreatic cancer, in which pancreatitis increases the risk of tumor development and K-ras mutations are frequently found. In a mouse genetic model of pancreatic cancer, adult mice were resistant to K-ras pancreatic carcinogenesis [5]. However, when mild chronic pancreatitis was induced in these mice, pancreatic intraepithelial neoplasia and invasive ductal carcinoma developed [5]. Thus, while ras/raf oncogenes may drive some cancer-promoting inflammation, an extrinsic inflammatory condition (pancreatitis) is required to drive carcinogenesis in the mouse and presumably human pancreatic cancer.

Finally, going back to one of the first experiments to make a link between inflammatory cytokines and cancer, pre-invasive papillomas were induced on mouse skin by a single topical application of the carcinogen DMBA, causing a ras mutation, and then skin inflammation induced by repeated doses of TPA. Alone, neither of these can cause these benign skin cancers but together they provide a powerful model of initiation and promotion. However, TNF-α knockout mice were profoundly resistant to this papilloma development [26].

Cancer-Related Inflammation in Experimental Pre-invasive Lesions

To my knowledge, there is no human or murine malignancy that does not have histologic evidence of 'inflammatory' stroma – some form of leukocyte infiltrate and tumor-associated fibroblasts in some areas of the tumour – but the extent and phenotype is variable. Genetic mouse cancer models have permitted investigation of the critical chemical mediators such as cytokines and transcription factors as well as the cellular components of this microenvironment. Mice can be examined at all stages of development of malignancy, but especially the earliest pre-invasive lesions.

In the K14-HPV16 model of squamous carcinogenesis, B cells and humoral immunity foster the development of dysplastic lesions by activating Fcγ receptors on resident myeloid cells in premalignant skin [27, 28]. The inflammatory microenvironment that precedes the pre-malignant lesions, and the subsequent dysplasia/malignancy, is strongly inhibited when these mice are crossed to B cell deficient or Fcγ knockout mice. However, in other genetic models of cancer e.g. breast cancer, T cells were found to be major players in tumour-promoting inflammation, at least in terms of promoting metastasis from primary lesions [29].

In genetic models of colitis-induced cancer and hepatocellular carcinoma, deletion of NF-κB transcription factors in cells of the myeloid lineage inhibited development of pre-invasive lesions [19, 22]. Macrophages are also strongly implicated in the progression to invasive metastatic lesions in a genetic model of breast cancer [30].

In the APC^{min} model of colon adenomatous polyposis, endogenous T regulatory cells, Treg, enhanced in vivo mast cell differentiation and a tumour-promoting microenvironment [31, 32]. This positive feedback loop seems to allow mast cells to reprogramme Treg towards inflammation and these cells in turn attract additional mast cells to the premalignant lesions.

Along with leukocytes, there are other stromal cells, such as fibroblasts, in the tumour microenvironment that can contribute to the inflammatory milieu. Research into links between cancer-related inflammation and cancer-associated fibroblasts, CAFs, has not been so extensive, but it has been accepted for many years that these cells are phenotypically and functionally different from normal tissue fibroblasts, and that they can have tumour-promoting activity [33]. Recent experiments using the K14-HPV16 skin carcinoma model described above [27] have focused on the role of CAF in hyperplastic and dysplastic lesions. CAFs purified from such lesions show a distinctive pro-inflammatory gene profile that includes upregulation of genes such as IL-1β, IL-6, CCL1, CCL5 and CXCL2 [34]. Similar profiles were seen in CAFs isolated from human malignancies. This CAF pro-inflammatory gene signature was a very early event in the K14-HPV16 model but was maintained in invasive carcinomas and was implicated in development of tumour vasculature. The sequence of cell involvement proposed in this model was that the initiated cells at the earliest stages of malignancy recruited

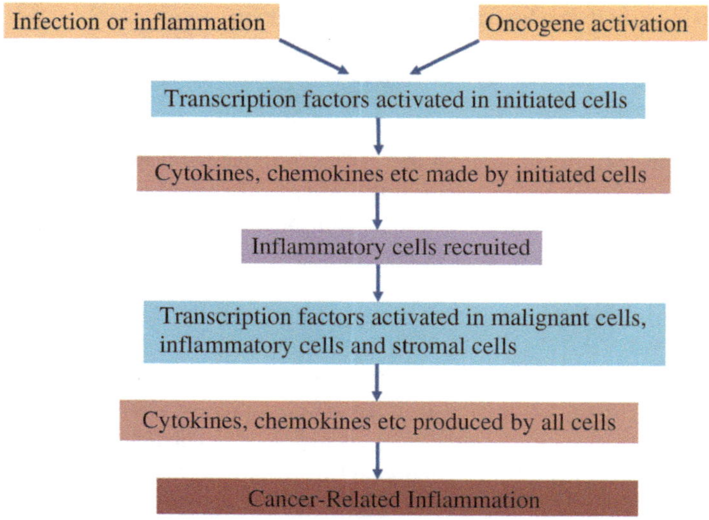

Fig. 2.1 Pathways of cancer-related inflammation (adapted from [1])

resident immune cells that in turn activated normal fibroblasts into CAFs via NF-κB signaling [34].

It is also relevant that in the first study of gene expression in microdissected stroma from human Barrett's oesophagus metasplasia and oesophageal carcinoma, inflammatory pathways, and genes such as IL-6 were upregulated during cancer progression [35].

These examples of the research in this area, taken together with many other studies on depletion of inflammatory cytokines and inflammatory transcription factors in genetic, inflammation-induced and transplantable tumour models (reviewed in [1]), show us that inflammatory mediators and cells are 'hard-wired' into the evolution of pre-invasive cancers, as summarized in Fig. 2.1.

Translating this Knowledge into Clinical Management of Pre-invasive Malignancy

Clinical trials that target the cytokines and chemokines characteristic of cancer-related inflammation are still at an early stage and are mainly focused on patients with advanced malignancy [36]. However principles learnt from this clinical research with cytokine and chemokine antagonists may eventually be useful in devising novel approaches to the management of pre-invasive cancers [37].

There are also compelling epidemiologic and clinical data that NSAIDs can protect against development of pre-invasive and invasive lesions in colorectal carcinoma and possibly other cancers such as breast, prostate, lung stomach and oesophageal [38–40]. However, there are insufficient data on the risk-benefit profile for cancer prevention to make any therapeutic recommendations [41]. Aspirin is the most studied NSAID but 10 years exposure is required before benefit is seen. As the main side effect of aspirin is peptic ulcers co-administration with a proton-pump inhibitor is currently being studied in clinical trial [41]. Other NSAIDs and selective COX-2 inhibitors are given to patients at high risk of colorectal cancer [42]. Many other agents of potential in cancer prevention e.g. curcumin [43], green tea [44], are also anti-inflammatory.

Conclusion

This chapter has described a role for inflammatory processes in the earliest stages of malignancy and identified a number of mouse models where this can be manipulated. While the mediators and cells that drive cancer-related inflammation may vary with oncogenic pathway and tissue of origin, there are some common pathways and leading to development of a tumour-promoting microenvironment. There is now a need for systematic study of anti-inflammatory approaches that may either inhibit or re-align the cancer-promoting microenvironment that is an important driver of pre-invasive malignancies. These approaches have great potential for prevention and treatment of pre-invasive disease.

References

1. Mantovani A, Allavena P, Sica A, Balkwill F (2008) Cancer-related inflammation. Nature 454:436–444
2. Ruffell B, DeNardo DG, Affara NI, Coussens LM (2010) Lymphocytes in cancer development: polarization towards pro-tumor immunity. Cytokine Growth Factor Rev 21:3–10
3. Borrello MG, Alberti L, Fischer A, Degl'innocenti D, Ferrario C, Gariboldi M, Marchesi F, Allavena P, Greco A, Collini P et al (2005) Induction of a proinflammatory program in normal human thyrocytes by the RET/PTC1 oncogene. PNAS 102:14825–14830
4. De Falco V, Gastellone MD, De Vita G, Cirafici AM, Hershman JM, Guerrero C, Fusco A, Melillo RM, Santoro M (2007) RET/papillary thyroid carcinoma oncogenic signaling through the Rap1 small GTPase. Cancer Res 67:381–390
5. Guerra C, Schuhmacher AJ, Canamero M, Grippo PJ, Verdaguer L, Perez-Gallego L, Dubus P, Sandgren EP, Barbacid M (2007) Chronic pancreatitis is essential for induction of pancreatic ductal adenocarcinoma by K-Ras oncogenes in adult mice. Cancer Cell 11:291–302
6. Sparmann A, Bar-Sagi D (2004) Ras-induced interleukin-8 expression plays a critical role in tumor growth and angiogenesis. Cancer Cell 6:447–458
7. Shchors K, Shchors E, Rostker F, Lawlor ER, Brown-Swigart L, Evan GI (2006) The Myc-dependent angiogenic switch in tumors is mediated by interleukin 1beta. Genes Dev 20:2527–2538
8. Soucek L, Lawlor ER, Soto D, Shchors K, Swigart LB, Evan GI (2007) Mast cells are required for angiogenesis and macropscopic expansion of Myc-induced pancreatic islet tumors. Nat Med 13:1211–1218

9. Galban S, Fan J, Martindale JL, Cheadle C, Hoffman B, Woods MP, Temeles G, Brieger J, Decker J, Gorospe M (2003) von Hippel–Lindau protein-mediated repression of tumor necrosis factor alpha translation revealed through use of cDNA arrays. Mol Cell Biol 23:2316–2328
10. Staller P, Sulitkova J, Lisztwan J, Moch H, Oakeley EJ, Krek W (2003) Chemokine receptor CXCR4 downregulated by von Hippel–Lindau tumour suppressor pVHL. Nature 425: 307–311
11. Bierie B, Stover DG, Abel TW, Chytil A, Gorska AE, Aakre M, Forrester E, Yang L, Wagner K-U, Moses HL (2008) Transforming growth factor-b regulates mammary carcinoma cell survival and interaction with the adjacent microenvironment. Cancer Res 68:1809–1819
12. Balkwill, F. (2009). TNF and Cancer: A Timeline. Nat Reviews Cancer, in press.
13. Dinarello CA (2009) Interleukin-1beta and the autoinflammatory diseases. N Engl J Med 360:2467–2470
14. Naugler WE, Karin M (2008) The wolf in sheep's clothing: the role of interleukin-6 in immunity, inflammation and cancer. Trends Mol Med 14:109–119
15. Mantovani A, Savino B, Locati M, Zammataro L, Allavena P, Bonecchi R (2010) The chemokine system in cancer biology and therapy. Cytokine Growth Factor Rev 21:27–39
16. Balkwill F (2004) The significance of cancer cell expression of CXCR4. Semin Cancer Biol 14:171–179
17. Iliopoulos D, Hirsch HA, Struhl K (2009) An epigenetic switch involving NF-kappaB, Lin28, Let-7 MicroRNA, and IL6 links inflammation to cell transformation. Cell 139:693–706
18. Balkwill F, Mantovani A (2001) Inflammation and cancer: back to Virchow? Lancet 357: 539–545
19. Maeda S, Kamata H, Luo JL, Leffert H, Karin M (2005) IKKbeta couples hepatocyte death to cytokine-driven compensatory proliferation that promotes chemical hepatocarcinogenesis. Cell 121:977–990
20. Naugler, W. E., Sakurai, T., Kim, S., Maeda, S., Kim, K. H., Elsharkawy, A. M., and Karin, M. (2007). Gender disparity in liver cancer due to sex differences in MyD88-dependent IL-6 production. Science In press
21. Bollrath J, Phesse TJ, von Burstin VA, Putoczki T, Bennecke M, Bateman T, Nebelsiek T, Lundgren-May T, Canli O, Schwitalla S et al (2009) gp130-mediated Stat3 activation in enterocytes regulates cell survival and cell-cycle progression during colitis-associated tumorigenesis. Cancer Cell 15:91–102
22. Greten FR, Eckman L, Greten TF, Park JM, Li Z-W, Egan LJ, Kagnoff MF, Karin M (2004) IKKb links inflammation and tumorigenesis in a mouse model of colitis-associated cancer. Cell 118:285–296
23. Fox JG, Wang TC (2007) Inflammation, atrophy, and gastic cancer. J Clin Invest 117:60–69
24. Grivennikov SI, Karin M (2010) Dangerous liaisons: STAT3 and NF-kappaB collaboration and crosstalk in cancer. Cytokine Growth Factor Rev 21:11–19
25. Suganuma M, Kuzuhara T, Yamaguchi K, Fujiki H (2006) Carcinogenic role of tumor necrosis factor-a inducing protein of *Helicobacter pylori* in human stomach. J Biochem Mol Biol 39:1–8
26. Moore R, Owens D, Stamp G, East N, Holdworth H, Arnott C, Burke F, Pasparakis M, Kollias G, Balkwill FR (1999) Tumour necrosis factor – a deficient mice are resistant to skin carcinogenesis. Nat Med 5:828–831
27. Andreu P, Johansson M, Affara NI, Pucci F, Tan T, Junankar S, Korets L, Lam J, Tawfik D, DeNardo DG et al (2010) FcRgamma activation regulates inflammation-associated squamous carcinogenesis. Cancer Cell 17:121–134
28. de Visser KE, Eichten A, Coussens LM (2006) Paradoxical roles of the immune system during cancer development. Nat Rev Cancer 1:24–37
29. DeNardo DG, Barreto JB, Andreu P, Vasquez L, Tawfik D, Kolhatkar N, Coussens LM (2009) CD4(+) T cells regulate pulmonary metastasis of mammary carcinomas by enhancing protumor properties of macrophages. Cancer Cell 16:91–102

30. Lin EY, Nguyen AV, Russell RG, Pollard JW (2001) Colony-stimulating factor 1 promotes progression of mammary tumors to malignancy. J Exp Med 193:727–739
31. Colombo MP, Piconese S (2009) Polyps wrap mast cells and Treg within tumorigenic tentacles. Cancer Res 69:5619–5622
32. Gounaris E, Blatner NR, Dennis K, Magnusson F, Gurish MF, Strom TB, Beckhove P, Gounari F, Khazaie K (2009) T-regulatory cells shift from a protective anti-inflammatory to a cancer-promoting proinflammatory phenotype in polyposis. Cancer Res 69:5490–5497
33. Cunha GR, Hayward SW, Wang YZ, Ricke WA (2003) Role of the stromal microenvironment in carcinogenesis of the prostate. Int J Cancer 107:1–10
34. Erez N, Truitt M, Olson P, Hanahan D (2010) Cancer-associated fibroblasts are activated in incipient neoplasia to orchestrate tumor-promoting inflammation in an NF-kappaB-dependent manner. Cancer Cell 17:135–147
35. Saadi A, Shannon NB, Lao-Sirieix P, O'Donovan M, Walker E, Clemons NJ, Hardwick JS, Zhang C, Das M, Save V et al (2010) Stromal genes discriminate preinvasive from invasive disease, predict outcome, and highlight inflammatory pathways in digestive cancers. Proc Natl Acad Sci U S A 107:2177–2182
36. Garber K (2009) First results for agents targeting cancer-related inflammation. J Natl Cancer Inst 101:1110–1112
37. Balkwill F, Mantovani A (2010) Cancer and inflammation: implications for pharmacology and therapeutics. Clin Pharmacol Ther 87:401–406
38. Elwood PC, Gallagher AM, Duthie GG, Mur LA, Morgan G (2009) Aspirin, salicylates, and cancer. Lancet 373:1301–1309
39. Jacobs EJ, Thun MJ, Bain EB, Rodriguez C, Henley SJ, Calle EE (2007) A large cohort study of long-term daily use of adult-strength aspirin and cancer incidence. J Natl Cancer Inst 99:608–615
40. Markowitz SD (2007) Aspirin and colon cancer – targeting prevention? N Engl J Med 356:2195–2198
41. Cuzick J, Otto F, Baron JA, Brown PH, Burn J, Greenwald P, Jankowski J, La Vecchia C, Meyskens F, Senn HJ, Thun M (2009) Aspirin and non-steroidal anti-inflammatory drugs for cancer prevention: an international consensus statement. Lancet Oncol 10:501–507
42. Steinbach G, Lynch PM, Phillips RKS, Wallace MH, Hawk E, Gordon GB, Wakabayashi N, Saunders B, Shen Y, Fujimura T et al (2000) The effect of celecoxib, a cyclooxygenase-2 inhibitor, in familial adenomatous polyposis. N Engl J Med 342:1946–1952
43. Epstein, J., Sanderson, I. R., and Macdonald, T. T. (2010). Curcumin as a therapeutic agent: the evidence from in vitro, animal and human studies. Br J Nutr, 1-13.
44. Fujiki H, Suganuma M, Matsuyama S, Miyazaki K (2005) Cancer prevention with green tea polyphenols for the general population, and for patients following cancer treatment. Curr Cancer Ther Rev 1:109–114

Chapter 3
Hereditary Factors and Pre-invasive Disease

Paul D.P. Pharoah

Abstract Cancer tends to run in families, a fact that has been recognised since Roman times and Paul Broca's description of a multi-case, multi-generation breast cancer family is over 140 years old [29]. Since then much has been learned about the contribution of heritable factors to the incidence of many invasive cancers. In contrast, much less is known about the role of germline genetics in pre-invasive disease. In this chapter I will briefly describe the state of our current knowledge of the genetics of the common cancers, with reference to pre-invasive disease where relevant. I will then describe how this knowledge might be used to improve the efficiency and effectiveness of early detection screening modalities.

The Genetics of Cancer

Inherited predisposition is well established as a risk factor for most of the common cancers and for many rare cancers. Many epidemiological studies have shown that an individual with a family history of cancer is at increased risk of developing the same cancer. The familial relative risk (FRR or λ) is a measure of how much more likely an individual with a given family history will develop disease compared to an individual without a family history. In general, the FRR is greater the closer the affected relative [1], and increases with the number of affected relatives in the family [2]. If a cancer develops at an early age in an individual the relative risk in the first relatives of that person will be greater, with the relative risk being greatest in young relatives of young cases. This pattern of age-specific FRRs has been confirmed in most of the common cancers and is likely to be true for all cancers. The FRR associated with a single, affected first-degree

P.D.P. Pharoah (✉)
Departments of Oncology and Public Health and Primary Care, University of Cambridge, Cambridge CB1 8RN, UK
e-mail: paul.pharoah@srl.cam.ac.uk

R.C. Fitzgerald (ed.), *Pre-Invasive Disease: Pathogenesis and Clinical Management*, DOI 10.1007/978-1-4419-6694-0_3, © Springer Science+Business Media, LLC 2011

relative (λ_1) varies for different cancers, but for most of the common cancers λ_1 is between two and three [2]. The FRR for less common cancers tends to be higher.

Most of what we know of the familial basis of cancer relates to invasive disease and there are almost no data evaluating the familial risks of pre-invasive disease. Perhaps the primary reason for this is the difficulty of studying pre-invasive disease. In particular most epidemiological studies rely on study participants recall of disease in family members – pre-invasive disease is less likely to have been diagnosed in older family members when present, and even where such a diagnosis has been made, it is unlikely that it would be accurately recalled. Furthermore, diagnosis and recording of pre-invasive diagnoses are much less likely to be complete than for invasive disease.

In principle, familial aggregation of disease may either be the results of genes segregating within families or may be due to environmental and lifestyle exposures that tend to be shared within families. Both these factors are probably relevant for most cancers, but twin studies show that inherited genetic factors are generally more important [3].

Disease predisposition alleles can be broadly characterised by their frequency in the population and the magnitude of the risk of disease in risk allele carriers (penetrance). Predisposition alleles that are rare in the general population can potentially be low or high penetrance, but the science of genetic epidemiology is currently unable to identify rare, low-penetrance disease alleles. Such alleles are likely to exist and may even account for the majority of the genetic component of cancer risk. Common predisposition alleles cannot be highly penetrant. If they were the disease would be common in the population and even so called common cancers are relatively rare at the population level – the lifetime risk of breast cancer, the commonest cancer in women in western populations, is only about one in ten. Thus, cancer predisposition alleles are generally categorised as either rare, high-penetrance alleles, or common, low-penetrance alleles.

In principle, genetic susceptibility to invasive cancer could operate at any point in the process of malignant transformation from normal epithelium to metastatic cancer. Our understanding of the inherited basis of cancer is, with few exceptions, too limited to define precisely the point along the pathway that a given predisposition allele operates.

Rare, High Penetrance Cancer Susceptibility Alleles

Family based linkage studies followed by positional cloning was very successful in the 1980s and 1990s in identifying rare, highly penetrant alleles associated with cancer predisposition syndromes. Colorectal cancer is a major feature of several of these syndromes including familial adenomatosis polyposis (FAP) and hereditary non-polyposis colorectal cancer (HNPCC) or Lynch syndrome. In both these disorders colonic adenomas are present as precursor lesions to invasive disease.

The syndromes provide a paradigm for the clinical utility of testing for genetic predisposition for a pre-invasive lesion and subsequent intervention in at risk individuals to reduce the risk of morbidity from invasive disease. FAP is associated with germline mutations in *APC*. Individuals who carry these mutations develop hundreds or thousands of adenomatous polyps in the colon in adolescence and early adulthood. Untreated, 100% of carriers go on to develop invasive colorectal carcinoma. The mainstay of the clinical management of carriers is prophylactic colectomy. HNPCC occurs in individuals with mutations in genes involved in DNA mis-match repair – *MLH1*, *MSH2*, *MSH3*, *MSH6*, *PMS1* and *PMS2* (reviewed in [4]). Deleterious mutations in these genes predispose carriers to multiple malignancies including colorectal, endometrial, ovarian, and renal, stomach, pancreas, small bowel and brain cancers. Predisposition to colorectal cancer occurs as a result of predisposition to colorectal adenomas, but carriers typically develop these lesions in early middle age with far fewer lesions than seen in FAP (typically less than 100). Untreated, the lifetime risk of invasive colorectal cancer is around 60–80% [5]. The clinical management of carriers is based around early detection and resection of pre-invasive disease by colonoscopy.

FAP and HNPCC are both examples of how genetic predisposition to pre-invasive disease can be used to identify individuals at high risk and offer them interventions aimed at reducing morbidity and mortality from invasive disease. However, the effectiveness of this approach is the result of several features of the genes involved and the related disease phenotype. First, genetic predisposition to invasive disease occurs through predisposition to a clearly identifiable, pre-invasive stage of disease. Thus it is possible to identify individuals at high risk of pre-invasive disease using genetic testing. Second, it is possible to identify pre-invasive stage of disease in at risk individuals using colonoscopy. Finally it is possible to reduce the risk of invasive disease in those with pre-invasive disease by polypectomy or prophylactic colectomy.

There are many other rare, inherited familial cancer syndromes some of which include pre-invasive lesions as part of the characteristic phenotype. However, it is beyond the scope of this chapter to discuss them all in detail.

Common, Low-Penetrance Cancer Susceptibility

The common disease, common variant hypothesis states that spontaneous mutations occurring during meiosis may become common in the population, as a result of factors including selective advantage (people with the gene variant are more likely to survive and reproduce) and population bottlenecks or expansions. Some of these variants will be harmful because they predispose to common diseases; combinations of variants underlie differences in disease susceptibility within the population.

However, until recently little was known about common genetic variation and cancer susceptibility. The emergence of high-throughput genotyping platforms combined with ever increasing information about genetic variation throughout the genome has enabled scientists to carry out empirical studies that evaluate common genetic variation across the genome for disease susceptibility in genome-wide association studies (GWAS). The commonest form of genetic variation in the human genome is the single nucleotide polymorphisms (SNP) and the currently available genotyping platforms that capture common variation across the genome genotype 500 k to 1.2 M SNPs. The last 2 years has seen the publication of a plethora GWAS for common diseases including several common cancers, notably breast, prostate and colorectal cancers [6]. At the time of writing, 27 loci with common susceptibility alleles had been reported for prostate cancer, 13 for breast cancer and 11 for colorectal cancer. GWAS in lung cancer [7,8], pancreatic cancer [9], ovarian cancer [10], melanoma [11,12], non-melanoma skin cancer [12], leukaemia [13] and glioma [14] have also been published. With the exception of breast and colorectal cancer, these cancers do not have a well-defined, easily-detectable, pre-invasive disease stage.

The pre-invasive lesion of breast cancer is ductal carcinoma in situ (DCIS) and lobular carcinoma in situ (LCIS). However, the epidemiology and molecular biology of malignant transformation from in situ to invasive disease is not well understood in breast cancer. It is clear that DCIS predisposes to invasive disease, but it is also clear that many in situ lesions do not become invasive, and some may even regress. Little is known about the natural history of the disease. There are no known factors that predispose to invasive change, including inherited genetic factors, and clinicopathological features of in situ disease that predict invasive change are not well established. Furthermore, it is not known whether all invasive cancer progress through a pre-invasive stage, or how long the duration an invasive cancer spends in the pre-invasive state.

The 13, established breast cancer susceptibility loci have been identified using standard genetic association study designs in which the frequency of putative risk alleles is compared in cases with disease and disease free controls. The 13 breast cancer susceptibility loci with common risk alleles that have been identified to date are listed in Table 3.1. These alleles have several, notable common characteristics: They act under a co-dominant genetic model with increasing risk for each

Table 3.1 Common, low-penetrance breast cancer susceptibility alleles

Locus	Locus/nearest gene	SNP	Risk allele freq	Per-allele relative risk	References
10q26	FGFR2	rs2981582	0.38	1.26	[16]
16q12	TOX3	rs12443621	0.46	1.20	[16,24]
2q35	2q35	rs13387042	0.50	1.20	[19,24]
6p12	ESR1	rs2046210	0.40	1.20	[25]
5p12	5p12	rs4415084	0.40	1.19	[26]
1p11	NOTCH2	rs11249433	0.39	1.16	[27]
14q24	RAD51L	rs999737	0.76	1.15	[27]
2q33	CASP8	rs1045485	0.85	1.14	[18]
5q11	MAP3K1	rs889312	0.28	1.13	[16]
3p24	NEK10, SLC4A7	rs4973768	0.46	1.11	[28]
8q24	8q24	rs13281615	0.40	1.08	[16]
11p15	LSP1	rs3817198	0.31	1.07	[16]
17q	COX11	rs6504950	0.73	1.05	[28]

copy of the risk allele carried; the per-allele relative risks are modest – the allele with the biggest effect, rs2981582 at the FGFR2 locus, confers a per allele risk of just 1.26; and the risk allele is generally the minor allele. Some of the SNPs lie within, or close to known genes, and others lie is regions of the genome with no known genes. The molecular mechanism of action of the SNPs on gene function have not yet been identified for any of the SNPs [15]. It is not even clear that any of the SNPs identified are the causal variants themselves – they may simply be markers strongly correlated with the true causal variant. Once the causal variant is identified, it will still be hard to determine how they alter gene function as they may not even lie within a gene or close to the gene of interest.

All these studies have used cases of invasive breast cancer as the primary disease phenotype, and no study designed to specifically investigate genetic susceptibility to in situ disease or to investigate the genetic determinants of the (putative) transition between in situ and invasive disease have been published. There have been no susceptibility alleles identified through the primary study of pre-invasive disease. Genome-wide association studies of pre-invasive breast cancer have not been carried out. Identifying alleles with risks of this magnitude requires extremely large sample sizes. For example, the data reported by Easton and colleagues [16] was based on over 20,000 invasive breast cancer cases and 20,000 controls from 22 different studies. Part of the reason for this is that extremely stringent levels of statistical significance are required in genetic association studies in order to reduce the problem of false positive associations. Genome-wide significance is generally quoted at about $P < 10^{-8}$ [17]. It seems unlikely that the magnitude of the relative risk for putative susceptibility variants for pre-invasive disease will be very different, and until large cohorts of pre-invasive disease are assembled adequately powered studies of pre-invasive disease will not be possible.

Some of the studies cited in Table 3.1 also reported the effect of the risk allele on carcinoma in situ. In all cases the sample size was small, with less than 1,000 in situ cases with available genotype data, and detecting modest risks at stringent significance levels would not be possible. Nevertheless, for the polymorphisms at the FGFR2, 2q35, CASP8, MAP3K1, 8q24 and LSP1 loci there was no significant difference in the risk of invasive disease and in situ disease [16,18,19]. At the 16q12 locus the risk of in situ disease was reported to be significantly higher than that for invasive disease [16]. The effect of the other six loci on risk of in situ disease was not reported. Given our limited understanding of the biological mechanisms of the associations, it is not possible to speculate how these loci might affect the risk of pre-invasive disease.

The Clinical Utility of Polygenic Disease Risk Prediction

The clinical utility of testing for rare, high-penetrance alleles is not questioned. However, these alleles account for a small fraction of the familial risk of disease and only a small proportion of cases will be carriers of such mutations.

Consequently, the potential for reducing the burden of disease in the population by intervening in mutation carriers will be, at best, small.

Novel methods for identifying individuals with pre-invasive disease described in other chapters (for example Chaps. 9 (Biomarkers), 10 (Molecular Imaging), 14 (Lung), 16 (Barrett's oesophagus)) provide new opportunities for reducing morbidity from invasive disease. However, many of these methods will not be suitable for application in unselected populations and may only be clinically useful in sub-groups of the population at high risk of (pre-invasive) disease. It would be possible to identify individuals at high risk of disease by testing for common, low-penetrance alleles. The potential of such polygenic risk prediction in a clinical setting has been widely debated [20–22] but as yet there is no consensus about the likely clinical utility. In reality, the clinical utility will depend not only on the predictive performance of the genetic test, but also on the options for management of individuals deemed to be at high risk. As technology for detecting pre-invasive disease becomes more advanced and options for management of individuals with pre-invasive disease are developed (e.g. Endoscopic treatment discussed in Chap. 12), the clinical utility of genetic risk prediction will also change. I will discuss some of the issues with specific reference to polygenic testing for breast cancer, but the principles could equally be applied to any other cancer.

In general, single risk alleles are likely to have extremely limited clinical utility, as the risks they confer will be modest. For example, the relative risks of breast cancer compared with the average risk in the population (relative risk of unity) are 0.83 for carriers of two low-risk alleles (common allele homozygotes) of *FGFR2* rs2981582, 1.05 for carriers of one high and one low risk allele (heterozygotes), and 1.38 for carriers of two high risk alleles (rare allele homozygotes). These risks are based on the published per-allele relative risk of 1.26 with the genotype-specific risks adjusted to be relative to the average population risk. They correspond to lifetime risks of 9.8% for women who carry one risk allele (47% of the population) and 12.7% for women who carry two risk alleles (14% of the populations) compared with a population average lifetime risk of 9.4% in the United Kingdom. Using genotype at this locus as a test for increased risk and considering all women who carry one or two risk alleles (61% of the population) as "at risk", the test would have a sensitivity of 68% (probability that someone who will get disease is tests positive) and specificity of just 39% (probability that someone who will not get disease is test negative), with a positive predictive value of 10.5% (probability that someone who tests positive will get breast cancer or their average lifetime risk).

A test based on genotype at multiple loci would be expected to perform better and so have greater clinical utility. In combination multiple alleles at different loci appear to combine multiplicatively on the relative risk scale. This is the log-additive, polygenic model of disease susceptibility. It is therefore relatively straightforward to compute the genotype specific risk based on the combined genotypes for any individual. Based on the 13 loci described above there are almost 1.6 million possible different genotype combinations. Some of these will be very rare in the population – only two women in a billion would be expected to carry two high risk alleles at each locus. Under the log-additive, polygenic model the distribution of relative risk in the population will follow a log-normal distribution. Based on the predicted distribution

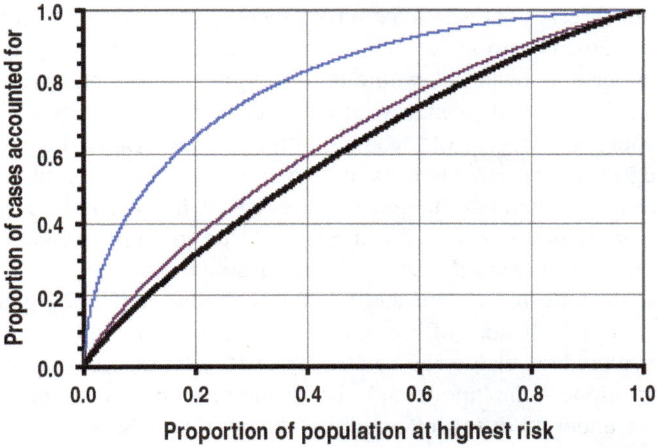

Fig. 3.1 The proportion of cases of breast cancer accounted for by the proportion of the population at highest risk. *Black line* – risk based on 13 known breast cancer susceptibility alleles; *purple line* – risk based on 13 known breast cancer susceptibility alleles and known lifestyle risk factors; *blue line* – risk based on all possible breast cancer susceptibility genes

of risk in the population, women on the lowest centile of risk will have a 59% reduction in risk (relative risk 0.41) compared to the population average (relative risk 1), whereas those on the top centile of risk will have an 115% increase in risk (relative risk 2.15). Ninety percent of women – those between the 5th and 95th centiles will have relative risks between 0.5 and 1.7. Women above the top centile would account for 2% of all cases, women above the 20th centile would account for 31% of cases and women in the top half of the risk distribution would account for 64% of all cases. Figure 3.1 shows the proportion of cases accounted for by proportion of population at highest risk. This is known as the receiver operator characteristic curve (ROC), and the area under this curve (AUC) gives a measure of the utility of a predictive test, where an AUC of 0.5 is no better than tossing a coin as a predictor of disease. The area under the curve for polygenic risk profiling is 0.60. For comparison, the figure shows the ROC curve if the effects of known lifestyle risk factors for breast cancer were added to the genetic factors (AUC=0.64), and the ROC curve that would be generated if all possible susceptibility genes were known (AUC=0.81) [23].

Thus, even using a combination of 13 loci the clinical utility of a polygenic test will be limited in predicting future disease for the individual – most women are at only slight increased risk, and the risk is only modest, even in the very small number at highest risk.

Nevertheless, polygenic risk profiles may provide useful risk stratification in the context of population-based screening programmes, particularly if combined with lifestyle risk factors [22]. The UK National Health Service breast screening program is currently offered to all women aged 50 and above, irrespective of family history or other risk factors. A 50 year old woman in the UK general population has a 2.3% chance of breast cancer within the next 10 years of her life. If we assume that 2.3% is the threshold at which the screening program has a net benefit, it makes sense to offer screening to all women with that level of risk, irrespective of age. Similarly, women at a lower risk would not be eligible for screening, also irrespective of age. A 40 year old woman with a 10-year risk of 2.3% would be offered screening, whereas a 55 year old woman with a 10-year risk of 1% would not. If such a strategy was implemented, the efficiency of the screening program would increase because it would be targeted at women at highest risk. The cost of a genetic test for purposes of risk profiling would be minimal compared with the costs of a lifetime screening program. Similar absolute risk arguments support the UK National Institute for Health and Clinical Excellence (NICE) guidelines for women with a family history of breast cancer, which recommend mammographic screening for women over the age of 40 if their 10-year risk is over 3% based on family history alone – the "moderate" risk group of women with an affected first degree relative under 40 or two affected first degree relatives, who account for less than 5% of the population.

It would be possible to offer every woman a personalized screening program in which age of starting screening would vary, based on her breast-cancer risk profile. A test using the 13 known loci would identify 10% of women with a relative risk of 1.55 or greater, which corresponds to a 10-year risk of 2.3% at age 40. Such women may benefit from additional screening outside the current NHS screening programme. There are, of course, many issues and questions that need to be addressed before such an approach became standard practice. For example, the simple models we describe make several assumptions, some of which may not be robust. The assumption that the benefit of mammographic screening for an individual woman is a simple function of absolute risk is clearly an oversimplification. The sensitivity of mammography is reduced in younger women and the true benefit is more likely to be a complex interaction between age and absolute risk. Furthermore, a population-oriented prevention program that is based on individual risk would be too complex for the marginal improvement in efficiency that it might bring. There would also be issues of patient and professional acceptance. Nevertheless, some companies are already offering polygenic testing and risk prediction and the age of personalised prevention based on personalised risk has already arrived.

Similar polygenic risk profiles could be used to identify individuals at increased risk of any cancer in order to identify a sub-group of the population that might benefit from enhanced screening that would include any screening modality that identifies individuals with pre-invasive disease.

Conclusion

There is a substantial inherited genetic component of the risk of most cancers and the molecular genetic basis for this is beginning to be unravelled. The potential benefit of genetic risk profiling is already evident, but may have real clinical utility with further developments in our understanding of the biology of pre-invasive disease. The next 10 years is likely to see continued developments in the genetic epidemiology of cancer. Large scale cohorts of patients with pre-invasive disease, such as those with in situ carcinoma of the breast and colorectal adenomatosis, are currently in progress and common genetic variants involved in susceptibility to pre-invasive disease and in the transformation from pre-invasive to invasive disease are sure to be identified. Next generation sequencing technologies may also make it possible to identify less common variants that confer low-penetrance susceptibility. Further research into the interface between risk and disease prevention is needed, but early disease detection programmes targeted at those at highest risk are a real possibility.

References

1. Amundadottir LT, Thorvaldsson S, Gudbjartsson DF et al (2004) Cancer as a complex phenotype: pattern of cancer distribution within and beyond the nuclear family. PLoS Med 1:e65
2. Houlston RS, Peto J (2004) Genetics and the common cancers. In: Eeles RA, Easton DF, Ponder BAJ, Eng C (eds) Genetic predisposition to cancer. Chapman and Hall, London, pp 235–247
3. Lichtenstein P, Holm NV, Verkasalo PK et al (2000) Environmental and heritable factors in the causation of cancer – analyses of cohorts of twins from Sweden, Denmark and Finland. N Engl J Med 343:78–85
4. Farrington SM, Dunlop MG (2004) Familial colon cacner syndromes and their genetics. In: Eeles RA, Easton DF, Ponder BAJ, Eng C (eds) Genetic predisposition to cancer. Arnold, London, pp 315–330
5. Vasen HF, Wijnen JT, Menko FH et al (1996) Cancer risk in families with hereditary nonpolyposis colorectal cancer diagnosed by mutation analysis. Gastroenterology 110:1020–1027
6. Easton DF, Eeles RA (2008) Genome-wide association studies in cancer. Hum Mol Genet 17:R109–R115
7. Hung RJ, McKay JD, Gaborieau V et al (2008) A susceptibility locus for lung cancer maps to nicotinic acetylcholine receptor subunit genes on 15q25. Nature 452:633–637
8. Thorgeirsson TE, Geller F, Sulem P et al (2008) A variant associated with nicotine dependence, lung cancer and peripheral arterial disease. Nature 452:638–642
9. Amundadottir L, Kraft P, Stolzenberg-Solomon RZ et al (2009) Genome-wide association study identifies variants in the ABO locus associated with susceptibility to pancreatic cancer. Nat Genet 41:986–990
10. Song H, Ramus SJ, Tyrer J et al (2009) A genome-wide association study identifies a new ovarian cancer susceptibility locus on 9p22.2. Nat Genet 41:996–1000
11. Brown KM, Macgregor S, Montgomery GW et al (2008) Common sequence variants on 20q11.22 confer melanoma susceptibility. Nat Genet 40(7):838–840
12. Gudbjartsson DF, Sulem P, Stacey SN et al (2008) ASIP and TYR pigmentation variants associate with cutaneous melanoma and basal cell carcinoma. Nat Genet 40(7):886–891
13. Papaemmanuil E, Hosking FJ, Vijayakrishnan J et al (2009) Loci on 7p12.2, 10q21.2 and 14q11.2 are associated with risk of childhood acute lymphoblastic leukemia. Nat Genet 41:1006–1010
14. Shete S, Hosking FJ, Robertson LB et al (2009) Genome-wide association study identifies five susceptibility loci for glioma. Nat Genet 41:899–904

15. Ghoussaini M, Pharoah PD (2009) Polygenic susceptibility to breast cancer: current state-of-the-art. Future Oncol 5:689–701
16. Easton DF, Pooley KA, Dunning AM et al (2007) Genome-wide association study identifies novel breast cancer susceptibility loci. Nature 447:1087–1093
17. Pe'er I, Yelensky R, Altshuler D, Daly MJ (2008) Estimation of the multiple testing burden for genomewide association studies of nearly all common variants. Genet Epidemiol 32: 381–385
18. Cox A, Dunning AM, Garcia-Closas M et al (2007) A common coding variant in CASP8 is associated with breast cancer risk. Nat Genet 39:352–358
19. Milne RL, Benitez J, Nevanlinna H et al (2009) Risk of estrogen receptor-positive and -negative breast cancer and single-nucleotide polymorphism 2q35-rs13387042. J Natl Cancer Inst 101:1012–1018
20. Gail MH (2008) Discriminatory accuracy from single-nucleotide polymorphisms in models to predict breast cancer risk. J Natl Cancer Inst 100:1037–1041
21. Janssens AC, van Duijn CM (2008) Genome-based prediction of common diseases: advances and prospects. Hum Mol Genet 17:R166–R173
22. Pharoah PD, Antoniou AC, Easton DF, Ponder BA (2008) Polygenes, risk prediction, and targeted prevention of breast cancer. N Engl J Med 358:2796–2803
23. Pharoah PDP, Antoniou A, Bobrow M et al (2002) Polygenic susceptibility to breast cancer: implications for prevention. Nat Genet 31:33–36
24. Stacey SN, Manolescu A, Sulem P et al (2007) Common variants on chromosomes 2q35 and 16q12 confer susceptibility to estrogen receptor-positive breast cancer. Nat Genet 39: 865–869
25. Zheng W, Long J, Gao YT et al (2009) Genome-wide association study identifies a new breast cancer susceptibility locus at 6q25.1. Nat Genet 41:324–328
26. Stacey SN, Manolescu A, Sulem P et al (2008) Common variants on chromosome 5p12 confer susceptibility to estrogen receptor-positive breast cancer. Nat Genet 40:703–706
27. Thomas G, Jacobs KB, Kraft P et al (2009) A multistage genome-wide association study in breast cancer identifies two new risk alleles at 1p11.2 and 14q24.1 (RAD51L1). Nat Genet 41:579–584
28. Ahmed S, Thomas G, Ghoussaini M et al (2009) Newly discovered breast cancer susceptibility loci on 3p24 and 17q23.2. Nat Genet 41:585–590
29. Broca PP (1866) Traites des tumeurs. Asselin, Paris

Chapter 4
Epigenetic Alterations as Contributors to the Pathogenesis, Detection, Prognosis and Treatment of Human Pre-invasive Neoplasia

Stefan David and Stephen J. Meltzer

Abstract The study of molecular processes driving human neoplasia development is achieving critical gains in terms of better detection and treatment. Current medicine already benefits from discovering genetic signatures of distinct cancers, and therapies have become more specifically targeted to the molecular aberrations defining particular cancers (e.g.: chronic myelogenous leukemia is now diagnosed by detecting the t(9;22)(q34;q11) translocation, and therapy is based on inhibitors of the aberrant *bcr-abl* kinase). Epigenetic processes complement the genetic determinants of the cellular phenotype, and their study is of great interest for cancer researchers.

The primary physiologic role of epigenetics is to govern cellular differentiation. Epigenetics have particular importance in organogenesis and also in maintaining the proper phenotypic profile of each cell in distinct organs and systems. The vast majority of current studies address DNA methylation changes pertinent to different tumor types. The global hypomethylation occurring in cancer results in genetic instability and may trigger enhanced expression of particular oncogenes. In contrast, aberrant promoter hypermethylation may reduce the expression of proteins that are critical for tissue homeostasis. This mechanism may reduce the expression of important tumor suppressor genes or the level of proteins critically involved in DNA maintenance and repair, cellular adhesion and intracellular signaling. Apart from methylation, neoplasia related perturbations were identified in virtually all of the epigenetic machinery. Proteins controlling DNA conformation (such as histone– modifying enzymes, or components of ATP-dependent remodeling and poly-ADP ribosylation) show reduced expression or activity in several distinct tumor types, providing evidence that epigenetics are critically involved in cancer development. The dynamic profile of epigenetic changes provides valuable background for clinical applications. Based on the particular epigenetic signatures described for different tumors, current studies focus on the development of epigenetic tests not only to diagnose cancer in early stages including pre-invasive disease, but also to identify patients at risk for tumor development. In addition, neoplasia-related

S. David (✉)
Department of Gastroenterology, Johns Hopkins School of Medicine, Baltimore, MD, USA
e-mail: Sdavida@jhmi.edu

R.C. Fitzgerald (ed.), *Pre-Invasive Disease: Pathogenesis and Clinical Management*,
DOI 10.1007/978-1-4419-6694-0_4,

epigenetic changes open a new therapeutic approach in human cancers, with drugs that undergo or have already passed clinical trials.

Epigenetics are therefore emerging as a promising field for both diagnostic and therapeutic approaches of human neoplasia and pre-invasive disease.

Introduction

All cells in the human organism share the same genotype. However, each cell type is characterized by a unique gene expression pattern. During cellular differentiation and maturation, the expression of certain sets of genes is silenced. The phenotypes of individual cell types are subsequently maintained throughout future generations. The gene expression profile of each cell type is programmed through changes in genomic DNA conformation, but not in DNA sequence (except for cells involved in immunoglobin synthesis).

Epigenetics describes heritable chromatin changes that exclude DNA sequence alterations [1]. A multitude of epigenetic events govern cellular phenotypic changes occurring along the normal – dysplasia – neoplasia axis. Studies of epigenetic modifications, especially methylation, elucidate cancer pathogenesis and contribute to the development of biomarkers in these devastating diseases. Discovering epigenetic modifications that occur in early cancer stages is therefore a key step in the identification of markers of pre-invasive disease. In the current chapter, we first describe different types of epigenetic events and explore their potential value in diagnosing cancer. In addition, because of the dynamic and reversible nature of epigenetic processes, we explore how the identification of particular epigenetic features in cancer may also hold therapeutic value.

Genomic DNA is wound around histone proteins to form a complex tertiary structure that can allow or impede transcription. Euchromatin (the "open" transcriptionally active state) grants transcription factors access to genomic DNA and facilitates gene expression. In contrast, heterochromatin (the compact form) silences gene transcription. The repeating unit of chromatin is termed the nucleosome. It comprises of 147 DNA base pairs wrapped around a basic protein octamer core. Two molecules of each of the core histones H2A, H2B, H3 and H4 co-associate to form this core. 50 base pairs of DNA sequence separate adjacent nucleosomes. Histone H1 binds to this 50-nucleotide linker sequence and stabilizes the complex between DNA and the histone octamer core. This interaction between DNA and histones is dynamic. Both DNA and histone proteins are subject to various modifications that affect their affinities for each other.

Dysregulated Epigenetic Mechanisms Occurring in Cancer

Several mechanisms act in a complementary fashion to dictate chromatin conformation. Of these, DNA methylation is currently the most widely studied. However, histone acetylation and methylation, poly-ADP ribosylation, and ATP-dependent chromatin remodeling also contribute to shaping chromatin spatial organization, with important effects on DNA repair and gene transcription.

ATP-Dependent Chromatin Remodeling

DNA packaging on histones is under the control of ATP-dependent chromatin remodeling complexes. Four classes of such chromatin remodelers have been described: switch/sucrose non-fermenting (SWI/SNF), imitation SWI (SWI), chromodomain-helicase-DNA-binding (CHD), and inositol/choline-responsive element-dependent gene activation mutant 80 (INO80). These classes all employ ATP hydrolysis to dynamically alter DNA-histone interactions. At the cellular level, chromatin remodeling ATPases participate in DNA repair, cell proliferation, and control and also help coordinate gene transcription [2]. Therefore, any modifications in their expression or function can significantly impact embryonic development and contribute to carcinogenesis.

The SWI/SNF family comprises two members: BRM (Drosophila protein Brahma homologue) and BRG1 (BRM/SWI2-related gene). Each of these proteins associates with BAFs (BRM/BRG1-associated factors) to form either BRM/BAF or BRG1/BAF complexes. BRM expression is decreased in gastric cancers, where BRM levels correlate with tumor histology and differentiation grade [3]. In prostate cancers, increased BRG1 levels are correlated with tumor size and invasiveness. Interestingly, BRM expression is inversely correlated with that of BRG1 in prostate cancer, suggesting different functions for each of these proteins in the development of prostatic neoplasia [4]. In contrast, the expression of both BRM and BRG1 is lost in 10% of lung cancers and correlates with decreased survival [5]. BAF proteins are designated by numbers, according to their molecular weight. BAF47 deletions were reported in blood dyscrasias (chronic myelogenous leukemia and in a subset of patients with Hodgkin Lymphoma) and in rhabdoid tumors of children [6–11]. Loss of BAF47 expression (through deletion of one allele and mutation or methylation of the second) is rare in rhabdoid tumors of adult patients.

ISWI (imitation switch) complexes are smaller than SWI/SNF chromatin remodelers. There are two classes of ISWI complexes, named after the ATPase they contain: Snf2h or Snf2l. Snf2h complexes are expressed in rapidly proliferating cells, in which they participate in chromatin assembly. In contrast, Snf2l complexes are present in differentiated cells, where they regulate gene transcription associated with the differentiation process. Increased expression of ISWI proteins has been reported in prostatic neoplasia [12].

CHD (chromodomain helicase DNA binding) ATPases are characterized by the presence of tandem chromodomains and of an SNF2-like helicase domain in their structure. Three subfamilies of CHD proteins have been described: the CHD1-CHD2, CHD3-CHD4, and CHD5-CHD9 subfamilies) [13]. Recent data indicate that CHD2 may function as a tumor suppressor, as CHD2-deficient mice develop lymhomas [14]. CHD3 and CHD4 associate with other proteins in large complexes termed NURDs (nucleosome remodeling and histone deacetylases), which alter chromatin conformation through both ATP-dependent remodeling and histone deacetylation. NURD complexes contain MTA (metastasis-associated) proteins. Of these, MTA1 promotes invasion in breast cancer [15]. CHD5 expression may be lost in human cancer, either via deletions or methylation. CHD5 deletion has been reported in neuroblastomas [16, 17]. Aberrant promoter hypermethylation is responsible for decreased CDH5 expression in gliomas, breast and colon cancers [18].

Histone Posttranslational Modifications

Changes in chromatin conformation are achieved not only by DNA modifications, but also by posttranslational changes in DNA-associated proteins. Histones can be posttranslationally modified via phosphorylation, ubiquitination, acetylation, or methylation. All these processes are interrelated and have important consequences on gene transcription, DNA stability and cell proliferation. Different patterns of posttranslational histone modifications correlate with distinct survival intervals in esophageal, breast, kidney and non-small-cell lung cancers [13–17]. Histone acetylation and methylation are the most widely studied of these modifications. Apart from differences in histone acetylation and methylation patterns, current studies in different tumors show modified expression or enzymatic activity of enzymes responsible for histone processing [1, 19, 20].

Histone acetylation occurs either on lysine groups located at amino-terminal tails or on the core domain or histones. Adding acetyl groups to these lysine residues neutralizes their positive charge and decreases interaction between histones and the negative phosphate groups on DNA. Enhanced histone acetylation in promoter regions may activate oncogene transcription. Conversely, decreased histone acetylation (e.g., as reported in prostate cancers) may silence the expression of tumor suppressor genes, such as p21 WAF1/Cip1 [21, 22]. Histone acetylation status depends on the ratio between the activities of histone acetyltransferases (HATs) and histone deacetylases (HDACs).

Four HAT classes have been described: the GNAT family (Gcn5-related N-acetyl transferase), the MYSF family (comprising the enzymes MOZ, YBF2/SAS3, SAS2 and TIP60) and the p300CBP family. HATs interact with proteins involved in critical cellular decisions (e.g., p53, Rb) or involved in important signaling pathways (e.g., Wnt) [23]. HAT overexpression has been reported in breast and ovarian tumors [24].

Genetic modifications of HATs significantly contribute to carcinogenesis. Mutations or translocations affecting CBP/p300 are linked to Rubinstein–Taiby syndrome, characterized by an increased predisposition to cancer. Numerous other translocations involving histone-processing enzymes have been described in acute myelogenous leukemia: T(8; 16)(p11; p13.3), resulting in a MOZ/CBP fusion protein; T(8; 22)(p11; q13) MORF/CBP fusion; T(10; 22)(q22; q13) MOZ/p300 chimeric protein, and inv (8)(p1 1q13.1), fusing MOZ to TIF2. HAT genetic aberrations have also been described in solid tumors as P300 missense or truncating mutation has been observed in colorectal and gastric cancers [25].

Histone deacetylation occurs through removal of acetyl groups in reactions catalyzed by histone deacetylases (HADCs). Currently, 18 different HDACs have been described. HDACs1-11 have Zn^{2+} dependent activity. HDAC1 is overexpressed in gastric, colon, prostate, and breast cancers [23–27]. HDAC2 overexpression is reported in gastric tumors [26]. HDAC6 expression is reduced in ERα-positive breast cancer, while HDAC1 levels are decreased in lung tumors [27, 28]. Genetic translocations may create chimeric proteins that result in defective HDAC recruitment. Previous studies of this class of modifications revealed T(15; 17) PML/RAR in promyelocytic leukemia and AML1/ETD in acute myelogenous leukemia [29, 30].

Sirtuins (Sirt1-7) comprise a distinct class of HDACs [24]. SIRT1, overexpressed in leukemias and glioblastomas, may alter apoptosis and cell growth [31, 32]. Enhanced SIRT7 levels have been observed in thyroid cancer [33, 34].

Histone methylation, occurring on either lysine or arginine residues in histone proteins, modifies the access of transcription factors to DNA. Divergent effects are exerted by this alteration, depending on methylation site. Generally, H3K4, H3K36 and H3K79 methylation exerts a permissive effect on gene transcription, while H3K9, H3K27 and H4K20 methylation is associated with transcriptional silencing [35]. Three classes of histone methyltransferases have been described: SET domain lysil methyltransferases, non-SET domain lysil methyltransferases, and arginine methyltransferases. *Enhancer of zeste homolog2* (EZH2, belonging to the SET domain lysil methyltransferase family) is an important component of polycomb complexes, which have a silencing effect on gene expression. Two classes of protein methyltransferases (PRMT I and PRMT II) are responsible for maintaining arginine methylation.

Histone methylation is a reversible process. Removal of methyl moieties is accomplished by histone demethylases. Lysine-specific demethylase 1 (LSD1) removes methyl groups from H3K4 by amine oxidation in a flavin adenine dinucleotide (FAD)-dependent reaction. LSD1 overexpression has been reported in poorly differentiated neuroblastoma [36]. In contrast, LSD1 expression is diminished in breast adenocarcinomas [37]. A second class of histone-demethylating enzymes comprises the Jumonji C (JmjC) domain demethylases, which remove methyl groups through an oxidative reaction. By removing the H3K27 methylation mark, JmjC domain demethylases prevent the polycomb PRC1 group of proteins from silencing gene transcription. Several JmjC domain demethylases have been linked to human neoplasia. JARID1B is overexpressed in esophageal, breast, prostate and testicular cancers [38, 39]. Demethylation of arginine-bound methyl groups is accomplished by petidylarginine deiminase 4 (PADI4) in a chemical reaction, which, instead of removing the methyl group, converts the methyl-arginine to citrulline [40, 41].

Polycomb/Trithorax Protein Function and DNA Methylation (Fig. 4.1)

Polycomb and Trithorax work antagonistically to maintain a stable gene expression pattern across multiple generations of cells. The balance between the activities of

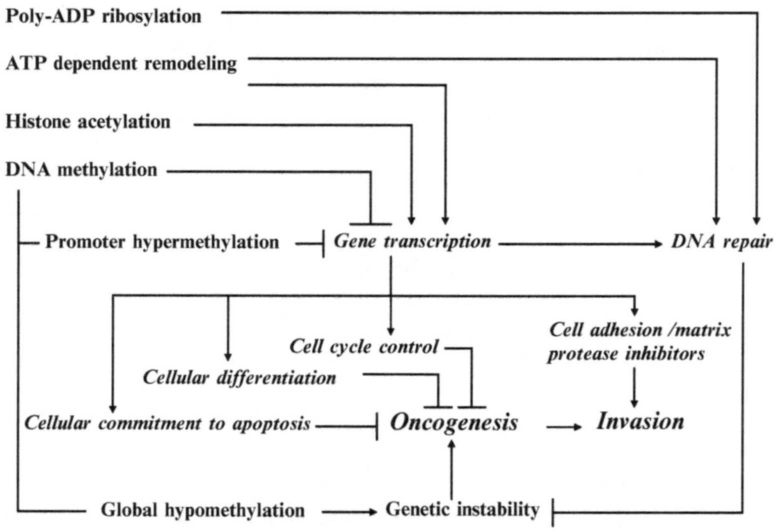

Fig. 4.1 Epigenetic processes and their involvement in basic oncogenesis mechanisms.

Polycomb and Trithorax proteins is important in maintaining stem cell identity and cellular differentiation [42–44].

Two different Polycomb complexes have been described: (1) the PRC1 complex, containing BMI1, MEL1 and CBX proteins; and (2) PRC2, comprising three components: *enhancer of zeste homolog2 (EZH2), suppressor of zeste 12 homolog (SUZ12), and embryonic ectodermal development (EED) [*45]. Proteins in each of the PRC complexes cooperate to achieve histone H3 lysine 27 trimethylation and to close the chromatin structure, functioning as marks that favor DNA methylation. The repressive function of PRC proteins on gene transcription has important consequences on cellular differentiation and cancer [46–48]. Several PRC2 components are overexpressed in different human cancers. EZH2 levels are increased in gastrointestinal cancers [49–51], tumors of the lung [52], skin [53, 54], breast [55, 56], prostate [53, 57–59], bladder [60], and endometrium [53], as well as in lymphomas [61] and myelomas [62]. SUZ12 overexpression has been reported in colon, breast and liver carcinomas [50, 63]. The PRC1 complex member Bmi1 is overexpressed in prostate [59], colon [64], and liver cancers [65]. Aberrant coexpression of EZH2 and BMI1 has been observed in liver cancer and in B-cell non-Hodgkin lymphomas, and their expression levels correlate with disease progression in the latter disease [50, 51, 60].

Poly-ADP ribosylation is a posttranslational modification in which homopolymers of ADP-ribose (PAR) are attached to various proteins by poly-ADP-ribose polymerase (PARP). The removal of PAR polymers from proteins is accomplished by poly-ADP-ribose glycohydrolase (PARG). When affecting histones, poly-ADP ribosylation converges with histone acetylation to relax the chromatin structure. PARP activity is associated not only with transcriptional control, but also with

DNA repair, cell cycle regulation, cell differentiation, and apoptosis [66]. Changes in poly-ADP-ribose polymer length and increased histone poly-ADP ribosylation have been reported in oral cancers. Multiple PARP enzymes have been identified. Most of the data regarding the role of PARP in cancer concerns PARP1. Interestingly, PARP1 levels vary widely in different cancer types. Thus, Ewing's sarcomas and malignant lymphomas, hepatocellular carcinomas, and early endometrial and colon cancers show increased PARP expression [67, 68]. In contrast, diminished PARP1 expression has been reported in breast, lung and laryngeal tumors [67, 69, 70].

DNA methylation is the most widely studied epigenetic mechanism in cancer. It comprises the covalent binding of a methyl group to the C5 of cytosines present in CpG dinucleotides. Although CpG dinucleotides represent only 1% of the entire genome, the 5′-ends of genes are particularly prone to DNA methylation, possessing a CpG content higher than 60%.

Aberrant hypermethylation of the CpG islands in gene promoters results in decreased gene expression. This methylation pattern is established during early development by DNMT3A and DNMT3B (de novo methylation) and is maintained in subsequent cell generations by DNMT1 [71, 72]. Methyl groups are transferred from S-adenosyl-methionine to cytosine. Aberrantly decreased methylation may result from decreased synthesis of S-adenosyl-methionine due to insufficient dietary intake of folate, methionine, vitamins B6 and B12 [73]. Aging and inflammation are the principal factors increasing CpG methylation during normal life [74, 75].

Methylation changes observed in neoplasia comprise global hypomethylation and promoter hypermethylation [76]. Decreased global methylation has a permissive effect on DNA point mutations and chromosomal instability [77]. Global hypomethylation is particularly relevant when it affects repetitive elements in the genomic DNA. As a result, parasitic sequences (LINE and SINE) can be activated and transcribed, leading to their elongation and movement. Another consequence of DNA demethylation is the reactivation of viral sequences integrated in the genome (e.g., hypomethylation of genomically integrated HPV16 DNA is correlated with cervical cancer progression) [78].

Numerous genes are silenced by aberrant promoter methylation. As a consequence, multiple cellular processes are disturbed, including DNA repair, cell cycle control, cellular commitment to apoptosis, and cell adhesion.

Aberrant promoter hypermethylation may contribute to cancer by inactivating tumor suppressor genes. Rb inactivation by multiple genetic hits, for example, provided the basis for Knudson's "two-hit hypothesis" [79]. However, while one copy of the gene is lost through gene deletion or mutation, silencing of the second copy may occur through aberrant promoter hypermethylation, resulting in loss of protein expression [80].

Specific gene sets have been suggested to become methylated either due to aging (type A genes), or related to cancer development (type C genes). The latter set has been used to define a "CpG Island Methylator Phenotype" (CIMP), initially described in gastric and colorectal cancers [81–83]. MLH1 and p16 are notable members of the type C group.

A distinct set of genes undergoing aberrant promoter hypermethylation cancer is involved in maintaining DNA integrity. Defective DNA mismatch repair resulting from reduced expression of DNA repair proteins has been well-documented in hereditary nonpolyposis colorectal cancer (HNPCC) [84, 85]. Decreased hMLH1 or hMSH2 expression due to promoter hypermethylation or mutation has been reported in breast, colorectal and gastric carcinomas and leukemias [86–90].

Dysfunctional cell cycle control is caused by reduced expression of proteins involved in mitotic checkpoints. Aberrant promoter hypermethylation of p16, p15 and p14 occurs in multiple human neoplasias and can correlate with clinical prognosis [91–98].

Methylation-induced silencing of genes involved in both the execution and regulation of apoptosis is another epigenetic feature of cancers. This process allows tumor cells to survive despite genetic errors, hypoxia, or other cell death-inducing conditions. A new concept of an "apoptotic methylation signature" has emerged in the progression of prostate tumors [99]. TNFα hypermethylation has been reported in a subset of T-cell lymphomas [100]. TRAIL signaling is dysregulated in ependymomas through aberrant methylation of proteins involved in this pathway [101]. Increased promoter methylation of DR4, a TRAIL receptor, reported in astroctymas and a subset of ovarian cancers, is considered to be responsible for cellular resistance to TRAIL-induced apoptosis [102, 103]. Aberrant hypermethylation of caspase-8 is a prominent feature of relapsing gliomas and mediates resistance to apoptosis in small cell lung cancers [104, 105]. Promoter hypermethylation of Bik, reported in renal carcinomas, suggests that pro-apoptotic regulators are also silenced through epigenetic mechanisms [106].

Another set of genes aberrantly hypermethylated in cancer is important in the control of cell migration and metastasis. Cadherins play important roles in cell adhesion, and their dysregulation may exert important consequences on cancer development [107]. The E-cadherin (CDH1) promoter is hypermethylated in colorectal, hepatic, breast, ovarian, and prostate carcinomas [108–114]. H-cadherin (CDH-13) undergoes promoter hypermethylation in esophageal breast, lung and colon cancers [115–119].

Cellular secreted proteases allow cell invasion and metastasis by degrading the intercellular matrix. Their actions are controlled by protease inhibitors, which may be silenced by aberrant methylation. Reduced expression of tissue inhibitor of matrix-metalloprotease 3 (TIMP3), occurring due to hypermethylation in cancer, permits easier dissemination of tumor cells [120].

Still another set of genes showing promoter hypermethylation encodes proteins involved in intracellular cell signaling. Wnt signaling is particularly important for cell proliferation and in the control of stem cell differentiation. We discuss the Wnt cascade not only because of its importance and complexity, but also due to its correlation with multiple signaling cascades and its interaction with proteins involved in cellular adhesion and differentiation. All of these factors converge to render the Wnt pathway particularly susceptible to being dysregulated through mutation or aberrant hypermethylation of proteins involved in its function and regulation. The central event in the canonical Wnt signaling cascade is β-catenin accumulation in the cytoplasm, followed by its translocation into the nucleus. Inside the nucleus, β-catenin binds TCF/LEF (T cell factor/lymphoid enhancer factor) to initiate transcription. In the cytoplasm, β-catenin is bound and phosphorylated in a protein complex comprising glycogen synthase kinase 3β (GSK-3β), casein kinase I (CKI), axin, and adenomatous polyposis coli (APC). Phosphorylated β-catenin is subsequently degraded through proteolysis. The binding of Wnt ligands to their cognate Frizzled receptor proteins activates the Disheveled family and subsequently inhibits the GSK-3β/CKI/axin/APC complex. The lipoprotein receptor-related protein (LRP5/6) also binds Wnt to allow activation of the signaling cascade. As a result of this binding, β-catenin is no longer degraded and, upon its cytoplasmic accumulation, it translocates to nucleus. Wnt signaling is regulated at both the intra- and extracellular levels. Inside the cell, apart from the GSK-3β/CKI/ axin/APC complex, Hint1, PKC1 and ICAT prevent β-catenin-initiated transcription. Extracellularly, Wnt inhibitory factor 1 (Wif-1) and soluble frizzled-related proteins (SFRPs) bind Wnt and prevent its interaction with Frizzled. Dickkopf proteins bind LRP5/6 to induce its endocytosis and prevent Wnt signaling [121]. APC methylation has been reported in multiple neoplasias, including esophageal, gastric, lung, breast, and prostate cancers [92, 110, 122–125]. APC, alone as part of a panel of methylated genes detected in serum, can be used to predict prognosis. Detection of APC methylation in serum is a poor prognostic factor in esophageal and prostate carcinomas [124, 126, 127]. Methylated APC and CDKN2A are markers of the progression of Barrett's esophagus (BE) to high-grade dysplasia (HGD) or esophageal adenocarcinoma (EAC) [120, 126, 128]. For the early detection of EAC, our group have demonstrated that additional genes (including RUNX3, HPP1, Reprimo, NELL1, TAC1, SST, AKAP12 and CDH13) undergo promoter methylation early in BE-associated neoplasia [115, 129–134]. As we will discuss below, these genes may serve as methylation biomarkers to identify BE patients at risk of developing future HGD or EAC.

Methylated APC and RASSF1A detected in serum also represent markers of circulating tumor cells and also correlate with advanced breast cancer stage [135]. Soluble Frizzle-Related Proteins (SFRPs) are important extracellular regulators of Wnt signaling. SFRP protein promoters are hypermethylated in gastrointestinal, lung, and genitourinary cancers, as well as in blood dyscrasias such as acute and chronic myelogenous leukemia, chronic lymphocytic leukemia, or multiple myeloma [4, 136–150].

Wif-1 shows promoter hypermethylation in hepatocellular carcinoma [151], gastrointestinal tumors [1, 152], lung cancer [98, 153], mesothelioma [154] and bladder cancer [143] Detection of methylated Wif-1 in pleural effusions may potentially complement the cytologic examination of pleural effusion to detect potential neoplastic origin [155].

Dickkopf proteins (DKK) represent an additional extracellular regulator of Wnt signaling, since they exhibit promoter hypermethylation in gastrointestinal and breast cancers and in acute myeloid leukemia [156].

A new set of candidate tumor suppressors comprises the RASSF genes, encoding proteins characterized by the presence of a Ras association domain. The presence of this domain allows these genes to function as negative effectors of Ras. As a result, RASSF proteins act by inhibiting proliferation and enhancing apoptosis [157]. RASFF1A hypermethylation has been detected in sera of patients with different types of neoplasia and is included in gene panels for which methylation is measured in diagnostic approaches [119, 158].

Another interesting finding is the presence of both aberrant methylation and mutation of HLA loci in gastric cancers and T-cell lymphomas, providing an insight into mechanisms mediating immune escape of tumor cells [159, 160].

Interestingly as well, hypomethylation of certain genes is also involved in human neoplasia. Promoter hypomethylation of multidrug resistance 1 gene (MDR1) is reported in tumors and sera of patients with invasive ductal breast carcinomas and correlates with tumor aggresivity [161]. Insulin-like growth factor 2 (IGF2) manifests promoter hypomethylation in osteosarcomas and cancers of the breast, colorectum, and liver and may potentially serve as a neoplasia biomarker [162–164].

Clinical Applications Related to Epigenetic Modifications Occurring in Neoplastic Disease

In addition to providing extremely valuable insights into the molecular mechanisms driving cancer development and progression, the study of epigenetic alterations has opened up a broad field for two important clinical applications. Because of the relative stability of the DNA molecule, the methylation status of different genes is a new category of test, which may serve as a powerful clinical biomarker. Another application currently under study is to develop new therapeutic agents based on disturbed epigenetic processes occurring in human cancer.

Biomarkers of Neoplastic and Pre-invasive Disease

A tremendous amount of information has accumulated with regard to epigenetic modifications occurring in cancer or preneoplastic lesions. The application of epigenetic markers has followed several avenues: (1) identifying the presence of a tumor, (2) predicting how aggressively the tumor will grow and spread, (3) predicting response to treatment, and (4) identifying patients at risk for a certain cancer even before the tumor occurs. As already discussed, numerous individual genes have emerged as strong candidates for methylation-related markers. We have discussed individual epigenetic events that characterize different tumors. To increase both the sensitivity and the specificity of a given epigenetic test, one new approach is to simultaneously investigate the methylation status in a panel of several genes and to eventually include other clinical parameters in the analysis, for both screening and prognosis-related purposes [165–170].

Various types of patient-derived samples have been studied, including tumor tissue and different body fluids, depending on the nature of the cancer studied. Numerous investigators are attempting to establish unique gene panels, which could potentially distinguish the presence of different tumor types by methylation levels of the investigated genes in patients' sera [143, 169, 171]. Methylation has also been studied for its ability to detect the presence of cancer cells in sputum samples from lung cancer patients [172–175]. Assessing the methylation status of difference genes in urine has value in identifying urinary tract cancers [176–179].

Increased desquamation of tumor cells within the gastrointestinal tract may provide a source of aberrantly methylated DNA that can be assessed to successfully identify tumors in stool specimens [180–182].

Early detection of any tumor is key to the success of any therapeutic strategy. Distinct sets of epigenetic events closely parallel phenotypic changes that occur during neoplasia development. Decreased H4K20 trimethylation occurs in precursor lesions of lung cancer [183]. As discussed, a much larger amount of information has accumulated concerning genes that undergo aberrant promoter hypermethylation in preneoplastic lesions and early in tumor development. Of particular interest for both understanding disease progression and for biomarker development, Barrett's esophagus represents a preneoplastic lesion that may or may not develop into cancer. BE is histologically characterized by the replacement of the squamous epithelial lining of the lower esophagus with intestinal-like metaplastic columnar epithelium [184]. The current strategy of clinically surveillance is to employ endoscopy for the periodically screening of BE patients. The dysplasia grade is assessed for identifying patients at risk for EAC development [184, 185]. However, the predictive value of dysplasia relatively is limited and tissue sampling (by the endoscopists) and interobserver variability (for the pathologists) add to the difficulty of classifying particular lesions [186]. The current screening approach also suffers from the discomfort imposed on patients and the high costs incurred by endoscopic surveillance. It is therefore stringently necessary to develop a more robust panel of biomarkers for assessing the BE patient's risk to progress to EAC.

Our group discovered a set of genes that undergo promoter hypermethylation early in the normal-dysplasia-neoplasia sequence [115, 129–134]. We have demonstrated that hypermethylation of CDKN2A, RUNX3 and HPP represent early epigenetic events occurring in progressing BE and that the methylation status of these genes correlates with patients' prognosis [129]. A subsequent study in our lab demonstrated Reprimo hypermethylation occurs early in EAC development and may serve as a neoplasia biomarker [130]. We additionally identified NELL1, TAC1, SST, AKAP12 and CDH13 as early methylated genes in EAC progression [115, 131–134]. Consolidating these findings, we havedeveloped a risk stratification model to predict which BE patients are at risk to progress to EAC [167, 168]. These studies suggest that assessing promoter hypermethylation of certain genes and correlating them with certain clinical parameters may improve detection from early, preinvasive stages of frank neoplasia to the identification of preneoplastic lesions prone to cancer progression.

These results provide a basis for developing panels consisting of both genes and clinical parameters, which may predict which patients progress from preneoplastic to frank neoplastic lesions (e.g., EAC), as well as their response to therapy [129, 167, 168, 187, 188].

Numerous techniques have been established to determine the methylation status of specific genes; each technique has its own strengths and weaknesses [189]. However, translating epigenetic discoveries into daily clinical practice will require much effort applied to validating biomarker-related findings and developing standardized techniques for obtaining, preparing/preserving, and processing samples, to allow comparison of epigenetic data obtained in different clinical settings.

Novel Therapeutic Approaches to Neoplastic Disease

In contrast to genetic modifications that occur in cancer, epigenetic changes may be reversed. Each epigenetic mechanism employs several classes of specific enzymes. As a result, a multitude of pharmacological inhibitors are under development, either as single or as adjuvant agents.

Depending on chemical structure, four classes of histone deacetylase inhibitors (HDACi) have been described: hydroxamic acid derivates (vorinostat, trichostatin, LAQ824, panobinostat, belinostat and ITF 2357), cyclic tetrapeptides (depsipeptide), benzamide (entinostat, MGCD0103) and short-chain aliphatic acids (valproic acid, phenylbutyrate and AN-9). Thus far, only vorinostat has obtained FDA approval, for treating cutaneous T-cell lymphoma (CTCL) [190]. Vorinostat, depsipeptide and MGCD0103 are currently in phase I and II clinical trials in both hematologic and solid tumors [191]. Histone methylation is also a susceptible target in cancer therapy. Both lysine and arginine methyltransferase inhibitors have been developed, and their activity is under study in different cancer models [20].

The potential use of PARP inhibitors in cancer therapy was suggested by the involvement of PARP in DNA repair. PARP inhibitors may work either alone (e.g., in tumors with deficient DNA repair mechanisms due to BRCA1 or BRCA2 deficiency) or in association with DNA-damaging chemo- or radiotherapeutic regimens [192, 193]. AGO14699 and INO-1001 have undergone phase I clinical trials in melanoma in combination with temozolomide [194, 195].

The demethylating agents 5-azacytidine and 5-aza-2′-deoxycytidine (decitabine) showed encouraging results in the treatment of myelodysplastic syndrome [196–198].

Conclusions

The study of epigenetic mechanisms that are dysregulated in cancer is a rewarding field. Not only does this study provide insights into cancer development, but it also furnishes clues to develop diagnostic and therapeutic tools. These efforts are far from over. However, by applying multiple gene panels, improved future diagnostic tools are now possible. In the therapeutic arena, multiple enzyme inhibitors are currently undergoing clinical trials, and a number of other new inhibitors have also been developed. A critical mass of information has been reached, and this milestone may lead to breakthroughs in the early diagnosis and treatment of human cancers.

References

1. Lafon-Hughes L, Di Tomaso MV, Mendez-Acuna L, Martinez-Lopez W (2008) Chromatin-remodelling mechanisms in cancer. Mutat Res 658:191–214
2. Keppler BR, Archer TK (2008) Chromatin-modifying enzymes as therapeutic targets – Part 2. Expert Opin Ther Targets 12:1457–1467
3. Yamamichi N, Inada K, Ichinose M, Yamamichi-Nishina M, Mizutani T, Watanabe H, Shiogama K, Fujishiro M, Okazaki T, Yahagi N, Haraguchi T, Fujita S, Tsutsumi Y, Omata M, Iba H (2007) Frequent loss of Brm expression in gastric cancer correlates with histologic features and differentiation state. Cancer Res 67:10727–10735
4. Cheng YY, Yu J, Wong YP, Man EP, To KF, Jin VX, Li J, Tao Q, Sung JJ, Chan FK, Leung WK (2007) Frequent epigenetic inactivation of secreted frizzled-related protein 2 (SFRP2) by promoter methylation in human gastric cancer. Br J Cancer 97:895–901
5. Reisman DN, Sciarrotta J, Wang W, Funkhouser WK, Weissman BE (2003) Loss of BRG1/BRM in human lung cancer cell lines and primary lung cancers: correlation with poor prognosis. Cancer Res 63:560–566
6. Grand F, Kulkarni S, Chase A, Goldman JM, Gordon M, Cross NC (1999) Frequent deletion of hSNF5/INI1, a component of the SWI/SNF complex, in chronic myeloid leukemia. Cancer Res 59:3870–3874
7. Yuge M, Nagai H, Uchida T, Murate T, Hayashi Y, Hotta T, Saito H, Kinoshita T (2000) HSNF5/INI1 gene mutations in lymphoid malignancy. Cancer Genet Cytogenet 122:37–42
8. Specchia G, Albano F, Anelli L, Storlazzi CT, Zagaria A, Liso A, Pannunzio A, Pastore D, Mestice A, Greco G, Liso V, Rocchi M (2004) Derivative chromosome 9 deletions in chronic myeloid leukemia are associated with loss of tumor suppressor genes. Leuk Lymphoma 45:689–694
9. DeCristofaro MF, Betz BL, Wang W, Weissman BE (1999) Alteration of hSNF5/INI1/BAF47 detected in rhabdoid cell lines and primary rhabdomyosarcomas but not Wilms' tumors. Oncogene 18:7559–7565
10. Versteege I, Sevenet N, Lange J, Rousseau-Merck MF, Ambros P, Handgretinger R, Aurias A, Delattre O (1998) Truncating mutations of hSNF5/INI1 in aggressive paediatric cancer. Nature 394:203–206
11. Biegel JA, Tan L, Zhang F, Wainwright L, Russo P, Rorke LB (2002) Alterations of the hSNF5/INI1 gene in central nervous system atypical teratoid/rhabdoid tumors and renal and extrarenal rhabdoid tumors. Clin Cancer Res 8:3461–3467
12. Mohamed MA, Greif PA, Diamond J, Sharaf O, Maxwell P, Montironi R, Young RA, Hamilton PW (2007) Epigenetic events, remodelling enzymes and their relationship to chromatin organization in prostatic intraepithelial neoplasia and prostatic adenocarcinoma. BJU Int 99:908–915
13. Marfella CG, Imbalzano AN (2007) The Chd family of chromatin remodelers. Mutat Res 618:30–40
14. Nagarajan P, Onami TM, Rajagopalan S, Kania S, Donnell R, Venkatachalam S (2009) Role of chromodomain helicase DNA-binding protein 2 in DNA damage response signaling and tumorigenesis. Oncogene 28:1053–1062

15. Kumar R, Wang RA, Bagheri-Yarmand R (2003) Emerging roles of MTA family members in human cancers. Semin Oncol 30:30–37
16. Thompson PM, Gotoh T, Kok M, White PS, Brodeur GM (2003) CHD5, a new member of the chromodomain gene family, is preferentially expressed in the nervous system. Oncogene 22:1002–1011
17. Fujita T, Igarashi J, Okawa ER, Gotoh T, Manne J, Kolla V, Kim J, Zhao H, Pawel BR, London WB, Maris JM, White PS, Brodeur GM (2008) CHD5, a tumor suppressor gene deleted from 1p36.31 in neuroblastomas. J Natl Cancer Inst 100:940–949
18. Mulero-Navarro S, Esteller M (2008) Chromatin remodeling factor CHD5 is silenced by promoter CpG island hypermethylation in human cancer. Epigenetics 3:210–215
19. Ellis L, Atadja PW, Johnstone RW (2009) Epigenetics in cancer: targeting chromatin modifications. Mol Cancer Ther 8:1409–1420
20. Spannhoff A, Hauser AT, Heinke R, Sippl W, Jung M (2009) The emerging therapeutic potential of histone methyltransferase and demethylase inhibitors. ChemMedChem 4:1568–1582
21. Goldsmith ME, Kitazono M, Fok P, Aikou T, Bates S, Fojo T (2003) The histone deacetylase inhibitor FK228 preferentially enhances adenovirus transgene expression in malignant cells. Clin Cancer Res 9:5394–5401
22. Banwell CM, Singh R, Stewart PM, Uskokovic MR, Campbell MJ (2003) Antiproliferative signalling by 1, 25(OH)2D3 in prostate and breast cancer is suppressed by a mechanism involving histone deacetylation. Recent Results Cancer Res 164:83–98
23. Lund AH, van Lohuizen M (2004) Epigenetics and cancer. Genes Dev 18:2315–2335
24. Mahlknecht U, Hoelzer D (2000) Histone acetylation modifiers in the pathogenesis of malignant disease. Mol Med 6:623–644
25. Muraoka M, Konishi M, Kikuchi-Yanoshita R, Tanaka K, Shitara N, Chong JM, Iwama T, Miyaki M (1996) p300 gene alterations in colorectal and gastric carcinomas. Oncogene 12:1565–1569
26. Song J, Noh JH, Lee JH, Eun JW, Ahn YM, Kim SY, Lee SH, Park WS, Yoo NJ, Lee JY, Nam SW (2005) Increased expression of histone deacetylase 2 is found in human gastric cancer. APMIS 113:264–268
27. Zhang Z, Yamashita H, Toyama T, Sugiura H, Omoto Y, Ando Y, Mita K, Hamaguchi M, Hayashi S, Iwase H (2004) HDAC6 expression is correlated with better survival in breast cancer. Clin Cancer Res 10:6962–6968
28. Osawa T, Chong JM, Sudo M, Sakuma K, Uozaki H, Shibahara J, Nagai H, Funata N, Fukayama M (2002) Reduced expression and promoter methylation of p16 gene in Epstein-Barr virus-associated gastric carcinoma. Jpn J Cancer Res 93:1195–1200
29. Grignani F, De Matteis S, Nervi C, Tomassoni L, Gelmetti V, Cioce M, Fanelli M, Ruthardt M, Ferrara FF, Zamir I, Seiser C, Lazar MA, Minucci S, Pelicci PG (1998) Fusion proteins of the retinoic acid receptor-alpha recruit histone deacetylase in promyelocytic leukaemia. Nature 391:815–818
30. Jones LK, Saha V (2002) Chromatin modification, leukaemia and implications for therapy. Br J Haematol 118:714–727
31. Huffman DM, Grizzle WE, Bamman MM, Kim JS, Eltoum IA, Elgavish A, Nagy TR (2007) SIRT1 is significantly elevated in mouse and human prostate cancer. Cancer Res 67:6612–6618
32. Liu G, Yuan X, Zeng Z, Tunici P, Ng H, Abdulkadir IR, Lu L, Irvin D, Black KL, Yu JS (2006) Analysis of gene expression and chemoresistance of CD133+ cancer stem cells in glioblastoma. Mol Cancer 5:67
33. de Nigris F, Cerutti J, Morelli C, Califano D, Chiariotti L, Viglietto G, Santelli G, Fusco A (2002) Isolation of a SIR-like gene, SIR-T8, that is overexpressed in thyroid carcinoma cell lines and tissues. Br J Cancer 86:917–923
34. Frye R (2002) "SIRT8" expressed in thyroid cancer is actually SIRT7. Br J Cancer 87:1479
35. Martin C, Zhang Y (2005) The diverse functions of histone lysine methylation. Nat Rev Mol Cell Biol 6:838–849

36. Schulte JH, Lim S, Schramm A, Friedrichs N, Koster J, Versteeg R, Ora I, Pajtler K, Klein-Hitpass L, Kuhfittig-Kulle S, Metzger E, Schule R, Eggert A, Buettner R, Kirfel J (2009) Lysine-specific demethylase 1 is strongly expressed in poorly differentiated neuroblastoma: implications for therapy. Cancer Res 69:2065–2071
37. Wang Y, Zhang H, Chen Y, Sun Y, Yang F, Yu W, Liang J, Sun L, Yang X, Shi L, Li R, Li Y, Zhang Y, Li Q, Yi X, Shang Y (2009) LSD1 is a subunit of the NuRD complex and targets the metastasis programs in breast cancer. Cell 138:660–672
38. Barrett A, Madsen B, Copier J, Lu PJ, Cooper L, Scibetta AG, Burchell J, Taylor-Papadimitriou J (2002) PLU-1 nuclear protein, which is upregulated in breast cancer, shows restricted expression in normal human adult tissues: a new cancer/testis antigen? Int J Cancer 101:581–588
39. Xiang Y, Zhu Z, Han G, Ye X, Xu B, Peng Z, Ma Y, Yu Y, Lin H, Chen AP, Chen CD (2007) JARID1B is a histone H3 lysine 4 demethylase up-regulated in prostate cancer. Proc Natl Acad Sci U S A 104:19226–19231
40. Cuthbert GL, Daujat S, Snowden AW, Erdjument-Bromage H, Hagiwara T, Yamada M, Schneider R, Gregory PD, Tempst P, Bannister AJ, Kouzarides T (2004) Histone deimination antagonizes arginine methylation. Cell 118:545–553
41. Wang Y, Wysocka J, Sayegh J, Lee YH, Perlin JR, Leonelli L, Sonbuchner LS, McDonald CH, Cook RG, Dou Y, Roeder RG, Clarke S, Stallcup MR, Allis CD, Coonrod SA (2004) Human PAD4 regulates histone arginine methylation levels via demethylimination. Science 306:279–283
42. Bird A (2007) Perceptions of epigenetics. Nature 447:396–398
43. Moehrle A, Paro R (1994) Spreading the silence: epigenetic transcriptional regulation during Drosophila development. Dev Genet 15:478–484
44. Ringrose L, Paro R (2007) Polycomb/Trithorax response elements and epigenetic memory of cell identity. Development 134:223–232
45. Lund AH, van Lohuizen M (2004) Polycomb complexes and silencing mechanisms. Curr Opin Cell Biol 16:239–246
46. Cao R, Zhang Y (2004) The functions of E(Z)/EZH2-mediated methylation of lysine 27 in histone H3. Curr Opin Genet Dev 14:155–164
47. Sparmann A, van Lohuizen M (2006) Polycomb silencers control cell fate, development and cancer. Nat Rev Cancer 6:846–856
48. Simon JA, Lange CA (2008) Roles of the EZH2 histone methyltransferase in cancer epigenetics. Mutat Res 647:21–29
49. Matsukawa Y, Semba S, Kato H, Ito A, Yanagihara K, Yokozaki H (2006) Expression of the enhancer of zeste homolog 2 is correlated with poor prognosis in human gastric cancer. Cancer Sci 97:484–491
50. Yonemitsu Y, Imazeki F, Chiba T, Fukai K, Nagai Y, Miyagi S, Arai M, Aoki R, Miyazaki M, Nakatani Y, Iwama A, Yokosuka O (2009) Distinct expression of polycomb group proteins EZH2 and BMI1 in hepatocellular carcinoma. Hum Pathol 40:1304–1311
51. Sasaki M, Ikeda H, Itatsu K, Yamaguchi J, Sawada S, Minato H, Ohta T, Nakanuma Y (2008) The overexpression of polycomb group proteins Bmi1 and EZH2 is associated with the progression and aggressive biological behavior of hepatocellular carcinoma. Lab Invest 88:873–882
52. Breuer RH, Snijders PJ, Smit EF, Sutedja TG, Sewalt RG, Otte AP, van Kemenade FJ, Postmus PE, Meijer CJ, Raaphorst FM (2004) Increased expression of the EZH2 polycomb group gene in BMI-1-positive neoplastic cells during bronchial carcinogenesis. Neoplasia 6:736–743
53. Bachmann IM, Halvorsen OJ, Collett K, Stefansson IM, Straume O, Haukaas SA, Salvesen HB, Otte AP, Akslen LA (2006) EZH2 expression is associated with high proliferation rate and aggressive tumor subgroups in cutaneous melanoma and cancers of the endometrium, prostate, and breast. J Clin Oncol 24:268–273
54. McHugh JB, Fullen DR, Ma L, Kleer CG, Su LD (2007) Expression of polycomb group protein EZH2 in nevi and melanoma. J Cutan Pathol 34:597–600

55. Collett K, Eide GE, Arnes J, Stefansson IM, Eide J, Braaten A, Aas T, Otte AP, Akslen LA (2006) Expression of enhancer of zeste homologue 2 is significantly associated with increased tumor cell proliferation and is a marker of aggressive breast cancer. Clin Cancer Res 12:1168–1174
56. Ding L, Kleer CG (2006) Enhancer of Zeste 2 as a marker of preneoplastic progression in the breast. Cancer Res 66:9352–9355
57. Varambally S, Dhanasekaran SM, Zhou M, Barrette TR, Kumar-Sinha C, Sanda MG, Ghosh D, Pienta KJ, Sewalt RG, Otte AP, Rubin MA, Chinnaiyan AM (2002) The polycomb group protein EZH2 is involved in progression of prostate cancer. Nature 419:624–629
58. Rhodes DR, Sanda MG, Otte AP, Chinnaiyan AM, Rubin MA (2003) Multiplex biomarker approach for determining risk of prostate-specific antigen-defined recurrence of prostate cancer. J Natl Cancer Inst 95:661–668
59. van Leenders GJ, Dukers D, Hessels D, van den Kieboom SW, Hulsbergen CA, Witjes JA, Otte AP, Meijer CJ, Raaphorst FM (2007) Polycomb-group oncogenes EZH2, BMI1, and RING1 are overexpressed in prostate cancer with adverse pathologic and clinical features. Eur Urol 52:455–463
60. Raman JD, Mongan NP, Tickoo SK, Boorjian SA, Scherr DS, Gudas LJ (2005) Increased expression of the polycomb group gene, EZH2, in transitional cell carcinoma of the bladder. Clin Cancer Res 11:8570–8576
61. van Kemenade FJ, Raaphorst FM, Blokzijl T, Fieret E, Hamer KM, Satijn DP, Otte AP, Meijer CJ (2001) Coexpression of BMI-1 and EZH2 polycomb-group proteins is associated with cycling cells and degree of malignancy in B-cell non-Hodgkin lymphoma. Blood 97:3896–3901
62. Croonquist PA, Van Ness B (2005) The polycomb group protein enhancer of zeste homolog 2 (EZH 2) is an oncogene that influences myeloma cell growth and the mutant ras phenotype. Oncogene 24:6269–6280
63. Kirmizis A, Bartley SM, Kuzmichev A, Margueron R, Reinberg D, Green R, Farnham PJ (2004) Silencing of human polycomb target genes is associated with methylation of histone H3 Lys 27. Genes Dev 18:1592–1605
64. Du J, Li Y, Li J, Zheng J. Polycomb group protein Bmi1 expression in colon cancers predicts the survival. Med Oncol 2009.
65. Xu CR, Lee S, Ho C, Bommi P, Huang SA, Cheung ST, Dimri GP, Chen X (2009) Bmi1 functions as an oncogene independent of Ink4A/Arf repression in hepatic carcinogenesis. Mol Cancer Res 7:1937–1945
66. Miwa M, Masutani M (2007) PolyADP-ribosylation and cancer. Cancer Sci 98:1528–1535
67. Masutani M, Nakagama H, Sugimura T (2005) Poly(ADP-ribosyl)ation in relation to cancer and autoimmune disease. Cell Mol Life Sci 62:769–783
68. Klenova E, Ohlsson R (2005) Poly(ADP-ribosyl)ation and epigenetics. Is CTCF PARt of the plot? Cell Cycle 4:96–101
69. Bieche I, de Murcia G, Lidereau R (1996) Poly(ADP-ribose) polymerase gene expression status and genomic instability in human breast cancer. Clin Cancer Res 2:1163–1167
70. Cao WH, Wang X, Frappart L, Rigal D, Wang ZQ, Shen Y, Tong WM (2007) Analysis of genetic variants of the poly(ADP-ribose) polymerase-1 gene in breast cancer in French patients. Mutat Res 632:20–28
71. Okano M, Bell DW, Haber DA, Li E (1999) DNA methyltransferases Dnmt3a and Dnmt3b are essential for de novo methylation and mammalian development. Cell 99:247–257
72. Issa JP (2004) CpG island methylator phenotype in cancer. Nat Rev Cancer 4:988–993
73. Duthie SJ, Narayanan S, Brand GM, Pirie L, Grant G (2002) Impact of folate deficiency on DNA stability. J Nutr 132:2444S–2449S
74. Jaenisch R, Bird A (2003) Epigenetic regulation of gene expression: how the genome integrates intrinsic and environmental signals. Nat Genet 33(Suppl):245–254
75. Kang GH, Lee HJ, Hwang KS, Lee S, Kim JH, Kim JS (2003) Aberrant CpG island hypermethylation of chronic gastritis, in relation to aging, gender, intestinal metaplasia, and chronic inflammation. Am J Pathol 163:1551–1556

76. Gronbaek K, Hother C, Jones PA (2007) Epigenetic changes in cancer. Apmis 115:1039–1059
77. Ballestar E, Esteller M (2008) Epigenetic gene regulation in cancer. Adv Genet 61:247–267
78. Badal V, Chuang LS, Tan EH, Badal S, Villa LL, Wheeler CM, Li BF, Bernard HU (2003) CpG methylation of human papillomavirus type 16 DNA in cervical cancer cell lines and in clinical specimens: genomic hypomethylation correlates with carcinogenic progression. J Virol 77:6227–6234
79. Knudson AG Jr (1971) Mutation and cancer: statistical study of retinoblastoma. Proc Natl Acad Sci U S A 68:820–823
80. Garinis GA, Patrinos GP, Spanakis NE, Menounos PG (2002) DNA hypermethylation: when tumour suppressor genes go silent. Hum Genet 111:115–127
81. Toyota M, Ahuja N, Ohe-Toyota M, Herman JG, Baylin SB, Issa JP (1999) CpG island methylator phenotype in colorectal cancer. Proc Natl Acad Sci U S A 96:8681–8686
82. Toyota M, Ahuja N, Suzuki H, Itoh F, Ohe-Toyota M, Imai K, Baylin SB, Issa JP (1999) Aberrant methylation in gastric cancer associated with the CpG island methylator phenotype. Cancer Res 59:5438–5442
83. Toyota M, Ho C, Ahuja N, Jair KW, Li Q, Ohe-Toyota M, Baylin SB, Issa JP (1999) Identification of differentially methylated sequences in colorectal cancer by methylated CpG island amplification. Cancer Res 59:2307–2312
84. Mueller J, Gazzoli I, Bandipalliam P, Garber JE, Syngal S, Kolodner RD (2009) Comprehensive molecular analysis of mismatch repair gene defects in suspected Lynch syndrome (hereditary nonpolyposis colorectal cancer) cases. Cancer Res 69:7053–7061
85. Imai K, Yamamoto H (2008) Carcinogenesis and microsatellite instability: the interrelationship between genetics and epigenetics. Carcinogenesis 29:673–680
86. Murata H, Khattar NH, Gu L, Li GM (2005) Roles of mismatch repair proteins hMSH2 and hMLH1 in the development of sporadic breast cancer. Cancer Lett 223:143–150
87. Gu M, Kim D, Bae Y, Choi J, Kim S, Song S (2009) Analysis of microsatellite instability, protein expression and methylation status of hMLH1 and hMSH2 genes in gastric carcinomas. Hepatogastroenterology 56:899–904
88. Mao G, Yuan F, Absher K, Jennings CD, Howard DS, Jordan CT, Gu L (2008) Preferential loss of mismatch repair function in refractory and relapsed acute myeloid leukemia: potential contribution to AML progression. Cell Res 18:281–289
89. Fleisher AS, Esteller M, Tamura G, Rashid A, Stine OC, Yin J, Zou TT, Abraham JM, Kong D, Nishizuka S, James SP, Wilson KT, Herman JG, Meltzer SJ (2001) Hypermethylation of the hMLH1 gene promoter is associated with microsatellite instability in early human gastric neoplasia. Oncogene 20:329–335
90. Fleisher AS, Esteller M, Wang S, Tamura G, Suzuki H, Yin J, Zou TT, Abraham JM, Kong D, Smolinski KN, Shi YQ, Rhyu MG, Powell SM, James SP, Wilson KT, Herman JG, Meltzer SJ (1999) Hypermethylation of the hMLH1 gene promoter in human gastric cancers with microsatellite instability. Cancer Res 59:1090–1095
91. Sato F, Harpaz N, Shibata D, Xu Y, Yin J, Mori Y, Zou TT, Wang S, Desai K, Leytin A, Selaru FM, Abraham JM, Meltzer SJ (2002) Hypermethylation of the p14(ARF) gene in ulcerative colitis-associated colorectal carcinogenesis. Cancer Res 62:1148–1151
92. Sarbia M, Geddert H, Klump B, Kiel S, Iskender E, Gabbert HE (2004) Hypermethylation of tumor suppressor genes (p16INK4A, p14ARF and APC) in adenocarcinomas of the upper gastrointestinal tract. Int J Cancer 111:224–228
93. Bernal C, Vargas M, Ossandon F, Santibanez E, Urrutia J, Luengo V, Zavala LF, Backhouse C, Palma M, Argandona J, Aguayo F, Corvalan A (2008) DNA methylation profile in diffuse type gastric cancer: evidence for hypermethylation of the BRCA1 promoter region in early-onset gastric carcinogenesis. Biol Res 41:303–315
94. Braggio E, Maiolino A, Gouveia ME, Magalhaes R, Souto Filho JT, Garnica M, Nucci M, Renault IZ. Methylation status of nine tumor suppressor genes in multiple myeloma. Int J Hematol 2009.
95. Krtolica K, Krajnovic M, Usaj-Knezevic S, Babic D, Jovanovic D, Dimitrijevic B (2007) Comethylation of p16 and MGMT genes in colorectal carcinoma: correlation with clinicopathological features and prognostic value. World J Gastroenterol 13:1187–1194

96. Guo XL, Sun SZ, Wang WX, Wei FC, Yu HB, Ma BL (2007) Alterations of p16INK4a tumour suppressor gene in mucoepidermoid carcinoma of the salivary glands. Int J Oral Maxillofac Surg 36:350–353
97. Brucher BL, Geddert H, Langner C, Hofler H, Fink U, Siewert JR, Sarbia M (2006) Hypermethylation of hMLH1, HPP1, p14(ARF), p16(INK4A) and APC in primary adenocarcinomas of the small bowel. Int J Cancer 119:1298–1302
98. Yoshino M, Suzuki M, Tian L, Moriya Y, Hoshino H, Okamoto T, Yoshida S, Shibuya K, Yoshino I (2009) Promoter hypermethylation of the p16 and Wif-1 genes as an independent prognostic marker in stage IA non-small cell lung cancers. Int J Oncol 35:1201–1209
99. Murphy TM, Perry AS, Lawler M (2008) The emergence of DNA methylation as a key modulator of aberrant cell death in prostate cancer. Endocr Relat Cancer 15:11–25
100. Zhang Q, Wang HY, Bhutani G, Liu X, Paessler M, Tobias JW, Baldwin D, Swaminathan K, Milone MC, Wasik MA (2009) Lack of TNFalpha expression protects anaplastic lymphoma kinase-positive T-cell lymphoma (ALK+ TCL) cells from apoptosis. Proc Natl Acad Sci U S A 106:15843–15848
101. Michalowski MB, de Fraipont F, Michelland S, Entz-Werle N, Grill J, Pasquier B, Favrot MC, Plantaz D (2006) Methylation of RASSF1A and TRAIL pathway-related genes is frequent in childhood intracranial ependymomas and benign choroid plexus papilloma. Cancer Genet Cytogenet 166:74–81
102. Elias A, Siegelin MD, Steinmuller A, von Deimling A, Lass U, Korn B, Mueller W (2009) Epigenetic silencing of death receptor 4 mediates tumor necrosis factor-related apoptosis-inducing ligand resistance in gliomas. Clin Cancer Res 15:5457–5465
103. Horak P, Pils D, Haller G, Pribill I, Roessler M, Tomek S, Horvat R, Zeillinger R, Zielinski C, Krainer M (2005) Contribution of epigenetic silencing of tumor necrosis factor-related apoptosis inducing ligand receptor 1 (DR4) to TRAIL resistance and ovarian cancer. Mol Cancer Res 3:335–343
104. Martinez R, Setien F, Voelter C, Casado S, Quesada MP, Schackert G, Esteller M (2007) CpG island promoter hypermethylation of the pro-apoptotic gene caspase-8 is a common hallmark of relapsed glioblastoma multiforme. Carcinogenesis 28:1264–1268
105. Hopkins-Donaldson S, Ziegler A, Kurtz S, Bigosch C, Kandioler D, Ludwig C, Zangemeister-Wittke U, Stahel R (2003) Silencing of death receptor and caspase-8 expression in small cell lung carcinoma cell lines and tumors by DNA methylation. Cell Death Differ 10:356–364
106. Sturm I, Stephan C, Gillissen B, Siebert R, Janz M, Radetzki S, Jung K, Loening S, Dorken B, Daniel PT (2006) Loss of the tissue-specific proapoptotic BH3-only protein Nbk/Bik is a unifying feature of renal cell carcinoma. Cell Death Differ 13:619–627
107. Jeanes A, Gottardi CJ, Yap AS (2008) Cadherins and cancer: how does cadherin dysfunction promote tumor progression? Oncogene 27:6920–6929
108. Kanazawa T, Watanabe T, Kazama S, Tada T, Koketsu S, Nagawa H (2002) Poorly differentiated adenocarcinoma and mucinous carcinoma of the colon and rectum show higher rates of loss of heterozygosity and loss of E-cadherin expression due to methylation of promoter region. Int J Cancer 102:225–229
109. Zou D, Yoon HS, Perez D, Weeks RJ, Guilford P, Humar B (2009) Epigenetic silencing in non-neoplastic epithelia identifies E-cadherin (CDH1) as a target for chemoprevention of lobular neoplasia. J Pathol 218:265–272
110. Prasad CP, Mirza S, Sharma G, Prashad R, DattaGupta S, Rath G, Ralhan R (2008) Epigenetic alterations of CDH1 and APC genes: relationship with activation of Wnt/beta-catenin pathway in invasive ductal carcinoma of breast. Life Sci 83:318–325
111. Rathi A, Virmani AK, Schorge JO, Elias KJ, Maruyama R, Minna JD, Mok SC, Girard L, Fishman DA, Gazdar AF (2002) Methylation profiles of sporadic ovarian tumors and nonmalignant ovaries from high-risk women. Clin Cancer Res 8:3324–3331
112. Graff JR, Herman JG, Lapidus RG, Chopra H, Xu R, Jarrard DF, Isaacs WB, Pitha PM, Davidson NE, Baylin SB (1995) E-cadherin expression is silenced by DNA hypermethylation in human breast and prostate carcinomas. Cancer Res 55:5195–5199

113. Kwon GY, Yoo BC, Koh KC, Cho JW, Park WS, Park CK (2005) Promoter methylation of E-cadherin in hepatocellular carcinomas and dysplastic nodules. J Korean Med Sci 20:242–247
114. Tamura G, Yin J, Wang S, Fleisher AS, Zou T, Abraham JM, Kong D, Smolinski KN, Wilson KT, James SP, Silverberg SG, Nishizuka S, Terashima M, Motoyama T, Meltzer SJ (2000) E-Cadherin gene promoter hypermethylation in primary human gastric carcinomas. J Natl Cancer Inst 92:569–573
115. Jin Z, Cheng Y, Olaru A, Kan T, Yang J, Paun B, Ito T, Hamilton JP, David S, Agarwal R, Selaru FM, Sato F, Abraham JM, Beer DG, Mori Y, Shimada Y, Meltzer SJ (2008) Promoter hypermethylation of CDH13 is a common, early event in human esophageal adenocarcinogenesis and correlates with clinical risk factors. Int J Cancer 123:2331–2336
116. Toyooka KO, Toyooka S, Virmani AK, Sathyanarayana UG, Euhus DM, Gilcrease M, Minna JD, Gazdar AF (2001) Loss of expression and aberrant methylation of the CDH13 (H-cadherin) gene in breast and lung carcinomas. Cancer Res 61:4556–4560
117. Toyooka S, Toyooka KO, Harada K, Miyajima K, Makarla P, Sathyanarayana UG, Yin J, Sato F, Shivapurkar N, Meltzer SJ, Gazdar AF (2002) Aberrant methylation of the CDH13 (H-cadherin) promoter region in colorectal cancers and adenomas. Cancer Res 62:3382–3386
118. Toyooka S, Toyooka KO, Maruyama R, Virmani AK, Girard L, Miyajima K, Harada K, Ariyoshi Y, Takahashi T, Sugio K, Brambilla E, Gilcrease M, Minna JD, Gazdar AF (2001) DNA methylation profiles of lung tumors. Mol Cancer Ther 1:61–67
119. Wang YC, Yu ZH, Liu C, Xu LZ, Yu W, Lu J, Zhu RM, Li GL, Xia XY, Wei XW, Ji HZ, Lu H, Gao Y, Gao WM, Chen LB (2008) Detection of RASSF1A promoter hypermethylation in serum from gastric and colorectal adenocarcinoma patients. World J Gastroenterol 14:3074–3080
120. Clement G, Braunschweig R, Pasquier N, Bosman FT, Benhattar J (2006) Methylation of APC, TIMP3, and TERT: a new predictive marker to distinguish Barrett's oesophagus patients at risk for malignant transformation. J Pathol 208:100–107
121. Bafico A, Liu G, Yaniv A, Gazit A, Aaronson SA (2001) Novel mechanism of Wnt signalling inhibition mediated by Dickkopf-1 interaction with LRP6/Arrow. Nat Cell Biol 3:683–686
122. Tsuchiya T, Tamura G, Sato K, Endoh Y, Sakata K, Jin Z, Motoyama T, Usuba O, Kimura W, Nishizuka S, Wilson KT, James SP, Yin J, Fleisher AS, Zou T, Silverberg SG, Kong D, Meltzer SJ (2000) Distinct methylation patterns of two APC gene promoters in normal and cancerous gastric epithelia. Oncogene 19:3642–3646
123. Esteller M, Sparks A, Toyota M, Sanchez-Cespedes M, Capella G, Peinado MA, Gonzalez S, Tarafa G, Sidransky D, Meltzer SJ, Baylin SB, Herman JG (2000) Analysis of adenomatous polyposis coli promoter hypermethylation in human cancer. Cancer Res 60:4366–4371
124. Richiardi L, Fiano V, Vizzini L, De Marco L, Delsedime L, Akre O, Tos AG, Merletti F (2009) Promoter methylation in APC, RUNX3, and GSTP1 and mortality in prostate cancer patients. J Clin Oncol 27:3161–3168
125. Brabender J, Usadel H, Danenberg KD, Metzger R, Schneider PM, Lord RV, Wickramasinghe K, Lum CE, Park J, Salonga D, Singer J, Sidransky D, Holscher AH, Meltzer SJ, Danenberg PV (2001) Adenomatous polyposis coli gene promoter hypermethylation in non-small cell lung cancer is associated with survival. Oncogene 20:3528–3532
126. Kawakami K, Brabender J, Lord RV, Groshen S, Greenwald BD, Krasna MJ, Yin J, Fleisher AS, Abraham JM, Beer DG, Sidransky D, Huss HT, Demeester TR, Eads C, Laird PW, Ilson DH, Kelsen DP, Harpole D, Moore MB, Danenberg KD, Danenberg PV, Meltzer SJ (2000) Hypermethylated APC DNA in plasma and prognosis of patients with esophageal adenocarcinoma. J Natl Cancer Inst 92:1805–1811
127. Henrique R, Ribeiro FR, Fonseca D, Hoque MO, Carvalho AL, Costa VL, Pinto M, Oliveira J, Teixeira MR, Sidransky D, Jeronimo C (2007) High promoter methylation levels of APC predict poor prognosis in sextant biopsies from prostate cancer patients. Clin Cancer Res 13:6122–6129

128. Wang JS, Guo M, Montgomery EA, Thompson RE, Cosby H, Hicks L, Wang S, Herman JG, Canto MI (2009) DNA promoter hypermethylation of p16 and APC predicts neoplastic progression in Barrett's esophagus. Am J Gastroenterol 104:2153–2160
129. Schulmann K, Sterian A, Berki A, Yin J, Sato F, Xu Y, Olaru A, Wang S, Mori Y, Deacu E, Hamilton J, Kan T, Krasna MJ, Beer DG, Pepe MS, Abraham JM, Feng Z, Schmiegel W, Greenwald BD, Meltzer SJ (2005) Inactivation of p16, RUNX3, and HPP1 occurs early in Barrett's-associated neoplastic progression and predicts progression risk. Oncogene 24:4138–4148
130. Hamilton JP, Sato F, Jin Z, Greenwald BD, Ito T, Mori Y, Paun BC, Kan T, Cheng Y, Wang S, Yang J, Abraham JM, Meltzer SJ (2006) Reprimo methylation is a potential biomarker of Barrett's-Associated esophageal neoplastic progression. Clin Cancer Res 12:6637–6642
131. Jin Z, Mori Y, Yang J, Sato F, Ito T, Cheng Y, Paun B, Hamilton JP, Kan T, Olaru A, David S, Agarwal R, Abraham JM, Beer D, Montgomery E, Meltzer SJ (2007) Hypermethylation of the nel-like 1 gene is a common and early event and is associated with poor prognosis in early-stage esophageal adenocarcinoma. Oncogene 26:6332–6340
132. Jin Z, Olaru A, Yang J, Sato F, Cheng Y, Kan T, Mori Y, Mantzur C, Paun B, Hamilton JP, Ito T, Wang S, David S, Agarwal R, Beer DG, Abraham JM, Meltzer SJ (2007) Hypermethylation of tachykinin-1 is a potential biomarker in human esophageal cancer. Clin Cancer Res 13:6293–6300
133. Jin Z, Mori Y, Hamilton JP, Olaru A, Sato F, Yang J, Ito T, Kan T, Agarwal R, Meltzer SJ (2008) Hypermethylation of the somatostatin promoter is a common, early event in human esophageal carcinogenesis. Cancer 112:43–49
134. Jin Z, Hamilton JP, Yang J, Mori Y, Olaru A, Sato F, Ito T, Kan T, Cheng Y, Paun B, David S, Beer DG, Agarwal R, Abraham JM, Meltzer SJ (2008) Hypermethylation of the AKAP12 promoter is a biomarker of Barrett's-associated esophageal neoplastic progression. Cancer Epidemiol Biomarkers Prev 17:111–117
135. Van der Auwera I, Elst HJ, Van Laere SJ, Maes H, Huget P, van Dam P, Van Marck EA, Vermeulen PB, Dirix LY (2009) The presence of circulating total DNA and methylated genes is associated with circulating tumour cells in blood from breast cancer patients. Br J Cancer 100:1277–1286
136. Zou H, Molina JR, Harrington JJ, Osborn NK, Klatt KK, Romero Y, Burgart LJ, Ahlquist DA (2005) Aberrant methylation of secreted frizzled-related protein genes in esophageal adenocarcinoma and Barrett's esophagus. Int J Cancer 116:584–591
137. Nojima M, Suzuki H, Toyota M, Watanabe Y, Maruyama R, Sasaki S, Sasaki Y, Mita H, Nishikawa N, Yamaguchi K, Hirata K, Itoh F, Tokino T, Mori M, Imai K, Shinomura Y (2007) Frequent epigenetic inactivation of SFRP genes and constitutive activation of Wnt signaling in gastric cancer. Oncogene 26:4699–4713
138. Qi J, Zhu YQ, Luo J, Tao WH (2006) Hypermethylation and expression regulation of secreted frizzled-related protein genes in colorectal tumor. World J Gastroenterol 12:7113–7117
139. Caldwell GM, Jones C, Gensberg K, Jan S, Hardy RG, Byrd P, Chughtai S, Wallis Y, Matthews GM, Morton DG (2004) The Wnt antagonist sFRP1 in colorectal tumorigenesis. Cancer Res 64:883–888
140. Bu XM, Zhao CH, Zhang N, Gao F, Lin S, Dai XW (2008) Hypermethylation and aberrant expression of secreted frizzled-related protein genes in pancreatic cancer. World J Gastroenterol 14:3421–3424
141. Suzuki H, Toyota M, Carraway H, Gabrielson E, Ohmura T, Fujikane T, Nishikawa N, Sogabe Y, Nojima M, Sonoda T, Mori M, Hirata K, Imai K, Shinomura Y, Baylin SB, Tokino T (2008) Frequent epigenetic inactivation of Wnt antagonist genes in breast cancer. Br J Cancer 98:1147–1156
142. Fukui T, Kondo M, Ito G, Maeda O, Sato N, Yoshioka H, Yokoi K, Ueda Y, Shimokata K, Sekido Y (2005) Transcriptional silencing of secreted frizzled related protein 1 (SFRP 1) by promoter hypermethylation in non-small-cell lung cancer. Oncogene 24:6323–6327
143. Urakami S, Shiina H, Enokida H, Hirata H, Kawamoto K, Kawakami T, Kikuno N, Tanaka Y, Majid S, Nakagawa M, Igawa M, Dahiya R (2006) Wnt antagonist family genes as biomarkers for diagnosis, staging, and prognosis of renal cell carcinoma using tumor and serum DNA. Clin Cancer Res 12:6989–6997

144. Veeck J, Geisler C, Noetzel E, Alkaya S, Hartmann A, Knuchel R, Dahl E (2008) Epigenetic inactivation of the secreted frizzled-related protein-5 (SFRP5) gene in human breast cancer is associated with unfavorable prognosis. Carcinogenesis 29:991–998
145. Lin YW, Chung MT, Lai HC, De Yan M, Shih YL, Chang CC, Yu MH (2009) Methylation analysis of SFRP genes family in cervical adenocarcinoma. J Cancer Res Clin Oncol 135:1665–1674
146. Takagi H, Sasaki S, Suzuki H, Toyota M, Maruyama R, Nojima M, Yamamoto H, Omata M, Tokino T, Imai K, Shinomura Y (2008) Frequent epigenetic inactivation of SFRP genes in hepatocellular carcinoma. J Gastroenterol 43:378–389
147. Jost E, Schmid J, Wilop S, Schubert C, Suzuki H, Herman JG, Osieka R, Galm O (2008) Epigenetic inactivation of secreted Frizzled-related proteins in acute myeloid leukaemia. Br J Haematol 142:745–753
148. Jost E, Gezer D, Wilop S, Suzuki H, Herman JG, Osieka R, Galm O (2009) Epigenetic dysregulation of secreted Frizzled-related proteins in multiple myeloma. Cancer Lett 281:24–31
149. Liu TH, Raval A, Chen SS, Matkovic JJ, Byrd JC, Plass C (2006) CpG island methylation and expression of the secreted frizzled-related protein gene family in chronic lymphocytic leukemia. Cancer Res 66:653–658
150. Pehlivan M, Sercan Z, Sercan HO (2009) sFRP1 promoter methylation is associated with persistent Philadelphia chromosome in chronic myeloid leukemia. Leuk Res 33:1062–1067
151. Ding Z, Qian YB, Zhu LX, Xiong QR (2009) Promoter methylation and mRNA expression of DKK-3 and WIF-1 in hepatocellular carcinoma. World J Gastroenterol 15:2595–2601
152. Taniguchi H, Yamamoto H, Hirata T, Miyamoto N, Oki M, Nosho K, Adachi Y, Endo T, Imai K, Shinomura Y (2005) Frequent epigenetic inactivation of Wnt inhibitory factor-1 in human gastrointestinal cancers. Oncogene 24:7946–7952
153. Mazieres J, He B, You L, Xu Z, Lee AY, Mikami I, Reguart N, Rosell R, McCormick F, Jablons DM (2004) Wnt inhibitory factor-1 is silenced by promoter hypermethylation in human lung cancer. Cancer Res 64:4717–4720
154. Batra S, Shi Y, Kuchenbecker KM, He B, Reguart N, Mikami I, You L, Xu Z, Lin YC, Clement G, Jablons DM (2006) Wnt inhibitory factor-1, a Wnt antagonist, is silenced by promoter hypermethylation in malignant pleural mesothelioma. Biochem Biophys Res Commun 342:1228–1232
155. Yang TM, Leu SW, Li JM, Hung MS, Lin CH, Lin YC, Huang TJ, Tsai YH, Yang CT (2009) WIF-1 promoter region hypermethylation as an adjuvant diagnostic marker for non-small cell lung cancer-related malignant pleural effusions. J Cancer Res Clin Oncol 135:919–924
156. Aguilera O, Fraga MF, Ballestar E, Paz MF, Herranz M, Espada J, Garcia JM, Munoz A, Esteller M, Gonzalez-Sancho JM (2006) Epigenetic inactivation of the Wnt antagonist DICKKOPF-1 (DKK-1) gene in human colorectal cancer. Oncogene 25:4116–4121
157. van der Weyden L, Adams DJ (2007) The Ras-association domain family (RASSF) members and their role in human tumourigenesis. Biochim Biophys Acta 1776:58–85
158. Tan SH, Ida H, Lau QC, Goh BC, Chieng WS, Loh M, Ito Y (2007) Detection of promoter hypermethylation in serum samples of cancer patients by methylation-specific polymerase chain reaction for tumour suppressor genes including RUNX3. Oncol Rep 18:1225–1230
159. Hirata T, Yamamoto H, Taniguchi H, Horiuchi S, Oki M, Adachi Y, Imai K, Shinomura Y (2007) Characterization of the immune escape phenotype of human gastric cancers with and without high-frequency microsatellite instability. J Pathol 211:516–523
160. Hiraki M, Kitajima Y, Sato S, Mitsuno M, Koga Y, Nakamura J, Hashiguchi K, Noshiro H, Miyazaki K. Aberrant Gene Methylation in the Lymph Nodes Provides a Possible Marker for Diagnosing Micrometastasis in Gastric Cancer. Ann Surg Oncol 2009
161. Sharma G, Mirza S, Parshad R, Srivastava A, Datta Gupta S, Pandya P, Ralhan R. CpG hypomethylation of MDR1 gene in tumor and serum of invasive ductal breast carcinoma patients. Clin Biochem 2009
162. Li Y, Meng G, Huang L, Guo QN (2009) Hypomethylation of the P3 promoter is associated with up-regulation of IGF2 expression in human osteosarcoma. Hum Pathol 40:1441–1447
163. Ito Y, Koessler T, Ibrahim AE, Rai S, Vowler SL, Abu-Amero S, Silva AL, Maia AT, Huddleston JE, Uribe-Lewis S, Woodfine K, Jagodic M, Nativio R, Dunning A, Moore G, Klenova E, Bingham S, Pharoah PD, Brenton JD, Beck S, Sandhu MS, Murrell A (2008) Somatically acquired hypomethylation of IGF2 in breast and colorectal cancer. Hum Mol Genet 17:2633–2643

164. Tang SH, Yang DH, Huang W, Zhou HK, Lu XH, Ye G (2006) Hypomethylated P4 promoter induces expression of the insulin-like growth factor-II gene in hepatocellular carcinoma in a Chinese population. Clin Cancer Res 12:4171–4177
165. Lee BB, Lee EJ, Jung EH, Chun HK, Chang DK, Song SY, Park J, Kim DH (2009) Aberrant methylation of APC, MGMT, RASSF2A, and Wif-1 genes in plasma as a biomarker for early detection of colorectal cancer. Clin Cancer Res 15:6185–6191
166. Su HY, Lai HC, Lin YW, Chou YC, Liu CY, Yu MH (2009) An epigenetic marker panel for screening and prognostic prediction of ovarian cancer. Int J Cancer 124:387–393
167. Jin Z, Cheng Y, Gu W, Zheng Y, Sato F, Mori Y, Olaru AV, Paun BC, Yang J, Kan T, Ito T, Hamilton JP, Selaru FM, Agarwal R, David S, Abraham JM, Wolfsen HC, Wallace MB, Shaheen NJ, Washington K, Wang J, Canto MI, Bhattacharyya A, Nelson MA, Wagner PD, Romero Y, Wang KK, Feng Z, Sampliner RE, Meltzer SJ (2009) A multicenter, double-blinded validation study of methylation biomarkers for progression prediction in Barrett's esophagus. Cancer Res 69:4112–4115
168. Sato F, Jin Z, Schulmann K, Wang J, Greenwald BD, Ito T, Kan T, Hamilton JP, Yang J, Paun B, David S, Olaru A, Cheng Y, Mori Y, Abraham JM, Yfantis HG, Wu TT, Fredericksen MB, Wang KK, Canto M, Romero Y, Feng Z, Meltzer SJ (2008) Three-tiered risk stratification model to predict progression in Barrett's esophagus using epigenetic and clinical features. PLoS ONE 3:e1890
169. Hsu HS, Chen TP, Wen CK, Hung CH, Chen CY, Chen JT, Wang YC (2007) Multiple genetic and epigenetic biomarkers for lung cancer detection in cytologically negative sputum and a nested case-control study for risk assessment. J Pathol 213:412–419
170. Brune K, Hong SM, Li A, Yachida S, Abe T, Griffith M, Yang D, Omura N, Eshleman J, Canto M, Schulick R, Klein AP, Hruban RH, Iacobuzio-Donohue C, Goggins M (2008) Genetic and epigenetic alterations of familial pancreatic cancers. Cancer Epidemiol Biomarkers Prev 17:3536–3542
171. Hoque MO, Feng Q, Toure P, Dem A, Critchlow CW, Hawes SE, Wood T, Jeronimo C, Rosenbaum E, Stern J, Yu M, Trink B, Kiviat NB, Sidransky D (2006) Detection of aberrant methylation of four genes in plasma DNA for the detection of breast cancer. J Clin Oncol 24:4262–4269
172. Chen JT, Chen YC, Wang YC, Tseng RC, Chen CY (2002) Alterations of the p16(ink4a) gene in resected nonsmall cell lung tumors and exfoliated cells within sputum. Int J Cancer 98:724–731
173. Wang YC, Lu YP, Tseng RC, Lin RK, Chang JW, Chen JT, Shih CM, Chen CY (2003) Inactivation of hMLH1 and hMSH2 by promoter methylation in primary non-small cell lung tumors and matched sputum samples. J Clin Invest 111:887–895
174. Destro A, Bianchi P, Alloisio M, Laghi L, Di Gioia S, Malesci A, Cariboni U, Gribaudi G, Bulfamante G, Marchetti A, Bosari S, Infante M, Ravasi G, Roncalli M (2004) K-ras and p16(INK4A)alterations in sputum of NSCLC patients and in heavy asymptomatic chronic smokers. Lung Cancer 44:23–32
175. Olaussen KA, Soria JC, Park YW, Kim HJ, Kim SH, Ro JY, Andre F, Jang SJ (2005) Assessing abnormal gene promoter methylation in paraffin-embedded sputum from patients with NSCLC. Eur J Cancer 41:2112–2119
176. Dulaimi E, Uzzo RG, Greenberg RE, Al-Saleem T, Cairns P (2004) Detection of bladder cancer in urine by a tumor suppressor gene hypermethylation panel. Clin Cancer Res 10:1887–1893
177. Battagli C, Uzzo RG, Dulaimi E, Ibanez de Caceres I, Krassenstein R, Al-Saleem T, Greenberg RE, Cairns P (2003) Promoter hypermethylation of tumor suppressor genes in urine from kidney cancer patients. Cancer Res 63:8695–8699
178. Yu J, Zhu T, Wang Z, Zhang H, Qian Z, Xu H, Gao B, Wang W, Gu L, Meng J, Wang J, Feng X, Li Y, Yao X, Zhu J (2007) A novel set of DNA methylation markers in urine sediments for sensitive/specific detection of bladder cancer. Clin Cancer Res 13:7296–7304
179. Woodson K, O'Reilly KJ, Hanson JC, Nelson D, Walk EL, Tangrea JA. The usefulness of the detection of GSTP1 methylation in urine as a biomarker in the diagnosis of prostate cancer. J Urol 2008;179:508–11; discussion 511–2

180. Lenhard K, Bommer GT, Asutay S, Schauer R, Brabletz T, Goke B, Lamerz R, Kolligs FT (2005) Analysis of promoter methylation in stool: a novel method for the detection of colorectal cancer. Clin Gastroenterol Hepatol 3:142–149
181. Huang ZH, Li LH, Yang F, Wang JF (2007) Detection of aberrant methylation in fecal DNA as a molecular screening tool for colorectal cancer and precancerous lesions. World J Gastroenterol 13:950–954
182. Wang DR, Tang D (2008) Hypermethylated SFRP2 gene in fecal DNA is a high potential biomarker for colorectal cancer noninvasive screening. World J Gastroenterol 14:524–531
183. Van Den Broeck A, Brambilla E, Moro-Sibilot D, Lantuejoul S, Brambilla C, Eymin B, Khochbin S, Gazzeri S (2008) Loss of histone H4K20 trimethylation occurs in preneoplasia and influences prognosis of non-small cell lung cancer. Clin Cancer Res 14:7237–7245
184. Cameron AJ (1998) Management of Barrett's esophagus. Mayo Clin Proc 73:457–461
185. Wang KK, Sampliner RE (2008) Updated guidelines 2008 for the diagnosis, surveillance and therapy of Barrett's esophagus. Am J Gastroenterol 103:788–797
186. Montgomery E (2005) Is there a way for pathologists to decrease interobserver variability in the diagnosis of dysplasia? Arch Pathol Lab Med 129:174–176
187. Hamilton JP, Sato F, Greenwald BD, Suntharalingam M, Krasna MJ, Edelman MJ, Doyle A, Berki AT, Abraham JM, Mori Y, Kan T, Mantzur C, Paun B, Wang S, Ito T, Jin Z, Meltzer SJ (2006) Promoter methylation and response to chemotherapy and radiation in esophageal cancer. Clin Gastroenterol Hepatol 4:701–708
188. Selaru FM, David S, Meltzer SJ, Hamilton JP (2009) Epigenetic events in gastrointestinal cancer. Am J Gastroenterol 104:1910–1912
189. Dehan P, Kustermans G, Guenin S, Horion J, Boniver J, Delvenne P (2009) DNA methylation and cancer diagnosis: new methods and applications. Expert Rev Mol Diagn 9:651–657
190. Duvic M, Vu J (2007) Vorinostat: a new oral histone deacetylase inhibitor approved for cutaneous T-cell lymphoma. Expert Opin Investig Drugs 16:1111–1120
191. Lane AA, Chabner BA (2009) Histone deacetylase inhibitors in cancer therapy. J Clin Oncol 27:5459–5468
192. McCabe N, Lord CJ, Tutt AN, Martin NM, Smith GC, Ashworth A (2005) BRCA2-deficient CAPAN-1 cells are extremely sensitive to the inhibition of Poly (ADP-Ribose) polymerase: an issue of potency. Cancer Biol Ther 4:934–936
193. Ratnam K, Low JA (2007) Current development of clinical inhibitors of poly(ADP-ribose) polymerase in oncology. Clin Cancer Res 13:1383–1388
194. Plummer R, Jones C, Middleton M, Wilson R, Evans J, Olsen A, Curtin N, Boddy A, McHugh P, Newell D, Harris A, Johnson P, Steinfeldt H, Dewji R, Wang D, Robson L, Calvert H (2008) Phase I study of the poly(ADP-ribose) polymerase inhibitor, AG014699, in combination with temozolomide in patients with advanced solid tumors. Clin Cancer Res 14:7917–7923
195. Bedikian AY, Papadopoulos NE, Kim KB, Hwu WJ, Homsi J, Glass MR, Cain S, Rudewicz P, Vernillet L, Hwu P (2009) A phase IB trial of intravenous INO-1001 plus oral temozolomide in subjects with unresectable stage-III or IV melanoma. Cancer Invest 27:756–763
196. Kaminskas E, Farrell A, Abraham S, Baird A, Hsieh LS, Lee SL, Leighton JK, Patel H, Rahman A, Sridhara R, Wang YC, Pazdur R (2005) Approval summary: azacitidine for treatment of myelodysplastic syndrome subtypes. Clin Cancer Res 11:3604–3608
197. Silverman LR, McKenzie DR, Peterson BL, Holland JF, Backstrom JT, Beach CL, Larson RA (2006) Further analysis of trials with azacitidine in patients with myelodysplastic syndrome: studies 8421, 8921, and 9221 by the Cancer and Leukemia Group B. J Clin Oncol 24:3895–3903
198. Kantarjian HM, O'Brien S, Shan J, Aribi A, Garcia-Manero G, Jabbour E, Ravandi F, Cortes J, Davisson J, Issa JP (2007) Update of the decitabine experience in higher risk myelodysplastic syndrome and analysis of prognostic factors associated with outcome. Cancer 109:265–273

Chapter 5
The Progression of Pre-invasive to Invasive Cancer

Souzan Sanati and D. Craig Allred

Introduction

Most human invasive carcinomas are thought to evolve through a series of increasingly abnormal "stages" over many years, decades in most cases. In general terms, the stages are often referred to as hyperplasia, atypical hyperplasia, and carcinoma in situ. The transition from one stage to the next is primarily dependent on the accumulation of random genetic mutations in epithelial cells, so progression is non-obligatory. It is becoming clear that other forces are also at play, such as alterations of epigenetic gene regulation, and adjacent stromal cells promoting tumor progression, among others, which we are only beginning to understand. Carcinoma in situ is a late stage of tumor progression, and the immediate precursor of invasive disease. In this setting, "carcinoma" means that there is an abnormal increase in the growth of tumor epithelial cells which accumulate in their normal environment (e.g. within ducts and lobules of the breast), but they do not invade out into the surrounding stroma or beyond. This chapter will discuss the development of invasive breast carcinomas (IBCs) as an example of the evolution of malignant epithelial neoplasms in general (Fig. 5.1). The general principles of the development and progression of invasive carcinomas are similar in many solid organs, although specific details may vary.

D.C. Allred (✉)
Department of Pathology and Immunology, Washington University School of Medicine, 660 South Euclid Avenue, Campus Box 8118, St. Louis, Missouri 63110, USA
e-mail: dcallred@path.wustl.edu

R.C. Fitzgerald (ed.), *Pre-Invasive Disease: Pathogenesis and Clinical Management*, DOI 10.1007/978-1-4419-6694-0_5,

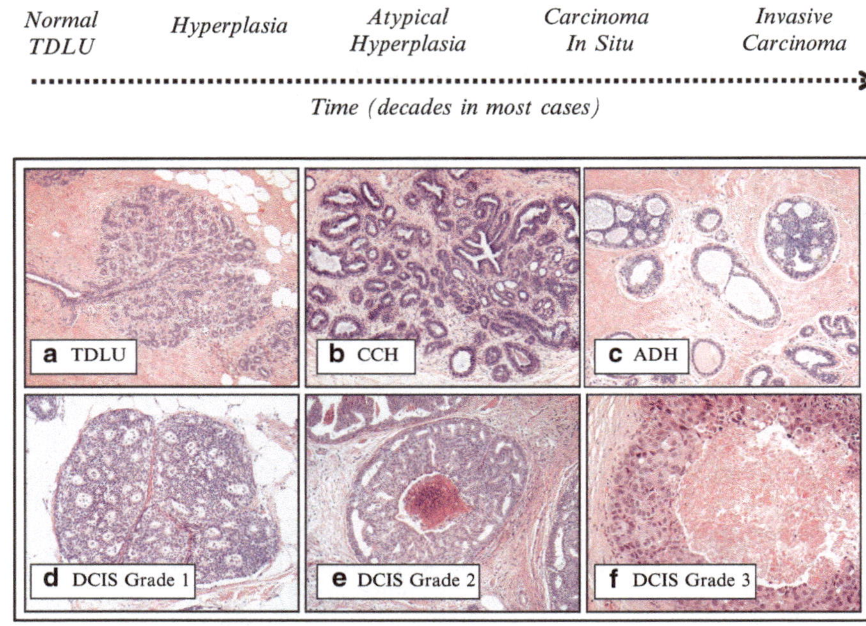

Fig. 5.1 Stages in the development and progression of premalignant (i.e. pre-invasive) breast cancer, including: (**a**) normal terminal duct-lobular unit (TDLU), (**b**) columnar cell hyperplasia (CCH), (**c**) atypical ductal hyperplasia (ADH), (**d**) ductal carcinoma in situ (DCIS), low-grade, (**e**) DCIS, intermediate-grade, and (**f**) DCIS, high-grade

The Evolution of Invasive Cancer in the Breast

Normal Epithelium

The human breast is capable of producing a large number of histologically defined abnormalities of growth. However, only a handful appears to have any significance as risk factors or precursors of breast cancer [1–3]. All of these abnormalities arise from normal breast epithelial cells within terminal duct-lobular unit (TDLU) (Fig. 5.1a). TDLUs are the smallest terminal branches of the ductal system ending in a grape-like cluster of acini whose primary function is to produce milk.

Recent studies have shown that histologically normal appearing breast epithelium are not always normal at the molecular level, and some of these morphologically silent genetic abnormalities (e.g. allelic imbalance, mutations) may predispose the cells to premalignant or malignant transformation. Although the overall frequency of abnormalities is quite low, it is significantly higher in normal cells adjacent to cancer cells than normal cells at a distance [4]. Some of these genetic defects may be shared with the adjacent cancer [4], although the majority are not and appear to be random [5].

Other studies have shown that breast tissue, especially in women at high risk for breast cancer, may contain regions of histologically normal appearing cells where activity of the p16 tumor suppressor gene is suppressed [6–8]. Compared to adjacent cells with normal p16 function, these cells show increased proliferation and elevated expression of cyclooxygenase 2 (COX2), and the latter appears to be associated with the development of many types of epithelial cancers. There are likely to be many other acquired and inherited molecular abnormalities in otherwise normal appearing cells to explain the broad range of risk of developing breast cancer between women.

Hyperplasia

Columnar cell hyperplasia (CCH) is the lesion thought to represent the earliest histologically identifiable potential precursor of breast cancer, which was suggested more than a century ago (Fig. 5.1b). CCH is characterized by expansion of lobular units by hyperplastic epithelial cells which are usually columnar in shape and show varying degrees of cytological stratification and atypia. These lesions are often multifocal, bilateral, and up to 100-fold larger (volume and numbers of cells) than the TDLUs they evolve from, representing a major alteration of growth [9]. The underlying causes of progression of normal mammary epithelium to CCH are mostly unknown. There is evidence for the role of estrogen in this process. For example, CCH is more common in pre-menopausal than post-menopausal breasts [3], and in cancerous compared to non-cancerous breasts [3, 10] where increased estrogen exposure is such a strong risk factor for developing breast cancer [11]. A recent study in mice over-expressing ERα in mammary epithelium noted the rapid development of hyperplasias which occasionally progressed to cancer [12], supporting the idea that elevated ERα may be partially responsible for the development and progression of CCH. Another recent study of Macaque monkeys with prolonged exposure to high levels of estrogen showed the rapid development of lesions histologically similar CCH in humans, occasionally progressed to more advanced precursors [13].

Several recent studies have shown highly elevated expression of ERα in the epithelial cells lining CCH [9, 14, 15]. Essentially all CCH express ERα in some cells and 80–90% show very high levels in nearly all cells, which is about threefold above normal [9]. There is also an increase in proliferation, and a decrease in apoptosis of similar (approximately threefold) magnitude, so the overall growth of CCH is due to an increase in cell number as well as a decrease in cell death. Since estrogen, mediated by ERα, stimulates proliferation [16] and suppresses apoptosis [17] in normal cells, elevated ERα in CCH may be a fundamental alteration leading to increased growth, although the cause of the elevation is unknown. Another recently discovered uniform molecular alteration in CCH compared to TDLUs is a decrease in epidermal growth factor (EGF) and an increase in amphiregulin (AREG) expression of very large magnitude [18–20]. These genes are important in the differentiation of adult breast, and embryonic breast development, respectively. Interestingly, they are both ligands for erbB1 TK receptor (also referred to as the epidermal growth factor receptor).

Because CCHs are so common in the population, and share important biological characteristics such as highly elevated ERα and changes in growth factors, their beginnings seem more likely to reflect alterations of development or differentiation rather than genetic mutations – perhaps adaptive in response to environmental stress such as increased estrogen exposure. Regardless, the end result is increased growth, creating fertile soil for accumulating random genetic defects leading to diversity and progression to other more advanced precursors of breast cancer.

Atypical Hyperplasia

The major type of atypical hyperplasia in the breast is referred to as atypical ductal hyperplasia (ADH) (Fig. 5.1c). ADH is rare, being found in only 2–3% of benign biopsies usually performed for unrelated reasons, and the incidence is probably even less in the population at large [3, 21, 22]. Histologically, ADH are characterized by small uniform mildly atypical hyperplastic epithelial cells which pile up on themselves, frequently in cribriform arrangements, mildly distending the ducts and acini they occupy, which are often found within or around CCH. By definition, ADH are very small (e.g. <2 mm).

Relatively little is known about the biological features of ADH, primarily because they are so rare and small, and because there are no representative animal models. However, a few things have been learned, primarily from IHC studies of formalin-fixed paraffin-embedded tissue (FFPET) samples from human patients. For example, IHC studies have shown that essentially 100% of ADH express high levels of ERα in nearly all cells, which is three- to fourfold higher than the average in normal cells [23, 24]. Average proliferation (about 5%) is also increased two- to threefold above that observed in normal cells [25, 26] and the majority of ERα-positive cells are proliferating [27, 28], which is unlike normal and similar to cancer cells. Preliminary studies also suggest that average apoptosis in ADH is decreased about two- to threefold relative to normal [29, 30], so growth appears to be accomplished through increased proliferation and decreased cell death. These characteristics are all very similar to CCH, which is not surprising in the sense that they are thought to be non-obligate precursors of ADH. The reciprocal changes in the expression of EGF and AREG observed in microarray studies of CCH are also present in ADH [18].

The ability of the epithelial cells in ADH to detach from the basement membrane and grow on top of themselves within ducts and acini probably represents a seminal event in the progression from a polyclonal (i.e. CCH) to a monoclonal (i.e. ADH) neoplasm, although the fundamental causes are unknown. This idea is reinforced by the relatively high incidence (>50%) of clonal allelic imbalances observed in ADH compared to CCH, many of which are shared with breast cancers, especially when they occur in the same breast, which makes sense if ADH is indeed a precursor of these lesions [1, 31–38].

In Situ Carcinoma

The most common type of in situ carcinoma in the breast is referred to as ductal carcinoma in situ (DCIS) (Figs. 5.1d–f). DCIS currently account for 20–25% of all newly diagnosed breast cancers [39, 40]. Most are detected by screening mammography, and they were rare (<5%) prior to screening [39–43]. DCIS show a continuum of histological diversity ranging from very well to very poorly differentiated [44–48] although, in clinical practice, they are often simply divided into two (e.g. non-comedo vs. comedo) or sometimes three (e.g. low vs. intermediate vs. high grade) categories, which fails to adequately convey their true diversity [48, 49]. Earlier precursors (CCH and ADH), as they are currently defined, are well differentiated, so substantial diversity appears to emerge primarily at the stage of DCIS during breast cancer evolution.

There are strong correlations between histological differentiation in DCIS and standard prognostic biomarkers in breast cancer. For example, nearly all well differentiated or low-grade DCIS express high levels of ERα and PgR in nearly all cells [24, 44–46, 50–59]. The proportion of cases expressing these receptors gradually declines to about 20% in the most poorly differentiated lesions, and there is also a decrease in the average proportion of positive cells [45]. Amplification and over-expression of erbB2 [42, 43, 45, 49, 50, 54, 60–71], and inactivating mutations of p53 [45, 50, 51, 56, 58, 59, 64, 71–79] are rare (5–10%) in well differentiated DCIS, but gradually increase to about 60% in the most poorly differentiated lesions. Average proliferation also gradually increases from <5% to nearly 40% from lowest to highest grade [45, 50, 59, 64, 67, 80, 81]. Apoptosis varies in the same direction from <1% to over 5% [29, 82, 83]. Apoptosis is quite low (average <1%) in normal cells and earlier precursors, and the elevated levels observed in higher grade DCIS, which have a large positive growth imbalance, demonstrates that the equilibrium between cell proliferation and death may not be accurately portrayed by the static methods used to measure these dynamic processes.

The correlations between histological differentiation and standard biomarkers in DCIS are nearly identical in IBCs, as well as in the DCIS component of IBCs, which is present in nearly all cases [45]. Thus, major diversity for these features appears to evolve first in DCIS and is later propagated to IBC, which was proposed at least a decade ago [84]. Although these features do not appear to influence the ultimate ability of DCIS to progress to invasive disease, they are associated with the rate of progression, as demonstrated by clinical studies showing a much higher rate of short-term local recurrence in higher-grade DCIS compared to lower-grade lesions treated by lumpectomy, although the rates converge with longer follow-up [85]. DCIS and IBCs have also been shown to be very similar at the high resolution of global gene expression evaluated by microarrays and other high throughput technologies, including similar distributions of luminal, basal, and erbB2 intrinsic molecular subtypes [45, 86–88].

Understanding the source, magnitude, and characteristics of the diversity in DCIS is important clinically because it may influence the rate of progression to IBC, the sensitivity to specific therapies, and point to new strategies for breast cancer prevention. One compelling hypothesis is that higher-grade DCIS gradually evolve from lower-grade DCIS and, thus, indirectly from ADH, by accumulating random genetic abnormalities over time. Furthermore, this "vertical" progression from low to high grade DCIS appears to be independent of the "lateral" progression to invasion. This is essentially the hypothesis of Darwinian clonal evolution, which is sometimes regarded as being contrary to the cancer stem cell hypothesis [89–91]. However, both ideas are based on persuasive evidence and, hopefully, future studies will reconcile some of the apparent inconsistencies [89, 90].

Studies of allelic imbalance by loss of heterozygosity and comparative genomic hybridization have shown that nearly all DCIS contain multiple clonal genetic abnormalities. The complexity of the imbalances is very large, involving at least 100 genetic loci on 17 chromosomes [31, 92–103], which rivals that observed in IBCs. Although this complexity suggests that there is a prominent randomness to the damage, there are hot spots on chromosomes 16q, 17p, and 17q where the overall incidence exceeds 40% [31, 93]. Interestingly, the specific identity of the majority of defects appears to be independent of histological differentiation, although the absolute number is substantially higher in more poorly differentiated lesions [31, 45, 93]. One of the hot spots (17p loss) spans the p53 locus, and DCIS with this defect show at least twice the frequency of imbalances as those without [45], suggesting that genetic instability and the passage of time are plausible mechanisms for the progression of lower grade to higher grade DCIS.

Invasive Carcinoma

The progression of in situ to invasive carcinoma (Fig. 5.2) is one of the most important steps in the progression of breast (or any other) type of carcinoma because it transforms an essentially harmless growth into a potentially lethal disease. The cellular and molecular alterations responsible for tumor invasion are a fascinating and evolving story. The vast majority of genetic and molecular alterations identified in the epithelium DCIS and IBCs are identical, which is surprising since invasion is such an enormous difference. Obviously, there must be differences responsible for invasion, but they have been surprisingly difficult to identify so far. One of the most important advances during the past decade was the understanding that surrounding stromal cells are playing an active role in tumor invasion [104]. There are many types of stromal cells in the breast, including fibroblasts, smooth muscle, endothelium, neurons, and macrophages, among others. Collectively, they perform many functions, including the production of extra-cellular matrix, which consists of many structural and regulatory proteins. In response to traumatic tissue injury, many of these cells and proteins are activated and involved in wound healing [105]. There are many similarities between the stroma of invasive carcinomas and healing wounds [106, 107]. For example, carcinoma-associated fibroblasts (CAFs) from several types of tumors, including breast cancer, show elevated expression of many growth factors involved in wound healing [108, 109]. CAFs can even promote

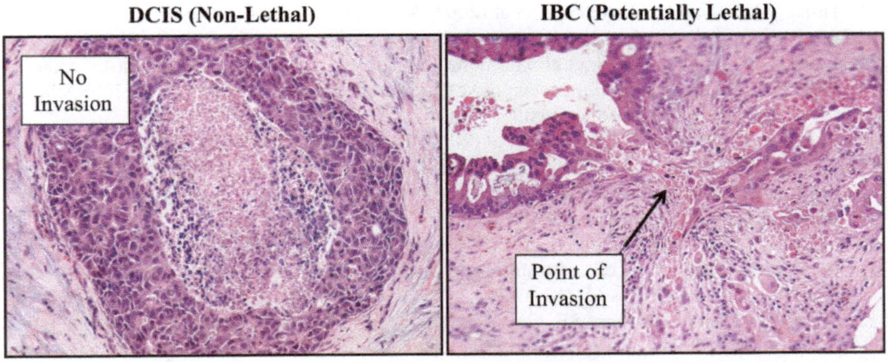

Fig. 5.2 The most compelling evidence that DCIS (*left panel*) is the immediate precursor of IBC is the presence of histologically identifiable points of invasion into the surrounding stroma (*right panel*)

benign epithelial cells to form invasive carcinomas in certain xenografts models [110], which is an unequivocal demonstration of the importance of stromal cells to tumor progression. Clonal genetic alterations (e.g. mutations, allelic imbalances, etc.) are essentially always found in the epithelium of invasive carcinomas [90, 111], but rarely in the adjacent stromal cells [111–113]. Genetic mutations in tumor epithelium are central to the development and progression of carcinomas, including progression to invasion, although the specific alterations which activate the stroma are largely unknown and the focus of considerable research today.

References

1. Allred DC, Hilsenbeck SG, Mohsin SK (2004) Biologic features of human premalignant breast disease. In: Harris JR, Lippman ME, Morrow M et al (eds) Diseases of the breast. Lippincott Williams & Wilkins, Philadelphia, pp 512–513
2. Wellings RR, Jensen HM (1973) On the origin and progression of ductal carcinoma in the human breast. J Natl Cancer Inst 50:1111–1118
3. Wellings SR, Jensen HM, Marcum RG (1975) An atlas of subgross pathology of the human breast with special reference to possible precancerous lesions. J Natl Cancer Inst 55:231–273
4. Deng G, Lu Y, Zlotnikov G et al (1996) Loss of heterozygosity in normal tissue adjacent to breast carcinomas. Science 274:2057–2059
5. Larson PS, de las Morenas A, Bennett SR et al (2002) Loss of heterozygosity or allele imbalance in histologically normal breast epithelium is distinct from loss of heterozygosity or allele imbalance in co-existing carcinomas. Am J Pathol 161:283–290
6. Bean GR, Bryson AD, Pilie PG et al (2007) Morphologically normal-appearing mammary epithelial cells obtained from high-risk women exhibit methylation silencing of INK4a/ARF. Clin Cancer Res 13:6834–6841
7. Crawford YG, Gauthier ML, Joubel A et al (2004) Histologically normal human mammary epithelia with silenced p16(INK4a) overexpress COX-2, promoting a premalignant program. Cancer Cell 5:263–273

8. Holst CR, Nuovo GJ, Esteller M et al (2003) Methylation of p16(INK4a) promoters occurs in vivo in histologically normal human mammary epithelia. Cancer Res 63:1596–1601
9. Lee S, Mohsin SK, Mao S, et al. Hormones, receptors, and growth in hyperplastic enlarged lobular units: early potential precursors of breast cancer. Breast Cancer Res 2005;8:http://breast-cancer-research.com/content/8/1/R6
10. Shaaban AM, Sloane JP, West CR et al (2002) Breast cancer risk in usual ductal hyperplasia is defined by estrogen receptor-alpha and Ki-67 expression. Am J Pathol 160:597–604
11. Martin AM, Weber BL (2000) Genetic and hormonal risk factors in breast cancer. J Natl Cancer Inst 92:1126–1135
12. Frech MS, Halama ED, Tilli MT et al (2005) Deregulated estrogen receptor alpha expression in mammary epithelial cells of transgeneic mice results in the development of ductal carcinoma in situ. Cancer Res 65:681–685
13. Wood CE, Hester JM, Appt SE, Geisinger KR, Cline JM (2008) Estrogen effects on epithelial proliferation and benign proliferative lesions in the postmenopausal primate mammary gland. Lab Invest 88(9):938–948
14. Simpson PT, Gale T, Reis-Filho JS et al (2005) Columnar cell lesions of the breast: the missing link in breast cancer progression? A morphological and molecular analysis. Am J Surg Pathol 29:734–746
15. Feeley L, Quinn CM (2008) Columnar cell lesions of the breast. Histopathology 52:11–19
16. Anderson E, Clarke RB (2004) Steroid receptors and cell cycle in normal mammary epithelium. J Mammary Gland Biol Neoplasia 9:3–13
17. Gompel A, Somai S, Chaouat M et al (2000) Hormonal regulation of apoptosis in breast cells and tissues. Steroids 65:593–598
18. Lee S, Medina D, Tsimelzon A et al (2007) Alterations of gene expression in the development of early hyperplastic precursors of breast cancer. Am J Pathol 171:252–262
19. Luetteke NC, Qiu TH, Fenton SE et al (1999) Targeted inactivation of the EGF and amphiregulin genes reveals distinct roles for EGF receptor ligands in mouse mammary gland development. Development 126:2739–2750
20. Troyer KL, Lee DC (2001) Regulation of mouse mammary gland development and tumorigenesis by the ERBB signaling network. J Mammary Gland Biol Neoplasia 6:7–21
21. Longacre TA, Bartow SA (1986) A correlative morphologic study of human breast and endometrium in the menstrual cycle. Am J Surg Pathol 10:382–393
22. Arpino G, Allred DC, Mohsin SK et al (2004) Lobular neoplasia on core-needle biopsy – clinical significance. Cancer 101:242–250
23. Schmitt FC (1995) Multistep progression from an oestorgen-dependent growth towards an autonomous growth in breast cancinogenesis. Eur J Cancer 31A:2049–2052
24. Barnes R, Masood S (1990) Potential value of hormone receptor assay in carcinoma in situ of breast. Am J Clin Pathol 94:533–537
25. De Potter CR, Praet MM, Slavin RE et al (1987) Feulgen DNA content and mitotic activity in proliferative breast disease: a comparison with ductal carcinoma in situ. Histopathology 7:1307–1319
26. Hoshi K, Tokunaga M, Mochizuki M et al (1995) Pathological characterization of atypical ductal hyperplasia of the breast. Jpn J Cancer Chemother 22(Supp 1):36–41
27. Clarke RB, Howell A, Potten CS et al (1997) Dissociation between steroid receptor expression and cell proliferation in the human breast. Cancer Res 57:4987–4991
28. Shocker BS, Jarvis C, Clarke RB et al (1999) Estrogen receptor-positive proliferating cells in the normal and precancerous breast. Am J Pathol 155:1811–1815
29. Bai M, Agnantis NJ, Sevasti K et al (2001) In vivo cell kinetics in breast carcinogenesis. Breast Cancer Res 3:276–283
30. Prosser J, Hilsenbeck SG, Fuqua SAW, et al. Cell turnover (proliferation and apoptosis) in normal epithelium and premalignant lesions in the same breast. Lab Invest 1997;76:119 [abstract 124A]
31. O'Connell P, Pekkel V, Fuqua SAW et al (1998) Analysis of loss of heterozygosity in 399 premalignant breast lesions at 15 genetic loci. J Natl Cancer Inst 90:697–703

32. Larson PS, de las Morenas A, Cerda SR et al (2006) Quantitative analysis of allele imbalance supports atypical ductal hyperplasia lesions as direct breast cancer precursors. J Pathol 209:307–316
33. Amari M, Suzuki A, Moriya T et al (1999) LOH analyses of premalignant and malignant lesions of human breast: frequent LOH in 8p, 16q, and 17q in atypical ductal hyperplasia. Oncol Rep 6:1277–1280
34. Chauqui RF, Zhuang Z, Emmert-Buck MR et al (1997) Analysis of loss of heterozygosity on chromosome 11q13 in atypical ductal hyperplasia and in situ carcinoma of the breast. Am J Pathol 150:297–303
35. Lakhani SR, Collins N, Stratton MR et al (1995) Atypical ductal hyperplasia of the breast: clonal proliferation with loss of heterozygosity on chromosomes 16q and 17p. J Clin Pathol 48:611–615
36. Rosenberg CL, de las Morenas A, Huang K et al (1996) Detection of monoclonal microsatellite alterations in atypical breast hyperplasia. J Clin Invest 98:1095–1100
37. Rosenberg CL, Larson PS, Romo JD et al (1997) Microsatellite alterations indicating monoclonality in atypical hyperplasias associated with breast cancer. Hum Pathol 28:214–219
38. Tsuda H, Takarabe T, Akashi-Tanaka S et al (2001) Pattern of chromosome 16q loss differs between an atypical proliferative lesion and an intraductal or invasive ductal carcinoma occurring subsequently in the same area of the breast. Mod Pathol 14:382–388
39. Ernster VL, Barclay J (1997) Increases in ductal carcinoma in situ (DCIS) of the breast in relation to mammography: a dilemma. Natl Cancer Inst Monogr 22:151–156
40. Ries LAG, Eisner MP, Kosary CL (2003) SEER cancer statistics review 1975–2000. National Cancer Institute, Bethesda
41. Society AC (2005) Breast cancer facts and figures 2005–2006. American Cancer Society, Inc., Atlanta
42. van de Vijver MJ, Peterse JL, Mooi WJ et al (1988) Neu-protein overexpression in breast cancer. Association with comedo-type ductal carcinoma in situ and limited prognostic value in stage II breast cancer. N Engl J Med 319:1239–1245
43. Allred DC, Clark GM, Molina R et al (1992) Overexpression of HER-2/neu and its relationship with other prognostic factors change during the progression of in situ to invasive breast cancer. Hum Pathol 23:974–979
44. Ottensen GL, Christensen IJ, Larsen JK et al (2000) Carcinoma in situ of the breast: correlation of histopathology to immunohistochemical markers and DNA ploidy. Breast Cancer Res Treat 60:219–226
45. Allred DC, Wu Y, Mao S et al (2008) Ductal carcinoma in situ and the emergence of diversity during breast cancer evolution. Clin Cancer Res 14:370–378
46. Leong AS, Sormunen RT, Vinyuvat S et al (2001) Biologic markers in ductal carcinoma in situ and concurrent infiltrating carcinoma. A comparison of eight contemporary grading systems. Am J Clin Pathol 115:709–718
47. Mack L, Kerkvliet N, Doig G et al (1997) Relationship of a new histological categorization of ductal carcinoma in situ of the breast with size and the immunohistochemical expression of p53, c-erb B2, bcl-2, and ki-67. Hum Pathol 28:974–979
48. Moreno A, Lloveras B, Figueras A et al (1997) Ductal carcinoma in situ of the breast: correlation between histologic classifications and biologic markers. Mod Pathol 10:1088–1092
49. Silverstein MJ, Cohlan BF, Gierson ED et al (1992) Duct carcinoma in situ: 227 cases without microinvasion. Eur J Cancer 28:630–634
50. Albonico G, Querzoli P, Feretti S et al (1996) Biophenotypes of breast carcinoma in situ defined by image analysis of biological parameters. Pathol Res Pract 192:117–123
51. Bose S, Lesser ML, Norton L et al (1996) Immunophenotype of intraductal carcinoma. Arch Pathol Lab Med 120:81–85
52. Chaudhuri B, Crist KA, Mucci S et al (1993) Distribution of estrogen receptor in ductal carcinoma in situ of the breast. Surgery 113:134–137

53. Giri DD, Dunda SAC, Nottingham JF et al (1989) Oestrogen receptors in benign epithelial lesions and intraduct carcinomas of the breast: an immunohistological study. Histopathology 15:575–584
54. Helin HJ, Helle MJ, Kallioneimi OP et al (1989) Immunohistochemical determination of estrogen and progesterone receptors in human breast carcinoma: correlation with histopathology and DNA flow cytometry. Cancer 63:1761–1767
55. Karayiannakis AJ, Bastounis EA, Chatzigianni EB et al (1996) Immunohistochemical detection of oestrogen receptors in ductal carcinoma in situ of the breast. Eur J Surg Oncol 22:578–582
56. Leal CB, Schmitt FC, Bento MJ et al (1995) Ductal carcinoma in situ of the breast. Histologic categorization and its relationship to ploidy and immunohistochemical expression of hormone receptors, p53, and c-erbB-2 protein. Cancer 75:2123–2131
57. Pallis L, Wilking N, Cedermark B et al (1992) Receptors for estrogen and progesterone in breast carcinoma in situ. Anticancer Res 12:2113–2115
58. Poller DN, Roberts EC, Bell JA et al (1993) p53 protein expression in mammary ductal carcinoma in situ: relationship to immunohistochemical expression of estrogen receptor and c-erbB-2 protein. Hum Pathol 24:463–468
59. Zafrani B, Leroyer A, Fourquet A et al (1994) Mammographically detected ductal in situ carcinoma of the breast analyzed with a new classification. A study of 127 cases: correlation with estrogen and progesterone receptors, p53, and c-erbB-2 proteins, and proliferative activity. Semin Diagn Pathol 11:208–214
60. Lodato RF, Maguire HC Jr, Greene MI et al (1990) Immunohistochemical evaluation of c-erbB-2 oncogene expression in ductal carcinoma in situ and atypical ductal hyperplasia of the breast. Mod Pathol 3:449–454
61. Barnes DM, Hanby AM, Gillett CE et al (1992) Abnormal expression of wild type p53 protein in normal cells of a cancer family patient. Lancet 340:259–263
62. Barnes DM, Meyer JS, Gonzalez JG et al (1991) Relationship between c-erbB-2 immunoreactivity and thymidine labeling index in breast carcinoma in situ. Breast Cancer Res Treat 18:11–17
63. Bartkova J, Barnes DM, Millis RR et al (1990) Immunohistochemical demonstration of c-erbB-2 protein in mammary ductal carcinoma in situ. Hum Pathol 21:1164–1167
64. Bobrow LG, Happerfield LC, Gregory WM et al (1994) The classification of ductal carcinoma in situ and its association with biological markers. Semin Diagn Pathol 11:199–207
65. De Potter CR, Foschini MP, Schelfhout AM et al (1993) Immunohistochemical study of neu protein overexpression in clinging in situ duct carcinoma of the breast. Virchows Arch A Pathol Anat 422:375–380
66. De Potter CR, Schelfhout A-M, Verbeeck P et al (1995) neu-Overexpression correlates with extent of disease in large cell ductal carcinoma in situ of the breast. Hum Pathol 26:601–606
67. Poller DN, Silverstein MJ, Galea M et al (1994) Ductal carcinoma in situ of the breast: a proposal for a new simplified histological classification association between cellular proliferation and c-erbB-2 protein expression. Mod Pathol 7:257–262
68. Ramachandra S, Machin L, Ashley S et al (1990) Immunohistochemical distribution of c-erbB-2 in in situ breast carcinoma: a detailed morphological analysis. J Pathol 161:7–14
69. Schimmelpenning H, Eriksson ET, Pallis L et al (1992) Immunohistochemical c-erbB-2 proto-oncogene expression and nuclear DNA content in human mammary carcinoma in situ. Am J Clin Pathol 97(Suppl):S48–S52
70. Somerville JE, Clarke LA, Biggart JD (1992) c-erbB-2 overexpression and histological type of in situ and invasive breast carcinomas. J Clin Pathol 45:16–20
71. Tsuda H, Iwaya K, Fukutomi T et al (1993) p53 mutations and c-erbB-2 amplification in intraductal and invasive breast carcinomas of high histologic grade. Jpn J Cancer Res 84:394–401
72. Chitemere M, Andersen TI, Hom R et al (1996) TP53 alterations atypical ductal hyperplasia and ductal carcinoma in situ of the breast. Breast Cancer Res Treat 41:103–109
73. Eriksson ET, Schmmelpenning H, Aspenblad U et al (1994) Immunohistochemical expression of the mutant p53 protein and nuclear DNA content during the transition from benign to malignant breast disease. Hum Pathol 25:1228–1233

74. O'Malley FP, Vnencak-Jones CL, Dupont WD et al (1994) p53 mutations are confined to the comedo type ductal carcinoma in situ of the breast: immunohistochemical and sequencing data. Lab Invest 71:67–72
75. Rajan PB, Scott DJ, Perry RH et al (1997) p53 protein expression in ductal carcinoma in situ (DCIS) of the breast. Breast Cancer Res Treat 42:283–290
76. Schmitt FC, Leal D, Lopes C (1995) p53 protein expression and nuclear DNA content in breast intraductal proliferations. J Pathol 176:233–241
77. Siziopikou KP, Prioleau JE, Harris JR et al (1996) Bcl-2 expression in the spectrum of preinvasive breast lesions. Cancer 77:499–506
78. Siziopikou KP, Schnitt SJ (2000) MIB-1 proliferation index in ductal carcinoma in situ of the breast: relationship to the expression of the apoptosis-regulating proteins bcl-2 and p53. Breast J 6:400–406
79. Walker RA, Dearing SJ, Lane DP et al (1991) Expression of p53 protein in infiltrating and in-situ breast carcinomas. J Pathol 165:203–211
80. Locker AP, Horrocks C, Gilmour AS et al (1990) Flow cytometric and histological analysis of ductal carcinoma in situ of the breast. Br J Surg 77:564–567
81. Meyer JS (1986) Cell kinetics of histologic variants of in situ breast carcinoma. Breast Cancer Res Treat 7:171–180
82. Bodis S, Siziopikou KP, Schitt SJ et al (1996) Extensive apoptosis in ductal carcinoma in situ of the breast. Cancer 77:1831–1835
83. Harn HJ, Shen KL, Yueh KC et al (1997) Apoptosis occurs more frequenty in intraductal carcinoma than in infiltrating duct carcinoma of human breast cancer and correlates with altered p53 expression: detected by terminal-deoxynucleotidyl-transferase-mediated dUTP-FITC nick end labelling (TUNEL). Histopathology 31:534–539
84. Gupta SK, Douglas-Jones AG, Morgan JM et al (1997) The clinical behavior of breast carcinoma is probably determined at the preinvasive stage (ductal carcinoma in situ). Cancer 80:1740–1745
85. Solin LJ, Kurtz J, Forquet A et al (1996) Fifteen-year results of breast-conserving surgery and definitive breast irradiation for the treatment of ductal carcinoma in situ of the breast. J Clin Oncol 14:754–763
86. Ma XJ, Salunga R, Tuggle JT et al (2003) Gene expression profiles of human breast cancer progression. Proc Natl Acad Sci U S A 100:5974–5979
87. Hannemann J, Velds A, Halfwerk JB et al (2006) Classification of ductal carcinoma in situ by gene expression profiling. Breast Cancer Res 8:R61
88. Porter D, Lahti-Domenici J, Keshaviah A et al (2003) Molecular markers in ductal carcinoma in situ of the breast. Mol Cancer Res 1:362–375
89. Polyak K (2008) Is breast tumor progression really linear? Clin Cancer Res 14:339–341
90. Polyak K (2007) Breast cancer: origins and evolution. J Clin Invest 117:3155–3163
91. Campbell LL, Polyak K (2007) Breast tumor heterogeneity: cancer stem cells or clonal evolution? Cell Cycle 6:2332–2338
92. Waldman FM, DeVries S, Chew KL et al (2000) Chromosomal alterations in ductal carcinomas in situ and their in situ recurrences. J Natl Cancer Inst 92:313–320
93. Hwang ES, DeVries S, Chew KL et al (2004) Patterns of chromosomal alterations in breast ductal carcinoma in situ. Clin Cancer Res 10:5160–5167
94. Smeds J, Warnberg F, Norberg T et al (2005) Ductal carcinoma in situ of the breast with different histopathological grades and corresponding new breast tumour events: analysis of loss of heterozygosity. Acta Oncol 44:41–49
95. Boecker W, Buerger H, Schmitz K et al (2001) Ductal epithelial proliferations of the breast: a biological continuum? Comparative genomic hybridization adn high-molecular-weight cytokeratin expression patterns. J Pathol 195:415–421
96. Aldaz CM, Chen T, Sahin A et al (1995) Comparative allelotype of in situ and invasive human breast cancer: high frequency of microsatellite instability in lobular breast carcinomas. Cancer Res 55:3976–3981
97. Chappell SA, Walsh T, Walker RA et al (1997) Loss of heterozygosity at chromosome 6q in preinvasive and early invasive breast carcinomas. Br J Cancer 75:1324–1329

98. Fujii H, Marsh C, Cairns P et al (1996) Genetic divergence in the clonal evolution of breast cancer. Cancer Res 56:1493–1497
99. Fujii H, Szumel R, Marsh C et al (1996) Genetic progression, histologic grade, and allelic loss in ductal carcinoma in situ of the breast. Cancer Res 56:5260–5265
100. Man S, Ellis IO, Sibbering M et al (1996) High levels of allele loss at the FHIT and ATM genes in non-comedo ductal carcinoma in situ and grade I tubular invasive breast cancers. Cancer Res 56:5484–5489
101. Munn KE, Walker RA, Varley JM (1995) Frequent alterations of chromosome 1 in ductal carcinoma in situ of the breast. Oncogene 10:1653–1657
102. Radford DM, Fair KL, Phillips NJ et al (1995) Allelotyping of ductal carcinoma in situ of the breast: deletion of loci on 8p, 13q, 16q, 17p and 17q. Cancer Res 55:3399–3405
103. Stratton MR, Collins N, Lakhani SR et al (1995) Loss of heterozygosity in ductal carccinoma in situ of the breast. J Pathol 175:195–201
104. Bissell MJ, Radisky D (2001) Putting tumours in context. Nat Rev Cancer 1:46–54
105. Tuxhorn JA, Ayala GE, Rowley DR (2001) Reactive stroma in prostate cancer progression. J Urol 166:2472–2483
106. Park CC, Bissell MJ, Barcellos-Hoff MH (2000) The influence of the microenvironment on the malignant phenotype. Mol Med Today 6:324–329
107. Barcellos-Hoff MH, Ravani SA (2000) Irradiated mammary gland stroma promotes the expression of tumorigenic potential by unirradiated epithelial cells. Cancer Res 60:1254–1260
108. Frazier KS, Grotendorst GR (1997) Expression of connective tissue growth factor mRNA in the fibrous stroma of mammary tumors. Int J Biochem Cell Biol 29:153–161
109. Kalluri R, Zeisberg M (2006) Fibroblasts in cancer. Nat Rev Cancer 6:392–401
110. Olumi AF, Grossfeld GD, Hayward SW et al (1999) Carcinoma-associated fibro blasts direct tumor progression of initiated human prostatic epithelium. Cancer Res 59:5002–5011
111. Allinen M, Beroukhim R, Cai L et al (2004) Molecular characterization of the tumor microenvironment in breast cancer. Cancer Cell 6:17–32
112. Hu M, Yao J, Cai L et al (2005) Distinct epigenetic changes in the stromal cells of breast cancers. Nat Genet 37:899–905
113. Qiu W, Hu M, Sridhar A et al (2008) No evidence of clonal somatic genetic alterations in cancer-associated fibroblasts from human breast and ovarian carcinomas. Nat Genet 40:650–655

Chapter 6
Contribution of the -Omics Era to Our Understanding of Preinvasive Disease and Progression to Cancer

Rita A. Busuttil and Alex Boussioutas

Abstract The term -omics refers to a biological field of study in which large scale network analysis techniques are used to interrogate various biological processes. Omics based technologies have been widely applied to studies of primary cancers. More recently, improvements in these techniques, such as increased sensitivity and decreased amounts of input sample has allowed their utilisation in the study of premalignant and preinvasive disease. Many premalignant lesions are known to persist for lengthy periods of time before progressing to cancer in only a small proportion of patients. Identification of the key genes and molecular mechanisms involved in progression may aid in identifying patients at high risk of progression and play a role in determining potential targets for prevention or treatment. This chapter outlines the current contribution of -omics technologies to our understanding of preinvasive and premalignant lesions of various types of adenocarcinomas.

Introduction

The completion of the human genome project in 2003 has generated large amounts of data which has potential use in the biomedical sciences. Identification of all genes in the human genome as well as the determination of their DNA sequences has facilitated the development of what has been termed the "-omics" era of science. New and more powerful genomics tools have been developed allowing researchers to interrogate the vast amounts of genomic information which is being

---

A. Boussioutas (✉)
Cancer Genomics and Predictive Medicine, Peter MacCallum Cancer Centre, East Melbourne 3002, Australia
and
Department of Medicine RMH/WH, University of Melbourne, Western Hospital, Footscray 3011, Australia
e-mail: alexb@unimelb.edu.au

R.C. Fitzgerald (ed.), *Pre-Invasive Disease: Pathogenesis and Clinical Management*,
DOI 10.1007/978-1-4419-6694-0_6,

generated. This allows for a more comprehensive and unbiased analysis of the events leading to the development of many disease types, including cancer.

There are four major types of "-omics"-based technologies, all capable of generating high throughput measurements and large amounts of data. Examples of those currently utilized and most commonly performed are: genomic SNP analysis (which detects single nucleotide polymorphisms); transcriptome analysis (a concurrent measure of the expression of all genes in a given tissue sample); proteomics (identification of all proteins in a given sample) and; metabolomics (quantitation and identification of all metabolites in a sample). Each of these four approaches offers its own insight into identifying variability in the components and function of a given sample. Each of these approaches also generates large amounts of data requiring powerful bioinformatic tools in order to perform analysis. The advent of whole genome sequencing is a further evolution of technology in the genomic and transcriptomic groups which adds data processing of some orders of magnitude to the technologies above.

Techniques facilitating genome wide analysis of DNA, RNA and proteins have been applied to research into most cancer types. These methods have provided researchers with the means to compare neoplastic samples with normal tissue and have resulted in the identification of gene expression patterns (also known as molecular signatures) helping advance our understanding of cancer biology. The information gained from these studies is now being applied to premalignant disease and pre-invasive disease. "Omics"-based studies have been performed for most cancer types however the study of premalignant diseases using these techniques has been very limited.

This chapter describes how "-omics"-based technologies have helped advance our understanding of the progression towards cancer with a few selected examples of cancers with well established pre-invasive and premalignant lesions such as adenocarcinoma of the esophagus, stomach and colon.

The -Omic Technologies

Transcriptomics

The transcriptome is the entire set of RNA transcripts which is produced by the genome at any one time. Transcriptomics is the global study of gene expression at the RNA level. Also known as genome-wide expression profiling or global analysis of gene expression this important tool has been instrumental in increasing our understanding of cell biology and the molecular mechanisms fundamental to both normal and defective biological processes. This technology has enabled researchers to identify new biomarkers of disease, targets for gene therapy and even drug development. One of the most widely used tools in this area is DNA microarrays. Recent technological advances allow the concurrent analysis of thousands of individual DNA sequences or probes on one array. Whilst these arrays have been widely used in the studies pertaining to RNA expression, arrays have now been developed for many other applications including, but not limited to, identifying changes in DNA copy number, epigenetic changes such as methylation as well as DNA mutations. Below is a brief description of some of the more widely used genomics platforms utilized in studies of pre-invasive and premalignant lesions.

Expression Analysis

Several high density DNA microarray platforms have been utilized in research. The most commonly used types of arrays are spotted arrays and in situ synthesized oligonucleotide arrays. Data from the first spotted array was published by Schena et al. in 1995 in a study examining the transcriptional activity of only 45 genes in yeast [1]. Technological advances since these early pioneering papers, as well as the completion of the human genome project, have resulted in arrays allowing the expression of genes in the full human genome to be studied. Much of the advance in technology has been fuelled by industry which sounded a death knell for institutional array services. Spotted arrays are prepared by robotic printing and can be further subdivided into two types: cDNA microarrays and oligonucleotide arrays. cDNA arrays use PCR amplified cDNA clones as the probe and thus can be generated without any prior sequence information. Disadvantages of this system are technical artifacts such as variable probe length and GC content between different clones. Oligonucleotide arrays, whereby long oligonucleotides of between 45 and 90 nucleotides in length, are deposited onto a slide are considered to be more reliable; however design of the oligonucleotides themselves requires prior sequence information. Both types of spotted arrays are prepared by mechanical deposition of the probes onto the surface of a glass slide using either robotic or inkjet based machinery. This process is usually imprecise and cDNA quantity can vary between print runs. In order to overcome these issues, co-hybridization of two targets, differentially labeled with fluorescent dyes (such as Cy3 and Cy5) is typically performed [2]. To allow comparisons to be made between large sample sets, the test samples are usually co-hybridized with a common reference as an internal control and then relative gene expression is determined. Pooled RNA from samples that have biological reference to the test samples are commonly used as the reference.

The principles of running two-color expression arrays involves extracting total RNA from the sample of interest as well as a reference sample and reverse transcribing into cDNA. Both the sample and the reference are then tagged with one of two dyes with spectrally distinct properties (i.e., Cy3 or Cy5). The samples are then pooled together and hybridized onto a single microarray. During this stage the labeled cDNA competitively binds to complementary sequences on the array. All remaining unbound and non-specific sample is then washed off the array and the array is scanned. Scanning is performed with a CCD or confocal based scanner. The laser excites the tagging dyes and the emissions are detected. The relative abundance of transcripts is measured by intensity of the probe after hybridization.

Commercial versions of expression arrays have been developed by several companies. One example is Affymetrix™ which is one of the largest commercial suppliers of microarrays. Affymetrix™ arrays are produced by direct synthesis of short oligonucleotides directly onto the substrate by a process known as photolithography. This mask-based fabrication process achieves a very high degree of reproducibility between slides and negligible variation in the printing procedure. This allows measurements of gene activity to be made without the need for an internal reference control. This one color (or single channel) detection system allows samples from two independent chips to be directly compared with each other. Technically the procedure is similar to that for spotted arrays, RNA is reverse transcribed to cDNA which is then labeled and hybridized to complementary nucleic acids attached to the chip. Fluorescence is still used to determine expression levels at a given location on the chip. An added advantage of these arrays is rather than having a single probe to represent each gene; each array contains a "probe set" consisting of a set of 25-mer oligonucleotides. Each probe set consists of both matching and mismatched sequences with the mismatched probes allowing for the control of non-specific hybridization and background. Over the years Affymetrix™ has been successful in decreasing feature size whilst increasing the information content available on their arrays.

Illumina is another provider of gene expression arrays; their technology is based on 3 μm silica beads which assemble in microwells on either fibre optic bundles or planar silica slides. Each bead is covered in many copies of an oligonucleotide which acts as a capture sequence. The process for determining gene expression levels of a given sample is very similar to that for other array types. A reverse transcription step of RNA is followed by an in vitro transcription step during which biotin labeled nucleotides are incorporated. This is followed by hybridization, blocking and washing steps and then staining with streptavidin conjugated Cy3. The fluorescence emission of Cy3 is the readout. Illumina have developed several variations of this protocol including one which allows for the analysis of partially degraded RNA and for RNA isolated from formalin fixed paraffin embedded sections.

Quantitative Real time polymerase chain reaction (qRT-PCR)

Real time PCR is commonly used for validating a small number of candidate genes identified in high throughput expression array studies. Commercially designed primers can be purchased or can be designed by the investigator and manufactured. This is a very sensitive method, requiring very low levels of input cDNA, which quantifies the relative abundance of mRNA present in the sample. The delta-delta Ct method of analysis allows the researcher to normalize the expression of each sample to an internal housekeeping gene (such as actin or GAPDH) and then to compare the expression of the gene of interest by comparing two independent samples to each other (i.e., normal and tumour). Real time PCR is generally highly prone to cross contamination and may also exhibit experimental variation between runs. These disadvantages can be minimized by the use of liquid handling robots to set up reactions. Alternatively, high throughput microfluidic cards in a 384 well format containing primers for a boutique list of genes supplied by the customer can be custom made and purchased. Real time PCR can also be used to validate copy number changes in genomic DNA sequences.

miRNA Screen

MicroRNAs (miRNAs) are short regulatory non-coding RNA molecules (16–29 nucleotides) which regulate gene expression. They are encoded by genes that are transcribed into primary transcripts which are then processed into pre-mRNA transcripts with a stem-loop structure by interaction with DICER (an endonuclease). DICER then cleaves the stem-loop structure forming two complementary short RNA molecules which are then incorporated into the RNA-induced silencing complex (RISC) which is then guided to the target mRNA. In conjunction with RISC, miRNAs then degrade the target mRNA (either by degradation or inhibiting translation) resulting in deregulated gene expression. It has been shown that miRNAs can act as tumour supressors or oncogenes and that their expression has been correlated with many human cancers (reviewed in [3]). miRNA expression can be detected by a variety of different methods which are variations of some of the techniques discussed above. Quantitative real time PCR assays have been developed whereby a modified reverse transcription protocol is followed by a real time assay and quantitation is via the routine delta delta Ct method. MiRNA microarrays and microfluidics chips specific for detecting miRNAs have also been developed by several companies (for example http://www.affymetrix.com and http://www.chem.agilent.com).

Genomic DNA Analysis

The term genomics refers to the comprehensive analysis of the function and structure of DNA. Genomic changes are known to play a role in the development of many diseases including cancer. Copy number gains have been linked to oncogene activation whilst copy number loss has been associated with inactivation of tumor suppressor genes. Several platforms for measuring copy number changes are currently being utilized and technology in this -omics field is constantly developing with new and improved variations on the current genomics platforms regularly being made available.

Array Comparative Genomic Hybridization (aCGH)

Comparative genomic hybridization (CGH) is a molecular cytogenetic method which can be used to identify changes in copy number occurring in chromosome specific regions of DNA. Array-CGH (aCGH) works on a combination of the principles of classical CGH and expression based arrays. Samples from test and reference samples which have been differentially labeled are hybridized to slides containing probes covering the entire genome and changes are detected by comparing the ratios of fluorescence detected for each of the test or reference samples. Copy number changes such as mutations and deletions can be detected by this method and its increased sensitivity over regular CGH allows the genomic location of each change to be more accurately mapped and identified. The advantage of this technique over the previously used karyotyping methods is that it is not necessary to prepare metaphase chromosomes from the "test" samples. This, along with the development and advancements in other techniques (such as micro-dissection and genomic DNA amplification) have made it possible to compare copy number changes in archived normal and "test" samples as well as those that are very small and heterogeneous.

The two types of aCGH arrays currently available are bacterial artificial chromosome (BAC) arrays and oligonucleotide based arrays. A more detailed performance comparison of the two techniques has been reported by Wicker et al. [4]. BAC arrays were the first type of array CGH to be introduced and are able to detect single copy changes with high sensitivity. They are prepared by spotting BAC clones into a slide which is subsequently processed by co-hybridizing fluorescently labelled test and reference samples as described earlier. The limitations with these arrays are the high cost associated with preparing the BAC clones as well as the limited resolution due to the large size of the BACS in comparison to oligonucleotide CGH arrays.

Oligonucleotide CGH arrays are prepared in much the same way as printed oligonucleotide expression arrays. They have the advantages of detecting changes with high resolution and are able to detect focal amplifications and deletions as small as 100 kb as well as single copy number change and loss. Overall they provide a more refined genomic profile than BAC arrays [5].

Single Nucleotide Polymorphism (SNP) Arrays

Single nucleotide polymorphisms (SNPs) are sequence variations occurring in the DNA of an individual when a single nucleotide in the genome is replaced with another. These types of changes occur approximately once every 100–300 bases with each individual harboring in excess of a million SNPs. They can occur in coding or non-coding regions of DNA and may not necessarily change the amino acid sequence of the resulting protein. However this is not always the case and SNP alleles have been reported to contribute to the development of disease. In addition they are known to serve as useful markers for some diseases.

SNP arrays provide two sets of information: SNP signal intensity and allelic imbalance. The SNP signal intensity provides copy number information whilst allelic imbalance allows for the detection of loss of heterozygosity (LOH). LOH occurs when one allele is already lost and the second is also deleted or mutated. Whole genome SNP arrays can be run at varying densities depending on the type of array chosen.

One of the major providers of genome arrays is Affymetrix™. This technology is designed for whole-genome SNP analysis. The procedure involves amplifying a subset of the human genome through a PCR based single primer amplification using input DNA which has been enzyme digested and ligated with an adaptor. Prior to hybridization to a GeneChip array the DNA is fragmented and labeled. Affymetrix™ provides arrays of varying densities ranging from the 10 K array covering the entire genome with 10,204 SNPs through to the SNP 6.0 array containing 906,600 SNPs as well as 946,000 additional non-polymorphic probes that are able to detect genetic differences such as copy number variation.

Another major provider of whole genome arrays is Illumina™. This is based on the same bead chip technology which was discussed earlier for expression analysis. Several different array types are available with the number of markers available on the array varying from about 650,000 to 1.1×10^6. The process involves two stages: the first is whole-genome amplification without the need for PCR or ligation steps and hybridization to the bead array. The second stage is an enzymatic single base extension which incorporates a labeled nucleotide for assay readout. One major advantage of this system is the low input amount of DNA required (200 ng) which makes it possible to analyze samples with low DNA yield. This is important for sample collection for some of these premalignant conditions which may be resected using small biopsies rather than surgically resected specimens (see later).

Proteomics

Proteomics involves the comprehensive study of proteins including their detection, characterization, identification, modification, function and regulation. The challenge of studying proteins is that their expression and stability (or half life) tends to vary in different cell types. Initial proteomics techniques include Western blot, enzyme-linked immuno-sorbent assay (ELISA), immunoprecipitation (IP) and use of immunohistochemistry (IHC) on tissue microarrays (TMAs). Evolving technologies for proteomic analysis have utilized Two-Dimensional Polyacrylamide Gel Electrophoresis (2D-PAGE), liquid chromatography and different mass spectroscopy devices to interrogate large numbers of proteins or peptides. More recently high throughput technologies have been incorporated in protein chemistry with the utilization of matrix assisted laser desorption/ionization – time of flight (MALDI-TOF) and surface enhanced laser desorption ionization – time of flight (SELDI-TOF) devices. These mass spectroscopy devices interrogate large numbers of peptides after appropriate separation usually based on peptide size or charge.

IHC is the process by which the presence and distribution of specific proteins or antigens in a cell or tissue can be determined. Briefly, the process involves the exposure of the tissue to a specific primary antibody to the antigen. A secondary antibody conjugated with an enzyme then binds to the primary antigen. The addition of chromagen and a substrate binds to the enzyme allowing visualization of the staining.

TMAs are paraffin blocks containing a large number of samples and allow high throughput and simultaneous analysis of samples interest to be observed on the same slide. They are prepared by identifying regions of interest from H&E slides of the required samples. Cores of 0.6 to 2 mm in diameter are then taken from conventional "donor" paraffin blocks using a hollow needle and placed into a recipient paraffin block [6, 7]. Sections can then be cut from the block and subject to a variety of processes including ISH, FISH and immunohistochemistry. TMAs have been widely used in the validation of many cancer studies [8, 9] including those using IHC to validate the expression of candidate genes in various preinvasive lesions in comparison to normal or tumour tissues.

Application of -Omics Technologies to Selected Preinvasive Diseases

As discussed in previous chapters a greater understanding of carcinogenic pathways from pre-invasive to invasive disease may enable the development of strategies to intervene in the natural history of the cancer.

In the following sections we discuss the current status of "-omics"-based studies relating to some well known precursor lesions which lead to adenocarcinomas as an endpoint and how this information might be applied clinically in the future.

Barrett's Esophagus/Dysplasia/Esophageal Adenocarcinoma

Barrett's esophagus (BE) is the precursor lesion for esophageal adenocarcinoma as discussed in Chap. 16 and summarised in Fig. 6.1. One of the key clinical challenges is to predict the patients most at risk of malignant progression. Most of our knowledge on the natural history of Barrett's carcinogenesis has come from a study of candidate genes, selected because of their established role in cancer, at different

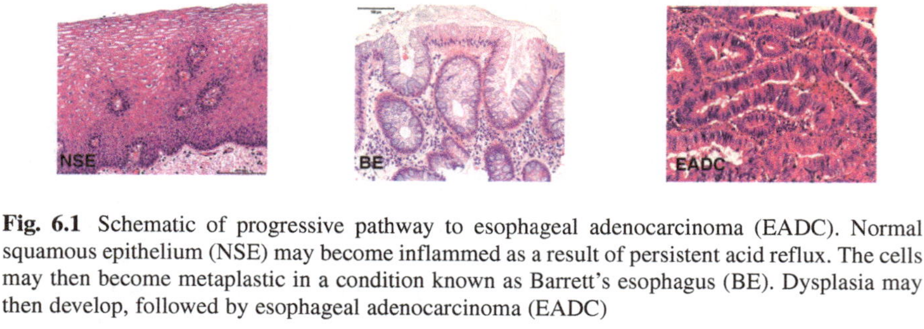

Fig. 6.1 Schematic of progressive pathway to esophageal adenocarcinoma (EADC). Normal squamous epithelium (NSE) may become inflammed as a result of persistent acid reflux. The cells may then become metaplastic in a condition known as Barrett's esophagus (BE). Dysplasia may then develop, followed by esophageal adenocarcinoma (EADC)

stages in the metaplasia-dysplasia-carcinoma sequence. However, more recently use of the -omic technologies has enhanced our understanding and the genes identified form these studies are summarised in Table 6.1.

A number of -omics based studies have been dedicated to the investigation of BE. One of the earliest studies published in 2002 by Selaru et al. [10] used cDNA microarrays to perform gene expression analysis on seven BE and six esophageal carcinoma samples of varying subtypes (squamous cell carcinoma, adenocarcinoma and one signet-ring carcinoma). Although the total number of samples used in the study was very small, of interest was the observation that the esophageal adenocarcinoma (EADC) samples tended to cluster more closely with other carcinoma samples rather than the BE samples from which they are thought to originate. Although a rudimentary analysis, this finding, not surprisingly, suggests there are significant gene expression changes between BE and established EADC [10]. This group also used artificial neural networks (ANN) to investigate differences in these groups. ANN is a supervised classification technique which is useful for analyzing more complex data. Their study shows that ANN is capable of distinguishing between BE and EADC [11].

This finding was further explored in a subsequent paper from the same group. This time the cohort consisted of 51 samples; 24 of which were normal esophageal mucosa (squamous), 18 were BE and the remaining nine were EADC samples [12]. In a comparison between normal esophagus and BE a total of 295 genes were differentially expressed with 162 of these genes up-regulated and the remaining 133 down-regulated. However, only 36 genes were differentially expressed when comparing BE samples with EADC samples suggesting that BE has more in common on a transcriptional level with EADC than it has with normal mucosa. These authors postulate that this finding supports the hypothesis that BE is an intermediate stage in esophageal carcinogenesis [12], however the differences detected may simply be highlighting the differences between normal mucosa and the properties of the new metaplastic BE cells. These authors also report 212 genes that were commonly differentially expressed in BE and EADC samples when compared to normal mucosa. These changes in expression are most likely to have occurred during the period of transition from BE to EADC [12].

In an attempt to identify potential biomarkers specific to BE these authors also compared the expression profile of BE samples from patients with (BE+EADC) and without (BE−EADC) concurrent EADC. Only three genes were found to be differentially expressed. *CXCL3*, *TNFRSF12A (Fn14)* and *MYADM* were all up-regulated in the BE+EADC samples. When this analysis was extended by grouping the BE+EADC samples with the EADC samples and then looking for differentially expressed genes in comparison with the BE−EADC samples 12 genes were found to be differentially expressed with nine of these being up-regulated and the remainder down-regulated. Four of these were selected for validation by quantitative real time PCR (qRT-PCR). *CXCL3*, *TNFRSF12A* and *MMP7* were found to exhibit a progressive increase in expression corresponding to the progressive stages of the pathway. Additionally, in concordance with the microarray results, expression of *C10orf116* was found to progressively decrease in expression from normal mucosa

Table 6.1 Summary of key candidate genes/loci which are changed in precursor lesions of Esophageal Adenocarcinoma

	RNA	miRNA	DNA	Proteomics
Genes/loci differentially expressed/gained in positive direction	CXCL3[a] [12]	miR-196[e] [32]	8q[e, f, g] [34]	MLCB[d] [44]
	TNFRS12A[a] [12]		6p[e, f, g] [34]	TPM2 [44]
	MMP7[a, b] [12]		20q[f, g] [34]	AKR1B10[d] [44]
	MYADM [12]		2p[f, g] [34]	HNRPK [44]
	DUSP2 [12]		10q[f, g] [34]	
	SC65 [12]		15q[f, g] [34]	
	PLAUR [12]		17q[f] [34]	
	PRG1[12]		7q[g] [34]	
	ANXA4 [19]			
	ARPC1B [19]			
	BIN1 [19]			
	CTSS [19]			
	GATA6[a] [26,28]			
	HLA-F [19]			
	HOXB7[a] [19]			
	IFI30 [19]			
	KIAA0062 [19]			
	KIF3B [19]			
	NICAL [19]			
	RAB20 [19]			
	RRBP1 [19]			
	TCF3[a] [19]			
	UCP2 [19]			
	COL6A1 [27]			
	COL12A1 [27]			
	COL3A1 [27]			
	COL5A2[c] [27]			
	CSPG2 [27]			
	POSTN[c] [27]			
	IL1R2 [20]			
	CCL20 [20]			
	CCL18 [20]			
	IL4R [20]			
	IFNAR2 [20]			
	ADH1B [20]			
	DGKQ [20]			
	MU2C [21]			
	MUC5AC[a] [29,35]			
	MUC6 [21]			
	TFF1[a, b] [29,35]			
	TFF3 [21]			
	HOXB5 [21]			
	HOXB6 [21]			
	FOXA3 [21]			
	TCF2 [21]			

(continued)

	RNA	miRNA	DNA	Proteomics
	NR1H3 [21]			
	NR1L2 [21]			
	MUC3B [21]			
	villin [21]			
Genes/loci differentially expressed/gained in negative direction	C10orf116[a] [12]		18q[e, g] [34]	S100A6 [44]
	HSPE1 [12]		Y[e, f, g] [34]	S100A8 [44]
	EREG [12]			DRP2 [44]
	CNN3 [12]		9p[f, g] [34]	TXN [44]
			7q[f] [34]	TXN2 [44]
	CALML3 [19]		14q[f, g] [34]	S100A9[d, b] [53,35]
	ZNF185 [19]			RPS15A[d] [44]
	KANK [19]		4q [35]	ATP5D [44]
	FCER1A [19]		5q [35]	LSM1 [44]
	BNIP3 [19]			UBE2V2[d] [44]
	FLJ2259 [19]		9p21 [40]	EIF5A[d] [44]
	S100A2[a] [19]		3p14 [40]	NM23[d] [44]
	SCCA1[a] [19]		13q22 [40]	STMN1[d] [44]
	SPRR3[a] [19]			CBX3[d] [44]
				CMPK [44]
				ARHGDIB[d, b] [44]
				ARHGDIA [44]
				PSMB4[d] [44]
				PSMA2[d] [44]
				ATP6V1E1 [44]
				GSTO1 [44]
				PSMA1[d] [44]
				PP[d] [44]
				TPM1[d] [44]
				ENO1[d, b] [44]
				LMNA[d, b] [44]

[12] – reference compares BE+EADC and EADC vs. BE–EADC
[19] – reference compares the progression of BE and EADC vs. normal squamous epithelium
[27] – reference compares BE vs. normal squamous epithelium
[20] – reference compares BE vs. normal squamous epithelium
[21] – reference compares BE vs. normal squamous epithelium
[34] – reference compares BE+HGD vs. normal squamous epithelium
[44] – reference compares BE vs. EADC
N/A – Not applicable
[a]Validated by qRT-PCR
[b]Validated by IHC
[c]Validated by ISH
[d]Protein and mRNA levels were correlated
[e]Change occuring in BE
[f]Change occuring in LGD
[g]Change occuring in HGD

through to EADC. *MMP7* has also been reported to be overexpressed in gastric and colorectal cancers [13, 14]. There is some evidence suggesting MMP7 could be a target in the Wnt signalling pathway which is known to play a role in cancer formation. In addition the MMPs are known to play a role in the breakdown of the extracellular matrix which can affect tumor growth. TNFRSF12A has been implicated in invasion [15], migration [16] and angiogenesis [17] whilst overexpression of CXCL3 in EADC has been confirmed by other groups using both microarray and immunohistochemistry methods [18]. CXCL3 and TNFRSF12A are both involved in cytokine–cytokine receptor interaction, which is a cancer related pathway [12].

A study by Kimchi et al. [19] using Affymetrix™ U133A genechip arrays examined samples of normal squamous mucosa, BE and EADC samples each collected from 24 patients. They identified 351 genes which were differentially expressed only in EADC samples and 104 expressed only in BE samples when compared to normal squamous mucosa. They identified a further 96 genes that were differentially expressed in both BE and EADC samples and proposed that these genes may potentially serve as prognostic or diagnostic markers. Further analysis of the data filtered this gene list down to 21 genes which were validated by qRT-PCR. Six of these genes are known to play a role in epidermal differentiation. Of these *GATA6*, *HOXB7* and *TCF3* were found to be up-regulated in the progression from squamous esophagus to BE to EADC. In contrast *S100A2*, *SCCA1* and *SPRR3* were progressively down-regulated. Further investigation showed that whilst each of these genes can be used on its own to discriminate between normal mucosa and EADC only HOXB7 expression levels can differentiate between normal mucosa and BE. The expression level of no single gene was able to accurately distinguish normal mucosa, BE and EADC into three subgroups.

These authors then looked at combinations of these genes and found that calculating the ratios of *GATA6* and *SPRR3* expression allows them to differentiate between normal mucosa (lowest), BE (moderate) and EADC (highest). They suggest that this marker combination may be useful for determining the risk of progression from BE to EADC, however further studies with a larger sample size would be needed to confirm this. There has not been further investigation on the potential role these genes play in the mechanism of carcinogenesis. The results of these studies remain associations between expression and stages of disease.

Another gene expression based study performed by Hao et al. using in house cDNA arrays had a sample cohort consisting of 48 biopsy samples obtained from 17 patients. From each patient biopsies were taken from normal esophagus, BE, EADC (if present) as well as duodenum. This group identified 648 genes with a fourfold difference in expression between BE and normal esophageal mucosa. Further analysis of these genes using a software package called PAM, which works by performing sample classification of gene expression data predicted that expression of AGR2 was sufficient to distinguish the difference between BE and normal samples. Thirty seven stromal genes including collagens (*COL6A1, COL12A1, COL3A1 and COL5A2*), *CSPG2* and *POSTN* were found to be highly expressed in BE and EADC in comparison with normal mucosa. Of these, expression of *COL5A2* and *POSTN* were validated using in situ hybridization. The authors postulate that the high expression of these stromal genes prior to dysplasia and EADC suggests that modification of the extracellular matrix is an early event in the development of EADC. In addition to normal esophageal mucosa, BE and EADC samples these authors included duodenum samples in their analysis as a control for the intestinal metaplasia phenotype observed in BE. These samples clustered closely to the BE samples and this similarity indicates the effects that cell lineage has on the clustering of samples.

A comprehensive study which compared expression levels of ten BE and five EADC samples as well as gastric samples including intestinal metaplasia (IM) of the stomach ($n=9$) (similar to BE and discussed in more detail in the next section) and intestinal type gastric cancer ($n=12$) was performed by Gomes et al. [20]. This group performed an analysis of functional modules which identified glycerolipid metabolism and cytokine/cytokine receptor modules to be active in greater than 50% of BE and IM samples. Further examination of these modules implicated several key genes within each module which are responsible for their activation. Within the glycerolipid metabolism module *IL1R2, CCL20, CCL18, IL4R* and *IFNAR2* were more highly expressed in BE and IM samples whilst *ADH1B* and *DGKQ* appeared to be key activators of the cytokine/cytokine receptor module. No validation was performed for any of these genes.

Greenawalt et al. performed a comprehensive analysis of gene expression profiles in a cohort of 128 samples including: normal mucosa, BE, EADC and SCC samples [21]. Gene ontology analysis was used to identify specific gene functions which are differentially expressed between the four groups. The samples were found to separate into four distinct clusters with BE and EADC samples (both of which exhibit a columnar phenotype) clustering separately from the normal and SCC samples which have a more squamous phenotype. The data obtained from this, and other studies indicate that genes which play a role in tissue development including those involved in keratinization, intercellular junctions, calcium-ion binding and endopeptidase activity were over represented in the comparison of BE and EADC samples compared to normal mucosa [12, 21]. Over-representation of genes involved in immune and inflammatory response and proteolysis were found specifically in EADC samples whilst genes involved in alcohol and digestive metabolism were found to be overrepresented only in BE samples [21]. Many of these pathways have been previously reported in the study by Wang et al. [12] and were discussed previously, however there was little overlap in the key genes identified in the two studies.

Greenawalt et al. also performed hierarchical clustering analysis of differentially expressed genes [21]. Several distinguishing clusters were identified. One of these clusters contained genes which were upregulated in SCC, EADC and BE samples in comparison to normal mucosa (squamous epithelium). Most of the genes are plasma membrane related and more specifically included MHC class I receptors and immune response genes. The second of the clusters contained genes which were specific to esophageal cancers and which the authors refer to as the "esophageal cancer cluster" and were differentially expressed in SCC and EADC samples only. This cluster consisted of several overlapping subclusters including the "SPARC" cluster, proliferation cluster and immune response cluster.

SPARC is an extracellular matrix protein known to be expressed in many advanced cancers including EADC [22]. It plays a role in extracellular matrix remodeling and could contribute to invasion by causing stromal de-adhesion [23, 24]. Indeed SPARC expression was found by one group to increase with the onset of BE and further increase with the development of dysplasia although this was limited to studying expression of mRNA by RT-PCR [22]. This is further evidence for the intermediate position of BE in the progression to EADC discussed by Wang et al. [12].

The proliferation cluster specifically contains genes involved in the M phase of the cell cycle whilst the immune response cluster contains MMP3 and MMP10 as well as PTGS2 (COX2) which has been linked to inflammation and proliferation. COX2 held significant promise as a target for intervention studies to try and mitigate the progression from BE to EADC. Treatment of a mouse model of BE with an inhibitor of COX2 was found to reduce incidence of progression to EADC [25]. Unfortunately a Phase IIb clinical trial of Celecoxib, a selective COX-2 non-steroidal anti-inflammatory drug (NSAID) failed to prevent progression from BE to EADC in humans [26].

Genes that were differentially expressed only in the EADC and BE samples compared to normal and squamous cell carcinoma samples consist mainly of genes which differentiate between squamous and columnar phenotypes. More specifically up-regulated genes include the mucins (*MUC2*, *MUC5AC* and *MUC6*) as well as mucin associated genes (*TFF1* and *TFF3*). A transcription factor cluster was also identified including *HOXB5* and *6*, *FOXA3* and *GATA6*, which is consistent with the Kimchi study described earlier [19].

These authors also identified differentially expressed genes which are specific only to BE. Up-regulated genes were specific to mitochondria, cellular lipid metabolism and oxidoreductase activity suggesting that these pathways may play an early role in the transition to EADC.

Although the Greenawalt study identified many genes that may play a role in the progression pathway through to EADC, none of these findings were validated. It is encouraging however that some of these genes have also been identified as candidates in other studies and have undergone further validation by other groups.

Microarray data obtained from several of the studies described above by Hao et al. [27] and Greenawalt et al. [21] as well as a study by Boussioutas et al. [28], which looked at gene expression in gastric samples (and which is discussed in more detail in the intestinal metaplasia section below) were interrogated by Lao-Sirieix and colleagues [29]. Their aim was to identify putative biomarkers with the ability to discriminate BE from normal esophageal or gastric mucosa for use in a non-invasive, non-endoscopic cytological screening device called a capsule sponge. This screening method involves the patient swallowing a capsulised sponge attached to a string. Once swallowed the capsule dissolves and the sponge can be retrieved by pulling the string allowing sampling from the esophagus on withdrawal. Cells can them be isolated from the sponge, embedded in paraffin and subsequently be analysed by IHC. Following validation of the 14 candidate genes identified by qRT-PCR and IHC, TFF3 was found to be both BE specific and highly expressed on the luminal surface epithelium of BE at the protein level indicating that TFF3 could potentially be used as a marker for BE. A validation study using TFF3 applied to the capsule sponge specimens in patients with known BE ($n=47$) compared to healthy controls ($n=99$) suggested a sensitivity of 78% and a specificity of 94% [29] (see also Chap. 16).

Determination of microRNA expression has also been used as a tool to study differences between various stages in the carcinogenic pathway leading to EADC. The trends observed in a study by Feber et al. [30] using Illumina bioarrays mimicked those observed in the study of total RNA expression. Each pathological subgroup was separated using microRNA profiles. BE ($n=5$) and EADC ($n=10$) subgroups appeared to be more similar to each other rather than the normal squamous mucosa ($n=9$). No specific miRNAs were found to be specific to BE. In contrast, a study by Luthra et al. reported that miR-196a levels were up-regulated in EADC samples compared with normal mucosa and that ANXA1 (a potential tumor suppressor gene) is a direct target of this microRNA [31]. A subsequent study by the same group identified three potential in silico targets of miR-196a based on their reported down-regulation in the progression from BE to EADC [32]. Their results show that increased expression of miR-196a in the progression from normal mucosa, BE, LGD, HGD and then EADC is correlated with decreasing expression of *KRT5*, *SPRR2C* and *S100A9*. These authors suggest that these genes are direct targets of miR-196a and that expression levels of miR-196a may be a useful marker for predicting progression from BE to EADC. Interestingly, other predicted in silico targets of miR-196a included GATA6 and HOXB7 which have been previously identified as being progressively up-regulated in the progression from normal mucosa to BE and then to EADC as discussed above [19]. Further analysis did not indicate any negative correlation between miR-196a expression levels and those of GATA6 or HOXB7 leading the authors to postulate that miR-196a is most likely not involved in the regulation of these genes [32]. It is encouraging that there is consistency between these reports and earlier studies showing differential expression of similar genes (*SPRR2C* and *S100A9*).

As well as changes in expression, several studies have also attempted to identify copy number changes occurring during the progression from precursor changes to EADC. A study by Walch et al. used CGH to characterize chromosomal changes in EADC and its precursor changes [33]. The study cohort consisted of 30 tumour samples and 25 precursor lesions (consisting of 11 HGD, 8 LGD and 6 metaplasias). They observed a step wise increase in the number of aberrations detected at each progressive stage from BE (seven chromosomal imbalances per case) to LGD (10.8) to HGD (13.4) and finally EADC (13.3). The most common changes (>25% of samples) observed in BE were gains on 8q and 6p and losses on 18q and the Y chromosome [33]. Gains were commonly observed on 8q, 20q, 2p, 10q, 6p, 15q and 17q in LGD with losses occurring 9p, 7q, 14q and Y. The number of chromosomal changes per sample increased again for HGD with gains on 8q, 20q, 2p, 7q, 10q, 6p and 15q. Deletions occurred on 4q, 5q, 9p, 18q, 14q and chromosome Y. The same changes occurred in EADC samples with additional regions having gains on 17q and loss on 7q [33]. The implication of Y chromosome aberrations (50% of BE cases, 100% LGD cases and 90% HGD cases) is interesting in the setting of well recognized gender differences in EADC incidence favoring males by 2:1.

A similar study by Riegman et al. reported the same trend of increasing number of chromosomal aberrations with increasing stepwise progression through the metaplasia-dysplasia-adenocarcinoma sequence, however they did not detect any copy number changes in their cohort of 6 BE samples [34]. These authors acknowledge that their data is not in agreement with the reports of others who have also detected chromosomal imbalance in BE samples [35–37] and have suggested that criteria used in sample selection may account for these discrepancies, although it is also feasible that the inconsistencies observed may be the result of low sample number. Another study by Croft et al. using CGH was unable to detect any significant chromosomal changes even in LGD samples [38]. It is clear however that common regions of LOH have been found in multiple studies including deletions in 5q which contains candidate genes APC and MCC [34].

To date there has been only one published report utilizing SNP analysis to study genomic changes in precursor lesions that lead to EADC [39]. Their results confirm that 5K BAC arrays and an Affymetrix™ 50K array are able to detect most of the same changes provided that the change is greater than 1 Mb in size, however smaller copy number changes were only detectable using the higher resolution Affymetrix™ array. Whilst between 73 and 1,860 copy number changes were detected in each of the BE biopsy samples studied most of the regions were unique to one of the six samples suggesting that they are not necessarily required changes for progression [39]. Three main regions of loss were detected: losses on chromosome 9p21 and 3p14 were detected in five of the six samples studied and of these 5 samples 3 had an additional deletion on chromosome 13q22. The observed deletion on 9p21 (also observed in the Walch study) is not surprising since the cohort was selected to enrich for samples exhibiting loss at the CDKN2A (p16) locus. Allelic loss of this locus and mutations in the CDKN/p16 gene has been previously implicated in early progression to EADC [40–42].

Further studies of the pre-neoplastic lesions of EADC using high resolution "-omic" techniques with a greater sample size and controlling for sample selection bias, may provide further information of the relationship of copy number change and the progression pathway.

Proteomics techniques were used by Zhao et al. to identify proteins which are differentially expressed between BE and EADC which may potentially act as candidate markers for the progression from BE to EADC [43]. They obtained paired samples from six patients and utilized liquid phase separation in the first dimension and NPS-RP HPLC in the second dimension followed by ESI-TOF mass spectrometry to identify 38 candidate proteins. Interestingly only around 50% of these were found to have similar expression levels at the mRNA level as determined by Affymetrix U133 arrays. Increased protein and mRNA expression in EADC compared to BE was also validated by IHC for ARHDIGB, Lamin A (LMNA) and Alpha-Enolase 1(ENO1) [43].

Intestinal Metaplasia/Dysplasia/Gastric Adenocarcinoma

As discussed in Chap. 17 gastric cancer (GC), particularly of the Intestinal type (IGC) has well defined premalignant stages that were initially found in an

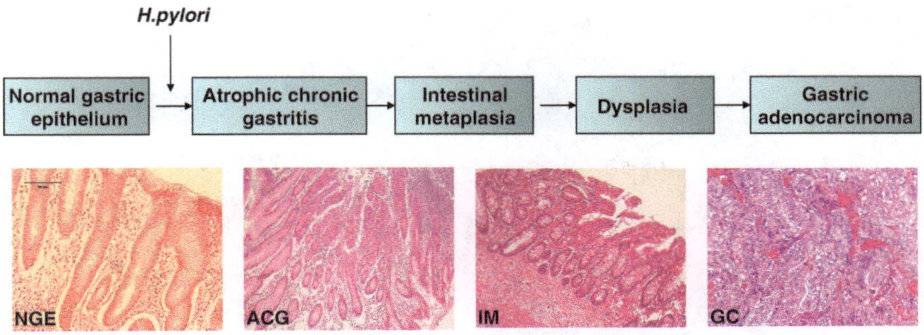

Fig. 6.2 Schematic diagram of premalignant lesions in gastric cancer. *H. pylori* has been associated with the development of atrophic chronic gastritis (ACG) from normal gastric epithelium (NGE). This may trigger a metaplastic process in which the cells take on characteristics of the intestine, a condition known as intestinal metaplasia (IM). This may then progress into dysplasia and then gastric adenocarcinoma (GC)

epidemiologic association as described by Correa [44]. The risk of progression from gastric IM to carcinoma has been difficult to quantify and is dependent on host and environmental factors. In a study from a high risk environment (East Asia) there was significant progression to more advanced lesions once IM was established [45].

The premalignant cascade first proposed by Correa is thought to be initiated by chronic infection with the bacterium *Helicobacter pylori* through a sequence of changes consisting of chronic atrophic gastritis (CG), intestinal metaplasia (IM), dysplasia and invasive neoplasia each of which is easily distinguished using histological techniques (Fig. 6.2).

There is relatively little known about the key genetic events in IM however genomics studies have helped to identify key genes involved in the progression from normal mucosa via the intermediates of IM and dysplasia to GC. A summary of the key changes observed in the premalignant stages of GC are listed in Table 6.2.

The first reported microarray gene expression profiling study looking at expression levels of premalignant vs. tumor samples was performed in our laboratory [28]. This study compared gastric cancer and precursor lesions in samples sourced from Australian (n=91) and Chinese patients (n=33). Tumor and adjacent non-neoplastic mucosal samples were collected from patients with GC at the time of resection. Non-neoplastic samples were classified as normal (n=9), chronic gastritis (n=27) or IM (n=22). Unsupervised clustering of the data classified the samples into distinct groups of malignant and non-malignant. The same unsupervised analysis also distinguished the different histological groups within the premalignant (Chronic gastritis and IM) and malignant subgroups. Chronic gastritis was characterized by a mitochondrial gene expression signature with up-regulated genes such as cytochrome c oxidase (COX) and NADH dehydrogenase (NDUF) [28]. It is proposed that this gene signature was linked to the presence of H. pylori which tends to colonize gastritic mucosa in preference to IM or malignant mucosa.

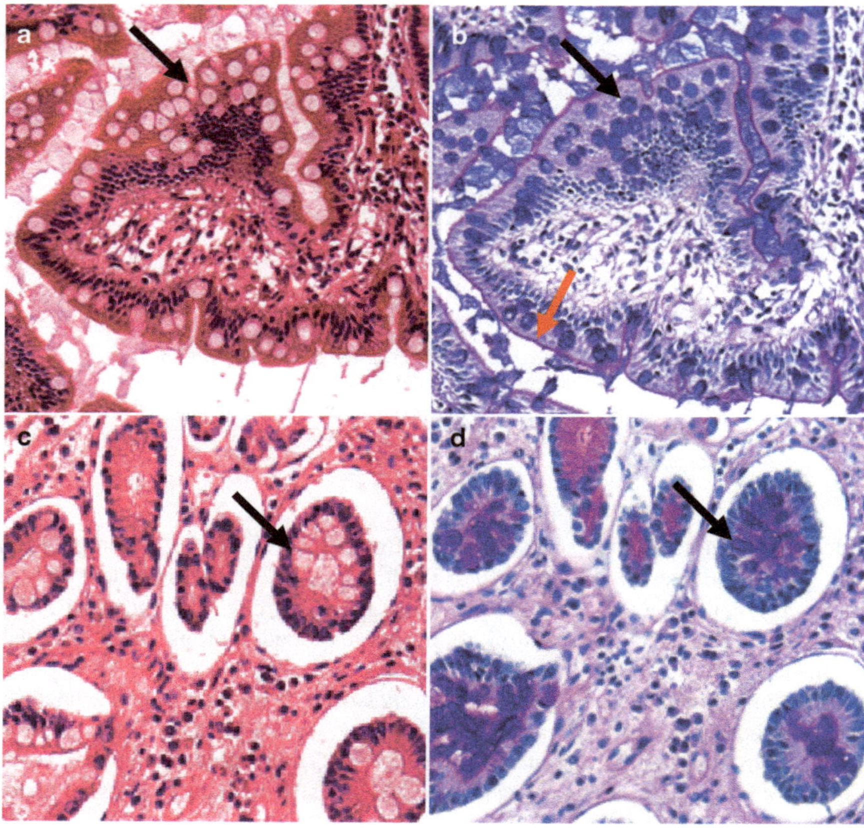

Fig. 6.3 H&E and Alcian-blue periodic acid Schiff staining of human IM (×200) (**a**) H&E and (**b**) AB/PAS of complete type IM. (**c**) H&E and (**d**) AP/PAS of incomplete type IM. *Black arrows* represent goblet cells and *red arrows* indicate presence of a brush border

Analysis of IM samples identified elevated expression of genes characteristic of the intestine and consistent with a transdifferentiation of the mucosa from a gastric to an intestinal phenotype (see Fig. 6.3). Genes that are involved in differentiation of the intestinal phenotype include CDX1, a homeodomain transcription factor whose expression is normally localized to the mucosa of the colon and Villin1 (a structural protein involved in the formation of microvilli in the small intestine). Villin 1 has also been reported to be up-regulated in chronic gastritis [46]. Other genes of interest which were consistently up-regulated in IM are FAT, a tumor suppressor that is related to the cadherin family of genes and TFF1 (Trefoil factor 1) which is also found to be a tumor suppressor and down-regulated in GC [47–49].

A similar study was performed by Meireles et al. [50] who used custom cDNA arrays created to enrich for genes either known to be differentially expressed in GC or other cancers. Their data was able to discriminate between each of the

Table 6.2 Summary of key candidate genes/loci which are changed in precursor lesions of Gastric Adenocarcinoma

	RNA	miRNA	DNA	Proteomics
Genes/loci differentially expressed/gained in positive direction	cdx1[a] [36]	N/A	N/A	Pepsin A [81]¥
	villin1 [36]			Pepsin B [81]¥
	FAT [36]			Gastric lipase [81]¥
	TFF1[b] [36]			
	MYO1A [36]			α1-antitrypsin [81]@
	MTP [36]			
	cholecystokinin [36]			
	PSG [36]			
	KLF-4 [36]			
	TGFalpha [36]			
	COL1A1 [75]@			
	FN1 [75]@			
	CTSB [75]@			
	COL1A2 [75]@			
	Hs.17781 [75]@			
	DAF [75]@			
	VIM [75]@			
	KRT20 [75]§			
	TUBB [75]§			
	KRT19 [75]§			
	CDH1 [75]§			
	KRT17 [75]§			
	DAF [75]§			
	CTSB [75]§			
Genes/loci differentially expressed/gained in negative direction	PRPF8 [75]@	N/A	N/A	
	Hs.327751 [75]@			
	VHL [75]@			
	LCK [75]@			
	BAD [75]@			
	VEGFB [75]@			
	POLR2h [75]@			
	PTSGS2 [75]§			

[36] – reference compares IM vs. normal gastric mucosa
[75][@] – reference compares the progression of IM and IGC vs. normal gastric mucosa
[75][§] – reference compares IM vs. normal gastric mucosa
[81][¥] – reference compares IM vs. GC (gastric juice)
[81][@] – reference compares the progression of IM and IGC vs. normal gastric mucosa (gastric juice)
N/A not applicable
[a]Validated by qRT-PCR
[b]Validated by IHC

histological subtypes with more genes being differentially expressed between tumors when compared to normal stomach than in IM vs. normal which is consistent with the Boussioutas et al. data set. They were unable to identify any genes which were differentially expressed between normal and chronic gastritis samples but this could be explained by the way they curated their genes for their array. A further analysis aimed to identify any genes which are differentially expressed in the Correa pathway from normal through to IM and then to IGC. They identified *COL1A1*, *FN1*, *CTSB*, *COL1A2*, *Hs.177781*, *DAF* and *VIM* as the seven top genes with highest increased expression and *PRPF8. Hs.327751*, *VHL*, *LCK*, *BAD*, *VEGFB* and *POLR2H* were the seven genes with decreased expression pattern. This analysis excluded tumors of the diffuse type. Tissue microarrays were used to validate findings in this study [50]. It is encouraging to see different datasets produce the same results when comparing IM. Many of the genes that were characteristic of IM were differentiation markers for the intestinal phenotype. However, the Meireles study found differential gene expression in IM despite using genes that were selected for cancer.

To date there have not been any studies of microRNA expression levels involving IM samples however in comparison to normal gastric mucosa multiple miRs have been found to be differentially expressed in GC [51, 52].

Whilst there have been several publications investigating genomic changes between normal tissues and GC [53, 54], at this stage there have not been any specific studies examining IM at the genomic level. It is conceivable that IM may harbor genomic aberrations in the form of DNA amplifications and/or deletions which are cumulative in IM and precede the transformation into GC although these are more likely to arise in dysplastic tissue.

One of the limitations of studies involving IM whether they are -omics based or otherwise is they rarely distinguish subtypes of IM (reviewed in [55]). It is possible that differences exist between these subgroups at the transcriptome, genome or protein level that may warrant further investigation. In addition it is possible that combining the data from the two subtypes (which may in fact be distinct from each other) could dilute out any interesting or relevant -omics based changes which would become apparent if they were analyzed as separate entities. This would require larger numbers of samples to allow significant distinction between the subtypes which are only subtly different histomorphologically.

Proteomics based studies in IM have been limited. One study used 2DGE to identify proteins which were present in the gastric juices of patients with varying stages of gastric disorders [56]. They observed that pepsin A and B as well as gastric lipase were common in the gastric juices of patients with normal mucosa and IM as well as ChG but were absent in about 60% of tumor samples in their cohort. Conversely α_1-antitrypsin exhibited increasing levels with progression and was detected in about 60% of the tumor samples. Further analysis by MALDI-TOF MS and nanoelectrospray MS/MS showed that the form of α_1-antitrypsin found in gastric juices varies slightly from that found in plasma. These authors suggest that α_1-antitrypsin may be a suitable prognostic marker for GC however no further validation of this hypothesis has been reported.

Adenoma/Dysplasia/Colorectal Carcinoma

v to the upper GI tract discussed previously, CRC is a potentially curable disease if detected and treated early. It is understood to develop via a stepwise progression termed the "adenoma-carcinoma" sequence first proposed by Fearon and Vogelstein in 1990 [57] and as discussed in Chaps. 5 and 18. In this pathway normal colonic mucosa proceeds to adenocarcinoma via an adenoma, which is defined as a dysplastic polyp in the colon (Fig. 6.4). This process is believed to take as long as 10 years allowing ample time for early detection and intervention [58].

Even though the pathway leading to CRC has been well described, information relating to the molecular mechanisms is still lacking. Table 6.3 summarizes some of the data obtained using -omics based technologies to study premalignant stages of CRC.

Notterman et al. [59] used Affymetrix™ RNA expression arrays to identify changes between normal colonic mucosa ($n=18$), adenomas ($n=4$) and adenocarcinomas ($n=18$). They reported that several changes observed in the carcinomas were also present in the adenomas suggesting that they are early changes in the progression pathway. These changes included increases in M_1 100,000 coactivator, *BIGH3*, *ckshs2*, *MGSA* and *matrilysin*, Genes found to be up-regulated in adenomas in comparison to adenocarcinomas are guanylin, down-regulated in adenocarcinoma and hevin. Several genes including transcription factors (*XBP-1, SSRP-1, ETS-2* and *SOX9*) as well as ribosomal proteins (s9 and S29) were mostly highly expressed in the adenoma group. The authors suggest that increased expression of these genes may be important in the transition between adenoma and adenocarcinoma [59]. The data from this study must however be interpreted with caution as the sample number for the adenoma group was low ($n=4$) and two different Affymetrix™ platforms were

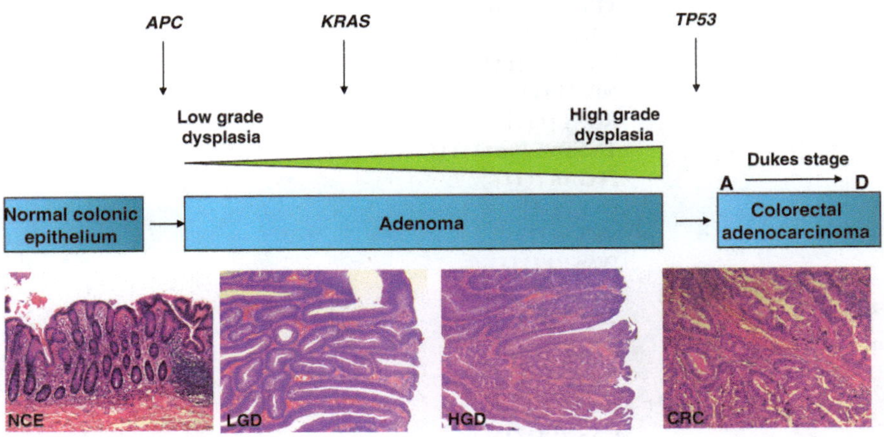

Fig. 6.4 Progressive pathway to colorectal adenocarcinoma. This pathway first described by Vogelstein details the role of mutations in the APC, KRAS and TP53 genes which trigger a malignant cascade from normal colonic epithelium (NCE) via adenoma, which becomes increasingly dysplastic finally leading to colorectal adenocarcinoma (CRC) as an end-point

Table 6.3 Summary of key candidate genes/loci which are changed in precursor lesions of Colorectal Adenocarcinoma

	RNA	miRNA	DNA	Proteomics
Genes/loci differentially expressed/gained in positive direction	M1 100,000 coactivator [88]@	miR-17 [93]	17p [96]	N/A
	BIGH3 [88]@	miR-19a [93]	13q [96]	
	ckshs2 [88]@	miR-20a [93]		
	MGSA [88]@	miR-19b-1 [93]	7 [97]	
	Matrilysin [88]@	miR-92a-1 [93]	20q [97]	
			13 [97]	
	Guanylin [88]¥	**miR-21 [112]**		
	Downregulated in adenocarcinoma [88]¥	**miR-181b [112]**		
	Hevin [88]¥			
	XBP-1 [88]‡			
	SSRP-1 [88]‡			
	ETS-2 [88]‡			
	SOX9 [88]‡			
	s9 [88]‡			
	s29 [88]‡			
	GPX2 [92]			
	PPIA [92]			
	GAPD [92]			
	ANXA2 [92]			
	ALDH1 [92]			
	ADAR [92]			
	TFF1[a, b] [110]			
	CTSA[a, b] [110]			
	PLAG2A [111]			
	NPM1 [111]			
	ROS1 [111]			
	TNFRSF10A[a] [111]			
	ITGA6 [111]			
	FAT [111]			
	VSX1 [111]			
	WASF2 [111]			
	HDAC1 [111]			
	SPINK1 [111]			
	RHEB [111]			
	IFITM1 [111]			
	WEE1 [111]			
	CASP1 [111]			
	EPHB3 [111]			
	PHB [111]			
	SOD1 [111]			

(continued)

Table 6.3 (continued)

	RNA	miRNA	DNA	Proteomics
Genes/loci differentially expressed/gained in negative direction	PGK1 [92]	N/A	17p [96]	N/A
	LDHA [92]		11q [96]	
	PSMD7 [92]			
	PSMB8 [92]			
	C20orf24 [100]			
	AURKA [100]			
	RNPC1 [100]			
	THL1 [100]			
	ADRM1 [100]			
	C20orf20 [100]			
	TCFL5 [100]			
	SIAT7D [111]			
	RARA[a] [111]			
	CSK [111]			
	BENE[a] [111]			
	RGS19IP1 [111]			
	VDR [111]			
	UGDH [111]			

[88]@ – reference compares the progression of adenoma and CRC vs. normal colonic mucosa
[88]¥ – reference compares adenoma vs. CRC
[88]‡ – reference compares adenoma vs. normal colon and CRC
[92] – reference compares adenoma vs. CRC
[100] – reference compares adenoma vs. CRC (thought to occur as a consequence of gain on Chr. 20)
Changes in bold represent changes in SSA vs. normal
N/A not applicable
[a]Validated by qRT-PCR
[b]Validated by IHC

used to compare adenocarcinoma with paired normals (Affymetrix™ 6500 GeneChip set) and adenoma with their matched normals (Affymetrix™ 6800 Genechip set).

A more substantial study by Nosho et al. looked at gene expression of 34 adenomas and 14 early invasive carcinomas each with a matched paired normal sample using cDNA arrays [60]. Cell signaling genes made up the majority of the genes which were up-regulated in adenomas compared to the carcinomas. Interestingly two of the genes found more highly expressed in the carcinomas are tumor suppressor genes (Smad4 and nm23) however both of these genes have previously been reported to be inactivated or down-regulated in late stage CRC samples [61, 62]. Nosho et al. suggest that this discrepancy may be due to the fact that the carcinomas in their study were early stage carcinomas and did not exhibit any invasion or metastasis [60].

Another cDNA based study by Yin et al. looked at 9 adenomas, 11 adenocarcinomas and matched normal tissue from each patient [63]. They identified 51 genes commonly up-regulated in both adenomas and adenocarcinomas. These genes encode for proteins involved in RNA/protein processing, cell adhesion molecules, oncogenes, cell cycle control, transcription factors and tumor associated molecules [63]. Commonly down-regulated genes include genes involved in programmed cell death, tumor suppression, immunity, cell adhesion molecules and growth suppression [63]. When directly comparing genes differentially expressed between adenomas and adenocarcinomas these authors found that genes involved in adaptation to low oxygen conditions (*GPX2, PPIA, GAPD, ANXA2, ALDH1, ADAR*) were highly expressed in adenomas. Genes known to be either induced or known to accumulate under conditions of hypoxia (*PGK1, LDHA, PSMD7* and *PSMB8*) were found to be expressed more highly in the adenocarcinoma cells [63].

Over-expression and down-regulation of specific miRNAs have been reported to play a role in both the development and progression of CRC. Over-expression of all of the genes comprising the mIR-17-92 cluster (miRs -17, -18a, -19a, -20a, 19b-1, 92a-1) with the exception of miR-18a has been correlated with copy number gain on chromosome 13q31 and expression has been shown to increase with progression from adenoma to CRC [64]. It has previously been shown that this miR cluster is regulated by c-myc which is located on chromosome 8q24. A recent review by Aslam et al. has extensively discussed the possible role of specific miRNAs in the early detection and therapy of CRC as well as in determination of patient prognosis, however these will not be discussed here in any more detail [65].

The Vogelstein model proposes that colorectal carcinogenesis occurs via a series of intermediate stages as a result of mutation accumulation in key regulatory genes. The sequential acquisition of specific genetic changes is directly related to the progression via the adenoma-carcinoma sequence. These changes have been well described and were characterized well before the advent of the -omics era using karyotyping techniques. Mutation in the *APC* gene is believed to be the first change which initiates the progressive pathway and occurs in up to 80% of adenomas and adenocarcinomas. This tumor suppressor gene encodes a protein which acts by binding to β-catenin. A mutation in this gene or this pathway results in defective Wnt signalling. The second key mutation in Vogelstein's progression pathway occurs in the *KRAS* gene (a well known oncogene). KRAS mutations are also an early event in the sequence but are found in only a low percentage of CRCs. The final stage in the progressive pathway is mutation or LOH in the p53 gene (Fig. 6.4).

Whilst the adenoma-carcinoma model suggests that mutation (or LOH) of the tumour suppressor genes APC and TP53 as well as mutation of the KRAS oncogene are required in order for colorectal carcinogenesis to occur several groups have argued that this is an overly simplistic hypothesis and have demonstrated that mutations in TP53 and KRAS very rarely both occur in the same tumor [66, 67]. CGH based studies have identified several chromosomal changes which occur even more frequently than these mutations. For example, a study looking at the frequency of chromosomal aberrations as well as APC, KRAS and TP53 mutations in adenomas they showed that whilst APC mutations were the most common single event, gains in 7p and 13q as well as losses on 17p and 11q occurred with a higher frequency than KRAS mutations [68]. This suggests a role for these aberrations in the development of CRC. Another study detected gains on chromosome 7, 13 and 20q in adenoma samples [69] as well as in adenocarcinoma samples and liver metastases.

More recently, several groups have performed correlative studies which aimed to identify common genetic changes occurring in colon cancer and then identifying genes residing within these regions. This is important as tumor suppressor genes are likely to be inactivated by a deletion whereas oncogenes can be activated by copy number amplification. Tsafrir et al. [70] demonstrated that >60% of differentially expressed sites are associated with gain or loss in the corresponding genomic region in CRC. Sheffer et al. [71] performed an elaborate study comparing SNP data generated using Affymetrix™ 50K arrays with expression data from Affymetrix™ U133A arrays from samples at varying stages of the adenoma-carcinoma sequence. The analysis of the data focused mainly on the changes occurring in tumor samples however they did identify significant copy number changes on chromosomes 14q, 20q, 20p and 8q between adenomas and Stage I CRC tumors, which are being interpreted as early events. Consistent with other studies amplification on chromosomal arm 20q was the most frequently occurring change and was observed in 91% of tumors and in some adenomas [71]. Gains on 20q have been observed in other tumor types and have been previously implicated with poor outcome in patients with CRC as well as GC.

In order to identify genes which may be differentially expressed as a result of copy number amplification on chromosome 20, Carvalho et al. performed copy number and gene expression analysis on early and advanced stage adenoma samples as well as colorectal adenocarcinomas [72]. They identified seven genes as putative oncogenes that were over-expressed in carcinomas as a consequence of copy number gain on chr20. They then proposed that these genes (C20orf24, AURKA, RNPC1, THL1, ADRM1, C20orf20 and TCFL5) are implicated in the progression from adenoma to CRC and suggest that they may potentially serve a role as biomarkers for progression [72]. This assertion remains untested in an independent cohort and would ideally require a prospective trial to determine progression.

Proteomic techniques have been utilized by several groups in an attempt to identify proteins involved in the CRC using either tumor issue or serum samples from cancer patients with varying degrees of success. To our knowledge, there is no literature available that describes proteins which are differentially regulated in adenomas.

Colon cancers themselves are often classified using the Dukes or TNM staging systems which are pathological assessments of tumor extent and give very good prognostic information [73]. The Dukes stages indicate more advanced disease from Dukes A (cancer confined to mucosa) through to Dukes D (cancer infiltrating adjacent organ or with distant metastases). A study by Birkenkamp-Demtroder et al. used Affymetrix™ genechip microarrays to identify candidate tumor supressors and oncogenes which may play a role in the progression of CRC through the Dukes stages [74]. They were also able to identify candidate genes specific to only one or two stages of the Dukes classification system. These genes could subsequently be used to identify specific stages of the disease however these were not extensively discussed in the manuscript [74].

These authors identified 226 known genes which were differentially expressed from normal colonic epithelium to CRC. Of these, 70 were candidate tumor suppressors which were found to be down-regulated in the cancer specimens and 88 genes were oncogenes and were over-expressed in the cancer samples. Interestingly genes which were over-expressed in cancers encoded for proteins which are involved in methylation, metabolism, cell cycle, cell adhesion and translation. Genes which were down-regulated in cancers encoded for proteins involved in membrane and protein trafficking, lipid metabolism and membrane proteins as well as kinases and phophorylases [74]. Most of the changes in gene expression occurred during the transition between normal colonic mucosa ($n=6$) to Dukes A cancers ($n=5$) and very few changes of expression during the progression through the Dukes stages (Dukes B $n=6$, Dukes C $n=4$). These authors postulate that tumors acquire their basic properties early on and that the subsequent changes are probably not required till later stages [74]. A similar study by Frederiksen et al. was able to further characterize five each of Dukes B and C tumors reporting a decreased expression in nuclear encoded mitochondrial genes in Dukes B compared to normal samples ($n=5$). This decrease in expression was further attenuated in the Dukes C samples. Genes which were found to be progressively increased in Dukes B and C when compared to normal samples were mainly stromal related genes and include thrombospondin 2 and platelet derived growth factor (PDGF) [75].

Several recent studies have exploited the fact that cells in the colon are consistently shed into the lumen and replenished. These cells are potentially detectable in stool samples. It is possible to extract DNA from these cells and subsequently perform genomic analysis as a means of screening for genomic events known to be implicated in CRC. The most common genetic markers used to-date includes KRAS, APC and TP53 which are often mutated in CRC. Since each of these mutation types occur in only a small amount of CRC they individually confer low specificity. Using several markers in combination tends to give better accuracy. This screening method has been successful to some extent with several groups developing assays containing a panel of target genes; the specificity of the tests is currently up to 90%. Whilst these tests appear to be relatively successful in the identification of CRC they are usually not as sensitive in their ability to detect the premalignant adenoma. A recent publication by Glockner et al. has identified *TFPI2* as a gene which has promoter hypermethylation in CRC as well as its precursor lesions [76]. This gene is believed to act as a tumour suppressor gene and is known to inhibit tumor proliferation in vitro. During the adenoma-carcinoma sequence hypermethylation of the promoter of this gene results in its expression being silenced which may confer pro-invasive properties to the cell. This group has validated its ability to detect hypermethylation of the TFPI2 promoter in stool samples and propose that it could be a used as an epigenetic marker which could identify patients with CRC or its precursor lesions at early stage [76]. Other genes which have been investigated as potential single gene epigenetic markers for CRC and its precursors, and which are also detectable in stool, include SFRP2 [77] and vimentin [78].

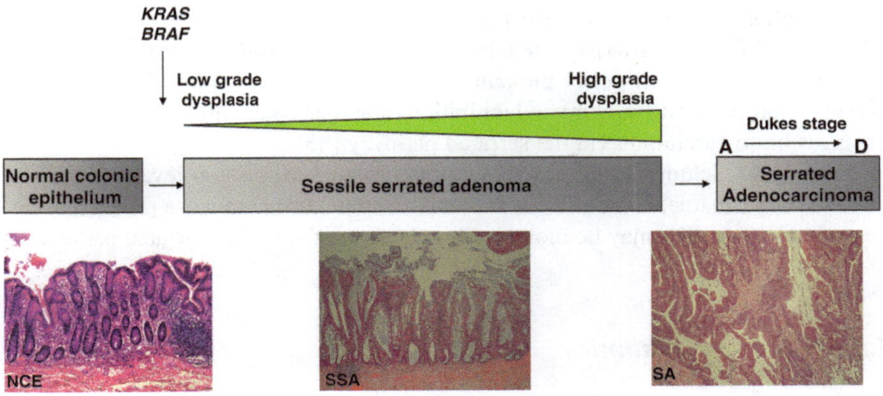

Fig. 6.5 Progressive pathway to serrated adenocarcinoma. This alternative pathway of CRC is characterised by mutations in the KRAS or BRAF genes which trigger a malignant cascade from normal colonic epithelium (NCE) via sessile serrated adenoma (SSA), which becomes increasingly dysplastic finally leading to serrated adenocarcinoma (SA) as an end-point cells and *red arrows* indicate presence of a brush border

In addition to the well-characterized Vogelstein pathway described above, there has been increasing interest in an alternative pathway of progression to CRC known as the serrated pathway (Fig. 6.5) [79]. Proponents of this pathway of colorectal carcinogenesis suggest a proportion of colorectal cancer may arise through a particular type of hyperplastic polyp as precursor lesion. Although these lesions have previously been considered harmless there is increasing evidence that a specific subtype known as sessile serated adenomas (SSA) have malignant potential and that these lesions may play a role in the development of colorectal adenocarcinomas. Histologically SSA are usually large and exhibit abnormal architecture and excessive mucin secretion and are characterized by somatic mutation of the BRAF gene (V600E) as well as methylation [80]. Although the serrated pathway of CRC is most often associated with a genetic predisposition there is evidence that it can occur in sporadic lesions [81].

To date the number of -omics based studies investigated key genes and pathways involved in the serrated pathway are few. A recent study by Caruso et al. used in-house cDNA arrays to identify genes differentially expressed between SSA and tubular adenomas [82]. The top two genes *TFF1* and *CTSE* were then validated by qRT-PCR and IHC. Expression of CTSE was found to be upregulated in SSA in comparison to normal mucosa with 50% of samples showing a 25- to 96-fold increase in expression. TFF1 was also found to be overexpressed up to 44-fold in the SSA samples. The potential use of these genes as biomarkers is promising but requires further validation.

A comparison of gene expression levels in serrated adenomas compared to normal colonic mucosa performed by Kim et al. identified 73 genes which were up-regulated by at least twofold and 51 genes down-regulated more than 50% [83]. The 24 most highly expressed genes (up- or down-regulated) are listed in Table 6.3.

These authors chose to validate expression of three of these genes (*TNFRSF10A/TRAIL*, *BENE* and *RARA*) by qRT-PCR. After considering the functions of the differentially expressed genes the authors propose that activation of proliferation signals, modified cell structure and inhibition of apoptosis are all early events in the progression to carcinoma via the serrated pathway [83].

A study by Schmitz et al. has shown that elevated expression levels of miR-21 miR-181b are characteristic of SSA in comparison to normal mucosa [84]. This suggests that these miR's may be biologically relevant in the sessile serrated pathway.

Limitations to Genomics

Whilst -omics based studies have been found to contribute to our knowledge of preinvasive lesions and their corresponding cancers it is also apparent that each technique has its own limitations. In addition it is very difficult to make direct comparisons between studies as a result of differences in platforms, methods of analysis and study design. Below are a few examples of such issues which should be considered when designing and performing experiments as well as while interpreting findings from the available literature.

Care should be taken at the very early stage of sample selection. It is necessary to select a study cohort which is randomized (as much as is reasonably possible) and in which known confounders (such as age, sex, tumor stage) are equally represented to account for potential sample bias.

In cases where DNA and RNA need to be extracted, immediate collection in liquid nitrogen and subsequent storage in liquid nitrogen or −80°C is required. This is not often feasible in a surgical setting where there is a delay between a sample being removed from the patient and being accessed by the researcher. Often this occurs when there is a need for pathological review of the entire sample before being released for research use. Improper tissue collection and storage may compromise RNA and/or DNA integrity and may result in poor quality data.

Preparation of samples for analysis is also important. Tumors and biopsy samples of tissues of interest are recognized as heterogeneous. In order for a researcher to ensure that they are analyzing a "pure" sample it is important to control for contamination by normal host tissue such as stromal and inflammatory components. The total percentage of the tissue being studied in a sample should also be taken into consideration, with many studies imposing a minimum of 70–80% sample tissue content for selection into -omics experiments. In the case of studies involving the study of pre-invasive lesions similar cutoffs/criteria for sample selection would also be necessary. For example in IM of the stomach only a certain number of glands within a sample may be affected and, if samples are not selected or prepared correctly it is possible that the effect of IM in these samples may be diluted out or disguised by the presence of larger amounts of normal glands. Selection for particular cell types within a sample may be facilitated by the use of some recent advances in techniques and technologies including needle microdissection as well as laser capture microscopy (LCM). LCM is useful for isolating homogeneous cell populations within a sample but has the disadvantages of increased sample processing time as well as having high costs associated with purchase and maintainence of the equipment. Alternatively, the "contamination" by other cell types may be characteristic of that disorder and may be an important factor to profile with -omics technologies. This makes the deconvolution of the data more onerous for the bioinformaticians but could lead to important avenues of research into pathogenesis.

Experimental variation may also be a factor, which needs to be taken into account during data analysis and experimental design. Array to array variation may occur between batches of arrays. Additionally batch to batch variation can occur when samples which are to be analyzed together are prepared and hybridized on different days. Ideally all samples within a study should be prepared and hybridized on the same day however this is often not feasible especially where the sample number is large. Some analysis software now applies algorithms which can take into account and remove batch effect during the analysis procedure.

A major criticism that we have of several publications reviewed during the process of preparing this chapter is the number of studies involving small numbers of samples. This may in some cases be attributed to the high cost associated with these experiments. Indeed the cost of arrays has been significant and is a limiting factor in several studies. Alternatively small sample size may be the result of lack of available samples either for the preliminary analysis or for validation of the findings. Findings from these studies need to be interpreted with caution as low sample number may introduce data bias.

The use of archival formalin fixed paraffin embedded (FFPE) samples would serve many advantages in studies of the progression of premalignant/preinvasive lesions. As well as having a long history of clinical data from these patients it is also likely that biopsies may be available for different stages of progression in the same patient which would allow genomic changes to be identified between each stage without having to take into consideration person to person variation. To date, use of FFPE samples has been restricted as DNA and RNA extracted from these samples has been of low abundance and/or poor quality. More recently however techniques are being developed to circumvent these issues and limitations.

In addition to the limitations arising from experimental design and sample preparation there are also potential issues associated with data analysis and subsequent interpretation. These issues have been reviewed extensively elsewhere and will not be discussed here [85].

Conclusions

Trends in the use of -omics for the study of disease reveal that the early studies in a particular disease or biological process are observational or hypothesis generating and progress towards their use in more targeted hypothesis driven research. Currently, -omics based studies on premalignant lesions are in this early phase often with small sample sizes. Large amounts of data are generated with each of the -omics platforms and although many candidate genes are identified very few of these have been validated and even less have progressed to serve any clinical utility. One of the better examples of this would be the study by Lao-Sirieix et al. which was discussed in the Barrett's esophagus section of this chapter [29]. This shows how a genomics based approach was used to identify candidate genes that were validated and finally applied to a clinical cohort as a diagnostic test. This test has several benefits over existing endoscopy based screening techniques as it is non-invasive and significantly cheaper.

Theoretically the ability to identify candidate genes which might predict the progression of a patient to cancer would be of great benefit. The premalignant conditions described here present as metaplastic or dysplastic changes in the tissue that may subsequently become cancerous. It then needs to be determined whether the differentially expressed genes are genuine markers of progression or whether they reflect the differentiation state of the tissue and may simply be bystanders rather than drivers of the phenotype.

To date there have been very few extensive correlative studies published which use multiple -omics based techniques in the same cohort of samples. Although currently cost prohibitive, a well designed study that aims to identify and link copy number change, expression and miRNA profiles in samples derived from the same patient would be an invaluable resource. Any findings would be difficult to validate in a prospective study due to the difficulties in designing a prospective clinical trial that is long enough or large enough to see an effect on cancer as an outcome. One alternative would be to apply a range of -omics based platforms to animal model systems which mimic the human progression pathways to cancer via premalignant intermediates. This would allow sampling from the same animal at each of the stages of progression and at varying time points.

There is considerable effort and resources being invested in designing these trials to answer these important questions. The ability to predict which individuals will progress to cancer if they develop a particular premalignant lesion remains the "holy grail" for molecular preventative medicine. Once this goal is reached the benefits of early detection of cancer can only then be realized. This may require the combination of clinical, demographic, pathological and molecular factors.

Acknowledgements The authors thank Miss Christina Tucci, Dr Nicholas Clemons and Dr Catherine Mitchell for providing the images used in this manuscript.

References

1. Schena M, Shalon D, Davis RW et al (1995) Quantitative monitoring of gene expression patterns with a complementary DNA microarray. Science 270:467–470
2. Cheung VG, Morley M, Aguilar F et al (1999) Making and reading microarrays. Nat Genet 21:15–19
3. Esquela-Kerscher A, Slack FJ (2006) Oncomirs – microRNAs with a role in cancer. Nat Rev Cancer 6:259–269

4. Wicker N, Carles A, Mills IG et al (2007) A new look towards BAC-based array CGH through a comprehensive comparison with oligo-based array CGH. BMC Genomics 8:84
5. van den Ijssel P, Tijssen M, Chin SF et al (2005) Human and mouse oligonucleotide-based array CGH. Nucleic Acids Res 33:e192
6. Simon R, Mirlacher M, Sauter G (2005) Tissue microarrays. Meth Mol Med 114:257–268
7. Simon R, Mirlacher M, Sauter G (2004) Tissue microarrays. Meth Mol Med 97:377–389
8. Chen W, Foran DJ (2006) Advances in cancer tissue microarray technology: Towards improved understanding and diagnostics. Anal Chim Acta 564:74–81
9. Simon R, Mirlacher M, Sauter G (2003) Tissue microarrays in cancer diagnosis. Expert Rev Mol Diagn 3:421–430
10. Selaru FM, Zou T, Xu Y et al (2002) Global gene expression profiling in Barrett's esophagus and esophageal cancer: a comparative analysis using cDNA microarrays. Oncogene 21: 475–478
11. Xu Y, Selaru FM, Yin J et al (2002) Artificial neural networks and gene filtering distinguish between global gene expression profiles of Barrett's esophagus and esophageal cancer. Cancer Res 62:3493–3497
12. Wang S, Zhan M, Yin J et al (2006) Transcriptional profiling suggests that Barrett's metaplasia is an early intermediate stage in esophageal adenocarcinogenesis. Oncogene 25:3346–3356
13. Yamamoto H, Horiuchi S, Adachi Y et al (2004) Expression of ets-related transcriptional factor E1AF is associated with tumor progression and over-expression of matrilysin in human gastric cancer. Carcinogenesis 25:325–332
14. Hovanes K, Li TW, Munguia JE et al (2001) Beta-catenin-sensitive isoforms of lymphoid enhancer factor-1 are selectively expressed in colon cancer. Nat Genet 28:53–57
15. Watts GS, Tran NL, Berens ME et al (2007) Identification of Fn14/TWEAK receptor as a potential therapeutic target in esophageal adenocarcinoma. Int J Cancer 121:2132–2139
16. Tran NL, McDonough WS, Donohue PJ et al (2003) The human Fn14 receptor gene is up-regulated in migrating glioma cells in vitro and overexpressed in advanced glial tumors. Am J Pathol 162:1313–1321
17. Lynch CN, Wang YC, Lund JK et al (1999) TWEAK induces angiogenesis and proliferation of endothelial cells. J Biol Chem 274:8455–8459
18. Milano F, Jorritsma T, Rygiel AM et al (2008) Expression pattern of immune suppressive cytokines and growth factors in oesophageal adenocarcinoma reveal a tumour immune escape-promoting microenvironment. Scand J Immunol 68:616–623
19. Kimchi ET, Posner MC, Park JO et al (2005) Progression of Barrett's metaplasia to adenocarcinoma is associated with the suppression of the transcriptional programs of epidermal differentiation. Cancer Res 65:3146–3154
20. Gomes LI, Esteves GH, Carvalho AF et al (2005) Expression profile of malignant and nonmalignant lesions of esophagus and stomach: differential activity of functional modules related to inflammation and lipid metabolism. Cancer Res 65:7127–7136
21. Greenawalt DM, Duong C, Smyth GK et al (2007) Gene expression profiling of esophageal cancer: comparative analysis of Barrett's esophagus, adenocarcinoma, and squamous cell carcinoma. Int J Cancer 120:1914–1921
22. Brabender J, Lord RV, Metzger R et al (2003) Differential SPARC mRNA expression in Barrett's oesophagus. Br J Cancer 89:1508–1512
23. Said N, Najwer I, Motamed K (2007) Secreted protein acidic and rich in cysteine (SPARC) inhibits integrin-mediated adhesion and growth factor-dependent survival signaling in ovarian cancer. Am J Pathol 170:1054–1063
24. Barth PJ, Moll R, Ramaswamy A (2005) Stromal remodeling and SPARC (secreted protein acid rich in cysteine) expression in invasive ductal carcinomas of the breast. Virchows Arch 446:532–536
25. Buttar NS, Wang KK, Leontovich O et al (2002) Chemoprevention of esophageal adenocarcinoma by COX-2 inhibitors in an animal model of Barrett's esophagus. Gastroenterology 122:1101–1112
26. Heath EI, Canto MI, Piantadosi S et al (2007) Secondary chemoprevention of Barrett's esophagus with celecoxib: results of a randomized trial. J Natl Cancer Inst 99:545–557

27. Hao Y, Triadafilopoulos G, Sahbaie P et al (2006) Gene expression profiling reveals stromal genes expressed in common between Barrett's esophagus and adenocarcinoma. Gastroenterology 131:925–933
28. Boussioutas A, Li H, Liu J et al (2003) Distinctive patterns of gene expression in premalignant gastric mucosa and gastric cancer. Cancer Res 63:2569–2577
29. Lao-Sirieix P, Boussioutas A, Kadri SR et al (2009) Non-endoscopic screening biomarkers for Barrett's oesophagus: from microarray analysis to the clinic. Gut 58:1451–1459
30. Feber A, Xi L, Luketich JD et al (2008) MicroRNA expression profiles of esophageal cancer. J Thorac Cardiovasc Surg 135:255–260, discussion 60
31. Luthra R, Singh RR, Luthra MG et al (2008) MicroRNA-196a targets annexin A1: a microRNA-mediated mechanism of annexin A1 downregulation in cancers. Oncogene 27:6667–6678
32. Maru DM, Singh RR, Hannah C et al (2009) MicroRNA-196a is a potential marker of progression during Barrett's metaplasia-dysplasia-invasive adenocarcinoma sequence in esophagus. Am J Pathol 174:1940–1948
33. Walch AK, Zitzelsberger HF, Bruch J et al (2000) Chromosomal imbalances in Barrett's adenocarcinoma and the metaplasia–dysplasia-carcinoma sequence. Am J Pathol 156:555–566
34. Riegman PH, Vissers KJ, Alers JC et al (2001) Genomic alterations in malignant transformation of Barrett's esophagus. Cancer Res 61:3164–3170
35. Gonzalez MV, Artimez ML, Rodrigo L et al (1997) Mutation analysis of the p53, APC, and p16 genes in the Barrett's oesophagus, dysplasia, and adenocarcinoma. J Clin Pathol 50:212–217
36. Wu TT, Watanabe T, Heitmiller R et al (1998) Genetic alterations in Barrett esophagus and adenocarcinomas of the esophagus and esophagogastric junction region. Am J Pathol 153:287–294
37. Zhuang Z, Vortmeyer AO, Mark EJ et al (1996) Barrett's esophagus: metaplastic cells with loss of heterozygosity at the APC gene locus are clonal precursors to invasive adenocarcinoma. Cancer Res 56:1961–1964
38. Croft J, Parry EM, Jenkins GJ et al (2002) Analysis of the premalignant stages of Barrett's oesophagus through to adenocarcinoma by comparative genomic hybridization. Eur J Gastroenterol Hepatol 14:1179–1186
39. Lai LA, Paulson TG, Li X et al (2007) Increasing genomic instability during premalignant neoplastic progression revealed through high resolution array-CGH. Genes Chromosomes Cancer 46:532–542
40. Paulson TG, Galipeau PC, Xu L et al (2008) p16 mutation spectrum in the premalignant condition Barrett's esophagus. PLoS ONE 3:e3809
41. Barrett MT, Sanchez CA, Galipeau PC et al (1996) Allelic loss of 9p21 and mutation of the CDKN2/p16 gene develop as early lesions during neoplastic progression in Barrett's esophagus. Oncogene 13:1867–1873
42. Galipeau PC, Prevo LJ, Sanchez CA et al (1999) Clonal expansion and loss of heterozygosity at chromosomes 9p and 17p in premalignant esophageal (Barrett's) tissue. J Natl Cancer Inst 91:2087–2095
43. Zhao J, Chang AC, Li C et al (2007) Comparative proteomics analysis of Barrett metaplasia and esophageal adenocarcinoma using two-dimensional liquid mass mapping. Mol Cell Proteomics 6:987–999
44. Correa P (1988) A human model of gastric carcinogenesis. Cancer Res 48:3554–3560
45. Leung WK, Lin SR, Ching JY et al (2004) Factors predicting progression of gastric intestinal metaplasia: results of a randomised trial on *Helicobacter pylori* eradication. Gut 53:1244–1249
46. MacLennan AJ, Orringer MB, Beer DG (1999) Identification of intestinal-type Barrett's metaplasia by using the intestine-specific protein villin and esophageal brush cytology. Mol Carcinog 24:137–143
47. Wright NA, Hoffmann W, Otto WR et al (1997) Rolling in the clover: trefoil factor family (TFF)-domain peptides, cell migration and cancer. FEBS Lett 408:121–123
48. Lefebvre O, Chenard MP, Masson R et al (1996) Gastric mucosa abnormalities and tumorigenesis in mice lacking the pS2 trefoil protein. Science 274:259–262
49. Taupin D, Pedersen J, Familari M et al (2001) Augmented intestinal trefoil factor (TFF3) and loss of pS2 (TFF1) expression precedes metaplastic differentiation of gastric epithelium. Lab Invest 81:397–408

50. Meireles SI, Cristo EB, Carvalho AF et al (2004) Molecular classifiers for gastric cancer and nonmalignant diseases of the gastric mucosa. Cancer Res 64:1255–1265
51. Guo J, Miao Y, Xiao B et al (2009) Differential expression of microRNA species in human gastric cancer versus non-tumorous tissues. J Gastroenterol Hepatol 24:652–657
52. Du Y, Xu Y, Ding L et al (2009) Down-regulation of miR-141 in gastric cancer and its involvement in cell growth. J Gastroenterol 44:556–561
53. Tsukamoto Y, Uchida T, Karnan S et al (2008) Genome-wide analysis of DNA copy number alterations and gene expression in gastric cancer. J Pathol 216:471–482
54. Gorringe KL, Boussioutas A, Bowtell DD (2005) Novel regions of chromosomal amplification at 6p21, 5p13, and 12q14 in gastric cancer identified by array comparative genomic hybridization. Genes Chromosomes Cancer 42:247–259
55. Busuttil RA, Boussioutas A (2009) Intestinal metaplasia: a premalignant lesion involved in gastric carcinogenesis. J Gastroenterol Hepatol 24:193–201
56. Lee K, Kye M, Jang JS et al (2004) Proteomic analysis revealed a strong association of a high level of alpha1-antitrypsin in gastric juice with gastric cancer. Proteomics 4:3343–3352
57. Fearon ER, Vogelstein B (1990) A genetic model for colorectal tumorigenesis. Cell 61:759–767
58. Dove-Edwin I, Thomas HJ (2001) Review article: the prevention of colorectal cancer. Aliment Pharmacol Ther 15:323–336
59. Notterman DA, Alon U, Sierk AJ et al (2001) Transcriptional gene expression profiles of colorectal adenoma, adenocarcinoma, and normal tissue examined by oligonucleotide arrays. Cancer Res 61:3124–3130
60. Nosho K, Yamamoto H, Adachi Y et al (2005) Gene expression profiling of colorectal adenomas and early invasive carcinomas by cDNA array analysis. Br J Cancer 92:1193–1200
61. Muller N, Reinacher-Schick A, Baldus S et al (2002) Smad4 induces the tumor suppressor E-cadherin and P-cadherin in colon carcinoma cells. Oncogene 21:6049–6058
62. Suzuki E, Ota T, Tsukuda K et al (2004) nm23-H1 reduces in vitro cell migration and the liver metastatic potential of colon cancer cells by regulating myosin light chain phosphorylation. Int J Cancer 108:207–211
63. Lin YM, Furukawa Y, Tsunoda T et al (2002) Molecular diagnosis of colorectal tumors by expression profiles of 50 genes expressed differentially in adenomas and carcinomas. Oncogene 21:4120–4128
64. Diosdado B, van de Wiel MA (2009) Terhaar Sive Droste JS et al. MiR-17-92 cluster is associated with 13q gain and c-myc expression during colorectal adenoma to adenocarcinoma progression. Br J Cancer 101:707–714
65. Aslam MI, Taylor K, Pringle JH et al (2009) MicroRNAs are novel biomarkers of colorectal cancer. Br J Surg 96:702–710
66. Smith G, Carey FA, Beattie J et al (2002) Mutations in APC, Kirsten-ras, and p53-alternative genetic pathways to colorectal cancer. Proc Natl Acad Sci U S A 99:9433–9438
67. Leslie A, Pratt NR, Gillespie K et al (2003) Mutations of APC, K-ras, and p53 are associated with specific chromosomal aberrations in colorectal adenocarcinomas. Cancer Res 63:4656–4661
68. Leslie A, Stewart A, Baty DU et al (2006) Chromosomal changes in colorectal adenomas: relationship to gene mutations and potential for clinical utility. Genes Chromosomes Cancer 45:126–135
69. Habermann JK, Paulsen U, Roblick UJ et al (2007) Stage-specific alterations of the genome, transcriptome, and proteome during colorectal carcinogenesis. Genes Chromosomes Cancer 46:10–26
70. Tsafrir D, Bacolod M, Selvanayagam Z et al (2006) Relationship of gene expression and chromosomal abnormalities in colorectal cancer. Cancer Res 66:2129–2137
71. Sheffer M, Bacolod MD, Zuk O et al (2009) Association of survival and disease progression with chromosomal instability: a genomic exploration of colorectal cancer. Proc Natl Acad Sci U S A 106:7131–7136
72. Carvalho B, Postma C, Mongera S et al (2009) Multiple putative oncogenes at the chromosome 20q amplicon contribute to colorectal adenoma to carcinoma progression. Gut 58:79–89

73. AJCC (2002) Cancer staging manual, 6th edn. Springer, New York
74. Birkenkamp-Demtroder K, Christensen LL, Olesen SH et al (2002) Gene expression in colorectal cancer. Cancer Res 62:4352–4363
75. Frederiksen CM, Knudsen S, Laurberg S et al (2003) Classification of Dukes' B and C colorectal cancers using expression arrays. J Cancer Res Clin Oncol 129:263–271
76. Glockner SC, Dhir M, Yi JM et al (2009) Methylation of TFPI2 in stool DNA: a potential novel biomarker for the detection of colorectal cancer. Cancer Res 69:4691–4699
77. Oberwalder M, Zitt M, Wontner C et al (2008) SFRP2 methylation in fecal DNA – a marker for colorectal polyps. Int J Colorectal Dis 23:15–19
78. Chen WD, Han ZJ, Skoletsky J et al (2005) Detection in fecal DNA of colon cancer-specific methylation of the nonexpressed vimentin gene. J Natl Cancer Inst 97:1124–1132
79. Jass JR, Filipe MI (1979) A variant of intestinal metaplasia associated with gastric carcinoma: a histochemical study. Histopathology 3:191–199
80. Young J, Jass JR (2006) The case for a genetic predisposition to serrated neoplasia in the colorectum: hypothesis and review of the literature. Cancer Epidemiol Biomark Prev 15:1778–1784
81. Young J, Jenkins M, Parry S et al (2007) Serrated pathway colorectal cancer in the population: genetic consideration. Gut 56:1453–1459
82. Caruso M, Moore J, Goodall GJ et al (2009) Over-expression of cathepsin E and trefoil factor 1 in sessile serrated adenomas of the colorectum identified by gene expression analysis. Virchows Arch 454:291–302
83. Kim K, Park U, Wang J et al (2008) Gene profiling of colonic serrated adenomas by using oligonucleotide microarray. Int J Colorectal Dis 23:569–580
84. Schmitz KJ, Hey S, Schinwald A et al (2009) Differential expression of microRNA 181b and microRNA 21 in hyperplastic polyps and sessile serrated adenomas of the colon. Virchows Arch 455:49–54
85. Tinker AV, Boussioutas A, Bowtell DD (2006) The challenges of gene expression microarrays for the study of human cancer. Cancer Cell 9:333–339

Chapter 7
Somatic Evolution in Neoplastic Progression and Cancer Prevention

Carlo C. Maley, Eva Szabo, and Brian J. Reid

Abstract Cancers develop through a process of somatic evolution. Thus, cancer prevention can be viewed as an attempt to change the selective pressures on tissues to either prevent or delay cancer onset. However, chemoprevention efforts have met with mixed success to date. Most of the cancer prevention trials that have failed have been in high risk patients that are either late in progression or have had chronic mutagenic exposures like cigarette smoke. We hypothesize that some of these trials fail because they select for clones that are resistant to the intervention and actually benefit those clones by suppressing their competitors. The evolutionary understanding of neoplastic progression leads to a variety of predictions and prescriptions for cancer prevention: We should be measuring the selective impact of our interventions in order to discover and manage the evolution of resistance. Pre-clinical models with extensive intratumor genetic heterogeneity should be developed to better predict clinical outcomes. Resistance is less likely to develop prior to the evolution of genetic and epigenetic instability. We should develop measures of the dynamics of somatic evolution so that we can develop interventions to slow the process of neoplastic progression. Multidrug cancer prevention cocktails should be developed that require multiple alterations in order for cells to become resistant to the cocktail. Finally, we should develop cancer prevention interventions with the goal of preventing, channeling or managing somatic evolution. Because somatic evolution is at the heart of neoplastic progression, it must be at the heart of how we manage the disease.

C.C. Maley (✉)
Molecular and Cellular Oncogenesis Program, The Wistar Institute, 3600 Spruce St, Philadelphia, PA 19104, USA
e-mail: cmaley@alum.mit.edu

R.C. Fitzgerald (ed.), *Pre-Invasive Disease: Pathogenesis and Clinical Management*, DOI 10.1007/978-1-4419-6694-0_7,

Evolution and the Challenges of Cancer

Somatic cells in our bodies evolve by natural selection long before the emergence of malignancy [1, 2]. Somatic cells acquire epigenetic alterations as well as genetic lesions (point mutations, copy number changes, translocations and loss of heterozygosity) that they pass on to their daughter cells upon division. Some of those heritable changes affect the fitness (proliferation and survival) of the clones and so there is natural selection in our somatic tissues. In fact, all of the hallmarks of cancer [3] are phenotypes that increase the fitness of a mutant clone over competitor clones lacking the phenotype. Thus, natural selection drives neoplastic progression. Cancer prevention is properly seen to be an attempt to intervene in this evolutionary process, either through applying new selective pressures to the somatic cells or by slowing the evolutionary process. But does cancer prevention, like cancer therapy, select for resistant clones, and if so, how can we improve cancer prevention efforts?

Therapeutic Resistance and the Rationale for Cancer Prevention

Cancer survival rates have changed little over the last 30 years, despite intense efforts to develop cancer therapies [4, 5]. Many therapies only extend life by a matter of months until a resistant clone emerges, apparently deriving from resistant cells present in the neoplasm before therapy [6, 7]. In fact, resistance to interventions has plagued cancer therapy efforts since their inception [8]. In a tumor composed of billions of cells, harboring hundreds to thousands of mutations [9–11], it is no longer surprising that some of those mutant cells will be resistant to an intervention. Relapse is then a matter of selection at the cellular level. Resistance to an intervention provides an enormous survival advantage to the resistant clone. The somatic evolution of neoplastic clones is thus central to our difficulties in curing cancer.

The response to the challenges of eradicating this evolving disease has taken one of three forms. First, combining multiple drugs in a cocktail to reduce the probability of a resistant cell clearly works better than single drug therapies [12, 13], though it can lead to increased toxicity and it has not led to the breakthroughs in the common epithelial cancers that it has in HIV [14]. Second, early detection of cancer may allow for surgical removal of the neoplasm as well as reduce the number of cells in the neoplasm at time of therapy and thereby reduce the probability that the neoplasm contains a resistant clone. Third, treatment of preinvasive conditions (in other words, cancer prevention) is implicitly based on the belief that fewer mutations will have accumulated in pre-malignant tissue and so it will be less likely to contain a resistant clone compared to a malignant neoplasm.

The Nature of Neoplastic Progression

We now know that cancer arises in the context of a variety of lesions in proto-oncogenes and tumor suppressor genes and that neoplasms accumulate large numbers of genetic and epigenetic alterations (hereafter referred to as (epi)genetic alterations), but how can they do so in the short span of a human life? Loeb recognized that the probability of a cell accumulating even a handful of independent mutations necessary and sufficient for cancer was vanishingly small [15, 16]. There are two solutions to Loeb's paradox. First, the mutator hypothesis posits that the mutation rate (or rate of (epi)genetic alterations) in pre-malignant tissue may be dramatically elevated, compared to normal somatic mutation rates. There are several potential types of increased mutation rate, including chromosome instability, microsatellite instability, point mutations and epigenetic mutations. There is strong support for the presence of chromosome instability, which has been defined as an increased rate of gain or loss of whole chromosomes or large regions of chromosomes, and which develops early in colonic neoplastic progression as well as other cancers [17]. Microsatellite instability is a second, well established type of genomic instability [17]. Second, the mutations are not independent. If a mutation gives a clone a fitness advantage over other cells in and around a neoplasm, then that clone will expand, potentially to billions of cells. Again, this dramatically increases the chance of accumulating more mutations in that clone [18, 19].

The two solutions to Loeb's paradox are not mutually exclusive, and in fact, mirror the main ingredients necessary to generate natural selection: if there is heritable variation in the population, and some of that variation causes differences in relative fitness between cells, then natural selection will ensue. As a case in point, we found that the clonal expansion of a genetically unstable clone in Barrett's esophagus predicted progression to malignancy [20].

Heterogeneity in Neoplasms

There is extensive evidence for heterogeneity in the phenotypes, genotypes and epigenotypes within neoplasms and pre-malignant tissues. To the extent that the phenotypic heterogeneity is encoded by genetic and epigenetic differences between cells, that heterogeneity will be subject to natural selection. Thus, one of the fundamental questions in the study of epigenetics in cancer biology is whether the daughter cells inherit the parental cell's epigenetic state upon cell division. This is clearly true for methylation of CpG sites, due to the activity of methyltransferases. The low fidelity of epigenetic inheritance (high epigenetic mutation rate), relative to genetic mutation rates, suggests that much of the early dynamics of neoplastic progression may be driven by natural selection on epigenetic traits. However, this remains to be shown, and chromosome instability has also been reported early in progression [17].

Epigenetic heterogeneity within neoplasms has been demonstrated for specific loci in the genome. Shibata and Tavaré used such heterogeneity to infer an early clonal expansion followed by long term coexistance of clones in colon cancer [21]. Varley et al. demonstrated the presence of sub-clonal structure in endometrial neoplasms, based on the methylation state at the promoter of a DNA mismatch repair gene, MLH1 [22]. As this case shows, aberrant methylation can silence genes involved in genome maintenance, and so the generation of epigenetic heterogeneity is likely to lead to genetic heterogeneity in some cases.

Genetic heterogeneity has been demonstrated by almost every form of genetic assay used on a neoplasm. The earliest work used cytogenetics to detect different patterns of translocations and chromosomal alterations in hematopoietic neoplasms [23–28]. Because these neoplasms could be tracked longitudinally, investigators were able to observe the evolution of sub-clones, as a cytogenetically defined clone acquired new chromosomal alterations. This early work led to Nowell's original description of cancer as an evolutionary process [29]. Later investigators found a diversity of clones in neoplasms based on modern forms of cytogenetics (spectral karyotyping} [30], sequence mutations [31], microsatellite mutations [32–34], loss of heterozygosity (LOH) [35], copy number alterations in both single cells, by fluorescent in situ hybridization (FISH) [36], and in larger samples, by comparative genomic hybridization [37].

Evolution in Stem Cells

Most epithelial tissues are organized into a hierarchy of differentiation with tissue specific stem cells, transient amplifying cells, and fully differentiated cells. It is important to note that tissues can only accumulate somatic alterations over the long term if those alterations happen in self-renewing cells [38]. If the phenotypic heterogeneity observed in neoplasms and pre-malignant tissues is only a matter of different stages of differentiation, and the self-renewing cells are genetically and epigenetically homogeneous, then natural selection cannot occur in that tissue. Since self-renewal is a distinguishing characteristic of stem cells, this means that all of the heterogeneity relevant to neoplastic progression is the heterogeneity within the stem cells and any other cells that have acquired the abnormal ability to self-renew. For natural selection to occur, and for a neoplasm to progress, there must be heterogeneity within the self-renewing cell population.

Natural Selection in Neoplasms

Natural selection does occur in neoplasms and pre-malignant tissues. The signature of natural selection is a clonal expansion. Clonal expansions have been detected in the presence of the same point mutation, or loss of the same set of alleles across a region of a chromosome, in so many samples from a tissue that the pattern cannot be explained by chance (convergent evolution) [39, 40]. While there may be selection for inactivation of a gene that might cause convergent evolution in independent cells, the particular basepair that gets mutated, or the exact break points for a copy number alteration, are essentially arbitrary and they are extremely unlikely to be replicated in independent genetic lesions. Clonal expansions can also be detected by shared neutral genetic lesions that have no effect on fitness [39] and so should not be the subject of convergent evolution. In some cases, the clonal expansions can be quite small [41], but in other cases they can be extremely large, filling an entire lung [40, 42], covering the surface of a bladder [43, 44], or spreading across as many as 16 cm in the esophagus [39].

The rate of clonal expansion depends on the relative fitness differential between a clone and its competitors. In most of the cases where a clonal expansion has been documented, it has been associated with a lesion in TP53 (p53) or CDKN2A (p16). TP53 and CDKN2A are two of the most commonly lost tumor suppressor genes, and as cell cycle check points, there is good reason to believe that loss of those genes would give a clone a proliferative and/or survival advantage. However, the relative fitness of those clones have not yet been measured *in vivo*, and the exact fitness effects of their loss will depend on the microenvironment of the clones. By the same token, we should be able to manipulate the relative fitness of clones by manipulating the microenvironment. By reducing the fitness benefits of (epi)genetic lesions in neoplastic cells, or increasing the relative fitness of normal cells or benign clones [45], we should be able to slow progression and delay or prevent the onset of cancer.

Artificial Selection in Neoplasms

Cancer therapy and chemoprevention are forms of artificial selection on the neoplastic cell population. They are attempts to reduce the relative fitness of neoplastic cells in relation to normal cells. Most therapies generate a large fitness differential between sensitive cells and resistant cells, and thus select for therapeutic resistance. In most cases, therapy has been found to select for alterations in the gene target that make the neoplastic cells resistant to the agent. For example, 5-flurouracil and methotrexate select for gene amplification of their targets, TYMS and DHFR respectively [46–51]. Targetted therapies such as imatinib (Gleevec) and gefitinib select for point mutations in their targets, BCR-ABL and EGFR [52–55]. By studying longitudinal samples of chronic myeloid leukemia (CML) patients, investigators have been able to make rapid progress in both determining the mechanism of therapeutic resistance [6, 52], and in developing second line therapies, such as dasatinib, that are effective against imatinib-resistant CML [55]. Further work has shown that these second line therapies select for additional mutations that make the CML resistant to dasatinib [55].

The presence of (epi)genetic heterogeneity within pre-malignant tissues implies that cancer prevention interventions will also select for clones resistant to the intervention. However, to our knowledge, no one to date has studied the selective effects of cancer prevention agents on the (epi)genetics of the pre-malignant cells in order to determine why those interventions might fail.

Evolution and Cancer Prevention

When we change the microenvironment of a neoplasm or its precursor, as we do with any intervention, we change the selective pressures on those somatic cells. The goal of such interventions can be seen as an attempt to decrease the fitness of neoplastic cells, relative to normal or more benign cells, or to slow the process of somatic evolution. Unfortunately, to date, cancer prevention has not been informed by evolutionary biology, so the change of relative fitness of neoplastic and normal cells *in vivo* under a prevention intervention has not yet been measured.

Progress to date in cancer prevention has been mixed. There have been notable successes in breast and colon cancer, and notable failures in lung cancer, along with many non-significant results.

There are many reasons a cancer prevention trial might fail, most of them shared with any clinical trial. The study may not have adequate power to detect a significant effect; adequate controls for comparison might not have been included; the participants may not have been randomly assigned to the different conditions or sampling bias may have crept in due to exclusion/inclusion criteria; biological heterogeneity among participants may obscure effects in subgroups of the cohort; the chosen dose may not be optimal for prevention or the intervention may take longer to act than the time frame of the intervention. Finally, the intervention under study may be ineffective. This final concern has led to calls for more studies of cancer preventive agents in pre-clinical models to determine the mechanism of action and for early phase clinical trials to optimize agent delivery and to determine preliminary efficacy prior to engaging in large definitive efficacy phase III clinical trials. We propose that a prevention trial may fail due to an evolutionary mechanism, and actually accelerate the development of cancer, even when none of these previous conditions are met.

We hypothesize that a chemopreventive agent may increase the incidence of cancer when a neoplasm is composed of both benign, susceptible clones and at least one relatively resistant clone. In such a situation, the application of a chemopreventive agent will give a competitive advantage to the resistant clone by inhibiting or eliminating its competitor clones. Evolutionary theory predicts that neoplasms late in progression and those chronically exposed to mutagens are more likely to harbor resistant clones than neoplasms early in progression due to the development of genetic instability, an accumulation of mutations, and the presence of clonal heterogeneity [56]. Of note, this hypothesis predicts that an intervention may be successful at preventing cancer in early neoplasms before the development of extensive (epi)genetic heterogeneity, yet fail or even accelerate progress at a later stage when heterogeneity generates clonal competition. The hypothesis also predicts that the negative effects of the intervention may persist after the intervention is stopped if a new dominant aggressive clone has emerged as a result of the intervention. We therefore hypothesize that chemoprevention will tend to be more successful before the development of extensive clonal heterogeneity.

Interventions That Inadvertently Increased Cancer Incidence

Some of the most striking results in cancer prevention have been cases where a promising agent was shown to increase the incidence of cancer. In most cases, the cause of this increase remains unknown.

Beta-Carotene

Low levels of beta-carotene in serum and plasma were consistently associated with development of lung cancer [57–60]. Further, beta-carotene's protective effects were supported by results in experimental models [61, 62]. On the basis of this evidence, two prospective lung cancer prevention trials were initiated. Contrary to expectation, beta-carotene increased the risk of developing lung cancer by as much as 28% as well as increasing all cause mortality [63, 64]. The effect was worse in consumers of tobacco and alcohol [63, 64]. A similar trial evaluating the use of beta-carotene to prevent recurrence of colorectal adenomas found a protective effect in participants that neither smoked nor drank, though again, there were indications that it might exacerbate adenoma risk in tobacco and alcohol users [65]. These combined data suggest that the interaction of smoking and beta-carotene is responsible for enhanced carcinogenesis potentially in multiple organ sites, an effect that could not be easily ascertained by epidemiologic studies.

Retinoids

Retinoids, including Vitamin A and its derivatives, have shown promise as chemopreventive agents [66, 67]. Isotretinoin (13-*cis*-retinoic acid) was found to reverse oral premalignant lesions and prevented second primary tumors in the head and neck in initial studies [68–71]. Since head and neck cancer and the majority of lung cancer share a common pathogenesis related to tobacco exposure, it was hypothesized that isotretinoin could be effective in preventing lung cancer as well [66]. Unfortunately, isotretinoin had no significant preventive effect when compared to placebo in a phase III definitive efficacy clinical trial. However, smokers were significantly more likely to have recurrence of non-small cell lung cancer than nonsmokers when treated with isotretinoin [72].

For another retinoid, all-*trans*-retinoic acid, phase I and II trials showed a positive effect of the drug on cervical interepithelial neoplasia [73]. A phase III trial followed these results and found that application of all-*trans*-retinoic acid led to complete regression in 43% of women with moderate cervical dysplasia compared to 27% ($P<0.05$) in the placebo group. However, all-*trans*-retinoic acid had no significant effect on women with severe cervical dysplasia when compared to the placebo group [74]. Reduced efficacy of all-*trans*-retinoic acid in severe cervical dysplasia compared to moderate cervical dysplasia was also found in a more recent randomized, placebo controlled trial [75].

Use of fenretinide, a synthetic retinoid, to prevent second primary breast cancers initially resulted in no over-all effect, but secondary analyses and 15 years of follow-up revealed a 38% reduction in breast cancers in pre-menopausal women but (not quite statistically significant) evidence of a 23% increased risk of breast cancer in post-menopausal women ($n=867$, RR=1.23, 95% CI, 0.63–2.40). The younger the woman, the greater the protective effect [76].

Risk–Benefit Balance in Cancer Prevention

All health care interventions require an assessment of the balance between the potential benefits of treating the disease process and the potential risks and side effects from the intervention. Cancer prevention trials are further complicated by the fact that in the absence of the intervention, only a fraction of the participants will progress to cancer. In addition, the nature of neoplastic progression may well require chemoprevention applied over long periods of time, perhaps indefinitely. Thus, the risks associated with the intervention must be properly balanced with the risk of progressing to cancer. Cancer prevention trials therefore need to assess all cause mortality and morbidity from non-cancer diseases to account for the risks incurred by the intervention as well as any reduced risk of cancer. This issue was highlighted by the results from colorectal cancer trials showing that the cyclooxygenase-2 (COX-2) inhibitors rofecoxib and celecoxib increase cardiovascular disease occurrence despite significant efficacy in reducing colorectal adenoma recurrence [77, 78]. The routine use of these agents for colorectal cancer prevention is therefore not recommended.

Unfortunately, the early stages of progression that our theory predicts will be the most likely to respond to a cancer prevention intervention, are the stages with the smallest probability of progressing to cancer during the lifetime of the participant, and thus require the most stringent safety criteria for our interventions and much larger cohorts to detect an effect on cancer/mortality outcome. There are at least three approaches to this problem. First, we may intervene at early stages but focus on dietary or drug interventions that have been shown to have minimal risks. Second, we may focus on cohorts with a high risk of progressing to cancer that is not based on increased genetic instability. Some genetic predispositions, such as inactivation of Rb, may provide useful cancer prevention cohorts. Third, we may focus on high risk groups where the safety criteria are less stringent, but take steps to address the likely problem of resistance, such as using multi-drug cocktails [79–81], adding drugs that specifically target the common resistance phenotypes (e.g., dasatinib for imatinib resistant CML (55), or targeting the ATP-binding cassette transporters [82]), or boosting the fitness of benign cells in and around the neoplasm [45].

Making Progress in Cancer Prevention

The challenges of cancer prevention are well illustrated by the previously discussed trials. Most of them were preceded by promising pre-clinical evidence and, often, observational studies in humans. They serve as a reminder of the importance of testing promising agents in randomized, double-blind, placebo controlled trials. They also serve as a reminder of the importance of following participants to a cancer endpoint and measuring morbidity and mortality from other disease processes, to account for interventions that may cause more harm than good in participants, many of whom would never have developed cancer even in the absence of the intervention. All of these recommendations are standard in the field of cancer prevention. However, the evolutionary theory of cancer provides further guidance for the development of cancer prevention strategies.

Longitudinal Surveillance

The first recommendation is simply to take longitudinal tissue samples before, during and after the trial. Though not every trial will result in an intervention that can reduce cancer burden, every trial should be designed so that if it fails, it should be possible to discover the reason for failure. In order to study our impact on somatic evolution, we need to be able to survey the genetics and epigenetics of the tissue prior to the intervention and compare that to the population of cells that survive the intervention, as has been done in CML [55]. Additional assays may reveal the phenotypic and (epi)genetic characteristics of participants and their neoplasms that do not even initially respond to the intervention.

Identify (Epi)Genetic Causes of Resistance and Test for Them Prior to Intervention

By comparing the epigenetics and genetics of the cell population prior to therapy and at the end of the trial, it is possible to discover the cause of acquired resistance [54, 55]. Once those (epi)genetic lesions are identified, they should be used as biomarkers prior to intervention, to predict who is likely to benefit from a cancer preventive intervention.

Develop Markers for the Forms of (Epi)Genetic Instability That Tend to Generate Resistance to the Intervention

There are many types and manifestations of genomic instability including chromosome instability with large scale copy number alterations, and loss of heterozygosity, microsatellite instability, point mutations, small insertions and deletions, translocations, as well as epigenetic alterations such as hypo- and hypermethylation of gene promoters. Most of these have been implicated in some form of acquired therapeutic resistance [46, 53, 55, 83, 84]. The results of experiments to identify the cause of resistance should lead to assays not only for the resistance lesion itself, but also for the type of instability that may be easier to detect throughout a neoplasm than a very rare clone with the specific resistance lesion. Once we have measures for the degree of the relevant form of instability, then we can begin developing interventions to reduce that instability as alternate or adjuvant forms of cancer prevention. This would be a fundamentally different approach to cancer prevention than targeting a specific gene implicated as a driver of clonal expansions in progression.

Intervene Prior to Genomic Instability

There is a trade-off between intervening early, when the likelihood of a resistant clone having evolved is minimized, versus intervening in high risk individuals who are most likely to progress to cancer and thus stand to benefit from an intervention. Ideally we would intervene before initiation [85], as in the case of oncogenic virus vaccines [86, 87]. Failing that, evolutionary theory suggests that we should try to intervene in high risk individuals prior to the evolution of genomic instability, if possible. This may require the development of assays to detect such high risk individuals prior to genomic instability and the refinement of assays to detect genomic instability itself.

Test for Differential Effects on Low and High Risk Patients

The essence of our hypothesis is that high risk patients are likely to have more genetic diversity within their tissues and thus are more likely to harbor resistance mutations than low risk patients. Therefore, early trials of a cancer prevention intervention should include the full spectrum of the disease and be powered to detect differential effects on low versus high risk patients. In the ideal setting, separate trials would be designed for different risk groups, using interventions specifically tailored to each group.

Use Pre-clinical Models with Extensive Intratumor Genetic Heterogeneity

We predict that one reason promising pre-clinical results often do not translate into clinical benefit is that the pre-clinical models do not capture the intratumor genetic heterogeneity of a spontaneous human neoplasm. Thus, the pre-clinical models fail to predict the kind of resistance that evolves in the human trials. Better pre-clinical models would include extensive genetic and/or epigenetic heterogeneity within each neoplasm so that we can identify agents that are likely to work even in the face of that heterogeneity and we can also discover the mechanisms of acquired resistance even before an agent is tested in humans. While there is a role for genetically homogeneous pre-clinical models in the development of an agent, because they are more likely to produce reproducible results, it may be a mistake to move an agent into clinical trials until the nature and likelihood of resistance is understood.

Measure the Dynamics of Evolution and Develop Interventions That Slow Evolution

A general principle in both science and engineering is that it is difficult to control a system if you cannot measure it. Evolutionary theory suggests that a particularly effective form of cancer prevention would be to slow the process of somatic evolution (Fig. 7.1). The rate of evolution is determined by four parameters:

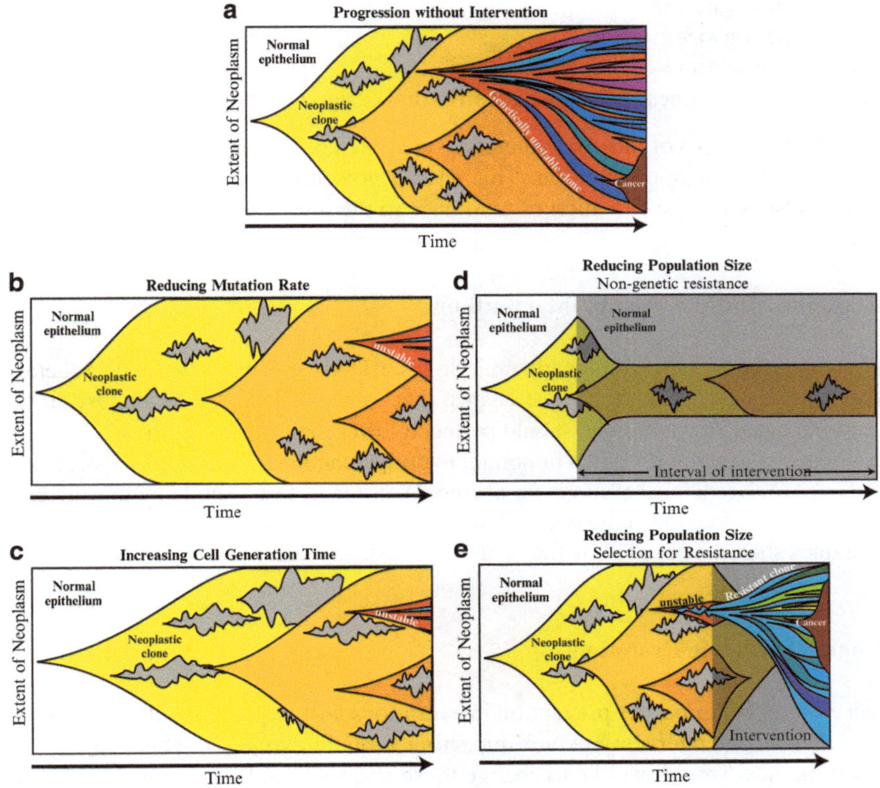

Fig. 7.1 A potential strategy for cancer prevention would be to slow the dynamics of somatic evolution. A mutation or epigenetic change can arise in normal epithelium. If it is selected, it will undergo clonal expansion ("neoplastic clone" in the figure). Additional mutations may be neutral (*gray clones*) or selectively advantageous and undergo further expansion. Expansion of a genetically unstable clone can produce many variants (*red and blue shaded clonal expansions*) that increase the risk of progression to cancer (*maroon*). (**a**) In the absence of an intervention, some individuals may progress to cancer. (**b**) If the mutation rate could be slowed, new clones would arise less frequently and the onset of cancer should be delayed substantially, perhaps for the lifespan of the individual. (**c**) If the generation time of the self-renewing cells in a neoplasm could be increased, both the mutation rate and the rate of clonal expansion would be reduced, thereby leading to risk reduction by substantially delaying the onset of cancer. (**d**) Most interventions (interval in gray) are designed to reduce the cell population size of a neoplasm. This should also be effective because it reduces the number of cells that can acquire new mutations and so effectively reduces the mutation rate. Neoplastic cells may remain if they are in locations inaccessible to the intervention (a form of non-genetic resistance). (**e**) An intervention may select for a resistant clone, which might be evolutionarily neutral in the absence of the intervention, but have a selective advantage in the presence of the intervention (*light blue*). Because an intervention suppresses competitor clones, and resistant clones are more likely to be generated by a genetically unstable clone, an intervention could, paradoxically, increase the rate of progression to cancer

(1) Mutation rate
(2) Population size
(3) Generation time
(4) The relative fitness effects of adaptive (epi)genetic lesions

If we had measures of those parameters *in vivo*, we could begin to develop interventions to slow somatic evolution. This should not only delay cancer onset, but it should also delay the evolution of resistance to the intervention.

Combine Multiple Agents/Interventions

The same logic that recommends multidrug cocktails in cancer (and HIV) therapy applies to cancer prevention. The chance that a neoplastic cell will be resistant to multiple agents/interventions should be much lower than the chance it will be resistant to a single agent [81]. It is important to design combination therapies that require different (epi)genetic alterations for acquired resistance, lest a single multidrug resistance lesion render the entire cocktail ineffective. Thus, the development of multidrug therapies should be guided by the nature of resistance likely to evolve to each agent.

Channel Somatic Evolution

Developing better cancer prevention interventions will require a better understanding of how our interventions are impacting somatic evolution. This leads to the question, how would we like to change those pressures and what would we like to select for? One potential answer is that we would like to select for benign cells, a strategy we have called benign cell boosters [45]. Alternatively, we could look for agents that select for quiescent or genetically stable cells, or perhaps cells that are easy to target with other agents (a.k.a., "the sucker's gambit") [45].

Conclusions

Neoplastic progression is fundamentally a somatic evolutionary process, and so cancer prevention is an exercise in controlling that evolution. Some of the failures of cancer prevention trials have led to calls for increased attention to the molecular mechanisms action for a proposed agent [88]. We also call for increased attention to the evolutionary mechanism of action. How does the intervention impact the population (epi)genetics of cells in and around a neoplasm?

It is no accident that the results for cancer prevention trials have mimicked the results for chemotherapy. The characteristics that make cancer hard to cure, the genetic instability and clonal evolution, arise long before the neoplasm becomes malignant. Our therapies tend to work on early stage cancers, when they can still be surgically removed, or relatively homogeneous cancers like childhood leukemia [89–91], which are less likely to harbor resistant clones. Similarly, we hypothesize that non-surgical interventions for pre-malignant neoplasms are less likely to work for neoplasms late in progression or chronically exposed to mutagens, like cigarette smoke, relative to neoplasms early in progression, because of the evolution of resistant clones. In particular, we suggest that the application of chemopreventive agents may actually increase the risk of cancer in some cases by biasing the clonal evolution within a neoplasm in favor of resistant, and likely genetically unstable clones.

There are many plausible reasons that one can find to explain the failure of any particular trial. The fact that in most cases we do not know why a cancer prevention trial did not succeed highlights the need to collect longitudinal tissue samples during trials. These repositories should be made available to the community to help determine how our interventions impact the evolution of neoplastic clones and potentially select for resistance.

Failures in cancer prevention trials do not imply that cancer prevention efforts should be abandoned. On the contrary, the original rationale for cancer prevention, that intervening early in progression should prove more efficacious than intervening in advanced stages of disease, is as strong as ever. It is our hope that a better understanding of the difficulties in cancer prevention efforts will help to guide and facilitate future trials. For example, careful identification of markers of (epi)genetic instability or the presence of an (epi)genetic lesion associated with resistance at baseline may help to focus efforts on subjects likely to benefit from a particular intervention. Accrual in chemoprevention trials may be facilitated if prospective participants may be enrolled in separate high risk and low risk cohorts, with the low risk cohorts followed to intermediate endpoints, ideally using valid measures of somatic evolution.

Attempts to influence the process of somatic evolution for cancer prevention may take the form of preventing the process from starting in the first place, by preventing initiation, or changing the selective pressures on the somatic cells through the introduction of an agent that changes the microenvironment of the cells. By focusing on our impact of our interventions on somatic evolution, we should be able to improve efforts in cancer prevention.

Acknowledgements We would like to thank Tom Paulson, Ernie Hawk, Rick Klausner, John Potter, Peter Nelson and Catherine Tangen for helpful discussions and advice. This work was supported by Commonwealth Universal Research Enhancement Program, Pennsylvania Department of Health, the Pew Charitable Trust, a McLean Contributionship, the Landon AACR Innovator Award for Cancer Prevention, and NIH grants R03 CA137811, P01 CA91955, P30 CA010815, R01 CA119224 and R01 CA140657.

References

1. Merlo LM, Pepper JW, Reid BJ, Maley CC (2006) Cancer as an evolutionary and ecological process. Nat Rev Cancer 6:924–935
2. Pepper J, Scott Findlay C, Kassen R, Spencer S, Maley C (2009) Cancer research meets evolutionary biology. Evol Appl 2:62–70

3. Hanahan D, Weinberg RA (2000) The hallmarks of cancer. Cell 100:57–70
4. Jemal A, Siegel R, Ward E, Murray T, Xu J, Thun MJ (2007) Cancer statistics, 2007. CA Cancer J Clin 57:43–66
5. Etzioni R, Urban N, Ramsey S et al (2003) The case for early detection. Nat Rev Cancer 3:1–10
6. Roche-Lestienne C, Preudhomme C (2003) Mutations in the ABL kinase domain pre-exist the onset of imatinib treatment. Semin Hematol 40:80–82
7. Mullighan CG, Phillips LA, Su X et al (2008) Genomic analysis of the clonal origins of relapsed acute lymphoblastic leukemia. Science 322:1377–1380
8. Chabner BA, Roberts TG Jr (2005) Timeline: chemotherapy and the war on cancer. Nat Rev Cancer 5:65–72
9. Stoler DL, Chen N, Basik M et al (1999) The onset and extent of genomic instability in sporadic colorectal tumor progression. Proc Natl Acad Sci U S A 96:15121–15126
10. Bielas JH, Loeb KR, Rubin BP, True LD, Loeb LA (2006) Human cancers express a mutator phenotype. Proc Natl Acad Sci U S A 103:18238–18242
11. Mardis ER, Ding L, Dooling DJ et al (2009) Recurring mutations found by sequencing an acute myeloid leukemia genome. N Engl J Med 361:1058–1066
12. Carrick S, Parker S, Thornton CE, Ghersi D, Simes J, Wilcken N. Single agent versus combination chemotherapy for metastatic breast cancer. Cochrane Database of Systematic Reviews 2009, Issue 2. Art. No.: CD003372. DOI: 10.1002/14651858.CD003372.pub3.
13. Delbaldo C, Michiels S, Syz N, Soria JC, Le Chevalier T, Pignon JP (2004) Benefits of adding a drug to a single-agent or a 2-agent chemotherapy regimen in advanced non-small-cell lung cancer: a meta-analysis. JAMA 292:470–484
14. The CASCADE Collaboration. Concerted Action on SeroConversion to AIDS and Death in Europe (2000). Survival after introduction of HAART in people with known duration of HIV-1 infection. Lancet 355:1158–1159.
15. Loeb LA (1991) Mutator phenotype may be required for multistage carcinogenesis. Cancer Res 51:3075–3079
16. Loeb LA, Springgate CF, Battula N (1974) Errors in DNA replication as a basis of malignant changes. Cancer Res 34:2311–2321
17. Rajagopalan H, Nowak MA, Vogelstein B, Lengauer C (2003) The significance of unstable chromosomes in colorectal cancer. Nat Rev Cancer 3:695–701
18. Luebeck EG, Moolgavkar SH (2002) Multistage carcinogenesis and the incidence of colorectal cancer. Proc Natl Acad Sci U S A 99:15095–15100
19. Tomlinson I, Bodmer W (1999) Selection, the mutation rate and cancer: ensuring that the tail does not wag the dog. Nat Med 5:11–12
20. Maley CC, Galipeau PC, Li X et al (2004) The combination of genetic instability and clonal expansion predicts progression to esophageal adenocarcinoma. Cancer Res 64:7629–7633
21. Siegmund KD, Marjoram P, Woo YJ, Tavare S, Shibata D (2009) Inferring clonal expansion and cancer stem cell dynamics from DNA methylation patterns in colorectal cancers. Proc Natl Acad Sci U S A 106:4828–4833
22. Varley KE, Mutch DG, Edmonston TB, Goodfellow PJ, Mitra RD (2009) Intra-tumor heterogeneity of MLH1 promoter methylation revealed by deep single molecule bisulfite sequencing. Nucleic Acids Res 37:4603–4612
23. de Grouchy J, de Nava C, Cantu JM, Bilski-Pasquier G, Bousser J (1966) Models for clonal evolutions: a study of chronic myelogenous leukemia. Am J Hum Genet 18:485–503
24. de Grouchy J, de Nava C (1968) A chromosomal theory of carcinogenesis. Ann Intern Med 69:381–391
25. Ford CE, Clarke CM (1963) Cytogenetic evidence of clonal proliferation in primary reticular neoplasms. Can Cancer Conf 5:129–146
26. Dawe CJ (1969) Phylogeny and oncogeny. Natl Cancer Inst Monogr 31:1–40
27. Yosida TH (1966) Relation between chromosomal alteration and development of tumors. Jpn J Genet 41:439–451
28. Hauschka TS (1961) The chromosomes in ontogeny and oncogeny. Cancer Res 21:957–974

29. Nowell PC (1976) The clonal evolution of tumor cell populations. Science 194:23–28
30. Heng HH, Stevens JB, Liu G et al (2006) Stochastic cancer progression driven by non-clonal chromosome aberrations. J Cell Physiol 208:461–472
31. Gonzalez-Garcia I, Sole RV, Costa J (2002) Metapopulation dynamics and spatial heterogeneity in cancer. Proc Natl Acad Sci U S A 99:13085–13089
32. Shibata D, Navidi W, Salovaara R, Li ZH, Aaltonen LA (1996) Somatic microsatellite mutations as molecular tumor clocks. Nat Med 2:676–681
33. Tsao JL, Tavare S, Salovaara R, Jass JR, Aaltonen LA, Shibata D (1999) Colorectal adenoma and cancer divergence. Evidence of multilineage progression. Am J Pathol 154:1815–1824
34. Tsao JL, Yatabe Y, Salovaara R et al (2000) Genetic reconstruction of individual colorectal tumor histories. Proc Natl Acad Sci U S A 97:1236–1241
35. Maley CC, Galipeau PC, Finley JC et al (2006) Genetic clonal diversity predicts progression to esophageal adenocarcinoma. Nat Genet 38:468–473
36. Murphy DS, Hoare SF, Going JJ et al (1995) Characterization of extensive genetic alterations in ductal carcinoma in situ by fluorescence in situ hybridization and molecular analysis. J Natl Cancer Inst 87:1694–1704
37. Harada T, Okita K, Shiraishi K, Kusano N, Kondoh S, Sasaki K (2002) Interglandular cytogenetic heterogeneity detected by comparative genomic hybridization in pancreatic cancer. Cancer Res 62:835–839
38. Cairns J (1975) Mutation selection and the natural history of cancer. Nature 255:197–200
39. Maley CC, Galipeau PC, Li X, Sanchez CA, Paulson TG, Reid BJ (2004) Selectively advantageous mutations and hitchhikers in neoplasms: p16 lesions are selected in Barrett's esophagus. Cancer Res 64:3414–3427
40. Franklin WA, Gazdar AF, Haney J et al (1997) Widely dispersed p53 mutation in respiratory epithelium. A novel mechanism for field carcinogenesis. J Clin Invest 100:2133–2137
41. Park IW, Wistuba II, Maitra A et al (1999) Multiple clonal abnormalities in the bronchial epithelium of patients with lung cancer. J Natl Cancer Inst 91:1863–1868
42. Dasgupta S, Yung RC, Westra WH, Rini DA, Brandes J, Sidransky D (2009) Following mitochondrial footprints through a long mucosal path to lung cancer. PLoS ONE 4:e6533
43. Czerniak B, Chaturvedi V, Li L et al (1999) Superimposed histologic and genetic mapping of chromosome 9 in progression of human urinary bladder neoplasia: implications for a genetic model of multistep urothelial carcinogenesis and early detection of urinary bladder cancer. Oncogene 18:1185–1196
44. Czerniak B, Li L, Chaturvedi V et al (2000) Genetic modeling of human urinary bladder carcinogenesis. Genes Chromosom Cancer 27:392–402
45. Maley CC, Reid BJ, Forrest S (2004) Cancer prevention strategies that address the evolutionary dynamics of neoplastic cells: simulating benign cell boosters and selection for chemosensitivity. Cancer Epidemiol Biomark Prev 13:1375–1384
46. Wang TL, Diaz LA Jr, Romans K et al (2004) Digital karyotyping identifies thymidylate synthase amplification as a mechanism of resistance to 5-fluorouracil in metastatic colorectal cancer patients. Proc Natl Acad Sci U S A 101:3089–3094
47. Schimke RT (1984) Gene amplification, drug resistance, and cancer. Cancer Res 44: 1735–1742
48. Curt GA, Carney DN, Cowan KH et al (1983) Unstable methotrexate resistance in human small-cell carcinoma associated with double minute chromosomes. N Engl J Med 308: 199–202
49. Carman MD, Schornagel JH, Rivest RS et al (1984) Resistance to methotrexate due to gene amplification in a patient with acute leukemia. J Clin Oncol 2:16–20
50. Horns RC Jr, Dower WJ, Schimke RT (1984) Gene amplification in a leukemic patient treated with methotrexate. J Clin Oncol 2:2–7
51. Trent JM, Buick RN, Olson S, Horns RC Jr, Schimke RT (1984) Cytologic evidence for gene amplification in methotrexate-resistant cells obtained from a patient with ovarian adenocarcinoma. J Clin Oncol 2:8–15

52. Gorre ME, Sawyers CL (2002) Molecular mechanisms of resistance to STI571 in chronic myeloid leukemia. Curr Opin Hematol 9:303–307
53. Engelman JA, Zejnullahu K, Mitsudomi T et al (2007) MET amplification leads to gefitinib resistance in lung cancer by activating ERBB3 signaling. Science 316:1039–1043
54. Azam M, Latek RR, Daley GQ (2003) Mechanisms of autoinhibition and STI-571/imatinib resistance revealed by mutagenesis of BCR-ABL. Cell 112:831–843
55. Shah NP, Skaggs BJ, Branford S et al (2007) Sequential ABL kinase inhibitor therapy selects for compound drug-resistant BCR-ABL mutations with altered oncogenic potency. J Clin Invest 117:2562–2569
56. Goldie G, Coldman A (1984) The genetic origin of drug resistance in neoplasms: implications for systemic therapy. Cancer Res 44:3643–3653
57. Ziegler RG (1989) A review of epidemiologic evidence that carotenoids reduce the risk of cancer. J Nutr 119:116–122
58. Peto R, Doll R, Buckley JD, Sporn MB (1981) Can dietary beta-carotene materially reduce human cancer rates? Nature 290:201–208
59. Dorgan JF, Schatzkin A (1991) Antioxidant micronutrients in cancer prevention. Hematol Oncol Clin N Am 5:43–68
60. Greenwald P (1993) NCI cancer prevention and control research. Prev Med 22:642–660
61. Krinsky NI (1989) Carotenoids and cancer in animal models. J Nutr 119:123–126
62. Bendich A, Olson JA (1989) Biological actions of carotenoids. FASEB J 3:1927–1932
63. Omenn GS, Goodman GE, Thornquist MD et al (1996) Effects of a combination of beta carotene and vitamin A on lung cancer and cardiovascular disease. N Engl J Med 330:1029–1035
64. Albanes D, Heinonen O, Taylor P et al (1996) Alpha-Tocopherol and beta-carotene supplements and lung cancer incidence in the alpha-tocopherol, beta-carotene cancer prevention study: effects of base-line characteristics and study compliance. J Natl Cancer Inst 88:1513–1515
65. Baron JA, Cole BF, Mott L et al (2003) Neoplastic and antineoplastic effects of beta-carotene on colorectal adenoma recurrence: results of a randomized trial. J Natl Cancer Inst 95:717–722
66. Mayne ST, Lippman SM (2005) Retinoids, carotenoids, and micronutrients. In: DeVita VT Jr, Hellman S, Rosenberg SA (eds) Cancer: principles and practice of oncology, 7th edn. Lippincott Williams & Wilkins, Philadelphia, pp 521–535
67. Okuno M, Kojima S, Matsushima-Nishiwaki R et al (2004) Retinoids in cancer chemoprevention. Curr Cancer Drug Targets 4:285–298
68. Hong WK, Endicott J, Itri LM et al (1986) 13-cis-retinoic acid in the treatment of oral leukoplakia. N Engl J Med 315:1501–1505
69. Hong WK, Lippman SM, Itri LM et al (1990) Prevention of second primary tumors with isotretinoin in squamous-cell carcinoma of the head and neck. N Engl J Med 323:795–801
70. Lippman SM, Batsakis JG, Toth BB et al (1993) Comparison of low-dose isotretinoin with beta carotene to prevent oral carcinogenesis. N Engl J Med 328:15–20
71. Vokes EE, Weichselbaum RR, Lippman SM, Hong WK (1993) Head and neck cancer. N Engl J Med 328:184–194
72. Lippman SM, Lee JJ, Karp DD et al (2001) Randomized phase III intergroup trial of isotretinoin to prevent second primary tumors in stage I non-small-cell lung cancer. J Natl Cancer Inst 93:605–618
73. Weiner SA, Surwit EA, Graham VE, Meyskens FL Jr (1986) A phase I trial of topically applied trans-retinoic acid in cervical dysplasia-clinical efficacy. Invest New Drugs 4:241–244
74. Meyskens FL Jr, Surwit E, Moon TE et al (1994) Enhancement of regression of cervical intraepithelial neoplasia II (moderate dysplasia) with topically applied all-trans-retinoic acid: a randomized trial. J Natl Cancer Inst 86:539–543
75. Ruffin MT, Bailey JM, Normolle DP et al (2004) Low-dose topical delivery of all-trans retinoic acid for cervical intraepithelial neoplasia II and III. Cancer Epidemiol Biomark Prev 13:2148–2152
76. Veronesi U, Mariani L, Decensi A et al (2006) Fifteen-year results of a randomized phase III trial of fenretinide to prevent second breast cancer. Ann Oncol 17:1065–1071
77. Bresalier RS, Sandler RS, Quan H et al (2005) Cardiovascular events associated with rofecoxib in a colorectal adenoma chemoprevention trial. N Engl J Med 352:1092–1102

78. Bertagnolli MM, Eagle CJ, Zauber AG et al (2006) Celecoxib for the prevention of sporadic colorectal adenomas. N Engl J Med 355:873–884
79. Kelloff GJ, Lippman SM, Dannenberg AJ et al (2006) Progress in chemoprevention drug development: the promise of molecular biomarkers for prevention of intraepithelial neoplasia and cancer – a plan to move forward. Clin Cancer Res 12:3661–3697
80. Potter JD (1997) beta-Carotene and the role of intervention studies. Cancer Lett 114:329–331
81. Potter J (1996) Chemoprevention: Pharmacology or biology. Oncology 10:1487–1488
82. Szakacs G, Paterson JK, Ludwig JA, Booth-Genthe C, Gottesman MM (2006) Targeting multidrug resistance in cancer. Nat Rev Drug Discov 5:219–234
83. Taplin ME, Rajeshkumar B, Halabi S et al (2003) Androgen receptor mutations in androgen-independent prostate cancer: Cancer and Leukemia Group B Study 9663. J Clin Oncol 21:2673–2678
84. Kobayashi S, Boggon TJ, Dayaram T et al (2005) EGFR mutation and resistance of non-small-cell lung cancer to gefitinib. N Engl J Med 352:786–792
85. Russo J, Mailo D, Hu YF, Balogh G, Sheriff F, Russo IH (2005) Breast differentiation and its implication in cancer prevention. Clin Cancer Res 11:931s–936s
86. The FUTURE II Study Group (2007) Quadrivalent vaccine against human papillomavirus to prevent high-grade cervical lesions. N Engl J Med 356:1915–1927
87. Paavonen J, Naud P, Salmeron J et al (2009) Efficacy of human papillomavirus (HPV)-16/18 AS04-adjuvanted vaccine against cervical infection and precancer caused by oncogenic HPV types (PATRICIA): final analysis of a double-blind, randomised study in young women. Lancet 374:301–314
88. Hong WK, Sporn MB (1997) Recent advances in chemoprevention of cancer. Science 278:1073–1077
89. DeAngelo DJ (2005) The treatment of adolescents and young adults with acute lymphoblastic leukemia. Hematology Am Soc Hematol Educ Program 2005:123–130
90. Ravindranath Y, Chang M, Steuber CP et al (2005) Pediatric Oncology Group (POG) studies of acute myeloid leukemia (AML): a review of four consecutive childhood AML trials conducted between 1981 and 2000. Leukemia 19:2101–2116
91. Radtke I, Mullighan CG, Ishii M et al (2009) Genomic analysis reveals few genetic alterations in pediatric acute myeloid leukemia. Proc Natl Acad Sci U S A 106:12944–12949

Part II
Model Systems and Clinical Approaches

Chapter 8
Precancer in Animal Models: Sequentially Acquired or Predetermined?

Robert D. Cardiff and Alexander D. Borowsky

The natural history of cancer is still not clear. The clinical starting point has been identified in precancerous intraepithelial neoplasms. We currently think of neoplastic progression as a multi-step continuum involving multiple somatic mutations. Early detection programs have had enormous effects on mortality rates of some cancers. However, some patient populations seem to elude our best treatment efforts. Studies of epithelial precancers in animal models support the notion that the biological potential of the neoplastic cells is fully encoded in the precancer. This implies that the subsequent events are primarily epigenetic and that the "code" will be better understood by examining the precancers rather than the end-stage cancer. In this review and opinion we will focus primarily on breast cancer and some of the experimental models of breast cancer because they offer the richest data sets for answering the question posed in the title: *Sequentially acquired or predetermined?* In large measure, this is the result of three critical components: (1) Longstanding efforts to stratify breast cancer and precancer for prognosis and therapy response; (2) An array of genetically engineered mouse (GEM) models of breast cancer; and (3) Experimental model systems including mouse transplantation technologies. There is emerging data which is similar, however, in other organ sites, both epithelial (prostate, pancreas, intestine) and non-epithelial (glia, lymphoid), that may lead to related conclusions [1–5].

History of Precancer

The idea that cancers emerge from pre-existing morphological change dates back to the pre-microscopic anatomical pathology era of the early nineteenth century [6]. The concept was promulgated and validated during the early era of microscopic

R.D. Cardiff (✉)
Department of Pathology and Laboratory Medicine, Center for Comparative Pathology, University of California, School of Medicine, Davis, California 95616, USA
e-mail: rdcardiff@ucdavis.edu

R.C. Fitzgerald (ed.), *Pre-Invasive Disease: Pathogenesis and Clinical Management*, DOI 10.1007/978-1-4419-6694-0_8, © Springer Science+Business Media, LLC 2011

pathology [7]. "Precancer", a term first used in the English literature by James Ewing [8], was recognized as a focal atypia associated with cancer in the early 1900s [9]. Eventually, cytological criteria were associated with precancer in the early twentieth century [10]. The predictive significance of cytological atypia was not fully realized until documented by Papanicolaou and Traut in the 1940s and was recommended by the American Cancer Society as a universal predictive tool in 1945. The concept and the test reduced the incidence of cervical cancer 73%, saving countless lives. This led to the universal acceptance of the "Pap" smear and other "early detection" crusades of the later twentieth century. These public health campaigns have reduced the cancer mortality from numerous epithelial neoplasms [11].

Precancerous hyperplasias were first described in the mouse in the early twentieth century [12]. As in human, the evidence was the remarkable association of cancer with multifocal atypical nodules in tumor-bearing mice [13]. Experimental carcinogenesis in the mouse and rabbit was also associated with a precursor lesion. Experimental carcinogenesis in the skin suggested a multistage progression with two steps, initiation and promotion [14] that was elegantly documented by Shubik and Berenblum [15–17]. Foulds, using the mouse mammary gland as an experimental model, wrote elegant essays and three monographs on neoplastic progression [18–21]. Other investigators found early morphological lesions in most organs of the mouse, rat and other laboratory animals [22–26]. In all cases, the focal atypias outnumbered the tumors, making it difficult to ascertain the exact relationship between them.

Foulds' monographs discuss neoplastic progression in all known animal and human tumors. These suggested a multi-stage model for every epithelial neoplasm. The multi-stage seems to be validated by epidemiological and clinical evidence of "multiple-hit" kinetics in most human cancers [27–29]. The more recent molecular analyses of colon cancer reinforced the notion that step-wise acquisition of morphological traits is associated with sequential acquisition of specific molecular lesions [30, 31]. We emerged from the twentieth century using a multi-stage, multi-step model with the sequential acquisition of genetic and morphological traits as a practical guide to neoplastic progression. The promise of the model is that treatment provided before the last "hit" in the sequence could prevent progression to the fatal disease.

Biological Predeterminism

Although the multi-stage, multi-step concept of neoplastic progression with sequential acquisition of gene alterations remains useful, it has never explained all of the natural history of cancer. For example, in 1951 Ian MacDonald was writing essays on biological predeterminism in breast and gastric cancer. MacDonald suggested that clinical outcome was more commonly determined by inherent or predetermined natural history than treatment [32–34]. Some patients seemed to start with aggressive or high mortality risk cancer phenotypes. Alternatively they may have simply progressed so quickly through a stepwise morphological continuum that many of the steps were not observable. In the current field of human breast cancer, the "triple negative" phenotype (estrogen receptor (*ER*) negative, progesterone receptor (*PR*) negative, and Her2/neu ERBB2 non-amplified) is associated with aggressive clinical progression [35]. Loss of ER/PR expression might be an acquired trait in the evolution of a breast cancer, but Her2/neu is the result of amplification of the ERBB2 genetic locus at multiple chromosomal insertion sites. Loss of this amplification seems unlikely, even if anti-ERBB2 specific antibody therapy (Traztusumab) resistance may be acquired. Meanwhile, the working clinical hypothesis in breast cancer is one of intrinsic subtypes which remain fixed, even as that subtype evolves to survive selective pressures such as anti-hormonal or anti-ERRB2 therapies. Are there similar "intrinsic subtypes" of other organ site cancers? The answer is "yes", some we have recognized by morphologic phenotype for many years, others, we are just beginning to understand. Can intrinsic subtypes evolve and adapt? Again the answer is "yes". Can the ability to adapt be predicted? This is the challenge before us, and it may involve the laws of probability as much as the biology of genetics and environment. The door is open to determining how much is programmed, how much can be manipulated, and how much is left to chance.

From select examples of cancer programmed at initiation it is not clear whether the sequential acquisition hypothesis is wrong, or if the exception "proved the rule". Following Karl Popper's famous negation rule, the hypothesis can be negated by a single example [36]. Many have come to believe that something is amiss with our concepts of multi-stage, multi-step progression with sequential acquisition but were understandably reluctant to accept the seemingly futile view of biological predeterminism [37].

The examples that have emerged have caused reexamination of the sequential acquisition hypothesis of cancer. Perhaps the best clinical example is cervical cancer. The confounding factor in human cervical cancer is the serotype of the human papilloma virus that has infected the woman's cervix years before emergence of an identifiable lesion [38]. The woman either has the HPV 16/18 serotype and progresses or she does not.

Other examples can be cited. Risk of progression in bladder cancer is more related to the p53 mutation than the cytology [39]. "Low grade" PIN is no longer considered to confer risk of prostate cancer [40]. Mathematical modeling of existing data concerning ductal carcinoma in situ (DCIS) of the breast and colorectal cancers better fit a parallel, rather than a sequential, model of neoplastic progression [41]. In vitro molecular models of human breast cancer suggest that the major changes in breast cancer occur *before* the emergence of DCIS [42]. Molecular analysis has failed to find any consistent changes associated with neoplastic progression in human DCIS to invasive breast cancer [43–46]. In other words, biological predeterminism is a viable model with molecular support.

Animal Models

The concept of biological predeterminism was developed in clinical cancer and vigorously attacked for lack of rigorous data [37]. With the lack of experimental data in humans, science has always turned to animal models. The inbred mouse has been the primary model for experimental cancer research since the early 1900s [47]. The development of the Jensen line provided the first in vivo transplantable cancer cell line in 1907, laying the foundation for experimental cancer research [47]. Many, if not all, of our concepts of neoplastic progression have been developed or tested in mouse models [48]. Precancer in animals was first documented by Apolant's hyperplastic alveolar nodules (HAN) in mice with tumors [12]. This type of "guilt-by-association" was confirmed and documented through numerous comparisons between tumor-free and tumor-prone mouse strains [49]. The virus (MMTV)-infected mice have many more "nodules" than malignancies. Surely, not all HAN advance at the same rate. This was a perplexing dilemma. Which HAN become tumors?

This problem was solved with the creation of the gland-free mammary fat pad technique. DeOme and colleagues proved by identification, isolation and transplantation that the mouse mammary HAN of Apolant and Haaland had a high risk of malignant change [23]. This technique led the way for experimental examination of individual HANs, documenting their heterogeneity and providing rigorous operational definitions of two steps of progression: nodulogenesis and tumorigenesis [50] (Fig. 8.1).

The biological potential of each nodule can be tested by transplantation (Fig. 8.1). The technique involves identifying the HAN in situ, surgically removing each nodule and transplanting them into gland-cleared mammary fat pads of syngeneic animals. The test-by-transplantation provided an operational definition of "preneoplasia" [23]. Studies in the subsequent 60 years have demonstrated that HAN are transformed, immortalized foci that can be serially transplanted and maintained in gland-cleared fat pads but, in contrast to malignancies, cannot grow in ectopic sites. These HAN transplants all are at high risk of developing malignancies at a predicable rate but each "line" has an individual, independent biology [51, 52]. Molecular analysis has shown that each HAN line is a unique clone [53–55]. These studies in the mammary gland have been recapitulated using other organ systems, establishing precancer lines in mice [56].

Fig. 8.1 (continued) in transplantation provides an operational definition of their biological potential. This test-by-transplantation uses the response of these tissues to normal growth controls to define each biological stage. Transplantation in orthotopic or ectopic sites provides an experimental definition for normal (**a**), hyperplasia (**b**), precancer (**c**), or cancer (**d**) mammary epithelial tissues. Fresh fragments of mammary tissue can be harvested from a "donor" mouse and transplanted into a "recipient" mouse, either in the orthotopic site – a gland cleared mammary fat pad – where the tissue proximal to the lymph node in the inguinal mammary stroma is removed at 3 weeks of age; or, in an ectopic site such as subcutaneous stroma. (**a**) *Normal mammary tissue* transplanted into the orthotopic site yields a normal branched ductal outgrowth, but does not grow in ectopic sites. After sequential "serial" transplant generations, the normal tissue will senesce, eventually resulting in no outgrowth. (**b**) *Hyperplasias*, in contrast, produce abnormal outgrowths and will not senesce after multiple serial transplant generations, but they still will not grow ectopically. (**c**) *Precancerous mammary tissues* are defined by immortal growth in serial transplantation in gland free fat pads, by lack of growth as ectopic transplants, and by eventual progression to malignancy that will grow ectopically. (**d**) *Malignant mammary tissues*, meanwhile, are able to grow consistently in either the orthotopic or ectopic site

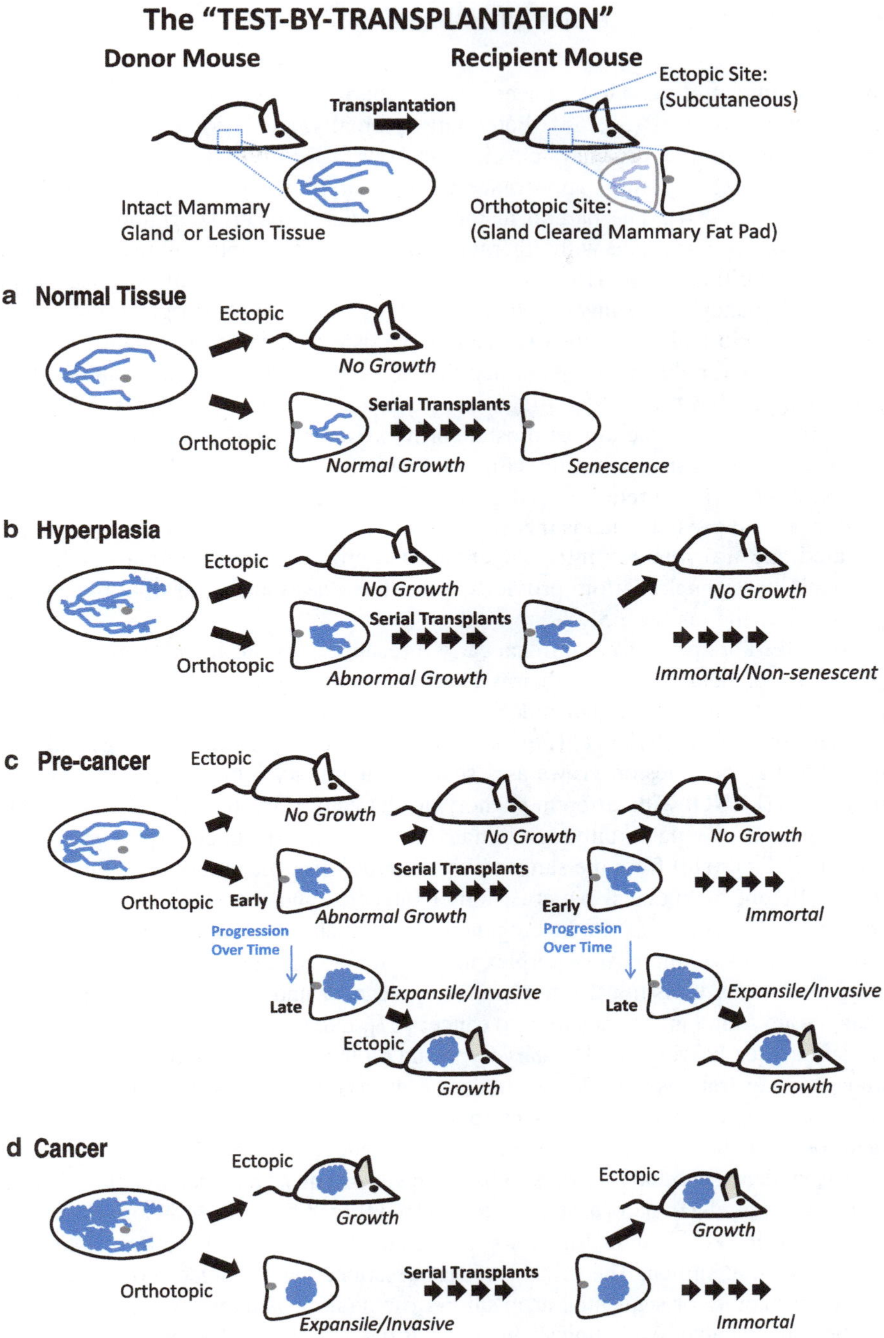

Fig. 8.1 The test-by-transplantation. A wide variety of mammary tissues types will grow in predictable patterns when transplanted into the gland-cleared (gland free) mouse mammary fat pad. Their behavior

Genetically Engineered Mouse Models

With the advent of genetic engineering, the repertoire of mouse models of human cancer has expanded [57, 58]. Potentially premalignant lesions have now been identified in different organ systems in numerous GEM [59]. The epithelial lesions are characterized by early appearance of focal atypical hyperplasia or dysplasia [59] (Figs. 8.2–8.4). The natural history of the disease can determine whether a given atypia is associated with emergence of cancer by simply following the time course in multiple mice. However, in the absence of evidence of progression to overt malignancy, many investigators are relying on the morphological distinction between in-situ and micro-invasive carcinoma as evidence of malignant potential [60]. Criteria for diagnosis of intraepithelial neoplasia have been established in several organs [59, 61]. The diagnosis for micro-invasion is more subtle. The recommendation for the mouse prostate provides sound principles [60].

The test-by-transplantation (Fig. 8.1) is the experimental alternative to morphological interpretation and guilt-by-association [62]. In the case of the mammary and prostate glands the focal atypias can be identified in situ, surgically isolated and transplanted into syngeneic or immunodeficient animals [63, 64]. The test-by-transplantation provides definitive assessment of the biological potential of the lesion [65].

The GEM are prone to multifocal early (precancer) lesions in any organ targeted [59] (Figs. 8.2 and 8.3). As in their wild type cousins, not all of the atypical lesions progress to malignancy. Atypical lesions from the same mammary gland have been isolated from the Tg(PyVmT) (Fig. 8.2) and serially transplanted [66] (Figs. 8.3 and 8.4). Each atypical lesion grows as a separate mammary intraepithelial neoplastic outgrowth (MINO) with different phenotypic characteristics [66] (Fig. 8.3). Even all MINOs from one gland, although initiated by the same oncogene, (polyoma virus middle T (PyVmT)) from the same mouse and the same mammary tree (Fig. 8.2c), have different histological patterns, tumor latencies and metastatic rates [64, 66] (Fig. 8.3). The origin of the heterogeneity from such a homogeneous genetic and molecular background is very perplexing. The major changes in expression pattern are found in the transition from normal to precancer and relatively few additional changes are found in the transition to cancer [67]. Each MINO is clonal with different and unique karyotypes. The karyotype and biology are very stable over multiple transplant generations [68]. These studies imply, as do studies with MMTV-infected HAN outgrowths, that the biological potential for each clone is pre-encoded and, therefore, genetically determined before the precancer emerges [69].

The evidence currently appears to be more consistent with a "parallel" rather than "sequential" model of neoplastic progression [69] (Fig. 8.5). Each MIN lesion isolated is uniquely encoded with its full biological potential by the time that a morphological lesion can be identified. The MINO system, described here, provides no evidence of genetic instability or sequential acquisition of mutations. Although the model might not be generalizable to all clinical situations, it fits with the mathematical predictions of Sontag and Axelrod and the culture-based model of Chin et al. [41, 42]. It suggests that cancer biology can be predetermined.

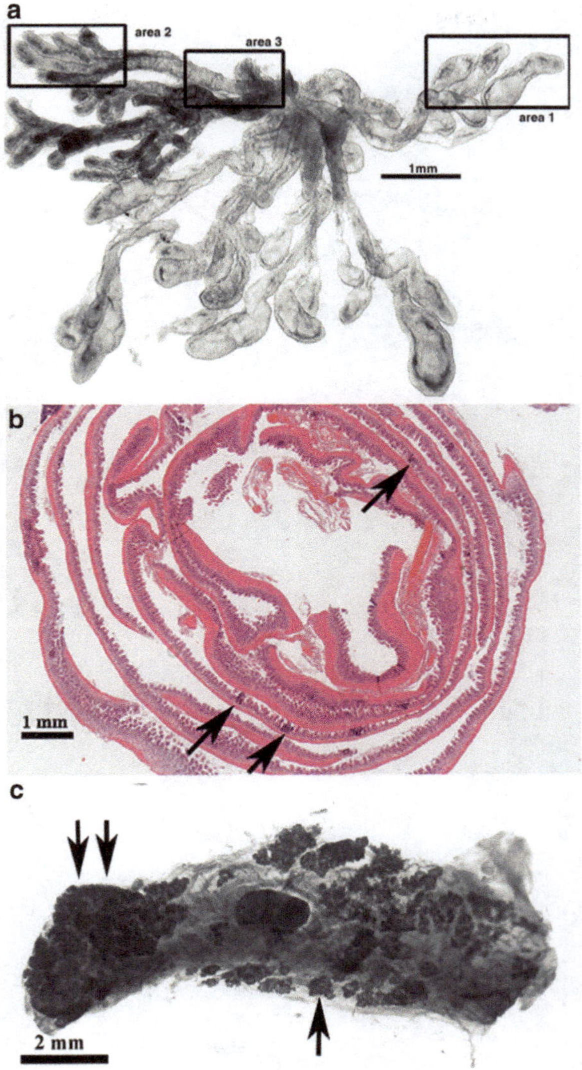

Fig. 8.2 Gross and low magnification images of multi-focal, preinvasive carcinoma. These images illustrate the principles of preinvasive cancer multifocality in (**a**) mouse prostate, (**b**) mouse small intestine and (**c**) mouse mammary gland. (**a**) Back lit photoimage of a dissected prostate from a Tg(SV40-Tag) (TRAMP) mouse showing the focal thickened epithelium scattered throughout the specimen. The diagnosis of precancer in the three areas marked was confirmed microscopically. (Photoimage courtesy of Drs. Danjacour and Cunha, UCSF). (**b**) H&E stained image of a "*Swiss Roll*" made from the intestinal tract of a Tg(APC) (MIN) mouse showing multiple *dark blue* dysplastic crypts throughout the intestine. The three *arrows* point to three of the many dysplastic crypts. One of the images is seen in Fig. 8.3i as a dysplastic crypt. (**c**) Mammary gland whole mount stained with hematoxylin to illustrate the multiple preinvasive mammary intraepithelial neoplasm (MIN) in a number 4 (inguinal) fat pad. The *double "down" arrows* point to a malignant tumor. The *single "up" arrow* points to one of the numerous foci of MIN

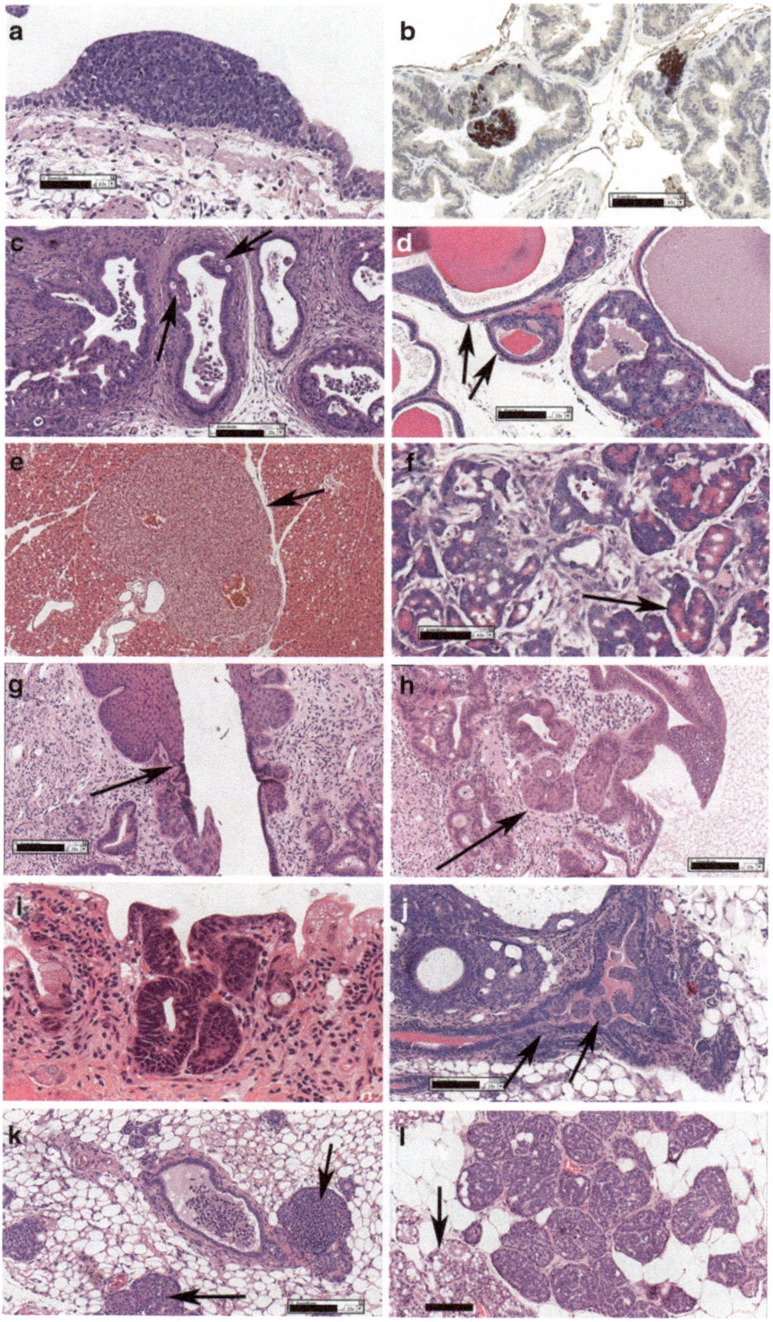

Fig. 8.3 Microscopic images of preinvasive cancers in various organs. High power images of preinvasive cancers. Note that all examples are focal atypias with adjacent, and frequently contiguous, normal epithelium. Fig. 8.1b is stained using anti-FoxA2 for immuno-histochemistry. All other

The implications of these observations are profound. First, the critical somatic mutations that determine the cell's fate occur before the appearance of the actual morphological lesion. If true, the understanding of the natural history of cancer will be based on the examination of the precursor cell. Once the code is understood, we should be able to predict outcome by examining the precancer cells. The fact is, this has already been done in human cervical cancer and HPV validates the concept. Second, the transition from precancer to invasive cancer is not necessarily caused by genetic instability but is more likely epigenetic. In gene expression analysis of DCIS and adjacent invasive ductal carcinomas, the cells of DCIS are essentially identical to the cells in the invasive cancer. In genomic content analysis there are few changes between the precancer and the invasive cancer, despite a typical finding that the DCIS harbors marked genetic change, copy number changes, amplifications, deletions and translocations. In the broad sense, epigenetics includes the environment, and interaction of the tumor or pretumor cells with the environment. It seems likely that the local DCIS environment influences progression to invasive carcinoma. More specifically, epigenetic modification of DNA may occur as a programmed response to the environment, and these changes may lead to progression. There is a long and growing list of epigenetically regulated genes implicated in cancer progression, chiefly tumor suppressors whose expression is down-regulated through promoter methylation [70].

Cancer Initiating Cells, Stem Cells and Precancer

If the pre-encoded model is accurate, we reasoned that a "cancer initiating cell" would be found in the MINO. Individual cells from enzymatically disassociated MINOs were isolated and placed in Matrigel. A small proportion of the individual

Fig. 8.3 (continued) samples are stained with hematoxylin and eosin. (**a**) Shows a small cluster of deep blue neuroendocrine cells in a TM(p53xCDN1$^{-/-}$) mouse. The neuroendocrine cells have small dense nuclei with scanty cytoplasm creating dense mass under the tall columnar respiratory epithelium. Note that the neoplastic cells do not extend beyond the basement membrane. (**b**) The anti-FoxA2 stain for neuroendocrine cells in a Tg(SV40-Tag) (TRAMP) mouse prostate showing small clusters of atypical neuroendocrine cells beneath the luminal epithelium but within the basement membrane. (**c**) Atypical epithelial clusters (*arrows*) within the lumens of mouse prostatic glands lined by otherwise normal epithelium from a Tm(Pten$^{-/-}$) mouse. (**d**) Small and large clusters of atypical foci in direct continuity with normal prostatic epithelium (*arrows*) from a Tm(NKT3.1$^{-/-}$) male. (**e**) An expansile mass (*arrow*) of neoplastic neuroendocrine cells in a "RIP-Tag" mouse. The mass contains a uniform population of insulin-producing cells. (**f**) An inflamed pancreatic lobule with a small focus atypical cells without the characteristic bright red zymogen granules (*arrow*) of the exocrine pancreas and large pleomorphic nuclei. (**g**) The squamo-columnar junction (*arrow*) from a Tg(HPV6) uterus. Note the cluster of large atypical cells at the junction. (**h**) The squamo-columnar junction in a Tg(HPV6) uterus showing atypical squamous metaplasia with gland involvement (*arrow*). (**i**) A high magnification image of a "dysplastic crypt" in a Tg(APC) mouse small intestine. Note how darkly stained the crypt cells are. (**j**) Atypical foci in mammary gland of Tm(STAT1$^{-/-}$). The atypical foci standout with large cells with abundant cytoplasm in the acini and along the otherwise normal ducts (*arrows*). (**k**) Atypical acini in a Tg(cNeu) mammary gland. They stand out from the background as solid nodules (*arrows*). (**l**) A cluster of atypical acini in at Tg(cNeux Cox2$^{-/-}$) mammary gland. Note that the adjacent mammary gland (*arrow*) is lactational

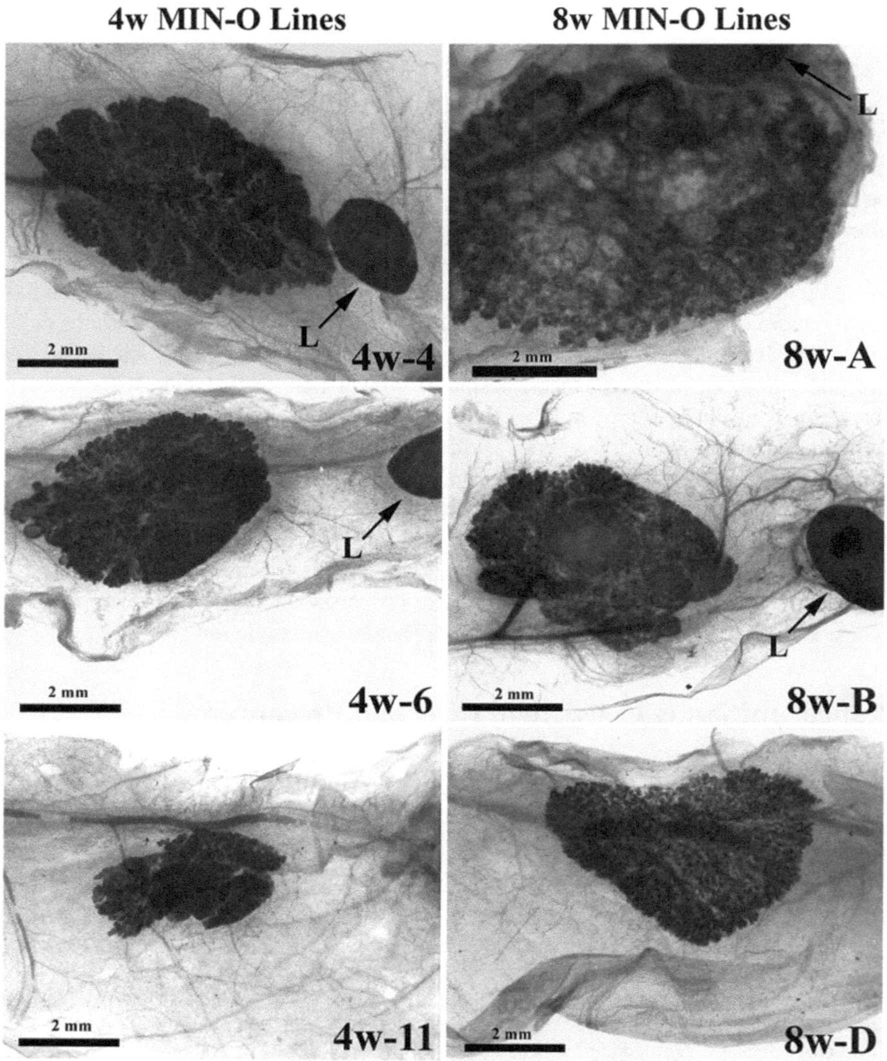

Fig. 8.4 Whole mount images of MINO transplant lines showing heterogeneity. Whole mounts of preinvasive mammary intraepithelial neoplasms (MIN) transplanted into the number 4 gland-cleared mammary fat pad. Note the lack of the normal branched ductal tree expected in transplants of normal mammary epithelium. Lines 4 came from transplants of three areas of the mammary bud in a 4 week old Tg(PyVmT) female. Lines 8 came from transplants of three MIN in the same mammary gland from a 8 week old Tg(PyVmT) female. All six transplants developed unique morphological, histological and biological properties upon serial transplantation (Images courtesy of Dr. J. Maglione, UCSD)

cells developed into epithelial spheres (MINOspheres) in Matrigel. Individual MINOspheres were transplanted into gland-cleared fat pads where they developed into hyperplastic MIN outgrowths that were consistent with the tissue of origin and developed malignancies at a predictable rate. The isolated MINO cells clearly recapitulated the entire biological scenario and outcome. Thus, cells with the pre-encoded biological outcome can be found in the precancer.

Cancer initiating cells may be referred to as "cancer stem cells" if they are capable of self renewal as well as asymmetric division (Table 8.1) to yield differentiated cells (and their precursors) which reconstitute the heterogeneity seen in the parent tumor [71]. The MINO experiments fulfill the self renewal criteria which is proved by additional serial transplantations which again result in the complete precancer phenotype comprised of multiple cell types, and a predictable transition to invasive carcinoma [72]. "Precancer stem cells" can therefore be defined as cells capable of self renewal as well as asymmetric division to yield the heterogeneous cell types constituting a precancer. Here, differentiation is a bit easier to define than in the cancer state. Here, there are distinct cell types which mimic more closely the cell types in the normal tissue. In the example of the mammary gland the clear division is between basal/ myoepithelial lineage, and luminal epithelial lineage.

Note that this definition of cancer stem cells does not require that a normal breast "stem cell" be the cell of origin of the tumor, although it has long been suspected that cancers do arise from precursor cells and *not* "terminally differentiated" cells. The cell of origin for cancers, including breast cancers, is very likely to be important with different cells of origin giving rise, perhaps, to different phenotypes (or "intrinsic subtypes") of cancer. In order to understand the relationship between the cell of origin and cancer phenotypes, several foundations are required, and, to date, many of these are not experimentally defined.

First, the tissue ontogeny must be known. What are the common and restricted precursors, and what is the complete spectrum of differentiated cells? In the mouse mammary gland, several proposed ontogenies have been described, with stem cells giving rise to both basal and luminal epithelia [73, 74]. Luminal epithelia clearly diverge into multiple functional cell types, including estrogen receptor positive and negative cells. It remains controversial, however, if the ER expression is fixed or plastic in an individual "terminally differentiated" luminal epithelial cell. Furthermore, it is becoming increasingly clear that the simple ontogenies do not reflect the true complexity.

Second, can differentiated cells "dedifferentiate" or go in reverse ontogeny? Cell tracking markers make these studies possible, but the question is currently unresolved. It is likely to be highly dependent on the context, i.e. the precise cell of origin. Some cells may be incapable of reverse differentiation, whereas others may do so commonly, even as a normal function. Some cell types may dedifferentiate only rarely as a result of rare accumulations of molecular changes.

Third, can each of the cell types in the normal ontogeny be identified with markers? If so, do these markers persist after transformation, are they altered in consistent ways, or are they gained or lost inconsistently. The mouse mammary gland has been reported to have stem cells marked by cell surface antigens, and these are reported to mark also the cancer stem cells in some GEM mammary carcinoma models [75–78]. The markers enrich for "stem like" behavior, which can only be tested via transplantation experiments using the precleared mammary fat pad, just as we have described for the MINO propagation. Because 100% of cells marked and tested in this biologic assay do *not* successfully give

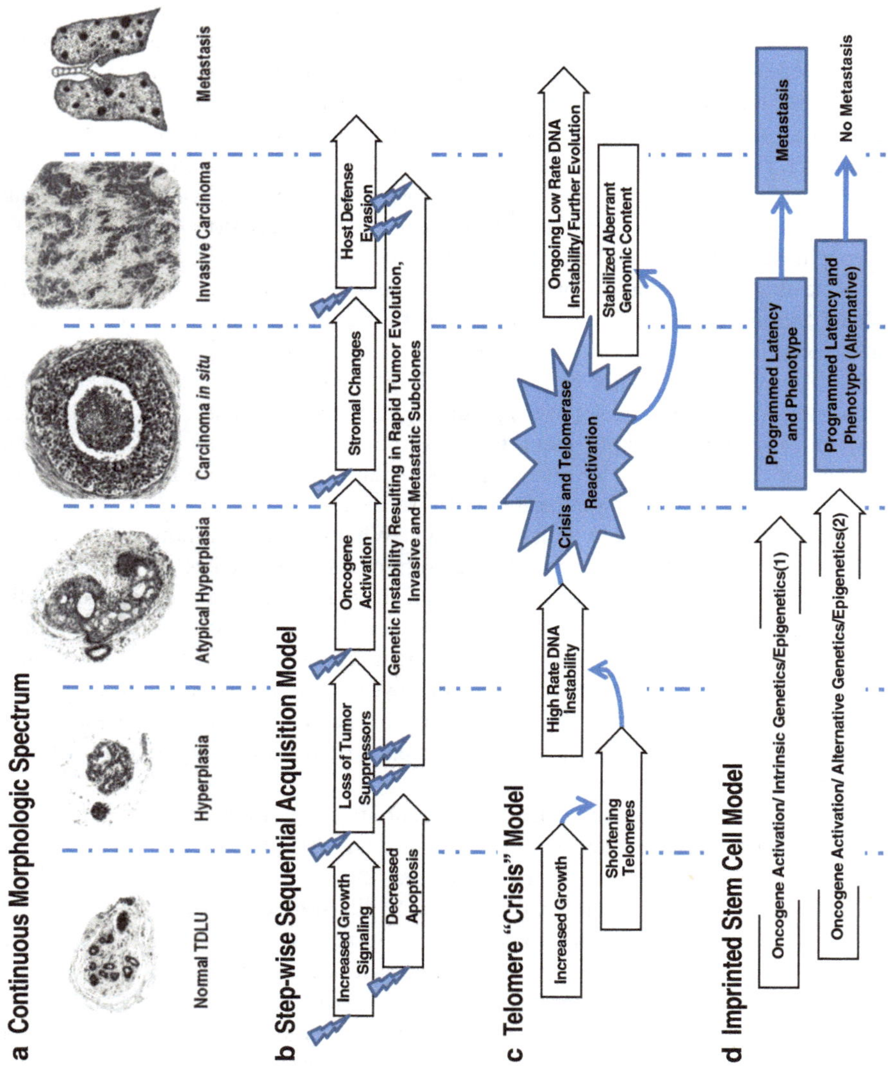

a Continuous Morphologic Spectrum
Normal TDLU
Hyperplasia
Atypical Hyperplasia
Carcinoma in situ
Invasive Carcinoma
Metastasis
b Step-wise Sequential Acquisition Model
Increased Growth Signaling
Decreased Apoptosis
Loss of Tumor Suppressors
Oncogene Activation
Stromal Changes
Host Defense Evasion
Genetic Instability Resulting in Rapid Tumor Evolution, Invasive and Metastatic Subclones
c Telomere "Crisis" Model
Increased Growth
Shortening Telomeres
High Rate DNA Instability
Crisis and Telomerase Reactivation
Stabilized Aberrant Genomic Content
Ongoing Low Rate DNA Instability/ Further Evolution
d Imprinted Stem Cell Model
Oncogene Activation/ Intrinsic Genetics/Epigenetics(1)
Oncogene Activation/ Alternative Genetics/Epigenetics(2)
Programmed Latency and Phenotype
Programmed Latency and Phenotype (Alternative)
Metastasis
No Metastasis

Table 8.1 Glossary of precancer and cancer concept terminology

Tumor initiating cell	A cell capable of re-establishing a tumor, usually defined experimentally by transplantation. Tumor initiation does not necessarily require self renewal, i.e. the stem population may be lost in the course of serial transplant generations
Cancer stem cell	A cell capable of re-establishing a tumor and self renewal
Precancer stem cell	A cell capable of re-establishing a precancer with self renewal. A precancer should obey some normal growth controls, growing within a defined normal space even if the morphology is not normal. To be a precancer, rather than atypical hyperplasia, the precancer must progress to the cancer phenotype which no longer obeys the normal growth controls
Stem-like behavior	Self-renewal and multilineage differentiation in symmetric and asymmetric cell division
Intrinsic subtype	A cancer with innate properties defined by gene expression. The subtype is defined at initiation, and does not transit to a different subtype over time
Symmetric cell division	Self-renewal through division to yield two new identical daughter cells
Asymmetric cell division	Cell division resulting in one cell identical to the original cell and a second cell with more differentiated properties
Differentiation	Cell specialization with normal cell type lineage properties
Dedifferentiation	Loss of normal lineage properties resulting in a more primitive cell
Multipotential	A cell which may differentiate along more than one lineage
Metaplastic carcinoma	A cancer of epithelial cell origin which changes its differentiation to a new lineage, such as a mesenchymal cell lineage
Epithelial mesenchymal transition (EMT)	A cancer which differentiates into a mesenchymal lineage, at least in a subset of cells. Metaplastic carcinoma is a rare form of EMT which is relatively complete in all of the cancer cells which remain mesenchymal, and do not re-transition from mesenchymal to epithelial differentiation (MET)
Plasticity	Cancers and cancer cells with greater plasticity are more readily able to adapt to their environment. EMT and MET maybe one form of cancer plasticity. Plasticity is likely to be a virulence factor for cancers

Fig. 8.5 Conceptual models of mammary cancer development. A morphologic spectrum of normal terminal duct-lobular units (TDLU), hyperplasia, atypia, ductal carcinoma in situ, and invasive and metastatic carcinoma suggests a stepwise progression (**a**). In the linear progression model, morphologic changes along the apparent spectrum are associated with the accumulation of molecular changes (**b**). In the telomere crisis model, the molecular changes occur much more rapidly as the cells approach telomere crisis. Cells which restabilize the telomere may survive and give rise to precancers with a permanent aberrant genetic profile. A lower level of ongoing instability may contribute to further progression (**c**). In the imprinted stem cell model, initiation may occur with or without genetic instability. Once an initiating oncogene or constellation of oncogenic changes are imprinted in the precancer stem cell generating an intrinsic subtype of cancer, progression is programmed, and is the result of conditioning of the microenvironment as the result of the precancer tissue and host interaction (**d**)

rise to either a normal mammary tree, (for normal stem cell assays) or reinitiated cancer (in cancer stem cell assays) there are two possible explanations which are not mutually exclusive. (1) The marker profile is incomplete, and results in a population which contains stem cells and non-stem cells and/or (2) the biologic assays are an under-estimate of individual cell potential. Cells in the bioassay are prone to lose their ability to grow, perhaps artifactually, but are very unlikely to gain the ability to grow if they did not initially have this potential.

Finally, the GEM technology is critical to the model of cell of origin. One of the major advances of the MINO mouse is that it isolates single cancer initiation foci in the transgenic mouse mammary gland where MMTV-LTR promoter/enhancer elements drive high level expression of an oncogene (PyVmT) throughout the mammary epithelia [66]. This result in multiple initiation foci in the GEM mouse. Alternative strategies, such as transplantation of the TP53 null mouse mammary epithelium result in heterogeneous phenotypes, perhaps in part because all of the cell types in this model carry the loss of p53 and subsequent susceptibility to genetic instability [79].

If there are cancer stem cells, are these cells the same, or different from the precancer stem cells? Do precancer stem cells evolve to become cancer stem cells, and if so what are the triggers? If not, what are the conditions under which the precancer stem cells give rise to invasive cancers?

Precancer Initiation and Genetic Instability

Significant somatic genome alterations, chromosome and allele amplifications and deletions, mutations, and microsatellite instability is the rule in many types of cancer, including breast cancer. Some have proposed that the initial alteration leading to cancer is a defect in DNA repair leading to a cell or cells with a "mutator phenotype" [80, 81], whereby mutations occur much more rapidly than normal yielding a statistical increase in the likelihood of a tumor initiating mutation or constellation of mutations. Extending this hypothesis is evidence that the rate of instability increases dramatically as proliferative cells reach "telomere crisis," a point where chromosome's telomeres are too short to protect the chromosome from significant alteration during DNA replication [42]. Cells which reactivate their telomerase restabilize their chromosomes and may survive the telomere crisis, and furthermore may have acquired tumor initiating chromosomal changes which are imprinted in the stabilized nascent cancer. Ongoing instability is common, but is reduced in its rate (Fig. 8.5b). Is the ongoing instability required for tumor progression? This is an important question. Many people think so, and this fits very well with the common conceptual model for cancer progression, progressive accumulation of molecular changes with corresponding progressive morphologic changes (Fig. 8.5a).

However, there is little evidence for the kind of direct linear model simplistically proposed. For example, there is no good evidence that hyperplastic lesions, or even atypical lesions in the breast are clonally related to DCIS lesions that occur in the same patients. In fact, there is more evidence that the "normal" appearing ducts are clonally related to the DCIS [82]. Some have assumed that these genetic markers, loss of heterozygosity and microsatellite length changes are early markers of premalignancy. It seems equally possible that changes might occur in the developing duct in childhood and during puberty, and that these changes might indicate an "at risk" branch of the mammary tree, but the changes occurred well prior to the onset of DCIS and are not causal. Additionally, patients with DCIS lesions do not typically show evidence of progression from low grade patterns of DCIS to high grade lesions. Instead, DCIS remains low grade even when it recurs much later. Lastly, the cancer phenotype is relatively fixed, and has been shown to have an intrinsic type. While this may be the result of different cells of origin, as described above, it is notable that even within the type, cancers retain their grade and differentiation over time and do not evolve to new phenotypes. This is not to say that cancers cannot be selected, under pressure, for example for chemotherapy resistance. The question is whether or not the ability to become resistant to therapy is, itself, an intrinsic property of the initiated cancer stem cell. Recent clinical evidence for the prognostic role of a "complete pathologic response" to chemotherapy, where patients treated with chemotherapy before local excision therapy showing no evidence of residual viable cancer have a much better prognosis than those who do have residual disease (even after dramatic shrinkage) suggests that it is an intrinsic property [83, 84]. Metastatic capacity is also likely to be intrinsically programmed. Evidence for a specific plasticity phenotype in some breast cancers is manifest as "epithelial to mesenchymal transition" EMT and correlates with metastatic capacity [72, 85].

Epigenetic Imprinting/Epigenetic Plasticity

The MINO mouse model of precancer proves that additional factors affect the program of the precancer beyond the initiating oncogene. The six individual MINO lines have distinct programs for latency to invasive carcinoma, and for metastatic capacity, despite the fact that they were isolated from the same mammary gland (Fig. 8.3). This could be an artifact of the model system, and it could even reflect slightly different cells of origin. The germline genetics and environment are controlled. It is also clearly possible that different patterns of DNA methylation were imprinted on each of the six lines, and these might account for the differences in programming.

Lastly, once other possibilities are excluded, such as accumulation of additional molecular "hits", or even differences in the oncogene expression level, how can we explain a precancer tissue transitioning to the invasive cancer phenotype. We hypothesize that the precancer phenotype, programmed from initiation, and reproduced by retransplantation of the programmed precancer stem cell results in a conditioning of the microenvironment. It is the feedback, then, from this conditioned microenvironment that induces the precancer to behave as an invasive cancer, and the invasive cancer then perpetuates the environmental conditioning (Fig. 8.5c). If this conceptual model is true, we would expect that the precancer stem cell could be recovered from the cancer, and, minus the conditioned environment would revert to the precancer phenotype. Similarly, the precancer might be induced to more rapidly transit to the invasive cancer phenotype if the cancer microenvironment were recombined with the precancer cells upon transplant. These hypotheses are currently being tested in experiments in our laboratory.

Conclusions and Implications

These views of precancer have profound experimental and clinical implications. Perhaps, the biological predeterminism of MacDonald is correct. Although the critics pointed out that the concept was never rigorously tested, the weight of the experimental data now suggests that the biology is predetermined in the stem cell population. With the emerging interest in stem cells and cancer initiating cells, we can find new hope for the futile cases of high risk cancers. ("It is in the stem cells, stupid!") If instead cancers can continue to evolve through genetic and epigenetic changes from one cancer subtype to another, specifically targeted therapies may never be effective. Fortunately, it appears that the intrinsic subtypes are just that, intrinsic. Even if adaptations occur, the cancer is still essentially the same cancer. In this context, it seems likely that the most successful (and lethal) cancers will be those with intrinsic adaptability or a plasticity phenotype. Epithelial to mesenchymal tumorigenesis is also characterized by mesenchymal to epithelial transition, a version of plasticity that has begun to be unraveled. One can anticipate that a book of codes, with a volume for each organ site, will be decoded, not by examining the final product that has undergone numerous secondary changes on the way to metastases, but in the precancer cells themselves. Once the signatures of fatality are known and recognized, they can be detected either in circulating cells or by fine needle biopsy of the precancers. Once detected and the signatures deciphered, we can develop new strategies to prevent their emergence or halt their progression.

Acknowledgements The authors would like cite funding from the National Center for Research resources (K26 RR0243037 (ADB), and U42 RR14905), and the National Cancer Institute (U01-CA105490 (RDC), and U01 CA141582). In addition support from the non-profit Center for Genomic Pathology is appreciated.

References

1. Alcantara Llaguno S, Chen J, Kwon CH, Jackson EL, Li Y, Burns DK, Alvarez-Buylla A, Parada LF (2009) Malignant astrocytomas originate from neural stem/progenitor cells in a somatic tumor suppressor mouse model. Cancer Cell 15:45–56
2. Esposito I, Seiler C, Bergmann F, Kleeff J, Friess H, Schirmacher P (2007) Hypothetical progression model of pancreatic cancer with origin in the centroacinar-acinar compartment. Pancreas 35:212–217
3. Tsao JL, Tavare S, Salovaara R, Jass JR, Aaltonen LA, Shibata D (1999) Colorectal adenoma and cancer divergence. Evidence of multilineage progression. Am J Pathol 154:1815–1824

4. Wang Y, Revelo MP, Sudilovsky D, Cao M, Chen WG, Goetz L, Xue H, Sadar M, Shappell SB, Cunha GR, Hayward SW (2005) Development and characterization of efficient xenograft models for benign and malignant human prostate tissue. Prostate 64:149–159
5. Warner JK, Wang JC, Hope KJ, Jin L, Dick JE (2004) Concepts of human leukemic development. Oncogene 23:7164–7177
6. Baillie M, Simms W (1806) Queries and responses from the medical committee of the society for investigating the nature and cure of cancer. Edinburgh Med Surg J 2:382–389
7. Rader KA (2004) Making mice: standardizing animals for American biomedical research, 1900–1955. Princeton University Press, Princeton, NJ
8. Woglom WH (1913) The study of experimental cancer research. A review. Columbia University Press, New York
9. Ewing J (1914) Precancerous diseases and precancerous lesions, especially in the breast. Med Rec 86:951–958
10. Papanicolaou GN, Traut HF (1943) Diagnosis of uterine cancer by the vaginal smear. The Commonwealth Fund, New York
11. NIH (1997) National Institutes of Health Consensus Development Conference statement on cervical cancer. Gynecol Oncol 66:351–361
12. Apolant H (1906) Die epithelialen Geschwülste der Maus. Arbeiten a.d. Koniglchn Inst F Expt Ther zu Frankfurt aM 1:7–68
13. Haaland M (1911) Spontaneous tumours in mice. In: Bashford EF (ed) Fourth scientific report on the investigations of the Imperial Cancer Research Fund. Imperial Cancer Research Fund, London, pp 1–113
14. Rous P, Kidd JG (1941) Conditioned neoplasms and subthreshold neoplastic states. J Exp Med 73:365–390
15. Berenblum I (1954) Carcinogenesis and tumor pathogenesis. In: Greenstein JP, Haddow A (eds) Advances in cancer research, vol 11. Academic Press, New York, pp 129–175
16. Berenblum I, Shubik P (1954) A new, quantitative approach to the study of the stages of chemical carcinogenesis in the mouse's skin. Br J Cancer 8:1–12
17. Shubik P (1950) Studies on the promoting phase in the stages of carcinogenesis in mice, rabbits and guinea-pigs. Cancer Res 10:15–17
18. Foulds L (1954) The experimental study of tumor progression: a review. Cancer Res 14:327–339
19. Foulds L (1957) Tumor progression. Cancer Res 17:355–356
20. Foulds L (1958) The natural history of cancer. J Chronic Dis 8:2–37
21. Foulds L (1959) Neoplastic development. Academic Press, London, New York
22. Beuving LJ, Faulkin LJ Jr, DeOme KB, Bergs VV (1967) Hyperplastic lesions in the mammary glands of Sprague-Dawley rats after 7, 12-dimethyl-benz[a]anthracene treatment. J Natl Cancer Inst 39:423–429
23. De Ome KB, Faulkin LJ, Bern HA, Blair PB (1959) Development of mammary tumors form hyperplastic alveolar nodules transplanted into gland-free mammary fat pads of female C3H mice. Cancer 24:1255–1258
24. Dunn TB (1945) Morphology and histogenesis of mammary tumors. In: Moulton FR (ed) Symposium on mammary tumors in mice. American Association for the Advancement of Science, Washington, DC, pp 13–38
25. Fekete E (1938) A comparative morphological study of the mammary gland in a high and a low tumor strain of mice. Am J Pathol 14:557–578
26. Foulds L (1949) Mammary tumors in hybrid mice: growth and progression of spontaneous tumors. Br J Cancer 3:345–375
27. Armitage P, Doll R (1957) A two-stage theory of carcinogenesis in relation to the age distribution of human cancer. Br J Cancer 11:161–169
28. Knudson AG Jr (1977) Mutation and cancer in man. Cancer 39:1882–1886
29. Pitot HC (1982) The natural history of neoplastic development: the relation of experimental models to human cancer. Cancer 49:1206–1211
30. Fearon ER, Hamilton SR, Vogelstein B (1987) Clonal analysis of human colorectal tumors. Science 238:193–197

31. Fearon ER, Vogelstein B (1990) A genetic model for colorectal tumorigenesis. Cell 61:759–767
32. Macdonald I (1951) Biological predeterminism in human cancer. Surg Gynecol Obstet 92:443–452
33. Macdonald I (1958) Individual basis of biologic variability in cancer. Surg Gynecol Obstet 106:227–229
34. Macdonald I, Kotin P (1954) Biologic predeterminism in gastric cancer as the limiting factor of curability. Surg Gynecol Obstet 98:148–152
35. Bauer KR, Brown M, Cress RD, Parise CA, Caggiano V (2007) Descriptive analysis of estrogen receptor (ER)-negative, progesterone receptor (PR)-negative, and HER2-negative invasive breast cancer, the so-called triple-negative phenotype: a population-based study from the California cancer Registry. Cancer 109:1721–1728
36. Weed DL (1985) An epidemiological application of Popper's method. J Epidemiol Community Health 39:277–285
37. Notkin LJ (1959) The theory of biologic predeterminism: its questionable usefulness and validity as a medical tool. Can Med Assoc J 81:190–191
38. Munger K, Scheffner M, Huibregtse JM, Howley PM (1992) Interactions of HPV E6 and E7 oncoproteins with tumour suppressor gene products. Cancer Surv 12:197–217
39. Fujimoto K, Yamada Y, Okajima E, Kakizoe T, Sasaki H, Sugimura T, Terada M (1992) Frequent association of p53 gene mutation in invasive bladder cancer. Cancer Res 52:1393–1398
40. Rekhi B, Jaswal TS, Arora B (2004) Premalignant lesions of prostate and their association with nodular hyperplasia and carcinoma prostate. Indian J Cancer 41:60–65
41. Sontag L, Axelrod DE (2005) Evaluation of pathways for progression of heterogeneous breast tumors. J Theor Biol 232:179–189
42. Chin K, de Solorzano CO, Knowles D, Jones A, Chou W, Rodriguez EG, Kuo WL, Ljung BM, Chew K, Myambo K, Miranda M, Krig S, Garbe J, Stampfer M, Yaswen P, Gray JW, Lockett SJ (2004) In situ analyses of genome instability in breast cancer. Nat Genet 36:984–988
43. Burstein HJ, Polyak K, Wong JS, Lester SC, Kaelin CM (2004) Ductal carcinoma in situ of the breast. N Engl J Med 350:1430–1441
44. Nishidate T, Katagiri T, Lin ML, Mano Y, Miki Y, Kasumi F, Yoshimoto M, Tsunoda T, Hirata K, Nakamura Y (2004) Genome-wide gene-expression profiles of breast-cancer cells purified with laser microbeam microdissection: identification of genes associated with progression and metastasis. Int J Oncol 25:797–819
45. Seth A, Kitching R, Landberg G, Xu J, Zubovits J, Burger AM (2003) Gene expression profiling of ductal carcinomas in situ and invasive breast tumors. Anticancer Res 23:2043–2051
46. Yao J, Weremowicz S, Feng B, Gentleman RC, Marks JR, Gelman R, Brennan C, Polyak K (2006) Combined cDNA array comparative genomic hybridization and serial analysis of gene expression analysis of breast tumor progression. Cancer Res 66:4065–4078
47. Cardiff RD, Kenney N (2007) Mouse mammary tumor biology: a short history. Adv Cancer Res 98:53–116
48. Foulds L (1975) Neoplastic development. Academic Press, New York, London
49. Deringer MK (1962) Development of tumors, especially mammary tumors, in agent-free strain DBA/2eB mice. J Natl Cancer Inst 28:203–210
50. De Ome KB, Nandi S, Bern HA, Blair PB, Pitelka DR (1962) The preneoplastic hyperplastic alveolar nodule as the morphological precursor of mammary cancer in mice. In: Severi L (ed) The morphological precursors of cancer. Division of Cancer Research, Perugia, pp 349–368
51. Medina D (2000) The preneoplastic phenotype in murine mammary tumorigenesis. J Mammary Gland Biol Neoplasia 5:393–407
52. Medina D (2002) Biological and molecular characteristics of the premalignant mouse mammary gland. Biochim Biophys Acta 1603:1–9
53. Cardiff RD (1984) Protoneoplasia: the molecular biology of murine mammary hyperplasia. Adv Cancer Res 42:167–190
54. Cardiff RD, Aguilar-Cordova E (1988) Protoneoplasia revisited: the molecular biology of mouse mammary hyperplasia. (review). Anticancer Res 8:925–933

55. Cardiff RD, Moghanaki D, Jensen RA (2000) Genetically engineered mouse models of mammary intraepithelial neoplasia. J Mammary Gland Biol Neoplasia 5:421–437
56. Cunha GR, Young P, Hom YK, Cooke PS, Taylor JA, Lubahn DB (1997) Elucidation of a role for stromal steroid hormone receptors in mammary gland growth and development using tissue recombinants. J Mammary Gland Biol Neoplasia 2:393–402
57. Cardiff RD, Ward JM, Barthold SW (2008) 'One medicine–one pathology': are veterinary and human pathology prepared? Lab Invest 88:18–26
58. Valli T, Barthold SW, Ward JE, Brayton C, Nikitin A, Borowsky AD, Bronson RT, Cardiff RD, Sundberg J, Ince T (2007) Over 60% of NIH extramural funding involves animal-related research. Vet Pathol 44:962–963, author reply 963–964
59. Cardiff RD, Anver MR, Boivin GP, Bosenberg MW, Maronpot RR, Molinolo AA, Nikitin AY, Rehg JE, Thomas GV, Russell RG, Ward JM (2006) Precancer in mice: animal models used to understand, prevent, and treat human precancers. Toxicol Pathol 34:699–707
60. Shappell SB, Thomas GV, Roberts RL, Herbert R, Ittmann MM, Rubin MA, Humphrey PA, Sundberg JP, Rozengurt N, Barrios R, Ward JM, Cardiff RD (2004) Prostate pathology of genetically engineered mice: definitions and classification. The consensus report from the Bar Harbor meeting of the Mouse Models of Human Cancer Consortium Prostate Pathology Committee. Cancer Res 64:2270–2305
61. Park JH, Walls JE, Galvez JJ, Kim M, Abate-Shen C, Shen MM, Cardiff RD (2002) Prostatic intraepithelial neoplasia in genetically engineered mice. Am J Pathol 161:727–735
62. Cardiff RD, Bern HA, Faulkin LJ, Daniel CW, Smith GH, Young LJ, Medina D, Gardner MB, Wellings SR, Shyamala G, Guzman RC, Rajkumar L, Yang J, Thordarson G, Nandi S, MacLeod CL, Oshima RG, Man AK, Sawai ET, Gregg JP, Cheung AT, Lau DH (2002) Contributions of mouse biology to breast cancer research. Comp Med 52:12–31
63. Chiaverotti T, Couto SS, Donjacour A, Mao JH, Nagase H, Cardiff RD, Cunha GR, Balmain A (2008) Dissociation of epithelial and neuroendocrine carcinoma lineages in the transgenic adenocarcinoma of mouse prostate model of prostate cancer. Am J Pathol 172:236–246
64. Maglione JE, McGoldrick ET, Young LJ, Namba R, Gregg JP, Liu L, Moghanaki D, Ellies LG, Borowsky AD, Cardiff RD, MacLeod CL (2004) Polyomavirus middle T-induced mammary intraepithelial neoplasia outgrowths: single origin, divergent evolution, and multiple outcomes. Mol Cancer Ther 3:941–953
65. Cardiff RD, Rosner A, Hogarth MA, Galvez JJ, Borowsky AD, Gregg JP (2004) Validation: the new challenge for pathology. Toxicol Pathol 32(Suppl 1):31–39
66. Maglione JE, Moghanaki D, Young LJ, Manner CK, Ellies LG, Joseph SO, Nicholson B, Cardiff RD, MacLeod CL (2001) Transgenic polyoma middle-T mice model premalignant mammary disease. Cancer Res 61:8298–8305
67. Namba R, Maglione JE, Young LJ, Borowsky AD, Cardiff RD, MacLeod CL, Gregg JP (2004) Molecular characterization of the transition to malignancy in a genetically engineered mouse-based model of ductal carcinoma in situ. Mol Cancer Res 2:453–463
68. Namba R, Maglione JE, Davis RR, Baron CA, Liu S, Carmack CE, Young LJ, Borowsky AD, Cardiff RD, Gregg JP (2006) Heterogeneity of mammary lesions represents molecular differences. BMC Cancer 6:275
69. Damonte P, Hodgson JG, Chen JQ, Young LJ, Cardiff RD, Borowsky AD (2008) Mammary carcinoma behavior is programmed in the precancer stem cell. Breast Cancer Res 10:R50
70. Vasilatos SN, Broadwater G, Barry WT, Baker JC Jr, Lem S, Dietze EC, Bean GR, Bryson AD, Pilie PG, Goldenberg V, Skaar D, Paisie C, Torres-Hernandez A, Grant TL, Wilke LG, Ibarra-Drendall C, Ostrander JH, D'Amato NC, Zalles C, Jirtle R, Weaver VM, Seewaldt VL (2009) CpG island tumor suppressor promoter methylation in non-BRCA-associated early mammary carcinogenesis. Cancer Epidemiol Biomarkers Prev 18:901–914
71. Clarke MF, Dick JE, Dirks PB, Eaves CJ, Jamieson CH, Jones DL, Visvader J, Weissman IL, Wahl GM (2006) Cancer stem cells–perspectives on current status and future directions: AACR workshop on cancer stem cells. Cancer Res 66:9339–9344
72. Damonte P, Gregg JP, Borowsky AD, Keister BA, Cardiff RD (2007) EMT tumorigenesis in the mouse mammary gland. Lab Invest 87:1218–1226

73. LaMarca HL, Rosen JM (2008) Minireview: hormones and mammary cell fate–what will I become when I grow up? Endocrinology 149:4317–4321
74. Woodward WA, Chen MS, Behbod F, Rosen JM (2005) On mammary stem cells. J Cell Sci 118:3585–3594
75. Abbey CK, Borowsky AD, Gregg JP, Cardiff RD, Cherry SR (2006) Preclinical imaging of mammary intraepithelial neoplasia with positron emission tomography. J Mammary Gland Biol Neoplasia 11:137–149
76. Alvi AJ, Clayton H, Joshi C, Enver T, Ashworth A, Vivanco MM, Dale TC, Smalley MJ (2003) Functional and molecular characterisation of mammary side population cells. Breast Cancer Res 5:R1–R8
77. Shackleton M, Vaillant F, Simpson KJ, Stingl J, Smyth GK, Asselin-Labat ML, Wu L, Lindeman GJ, Visvader JE (2006) Generation of a functional mammary gland from a single stem cell. Nature 439:84–88
78. Stingl J, Eirew P, Ricketson I, Shackleton M, Vaillant F, Choi D, Li HI, Eaves CJ (2006) Purification and unique properties of mammary epithelial stem cells. Nature 439:993–997
79. Jerry DJ, Kittrell FS, Kuperwasser C, Laucirica R, Dickinson ES, Bonilla PJ, Butel JS, Medina D (2000) A mammary-specific model demonstrates the role of the p53 tumor suppressor gene in tumor development. Oncogene 19:1052–1058
80. Loeb LA (1991) Mutator phenotype may be required for multistage carcinogenesis. Cancer Res 51:3075–3079
81. Loeb LA (1994) Microsatellite instability: marker of a mutator phenotype in cancer. Cancer Res 54:5059–5063
82. Euhus DM, Cler L, Shivapurkar N, Milchgrub S, Peters GN, Leitch AM, Heda S, Gazdar AF (2002) Loss of heterozygosity in benign breast epithelium in relation to breast cancer risk. J Natl Cancer Inst 94:858–860
83. Dorssers LC, Van der Flier S, Brinkman A, van Agthoven T, Veldscholte J, Berns EM, Klijn JG, Beex LV, Foekens JA (2001) Tamoxifen resistance in breast cancer: elucidating mechanisms. Drugs 61:1721–1733
84. Turton NJ, Judah DJ, Riley J, Davies R, Lipson D, Styles JA, Smith AG, Gant TW (2001) Gene expression and amplification in breast carcinoma cells with intrinsic and acquired doxorubicin resistance. Oncogene 20:1300–1306
85. Blanco MJ, Moreno-Bueno G, Sarrio D, Locascio A, Cano A, Palacios J, Nieto MA (2002) Correlation of snail expression with histological grade and lymph node status in breast carcinomas. Oncogene 21:3241–3246

Chapter 9
Biomarkers for Detection of Intra-epithelial Neoplasia

Kareem M. Shariff and Pierre Lao-Sirieix

Abstract Biological characteristics have been used for millennia to characterise and diagnose ailments and we now term these biomarkers. With the advent of the "omics" era the knowledge of the molecular events involved in carcinogenesis has increased greatly and this has been followed by the expectation that clinical practice could be revolutionised by novel molecular approaches. The National Institute of Health (NIH) has initiated a Biomarker workforce to clearly define biomarkers and the Early Detection Research Network Group offer guidelines for the development and validation of cancer biomarkers. The idea is that these more stringent guidelines will reduce the number of badly designed, underpowered biomarker studies so that quality data can be collected which will help bring biomarkers into clinical use. Although developed for invasive cancer these definitions and guidelines also apply to markers for intraepithelial neoplasia (IEN). The identification of these pre-malignant lesions may be central to reduction of cancer mortality since they are indolent and allow time for chemoprevention and/or treatment measures before cancer develops to an incurable stage. Biomarkers are needed to allow for detection of IENs and to predict which lesions are at highest risk of progression. The development and validation of cancer biomarkers is riddled with practical difficulties such as sample collection and identification of confounding factors and these are in many cases highly problematic in the case of IEN. Although a number of biomarkers are under evaluation for IEN, there are currently no biomarkers in clinical practice that were developed specifically for this purpose. Screening markers such as prostate serum albumin and faecal occult blood test do however also detect early cancers including a small proportion of IEN. There is a real clinical need for biomarkers in the field of preinvasive disease however it is likely that progress will only be made if strong collaborative links are forged between academia, industry and clinical practice.

P. Lao-Sirieix (✉)
Cancer Cell Unit, Hutchison-MRC Research Centre, Cambridge CB22 0XZ, UK
e-mail: pss@hutchison-mrc.cam.ac.uk

R.C. Fitzgerald (ed.), *Pre-Invasive Disease: Pathogenesis and Clinical Management*,
DOI 10.1007/978-1-4419-6694-0_9,

Introduction

The evolution of biomarkers is a remarkable story. Biomarkers were identified in easily accessible body fluids like the urine or the blood and as technology evolved the focus of biomarker identification changed to analysis of tissue itself. With the recent advances in proteomics and for purely pragmatic reasons, the focus has shifted back to easily accessible body fluids. Advances in technology have played a major role with each milestone of biomarker development.

While the term biomarker was first coined in the twentieth century, biomarkers have been used for millennia to diagnose ailments. The Ebers Papyrus, dated around 1600–1500 BC but thought to be a copy of a text written around 3000 BC, describes anatomical observations with surprising accuracy as well as treatments for various conditions. The presence of honey-sweet urine that attracted flies and ants was used as a specific sign for polyuria. It was in 1674 that Thomas Willis made the distinction between diabetes, characterised by the sweet urine, and other causes of polyuria, therefore using the presence of glucose in the urine as a biomarker. The description of a protein in the acidified urine of patients with multiple myeloma in 1846 heralded the advent of cancer biomarkers [1]. After a period of almost nine decades, little progress was made until acid phosphatase was highlighted as a marker for metastatic prostate cancer [2]. However, the low sensitivity and specificity of most early tests hindered the clinical use of biomarkers. The development of a sensitive and specific radioimmunoassay for the quantification of insulin in 1960 made it possible to measure small concentrations of solute in biological fluids and has paved the way for biomarker detection in body fluids [3]. Alpha fetoprotein, first discovered in 1956 [4], was identified in mice with hepatocellular cancer [5] and thence in humans [6]. Similarly carcinoembryonic antigen (CEA) first described in 1965 in human colon cancer tissue extracts [7] was later measured in serum using a sensitive radioimmunoassay technique [8]. Introduction of monoclonal antibodies in 1975 [9] initiated a phase of intense discovery of new tumour tissue antigens shed into the plasma like the cancer antigen 125 (CA 125) first reported in 1984 [10] and others such as CA 15.3, CA19.9 and PSA [11].

The 1970's were marked by rapid advances in the understanding of carcinogenesis and discovery of oncogenes led to identification of genetic mutations associated with cancer development [12]. Genetic changes were initially analyzed in tumour biopsies, but the reporting of DNA in serum of cancer patients in 1977 [13], using radioimmunoassay, opened up new avenues for screening. Cancer-associated mutations in *p53* and *RAS* were identified in the 1991 and 1992 in urine and stools of cancer patients [14, 15]. To detect these mutations micrograms of DNA were needed requiring a sensitive assay. In 2001 a dramatic improvement in technology with microarrays and mass spectrometry has led to an exponential increase in the publications of biomarkers [16] (Fig. 9.1).

In more recent years, it has become recognised that most epithelial tumours develop through a pre-invasive stage, often referred to as intra-epithelial neoplasia

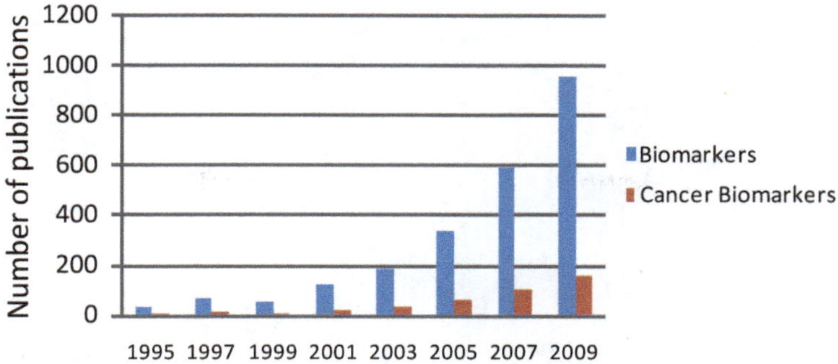

Fig. 9.1 Number of publications identified in Pubmed with "biomarker" or "cancer biomarker" as search terms in the title of articles since 1995

(IEN) [17]. In some ways, discovery of a biomarker to detect IEN has become a Holy Grail for early detection. Indeed, theses lesions are considered to be reversible. Their small size and the long lag period, from years to decades, before invasive cancer develops affords the opportunity for early detection and curative treatment. Volgenstein was the first to map the accumulation of molecular alterations required for colon cancer development [18]. Like colon cancers, most epithelial tumours develop through the accumulation of molecular alterations many of which precede the invasive phenotype. Most IEN lesions display profound molecular abnormalities than can be used for diagnosis and for patient management [17, 19] (Fig. 9.2) (and see disease specific Chapters).

With the advent of the "omics" era, the knowledge of the molecular events involved in carcinogenesis has increased greatly (see Chap. 6) and has been followed by the expectations that clinical practice could be revolutionised by novel molecular approaches. So far, few biomarkers have been approved by the FDA in the US [11] and even less are being developed for detection of IEN. The lack of novel clinical tools can be explained by a numbers of reasons [20]. First the perceived value of novel therapies is higher than that of diagnostic tests and treatments are therefore better reimbursed by many insurance companies. It is also perceived that novel diagnostics are evaluated more rigorously since a significant improvements over existing tests need to be proven together with complex economic modelling. In contrast a new therapy, to be successful, needs to be an improvement on a current one or needs to present less side effects. These two factors have detracted large pharmaceutical companies from developing diagnostics tests. Furthermore, the need to access human specimens for pre-clinical validation studies adds practical and feasibility issues. Guidelines have been published for the validation of biomarker assays. While these are not followed as strictly as the phases of development of therapeutics, regulatory agencies will require a high level of validation before any approval is granted [21].

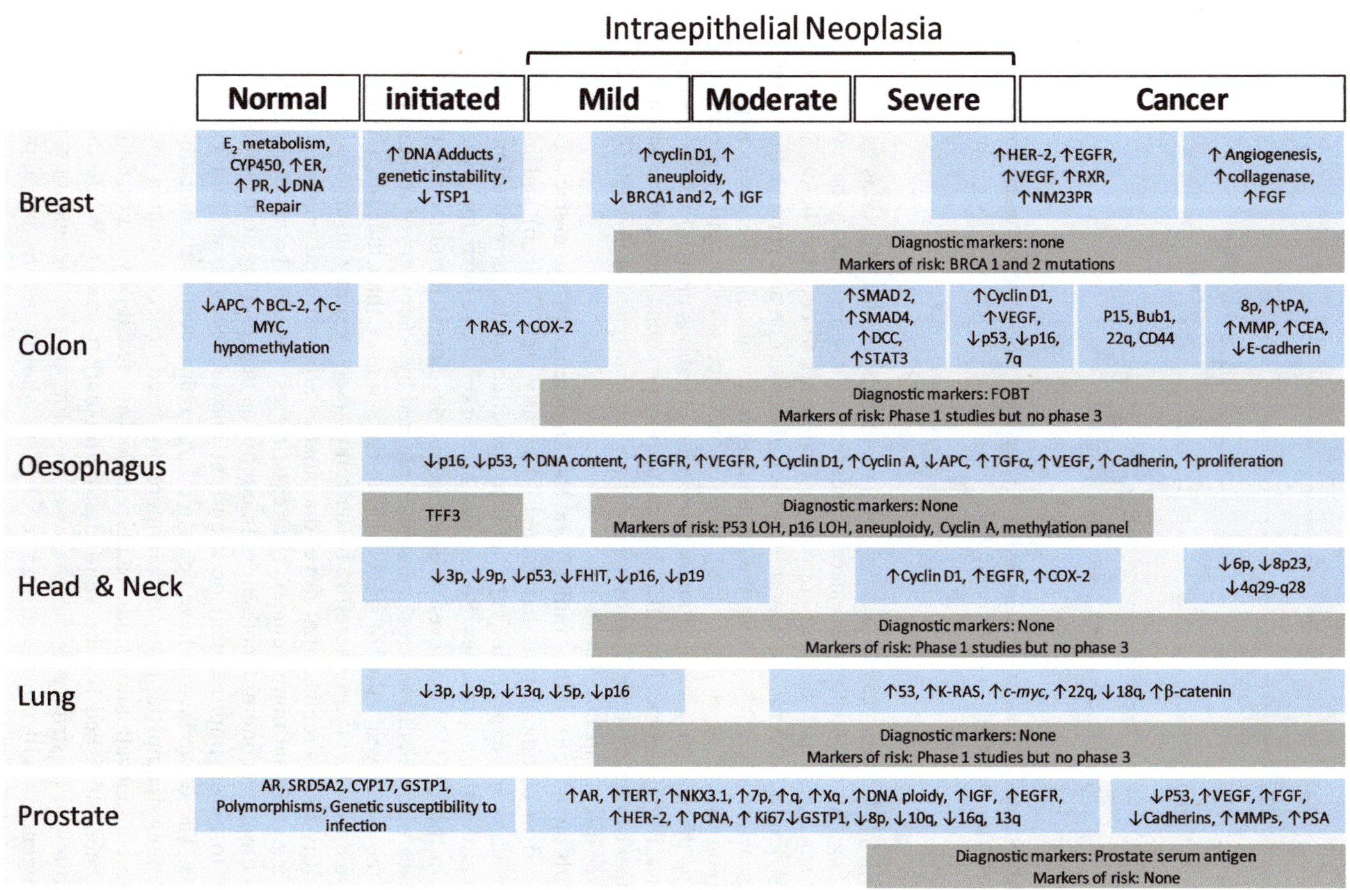

Fig. 9.2 Molecular alterations during carcinogenesis and biomarkers in clinical trial and in clinical use (adapted from Kelloff et al. [19]). For each tissue type, common molecular alterations are indicated in blue boxes and promising biomarkers are indicated in the grey boxes

Definitions

With the exponential increase in publications related to biomarkers in the last 15 years (Fig. 9.1), efforts have been made by the Biomarker Definition Working Group, under the initiative of the National Institute of Heath, to create standardised definitions and to classify biomarkers based on their application [22]. The following definitions were given by the Biomarker Definition Working Group:

- Biological markers (biomarker): a characteristic that is objectively measured and evaluated as an indicator of normal biological processes, pathogenic processes, or pharmacological responses to a therapeutic intervention".
- Clinical endpoint: A characteristic or variable that reflects how a patient feels, functions, or survives.
- Surrogate endpoint: A biomarker that is intended to substitute for a clinical endpoint. A surrogate endpoint is expected to predict clinical benefit (or harm or lack of benefit) based on epidemiologic, therapeutic, pathophysiologic, or other scientific evidence.

Clinical and surrogate endpoints will not be discussed here. In the context of this chapter, the term biomarker will be used in the sense of a biological marker as per the Biomarker Definition from the Working Group [22].

Biomarkers can be further sub-classified according to their intended use.

(1) Diagnostic markers: these markers inform on the presence or absence of cancer, or a premalignant condition, deserving clinical attention at a given point in time. Biomarkers can be used as adjuncts to diagnosis or a diagnostic modality on their own. For example measurement of the blood levels of α-fetoprotein is recommended for diagnosis of hepatocellular cancer in conjunction with abdominal ultrasound [23]. On the other hand, prostate specific antigen (PSA) is used for screening for prostate cancer and is one of the most widely used diagnostic biomarkers [11]. Though it has been approved by FDA for screening, its use still has limitations and remains controversial [24].
(2) Markers of progression: These markers are used to assess the risk a particular patient has to progress to cancer over a given period of time. The quantitative or qualitative assessment of risk of developing a cancer may rely on the use of mathematical or statistical modelling to predict the probability of developing cancer [25]. For example, the cumulative risk of carriers of BRCA1 and BRCA2 mutations, found in ductal carcinoma in situ [26], to develop breast cancer at age 70 was 57% (95% CI 47–66) and 49% (95% CI 40–57%) respectively [27]. Another example is the detection of mismatch-repair genes (primarily MLH1 and MSH2) mutations which can predict lifetime risk of colorectal cancer of about 80% in at risk families [28]. In keeping with this idea the low expression of MLH1 in normal colonic tissue has been suggested to predict, to some extent, the risk of developing adenomas [29].
(3) Prognostic marker: These are markers indicative of the probability of survival. Gene signatures were identified in breast and prostate cancer that outperformed

or provided additional value to the current clinical staging algorithms used to predict patient survival [30–32].

(4) Predictive markers: Markers predictive of therapeutic efficacy. Oestrogen receptor positivity is currently used as a predictor of response to targeted hormonal agent like tamoxifen [33] and HER2/NEU positivity for therapy with trastuzumab [34].

Diagnostic biomarkers and risk of progression markers are applicable to IEN and as this is the focus of the Monograph only these will be discussed further.

Sources of Biomarker Material

As mentioned earlier a potential biomarker can be tested from different specimens or sources which include blood or body fluids or ideally material from the lesion itself. However, the acquisition of human tissue, which can be done using a variety of techniques, such as biopsy, surgery, brushing, or scraping, remains a real hurdle to biomarker discovery and validation. In most cases, IENs with the most active biomarker research are those in which tissues are more readily accessible. These include IEN of the head and neck (oral and larynx), gastrointestinal tract (oesophagus, gastric and colonic), bronchus, cervix and skin (see disease specific chapters). The attraction of these is mainly practical. Even in situations where it is easy to obtain specimens, it is likely that there will be an associated morbidity. For example, endoscopic biopsying of the oesophagus or stomach carries a risk of perforation or bleeding of about 0.03%. Though this may seem uncommon, these small risks become significant when applied to a large number of individuals to test [35]. In other cases the very anatomical location of an organ makes it difficult to obtain tissue; for example the pancreas and ovaries require surgery or high risk procedures to collect tumour specimens.

Given the difficulties in accessing the tissues of interest directly, blood or body fluids are more appealing for the application of biomarkers as sample collection is less invasive, easier to perform and is the most cost-effective way to collect human samples [36]. Numerous biomedical studies have demonstrated that plasma protein levels reflect human physiological or pathological states and can be used for disease diagnosis and prognosis [16]. Various tumour products or products from pre-invasive tissue, like circulating cells, cell-free DNA and RNA, peptides, proteins and metabolites can be measured in the blood. However, these attractive sources of material have their own limitations. The chance of detecting a protein or any other solute specific to an IEN is likely to be small because of the total body volume and attempting to identify a specific biomarker in litres of blood, which contain abundant proteins, from a peripheral site will prove problematic [36]. In keeping with this there has been evidence of poor concordance between tissue and plasma concentration of variety of molecules [37–39]. Furthermore, the blood proteome is very sensitive to environmental changes and controlling for this has its own challenges. Depending on the localisation of the IEN, other body fluids such as nipple aspirate, urine, saliva, pleural

Table 9.1 Clinical condition affecting biomarker levels

Biomarker	Cancer type	Conditions affecting biomarker level
CA 125	Ovarian	Endometriosis [43] Heart failure [44] Hepatitis/Liver failure [42]
CA 19-9	Pancreatic	Chronic hepatitis [45] Cholestasis [42]
PSA	Prostate	Urinary tract infection [46] Benign prostatic hyperplasia [46]

effusion, ascites, bronchoalveolar lavage, synovial aspirate and cerebrospinal fluid [40] may be used. These are however likely to have the same limitations as blood.

Furthermore, cancer is often associated with inflammation and trying to tease out inflammatory markers from cancer markers may prove difficult [41] (see also Chap. 2). Diseases such as infections, hepatic and renal conditions, concomitant to the cancer may also influence the biomarker levels (Table 9.1). Benign tumours adjacent to an invasive tumour have also been reported to harbour increased expression of biomarkers. Life style factors like smoking and medical factors like medication including chemotherapy; instrumentation such as cystoscopy and laproscopy may influence the biomarkers [42]. It is therefore important to be aware of confounding factors when reporting test results.

In order to preserve the proteins and nucleic acid, in most instances, the tissue samples need to be flash frozen within minutes and stored at −80°C [47]. This may have cost implications, the timing of collection and preservation, method of extraction of nucleic acid, quantity of tissue may impact on sample quality and hence reliability of results [48, 49]. Measurements of α-fetoprotein, carcinoembryonic antigen and CA 125 are more readily affected by long-term frozen storage compared with frequent freezing-thawing, and CA 19-9 is generally relatively unstable [50]. The stability of PSA is critical and appropriate storage temperatures should be adhered to for reliable screening results [46].

Further to these purely practical hurdles, most countries require ethical approval for studies involving human participants and in many cases an integrated clinical team of research nurses and clinicians is required to streamline the collection process. This may prove very problematic for some scientists not actively involved in clinical collaborations.

Biomarker Development and Validation

Most biomarkers in current use were derived empirically and despite a large number of novel biomarkers proposed in the literature, very few have made it to the clinic. Indeed, the “omics” have streamlined the discovery process and opened the door to a wide variety of molecular markers ranging from genetic alterations (e.g. mutations, SNP, allelic loss, DNA content abnormalities, translocation) to epigenetic alterations (e.g. methylation, acetylation) and variation in expression of miRNA, mRNA or proteins (see Fig. 5, Chap. 16). Whether identified markers are single markers or signatures, stringent validation is required to ensure the clinical applicability of a given marker [37]. The more specific the design of the discovery experiment, the most likely it is to yield a biomarker test that will be validated across different centres and populations.

Phases of development of diagnostic biomarkers can be compared to some extent to drug discovery with a set of preclinical phases encompassing the discovery phase, internal and external validation phases usually in a retrospective setting and a set of clinical phases, usually prospective, testing the applicability of the test to the population of interest and to assess the health and economical benefits afforded. Under the impulsion of the National Institute of Health, the Early Detection Research Network (EDRN) there are published guidelines for the development of biomarkers of risk of progression to cancer [51] (Fig. 9.3). These guidelines, or rather their principles, can easily be applied to other types of biomarkers such as those described in Fig. 9.2.

As mentioned the discovery phase may be based on a candidate target approach or "omics" approach. The first validation phase in both cases assesses the presence of the marker in disease samples versus normal control samples or at different stages of the disease. Validation of diagnostic markers follows retrospective internal and external validation ideally in a multi-centred study to take into account regional or national variations. The prospective clinical phases assess the applicability of the test in the clinical setting of choice followed by a larger study testing the decrease in mortality afforded by the test. For predictors of risk biomarkers need to be assessed at different stages of disease progression (i.e. normal tissue, pre-malignant tissue and cancer tissue) and then in a case–control study in which patients who progressed to cancer are compared to non-progressors. This is followed by a prospective phase and then study one in which clinical management is modified depending on the results of the biomarker test.

Practical issues may hamper the development and validation of novel markers. For a biomarker to be clinically viable the technique used to measure it should be simple. Immunohistochemistry is used routinely in pathology departments across the world. Unfortunately technological issues way not permit the perfect biomarker to leave the confine of the research setting. For example, DNA content abnormalities, tetraploidy and aneuploidy, have been evaluated in a phase 4 study as defined by the

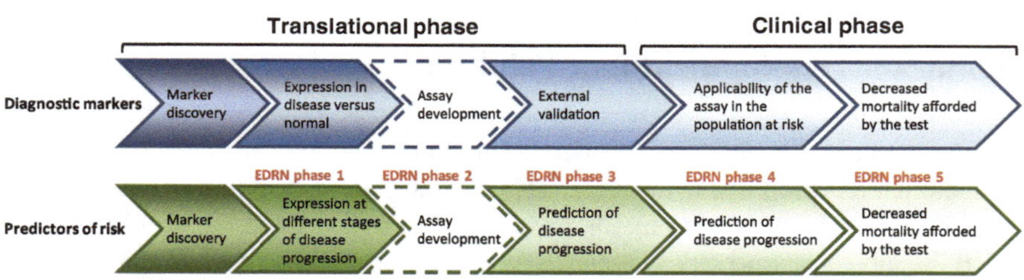

Fig. 9.3 Phases of biomarker development

EDRN and shown to accurately predict the risk of progression to adenocarcinoma in patient affected by its precursor, Barrett's oesophagus [52]. However, the methodology used to assess the markers is very technically demanding, expensive and requires state-of-the art research facilities. Unless alternative approaches are developed, these markers will not be used clinically despite their accuracy at assessing the risk of progression to cancer of patients with Barrett's oesophagus (see also Chap. 16). Cyclin D1 in the context of Barrett's oesophagus illustrates the point of external validation beautifully. Cyclin D1 overexpression was described as a marker of risk of progression in a relatively small cohort [53] and generated a lot of excitement in the Barrett's community. A few years later, the predictive risk of Cyclin D1 was not confirmed in a large population based cohort [54] (see also Chap. 16).

For a biomarker to be clinically useful the assays developed should be accurate and precise. An example of a complex clinical marker is epidermal growth factor receptor 2, *ERBB2* (referred to clinically as *HER2*). *HER2* is amplified in approximately 18–20% of breast cancers [55] (see also Chap. 20). *HER2* positivity predicts poor prognosis but also therapeutic response to trastuzumab treatment which improves time to progression and survival [34]. Given the significant cardiac events associated with trastuzumab [56] and the expenditure associated with such a drug, the accuracy of testing for *HER2* is essential for good patient management. Following FDA approval of testing for *HER2* by immunohistochemistry (IHC) and fluorescence *in-situ* hybridisation (FISH) based assays [11], the American Society of Clinical Oncology and College of American Pathologists has published guidelines for *HER2* testing [57, 58]. While both tests have merits, they also have disadvantages. Provided that the samples are preserved adequately [59], HER2 IHC is simple and straightforward; however patients with an intermediate score (2+) are considered equivocal thus requiring further confirmation of their status by FISH. FISH is more expensive and 3% of patients will have a score close to the accepted cut-off and will be considered equivocal [59]. The concordance between *HER2* gene amplification, FISH, and *HER2* protein overexpression assessed by IHC has been an issue and only 24% of specimens with 2+ immunostaining scores had HER2 amplification [60]. There are however disagreements with the current guidelines suggesting that because of concerns with tissue fixation and reproducibility of IHC, FISH should be the primary *HER2* test [61]. Furthermore, FDA also allowed pathology labs to develop their own assays, but around 26% of these assays at the local community testing do not correlate with the central labs [62].

Benefits of Biomarkers

Histopathology was and remains the "gold standard" for diagnosing established cancer and IEN. One of the main issues with pathological diagnosis is the delay in therapy. In more general terms, by the time a cancer becomes manifest on the standard histology slide, it has advanced far beyond the inception stage where the available curative therapies for cancer become ineffective. For IEN, the issues in pathology lie more with the difficulty in correctly diagnosing lesions. Very often, the lesions are small and associated with inflammation which may mask the extent of dysplasia. The grading of dysplasia is used to make important clinical decisions such as offering patients treatments that tend to be invasive and associated with a high physical or psychological morbidity such as oesophagectomy or prostatectomy. Worldwide, it has been recognised that early detection is central to reducing morality for many cancer types and that late presentation of patients which is a major cause for cancer mortality [63, 64]. Molecular alterations and secreted factors may allow for clinician to gauge the risk of a patient with a premalignant condition developing a cancer. In case of a high risk, the patient could be offered early, ideally non-invasive, treatment to eliminate the risk. Conversely, if the patient was considered to be at low risk, they could reassured and subsequently discharged from expensive clinical follow up, if appropriate. Barrett's oesophagus, the premalignant condition leading to oesophageal adenocarcinoma is a perfect example of this. Patients with Barrett's oesophagus are currently involved in an expensive and stressful clinical programme of repeated endoscopies to assess the presence of dysplasia and cancer [65]. However the low conversion rate of Barrett's to adenocarcinoma [66] means that most patients will never develop cancer but are still invited in two-yearly to yearly endoscopy. However, the recent development of a novel treatment called radiofrequency ablation, with low invasiveness compared to the standard of oesophagectomy, opens the possibility to offer treatment to patients with pre-invasive disease [67] (see also Chap. 12).

The development of screening tests, designed to detect IEN and/or early cancer in the population before symptom development, is also central to early diagnosis. Some of the screening tests rely on biomarkers such as PSA for prostate cancer [68], fecal occult blood for colorectal cancer [69] and so on. To be effective, screening tests need to be rolled out nationally and are as such regulated very tightly. Further to the development of the test per se, 23 stringent criteria, the Wilson-Jungner criteria, need to be met [70–72] (see Chap. 13).

Other biomarkers are used to offer additional information to the traditional histopathological assessment. For example α fetoprotein and human chorionic gonadotrophin in germ cell tumours are used in diagnosis but are also helpful in differentiating the type and stage of tumour [73]; and detection of BRAC 1 mutations is used both to inform on the risk of progression and for prognosis [74].

Despite the great promise of biomarkers to improve the diagnosis of cancers, very few have been approved by regulatory authorities and are in current clinical use.

Disease Specific Examples of Promising Biomarkers and Biomarkers in Clinical Use

Barrett's Oesophagus

There are currently no biomarkers in routine clinical use for the diagnosis of Barrett's oesophagus and associated cancers. A non-endoscopic screening test for

Barrett's oesophagus based on a novel sampling device called the Cytosponge and a biomarker, trefoil factor 3 (TFF3) is currently under assessment in a clinical trial based in the primary care (see also Chap. 16). This is the only biomarker in clinical trial in Barrett's oesophagus. However, during the last 20 years, there has been a wealth of interest in the identification of markers of risk of progression. No biomarker has made it to the clinic despite impressive data from the so-called "Seattle panel". This panel incorporates 9p and 17p LOH as well as DNA content abnormalities and patients harbouring all three of these have a relative risk of progression of 38.7 (95% CI 10.8–138.5; $p<0.001$) with a 5 year cumulative incidence of oesophageal adenocarcinoma of 79.1% compared to those with no abnormalities who had a 0% cumulative incidence of cancer [75]. The methodology used to assess the panel is not amenable to routine practice, however alternative approaches, such as the use of SNP array, are being developed [76, 77].

Prostatic Intraepithelial Neoplasia

Prostate-specific antigen (PSA) is an androgen-regulated serine protease, a member of the glandular kallikrein family. It is produced by normal prostate epithelial cells and its expression is confined to seminal fluid with concentrations 10^5 fold higher than in blood. During progression to cancer the architectural disruption of prostate gland leads to an increased release into the circulation to the same as in the semen [78]. The FDA approved PSA for monitoring patients after definitive treatment for prostate cancer in 1986 [78] and approval for diagnosis was granted in 1994 [78]. Not all patients enrolled in studies have prostate biopsies taken and since the number of biopsies taken during a single procedure influences the detection rate of cancer, calculating the precise sensitivity and specificity of PSA is difficult [78, 79]. A systematic review reported a sensitivity of 78–100% and specificity from 6 to 66% for total PSA, with the highest values being reported by the smallest studies [80]. A recent randomised control trial reported a positive predictive value of 24.1% (range, 18.6–29.6) [81]. Elevated levels have also been identified in cases with high-grade prostate intraepithelial neoplasia (HGPIN) [82]. In most cases, patients with HGPIN, are being followed up since up to 20% of these will develop a prostate cancer [82]. However, contrary to the oesophagus since prostate cancer are relatively slow to develop, there is no clinical pressure to detect all cases of HGPIN especially since, some argue that PSA for prostate cancer screening was adopted too early without strong enough scientific evidence [83] and it still remains unclear whether or not prostate cancer screening saves lives [84].

Colonic Adenomas

The detection of abnormal DNA and occult blood in stools are the most frequently used biomarkers for colorectal cancer screening. More than four different FDA approved faecal occult blood tests (FOBT) exist and are recommended by major societies for screening of colorectal cancer [85–87]. FOBT was recently demonstrated in a Cochrane Review to reduce mortality and incidence of colorectal cancer [88]. The sensitivity of faecal occult blood test ranges from 37.1 to 90.9% depending on the test used and on the size of lesion to detect [87]. The associated specificity is in the region of 90–95% [87]. A positive FOBT is generally followed by a colonoscopy during which any visible adenoma will be removed. The sensitivity of FOBT to detect adenomas of ≥10 mm ranges from 29.5 to 54.4%. It is not clear whether the practice of colonic adenoma removal reduces the risk of cancer development especially since a number of adenomas will be small, flat and undetectable.

Conclusions

The rapid expansion of potential biomarkers has driven a lot enthusiasm and hope for the early detection of many malignancies. To date, only a few tests have delivered on these promises and have been integrated into the clinical setting. Surprisingly, there are currently no biomarkers which were developed with the specific intent of diagnosing IEN which have been incorporated into routine clinical practice. The development of strict guidelines for the discovery and validation, akin to those available for the drug discovery, will lead to less empirical discovery and less application of improperly validated markers such as PSA. This will hopefully lead to higher quality data on biomarkers, but the worry is that researchers will be deterred from working in this area. Strong collaborative links between industry and academia will need to be developed to ensure a fast and reliable delivery of biomarkers. It is expected that the advent of targeted therapy will prime the major pharmaceutical companies to develop biomarkers side-by-side with their novel drugs or therapies.

Acknowledgements The authors are supported by the Medical Research Council, Cambridge Experimental Cancer Medicine Centre and the NIHR Cambridge Biomedical Research Centre.

References

1. Jones H (1848) On a new substance occuring in the urine of a patient with mollities ossium. Phil Trans R Soc Lond 138:55–62
2. Gutman A, Sproul E (1936) Significance of increased phosphatase activity of bone at the site of osteoblastic metastases secondary to carcinoma of the prostate gland. Am J Cancer 28:485–495
3. Yalow RS, Berson SA (1960) Immunoassay of endogenous plasma insulin in man. J Clin Invest 39:1157–1175
4. Bergstrand C, Czar B (1956) Demonstration of a new protein fraction in serum from the human fetus. Scand J Clin Lab Invest 8(2):174
5. Abelev G et al (1963) Production of embryonal alpha-globulin by transplantable mouse hepatomas. Transplantation 1:174–180

6. Tatarinov LS (1964) Detection of embryo-specific alpha-globulin in the blood serum of a patient with primary liver cancer. Vopr Med Khim 10:90–91
7. Gold P, Freedman SO (1965) Demonstration of tumor-specific antigens in human colonic carcinomata by immunological tolerance and absorption techniques. J Exp Med 121: 439–462
8. Thomson DM et al (1969) The radioimmunoassay of circulating carcinoembryonic antigen of the human digestive system. Proc Natl Acad Sci U S A 64(1):161–167
9. Kohler G, Milstein C (1975) Continuous cultures of fused cells secreting antibody of predefined specificity. Nature 256(5517):495–497
10. Bast RC Jr et al (1983) A radioimmunoassay using a monoclonal antibody to monitor the course of epithelial ovarian cancer. N Engl J Med 309(15):883–887
11. Ludwig JA, Weinstein JN (2005) Biomarkers in cancer staging, prognosis and treatment selection. Nat Rev Cancer 5(11):845–856
12. Hanahan D, Weinberg RA (2000) The hallmarks of cancer. Cell 100(1):57–70
13. Leon SA et al (1977) Free DNA in the serum of cancer patients and the effect of therapy. Cancer Res 37(3):646–650
14. Sidransky D et al (1991) Identification of p53 gene mutations in bladder cancers and urine samples. Science 252(5006):706–709
15. Sidransky D et al (1992) Identification of ras oncogene mutations in the stool of patients with curable colorectal tumors. Science 256(5053):102–105
16. Anderson NL, Anderson NG (2002) The human plasma proteome: history, character, and diagnostic prospects. Mol Cell Proteomics 1(11):845–867
17. O'Shaughnessy JA et al (2002) Treatment and prevention of intraepithelial neoplasia: an important target for accelerated new agent development. Clin Cancer Res 8(2):314–346
18. Fearon ER, Vogelstein B (1990) A genetic model for colorectal tumorigenesis. Cell 61(5):759–767
19. Kelloff GJ et al (2006) Progress in chemoprevention drug development: the promise of molecular biomarkers for prevention of intraepithelial neoplasia and cancer – a plan to move forward. Clin Cancer Res 12(12):3661–3697
20. Phillips KA et al (2006) Diagnostics and biomarker development: priming the pipeline. Nat Rev Drug Discov 5(6):463–469
21. Gutman S, Kessler LG (2006) The US Food and Drug Administration perspective on cancer biomarker development. Nat Rev Cancer 6(7):565–571
22. Biomarkers Definitions Working Group (2001) Biomarkers and surrogate endpoints: preferred definitions and conceptual framework. Clin Pharmacol Ther 69(3):89–95
23. Ryder SD (2003) Guidelines for the diagnosis and treatment of hepatocellular carcinoma (HCC) in adults. Gut 52(suppl 3):iii1–iii8
24. Punglia RS et al (2003) Effect of verification bias on screening for prostate cancer by measurement of prostate-specific antigen. N Engl J Med 349(4):335–342
25. Elmore JG, Fletcher SW (2006) The risk of cancer risk prediction: "What is my risk of getting breast cancer"? J Natl Cancer Inst 98(23):1673–1675
26. Smith KL et al (2007) BRCA Mutations in Women with Ductal Carcinoma In situ. Clin Cancer Res 13(14):4306–4310
27. Chen S, Parmigiani G (2007) Meta-analysis of BRCA1 and BRCA2 penetrance. J Clin Oncol 25(11):1329–1333
28. Markowitz SD, Bertagnolli MM (2009) Molecular origins of cancer: Molecular basis of colorectal cancer. N Engl J Med 361(25):2449–2460
29. Sidelnikov E et al (2009) MutL-Homolog 1 Expression and Risk of Incident, Sporadic Colorectal Adenoma: Search for Prospective Biomarkers of Risk for Colorectal Cancer. Cancer Epidemiol Biomark Prev 18(5):1599–1609
30. van de Vijver MJ et al (2002) A gene-expression signature as a predictor of survival in breast cancer. N Engl J Med 347(25):1999–2009
31. van 't Veer LJ et al (2002) Gene expression profiling predicts clinical outcome of breast cancer. Nature 415(6871):530–536

32. Glinsky GV et al (2004) Gene expression profiling predicts clinical outcome of prostate cancer. J Clin Investig 113(6):913–923
33. Early Breast Cancer Trialists' Collaborative Group (1998) Tamoxifen for early breast cancer: an overview of the randomised trials. Lancet 351(9114):1451–1467
34. Slamon DJ et al (2001) Use of chemotherapy plus a monoclonal antibody against HER2 for metastatic breast cancer that overexpresses HER2. N Engl J Med 344(11):783–792
35. Shaheen NJ et al (2002) Upper endoscopy as a screening and surveillance tool in esophageal adenocarcinoma: a review of the evidence. Am J Gastroenterol 97(6):1319–1327
36. Veenstra TD et al (2005) Biomarkers: mining the biofluid proteome. Mol Cell Proteomics 4(4):409–418
37. Hung KE, Yu KH (2010) Proteomic approaches to cancer biomarkers. Gastroenterology 138(1):46–51, e41
38. Hanash SM et al (2008) Mining the plasma proteome for cancer biomarkers. Nature 452(7187):571–579
39. Anderson L, Seilhamer J (1997) A comparison of selected mRNA and protein abundances in human liver. Electrophoresis 18(3–4):533–537
40. Hu S et al (2006) Human body fluid proteome analysis. Proteomics 6(23):6326–6353
41. Colotta F et al (2009) Cancer-related inflammation, the seventh hallmark of cancer: links to genetic instability. Carcinogenesis 30(7):1073–1081
42. Sturgeon CM et al (2009) Serum tumour markers: how to order and interpret them. BMJ 339:b3527
43. Muyldermans M et al (1995) CA125 and endometriosis. Hum Reprod Update 1(2):173–187
44. Duman C et al (2003) Elevated serum CA 125 levels in mitral stenotic patients with heart failure. Cardiology 100(1):7–10
45. Bertino G et al (2007) Meaning of elevated CA 19-9 serum levels in chronic hepatitis and HCV-related cirrhosis. Minerva Gastroenterol Dietol 53(4):305–309
46. Price CP et al (2001) Pre- and post-analytical factors that may influence use of serum prostate specific antigen and its isoforms in a screening programme for prostate cancer. Ann Clin Biochem 38(Pt 3):188–216
47. Tumor Analysis Best Practices Working Group (2004) Expression profiling – best practices for data generation and interpretation in clinical trials. Nat Rev Genet 5(3):229–237
48. Srinivasan M et al (2002) Effect of fixatives and tissue processing on the content and integrity of nucleic acids. Am J Pathol 161(6):1961–1971
49. Medeiros F et al (2007) Tissue handling for genome-wide expression analysis: a review of the issues, evidence, and opportunities. Arch Pathol Lab Med 131(12):1805–1816
50. Gao YC et al (2007) Effect of freeze-thaw cycles on serum measurements of AFP, CEA, CA125 and CA19-9. Scand J Clin Lab Invest 67(7):741–747
51. Sullivan Pepe M et al (2001) Phases of biomarker development for early detection of cancer. J Natl Cancer Inst 93(14):1054–1061
52. Chao DL et al (2008) Cell Proliferation, Cell Cycle Abnormalities, and Cancer Outcome in Patients with Barrett's Esophagus: A Long-term Prospective Study. Clin Cancer Res 14(21):6988–6995
53. Bani-Hani K et al (2000) Prospective study of cyclin D1 overexpression in Barrett's esophagus: association with increased risk of adenocarcinoma. J Natl Cancer Inst 92(16):1316–1321
54. Murray L et al (2006) TP53 and progression from Barrett's metaplasia to oesophageal adenocarcinoma in a UK population cohort. Gut 55(10):1390–1397
55. Slamon DJ et al (1987) Human breast cancer: correlation of relapse and survival with amplification of the HER-2/neu oncogene. Science 235(4785):177–182
56. Hayes DF, Picard MH (2006) Heart of darkness: the downside of trastuzumab. J Clin Oncol 24(25):4056–4058
57. Wolff AC et al (2007) American Society of Clinical Oncology/College of American Pathologists Guideline Recommendations for Human Epidermal Growth Factor Receptor 2 Testing in Breast Cancer. Arch Pathol Lab Med 131(1):18–43

58. Wolff AC et al (2007) American Society of Clinical Oncology/College of American Pathologists Guideline Recommendations for Human Epidermal Growth Factor Receptor 2 Testing in Breast Cancer. J Clin Oncol 25(1):118–145
59. Hicks DG, Kulkarni S (2008) HER2+ breast cancer: review of biologic relevance and optimal use of diagnostic tools. Am J Clin Pathol 129(2):263–273
60. Dybdal N et al (2005) Determination of HER2 gene amplification by fluorescence in situ hybridization and concordance with the clinical trials immunohistochemical assay in women with metastatic breast cancer evaluated for treatment with trastuzumab. Breast Cancer Res Treat 93(1):3–11
61. Sauter G et al (2009) Guidelines for Human Epidermal Growth Factor Receptor 2 Testing: Biologic and Methodologic Considerations. J Clin Oncol 27(8):1323–1333
62. Roche PC et al (2002) Concordance between local and central laboratory HER2 testing in the breast intergroup trial N9831. J Natl Cancer Inst 94(11):855–857
63. (2010) World Health Organisation, Screening and early detection of cancer: Early detection of cancer greatly increases the chances for successful treatment. http://www.who.int/cancer/detection/en/
64. Department of Health, Cancer Reform Strategy (2007) http://www.dh.gov.uk/en/Publicationsandstatistics/Publications/PublicationsPolicyAndGuidance/DH_081013
65. Reid BJ et al (2010) Barrett's oesophagus and oesophageal adenocarcinoma: time for a new synthesis. Nat Rev Cancer 10(2):87–101
66. Sikkema M et al (2010) Risk of esophageal adenocarcinoma and mortality in patients with Barrett's esophagus: A systematic review and meta-analysis. Clin Gastroenterol Hepatol 8:235–244
67. Shaheen NJ et al (2009) Radiofrequency ablation in Barrett's esophagus with dysplasia. N Engl J Med 360(22):2277–2288
68. (2008) Prostate cancer: diagnosis and treatment. http://guidance.nice.org.uk/CG58. Accessed 2 Mar 2010
69. Imperiale TF et al (2004) Fecal DNA versus fecal occult blood for colorectal-cancer screening in an average-risk population. N Engl J Med 351(26):2704–2714
70. Agency for Healthcare Research and Quality US Preventive Services Task Force (USPSTF) (2009) http://www.ahrq.gov/clinic/uspstfix.htm. Accessed 2 Dec 2009
71. Wilson JM, Jungner YG (1968) Principles and practice of mass screening for disease. Bol Oficina Sanit Panam 65(4):281–393
72. (2003) Structured review for the UK National Screening Committee – appraising the viability, effectiveness and appropriateness of an anal cancer screening programme. http://www.library.nhs.uk/screening/ViewResource.aspx?resID=60464. Accessed 23 Feb 2010
73. Bosl GJ, Motzer RJ (1997) Testicular germ-cell cancer. N Engl J Med 337(4):242–253
74. Robson ME et al (2004) A combined analysis of outcome following breast cancer: differences in survival based on BRCA1/BRCA2 mutation status and administration of adjuvant treatment. Breast Cancer Res 6(1):R8–R17
75. Galipeau PC et al (2007) NSAIDs modulate CDKN2A, TP53, and DNA content risk for progression to esophageal adenocarcinoma. PLoS Med 4(2):e67
76. Li X et al (2008) Single nucleotide polymorphism-based genome-wide chromosome copy change, loss of heterozygosity, and aneuploidy in Barrett's esophagus neoplastic progression. Cancer Prev Res (Phila Pa) 1(6):413–423
77. Paulson TG et al (2009) Chromosomal instability and copy number alterations in Barrett's esophagus and esophageal adenocarcinoma. Clin Cancer Res 15(10):3305–3314
78. Lilja H et al (2008) Prostate-specific antigen and prostate cancer: prediction, detection and monitoring. Nat Rev Cancer 8(4):268–278
79. Lin K et al (2008) Benefits and harms of prostate-specific antigen screening for prostate cancer: an evidence update for the U.S. Preventive Services Task Force. Ann Intern Med 149(3):192–199
80. Harvey P et al (2009) A systematic review of the diagnostic accuracy of prostate specific antigen. BMC Urol 9(1):14

81. Schroder FH et al (2009) Screening and prostate-cancer mortality in a randomized European study. N Engl J Med 360(13):1320–1328
82. Hekal IA (2008) The patients less than 50 years: is there a need to lower the PSA cutoff point? Prostate Cancer Prostatic Dis 12(2):148–151
83. Brawley OW (2009) Prostate Cancer Screening; Is This a Teachable Moment? J Natl Cancer Inst 101(19):1295–1297
84. Andriole GL et al (2009) Mortality results from a randomized prostate-cancer screening trial. N Engl J Med 360(13):1310–1319
85. Levin B et al (2008) Screening and Surveillance for the Early Detection of Colorectal Cancer and Adenomatous Polyps, 2008: A Joint Guideline from the American Cancer Society, the US Multi-Society Task Force on Colorectal Cancer, and the American College of Radiology. CA Cancer J Clin 58(3):130–160
86. Tumor Analysis Best Practices Working Group (2008) Screening for colorectal cancer: U.S. Preventive Services Task Force recommendation statement. Ann Intern Med 149(9):627–637
87. Whitlock EP et al (2008) Screening for colorectal cancer: a targeted, updated systematic review for the U.S. Preventive Services Task Force. Ann Intern Med 149(9):638–658
88. Hewitson P, et al (2007) Screening for colorectal cancer using the faecal occult blood test, Hemoccult. Cochrane Database Syst Rev (1):CD001216

Chapter 10
Molecular Imaging of Cancer and the Implications for Pre-invasive Disease

Scott K. Lyons and Kevin M. Brindle

Abstract The fluorescence microscope is a standard tool in any cell biology lab, enabling the visualisation of appropriately labelled probe molecules in the context of cell anatomy. These probe molecules can be used to image various aspects of cell physiology and biochemistry, for example, the levels of intracellular Ca^{2+}, the location, binding and mobility of specific proteins and, using gene reporter constructs, the transcriptional activity of specific genes. The techniques of molecular imaging allow similar measurements to be made deep inside the tissues of a living organism, for example in tumours in mouse models of cancer. Since many of the molecular imaging modalities that are employed in the laboratory can also be used clinically, the techniques of molecular imaging, in principle, also permit investigation of these fundamental aspects of tumour biology in the clinic. These techniques are set to play a key role in translational research, that is in translating our growing understanding of the cell biology of cancer and pre-invasive disease into new ways of detecting and treating the disease.

Introduction

Tumour detection and assessment of treatment response has, to date, relied principally on radiological measurements of tissue anatomy and tumour size respectively [1], using mainly X-ray computed tomography (CT) and magnetic resonance imaging (MRI). These measurements can lack sensitivity, often do not provide any prognostic information and, in the case of treatment response monitoring, cannot detect the

K.M. Brindle (✉)
Cancer Research UK, Cambridge Research Institute, Li Ka Shing Centre, Robinson Way, Cambridge CB2 0RE, UK
and
Department of Biochemistry, University of Cambridge, Tennis Court Road, Cambridge CB2 1GA, UK
e-mail: kmb1001@cam.ac.uk

R.C. Fitzgerald (ed.), *Pre-Invasive Disease: Pathogenesis and Clinical Management*, DOI 10.1007/978-1-4419-6694-0_10,

effects of those drugs which only arrest tumour growth rather induce tumour regression. The techniques of molecular imaging can provide more sensitive detection of a primary tumour and its possible metastases, can be used to stage and grade tumours and thus provide prognostic information and can detect treatment response long before there is any evidence of tumour regression [2–13].

The aim of "molecular imaging" is to transfer into a conventional image of tissue anatomy, information about underlying tissue biology and physiology. This may be accomplished, for example, by injection of an appropriately labelled probe molecule, which can then be imaged using a clinically applicable imaging modality, such as MRI, positron emission tomography (PET), single photon computed tomography (SPECT), ultrasound or some form of optical or near-infrared (NIR) imaging. The image of probe distribution can then be co-registered with an image of tissue anatomy, typically acquired using MRI or CT. In the case of a tumour this may, for example, involve a labelled probe molecule that binds to a receptor expressed on the tumour cell, whose expression may be increased by tumour progression and which may be down regulated following successful treatment. As our understanding of the molecular basis of cancer improves there will be further opportunities to design molecular imaging probes that report on specific aspects of a tumour's biology and the changes in this biology with tumour progression and treatment. This development has been facilitated by the availability of the clinical imaging modalities listed above in relatively high-resolution configurations that are suitable for imaging small animal models of disease, notably mice [14]. Techniques developed in the animal models can then be translated, fairly straightforwardly, to the clinic. This process of translation is also being helped by the development of mouse models of disease that more faithfully reproduce the molecular and physiological characteristics of the human disease [15]. Thus these models could be used both to develop new treatments and also the imaging methods that could then be used to determine whether these treatments are working in the clinic, possibly in an iterative way.

Molecular imaging techniques, particularly those that are MRI- or radionuclide-based, are relatively slow and expensive and it is unlikely that they will be used for patient screening, unless that patient population has already been heavily stratified, for example if genomic analyses indicate that the group is highly pre-disposed to develop a particular cancer. Instead molecular imaging is more likely to be used to locate tumour(s) in those patients that have already been identified as having disease, for staging and grading and for assessment of treatment response. In the latter case, by detecting early evidence of treatment response, imaging could be used to guide subsequent treatment, with ineffective treatments being discarded at an early stage allowing selection of the most effective treatment for the individual patient. However, for some molecular imaging techniques, for example optical and NIR imaging, and in some situations, it is feasible to use molecular imaging techniques to detect pre-invasive disease. Several optical endoscopy-based imaging methods have been used to screen and diagnose patients with tumours of the GI tract [16, 17] and lung [18]. For example, optical coherence tomography can be used to measure differential reflectance of infrared light to identify pre-malignant lesions on the luminal surface of the GI tract [16]. Autofluorescence and narrow-band imaging endoscopic methods have been used to detect pre-malignant oesophageal lesions in patients, either by measuring intrinsic differences in image contrast or differences in mucosal morphology between healthy and diseased tissue [17]. Novel tumour-specific fluorescent dyes have also been reported recently that can enhance endoscopic detection of dysplastic lesions in the colon. Regions of the colon that appear suspect under white light can be sprayed with these dyes and then washed, with pre-malignant lesions retaining the fluorescent label [19]. Prostate cancer can grow so slowly that many patients will die with the disease rather than of the disease, however if the cancer does metastasise then there is currently no cure and the cancer becomes lethal. MRI measurements of tissue morphology and ^{1}H MR spectroscopic imaging measurements of tissue metabolite levels have shown some promise for detecting the more aggressive tumours that are likely to metastasise [20]. This information can then be used to guide subsequent therapy.

Genomic analyses of tumour biopsies, including microarray analyses of mRNAs and miRNAs and tumour genome sequencing are already impacting prognosis and predicting individual patient responses to specific drugs [21]. Proteomic analyses of serum samples may help with the detection of disease and in predicting response to treatment [22]. These "omic" methods are complementary to those of imaging and indeed may assist in the identification of new molecular imaging targets that report on specific aspects of the disease, its progression and its response to treatment. Imaging, however, has some important advantages. The techniques are non-invasive and therefore allow longitudinal monitoring of disease development and treatment response at multiple disease foci. The imaging methods cover the entire tumour, which may often be grossly heterogeneous, and with higher resolution imaging techniques, such as MRI, information can be obtained from specific regions within a tumour. Obtaining this information by biopsy would be difficult, if not impossible, moreover the data may be biased by the selection of biopsy site within the tumour. The biopsy needle may even miss the tumour. In the prostate, for example, biopsy sampling error, even when ultrasound-guided, can lead to false negative rates as high as 40% [23].

In this review we outline the physical principles behind those molecular imaging techniques that have been used in the clinic and show, with examples, how they can be used to detect, stage and monitor the treatment response of tumours. We also discuss preclinical studies that should facilitate the development and translation of new imaging probes and molecular imaging techniques to the clinic. Radiology has traditionally been a discipline that images tissue anatomy, in the future, using the techniques of molecular imaging, it will also become a discipline that images tissue biology, biochemistry and physiology.

Magnetic Resonance Imaging and Spectroscopy

MRI can give excellent images of soft tissues, such as tumours (Fig. 10.1). The technique works by mapping, in 3D, the distribution and MR properties of tissue water protons, which are very abundant (60–70 M) and is a mainstay of any hospital Radiology Department. MRI was first described in the early 1970s [24] and its development led to the award of the Nobel Prize for Physiology and Medicine

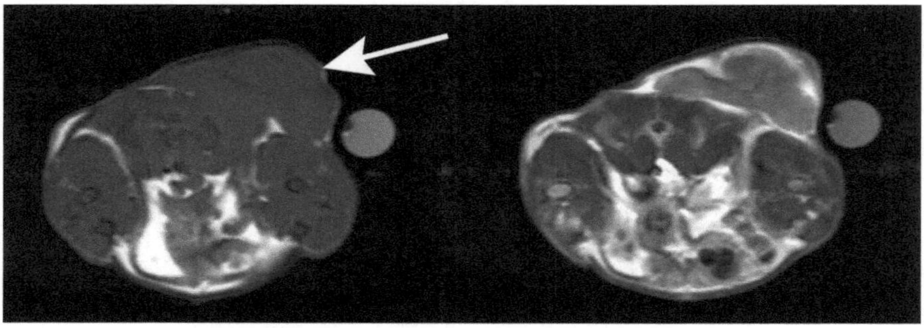

Fig. 10.1 The pre-contrast image on the *left* shows a tumour on the lower flank of a mouse (*arrowed*). The image on the *right* was acquired a few minutes after the intravenous injection of a Gd^{3+}-based contrast agent, which gives positive contrast. The low molecular weight agent readily exits the leaky vasculature, enhancing signal from the tumour. Images courtesy of Dr Mikko Kettunen

to Paul Lauterbur and Sir Peter Mansfield in 2003. Magnetic resonance, in the form of magnetic resonance spectroscopy (MRS), can also be used to detect non-invasively small molecule metabolites in tissues. These studies, which again began in the early 1970s, started with ^{31}P MRS measurements of ATP, Pi, phosphocreatine and sugar phosphates in skeletal muscle [25, 26]. There were also early ^{31}P MRS studies in tumours, which demonstrated that tumours had relatively high levels of the phosphomonesters, phosphocholine and phosphoethanolamine [27, 28], when compared to other tissues (a typical ^{31}P NMR spectrum of a tumour is shown in Fig. 10.2).

A detailed discussion of the physical principles of this technique is beyond the scope of this review and the reader is referred to some excellent textbooks in this area [29, 30]. However, a brief introduction is necessary if the reader is to understand the potential and also the limitations of the techniques of MRI and MRS.

Some atomic nuclei possess the property of spin. The combination of spin and charge results in a magnetic dipole and, when placed in a magnetic field, the spins will tend to align with field. However, it is such a weak interaction that there are nearly an equal number of spins aligned against the field. For spin ½ nuclei, such as ^{1}H, ^{31}P and ^{13}C, there are two allowed energy levels. The lower energy level corresponds to spins aligned with the field and the higher energy level against the field. There is a slight excess of spins in the lower energy level and as a result a net magnetization (M_z) or polarization that lies along the field direction (B_0) (Fig. 10.3). At the magnetic field strengths commonly used in the clinic (1.5–3 T; the earths magnetic field is ~60 μT) the excess of spins in the lower energy level amounts to only a few ppm and it is this very low level of polarization that is responsible for the insensitivity of magnetic resonance techniques when compared to the other imaging modalities.

The magnetic dipoles associated with the spins do not simply align with the applied magnetic field (B_0) but precess about it at a frequency (ω) that is a characteristic of the particular atomic nucleus, which is given by its gyromagnetic ratio (γ),

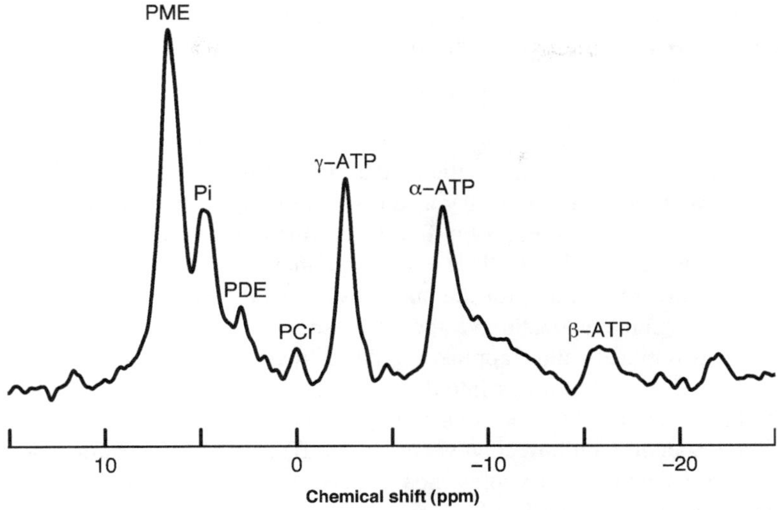

Fig. 10.2 Localised ^{31}P MR spectrum from an implanted tumour in a mouse. The spectrum shows signals from the γ-, α- and β-phosphates of nucleoside triphosphates (predominantly ATP), from phosphocreatine, which is from underlying muscle tissue, from phosphodiester compounds (PDE), such as glycerophosphorylcholine, from intracellular inorganic phosphate (the chemical shift or frequency of this resonance can be used to determine intracellular pH) and phosphomonoesters (PME), which are predominantly phosphocholine and phosphoethanolamine. The low intensity of the β-ATP resonance, which should be comparable in intensity to the other ATP resonances, is an artefact of the pulse sequence used to localise signal from the tumour. Data courtesy of Drs Mikko Kettunen and Mariagnese Barbera

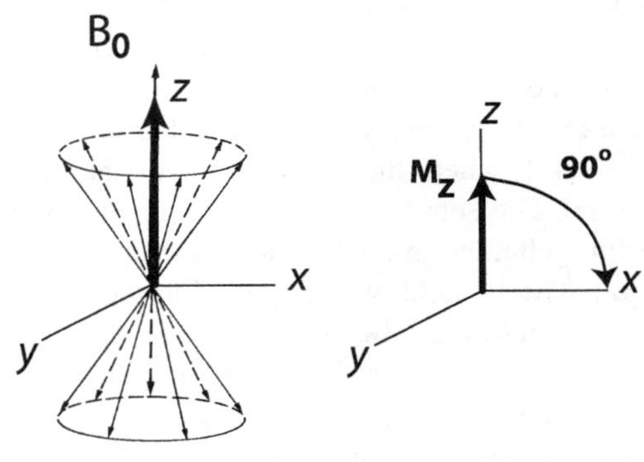

Fig. 10.3 Spin ½ nuclei can align with or against the field. There is a slight excess of spins aligned with the field (lower energy), which gives rise to a net magnetization (M_z) lying along the direction of the main magnetic field (B_0). Application of an oscillating magnetic field (B_1) at right angles to the main magnetic field, and resonant with the spin precession frequency, induces transitions between the two energy levels and tips the net magnetization (M_z) into the *x-y* plane

and which is a linear function of the applied magnetic field (B_0). At a field of 9.4 T, for example, ^1H spins precess at 400 MHz, ^{31}P at 162 MHz and ^{13}C at 100 MHz.

$$\omega = \gamma B_0$$

If we apply an oscillating magnetic field at right angles to the main field, B_0, and which rotates at the same frequency as the spin precession frequency (ω) i.e. it is resonant with the spin precession frequency, then we will induce transitions between the two energy levels. This is the phenomenon of nuclear magnetic resonance. It is more convenient, for the purposes of this discussion, to consider what happens to the net magnetization vector (M_z) associated with the ensemble of spins. This will now rotate about the applied oscillating magnetic field (see Fig. 10.3) and as a result we can tip this vector into the *x-y* plane, where it gives rise to a signal in the NMR receiver coil (this coil is also often used to apply the oscillating magnetic field, B_1). Depending on how long we apply the B_1 field will determine where the net vector associated with the spins ends up. The B_1 field is typically applied in the form of a pulse (called a radiofrequency or r.f. pulse); a 90° pulse will tip M_z fully into the *x-y* plane, while a 180° pulse (which is twice the length of the 90° pulse) will tip it along the $-z$ direction. When in the *x-y* plane the individual vectors will dephase, due to B_0 field inhomogeneties (the variations in B_0 will cause them to precess at different frequencies) and also to lose amplitude due to spin–spin interactions or spin–spin relaxation. This spin–spin relaxation is a first order process and is described by the time constant T_2, which is typically in the msec range. If T_2 is short then there is a rapid loss of signal in the *x-y* plane. The recovery of the magnetization along the M_z or B_0 field direction is also a first order process and is described by the spin lattice relaxation time T_1, which is typically in the sec range. This relaxation process is determined by dipole–dipole interactions between the spins and between the spins and their environment ($T_1 \geq T_2$).

The precessional frequency of the spins is modulated by their chemical environment. The surrounding electrons produce varying degrees of shielding of the B_0 field and hence relatively small changes in frequency. This is known as chemical shift and is expressed in ppm of the B_1 frequency. For ^1H the chemical shift range is typically 10 ppm (so for ^1H at 9.4 T, where the resonance frequency is 400 MHz, 10 ppm corresponds to 4,000 Hz). This sensitivity to chemical environment is what has made NMR such a powerful technique in analytical chemistry and for protein structure determination [31, 32]. The B_1 field, when applied in the form of a high intensity pulse, has a large bandwidth (the bandwidth, Δv, is $\approx 1/t_p$, where t_p is the pulse width, so a 10 μs pulse will have a bandwidth of ~100 kHz). Following the B_1 pulse all the resonances are excited simultaneously and their magnetization vectors will precess at different frequencies in the *x-y* plane and decay according to their T_1 and T_2 relaxation times. Fourier transformation of these signals, which are acquired simultaneously, turns this amplitude – time domain signal into an amplitude – frequency domain spectrum, where position on the *x* axis indicates frequency or chemical shift (Fig. 10.2). Because of the lack of sensitivity, the B_1 pulse may be repeated multiple times (depending on the time resolution and signal-to-noise required) and the resulting signals averaged to improve the signal-to-noise ratio, which increases as the square root of the number of scans. The peak intensities are proportional to the number of spins and the peak width at half maximum is $\approx 1/\pi T_2$.

Imaging works by frequency encoding space. Imagine a sphere of water in a homogeneous magnetic field (B_0) (Fig. 10.4). A ^{1}H spectrum of this sphere will give a single peak from the protons in the water molecules. If we superimpose on the main magnetic field, B_0, a linear magnetic field gradient across the sample, for example along the *z* axis (G_z), then since frequency is a linear function of the magnetic field strength the spins will resonate at different frequencies according to their position in this gradient. If we acquire a spectrum in the presence of this gradient then we will get a profile of the sphere in the *z* direction. This is the essence of all imaging and localised spectroscopy experiments. Images are acquired using a series of r.f. pulses and gradient pulses in the *x*, *y* and *z* directions. A fuller description of imaging is beyond the scope of this chapter and the reader is referred to an excellent and very readable text on this subject [30].

MRI has the advantages over X-ray CT that it doesn't use ionizing radiation and image contrast for soft tissues is much greater. Moreover, this contrast can be manipulated, by the use of appropriate r.f. pulse sequences, to interrogate some aspects of tissue biology. For example, deoxygenated haemoglobin is paramagnetic and its presence can be detected in T_2-weighted images, where it results in loss of signal intensity. The exploitation of this phenomenon in imaging of human brain function is well known (functional or fMRI) [33]. Increased neuronal firing, in response to some stimulus, causes an increase in blood flow to the region of the brain affected, without a corresponding increase in oxygen consumption. As a result there is a decrease in the level of deoxygenated haemoglobin in that region of the brain and consequently an increase in signal intensity in a T_2-weighted image. This has proved to be a very powerful method for mapping human brain activity in response

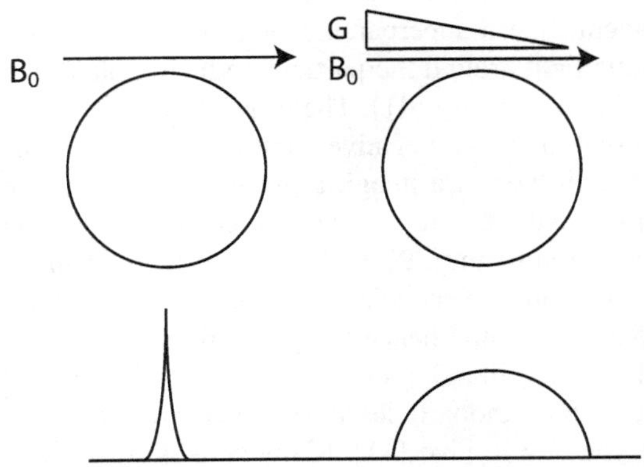

Fig. 10.4 Consider a sphere of water in a uniform magnetic field (B_0). This will give rise to a single resonance in the ^{1}H MR spectrum. If we superimpose a linear magnetic field gradient (G) on the main magnetic field, then the resulting ^{1}H MR spectrum will give a profile of the sphere of water in the direction of the gradient

to specific stimuli or mental tasks [34]. In tumours this so called BOLD (Blood Oxygen Level Dependent) effect can be used to detect changes in tumour blood flow, for example in response to carbogen breathing [35].

The MRI experiment is intrinsically sensitive to diffusion. If there is rapid diffusion of the water molecules during the imaging pulse sequence then this can lead to loss of signal intensity, an effect which is increased by the inclusion of diffusion-weighting magnetic field gradients within the pulse sequence [36]. By incrementing these gradient pulses it is possible to measure the apparent diffusion coefficient (ADC) of the water molecules. In a tumour these ADC measurements are sensitive to the cellularity of the tumour and can be used to detect a decrease in cellularity following a positive response to treatment [37, 38]. For example, in glioma patients ADC measurements were used to detect response to treatment before there was evidence of tumour regression [39].

Molecular imaging using ^{1}H MRI of tissue water can be accomplished using paramagnetically labelled probe molecules. These can be detected through the effects that they have on the water T_1 and T_2 relaxation times. A T_1 agent, like a Gd^{3+}-chelate (Gd^{3+} has seven unpaired electrons and is highly paramagnetic) can cause rapid T_1 relaxation of water protons. If signal is acquired rapidly, that is the next B_1 pulse is applied before the magnetization has had time to relax back along the z axis, then less signal will be obtained with the next and successive B_1 pulses and the signal becomes "saturated". The Gd^{3+}-chelate, by accelerating relaxation along the z axis, relieves this saturation and thus increases signal intensity in the image. It is a positive contrast agent (see Fig. 10.1). Since water molecules coordinated with the Gd^{3+} (inner sphere relaxation) exchange rapidly with the bulk water the effect is amplified and it has been estimated that as little as 100 μM contrast agent can be detected in this way in tissue [40]. Note, however, that this sensitivity is poor when compared with the pM sensitivity of radionuclide imaging (see below). The paramagnetic Gd^{3+} also increases T_2 relaxation, but the effects of this on image intensity can be minimised by appropriate choice of imaging pulse sequence. A T_2 agent, like a superparamagnetic iron oxide (SPIO) nanoparticle, distorts the magnetic field around the particle, inducing rapid dephasing in the x-y plane and loss of signal intensity [41]. The drawback of these agents as molecular imaging probes is that they give negative contrast, which in a tumour can be difficult to detect, although there are imaging pulse sequences that can turn this into positive contrast [42], and they are relatively large (10–50 nm). This large size can restrict tissue penetration of the SPIO-labelled probe molecule, even in a tumour where the vasculature can be very leaky, and perhaps more importantly clearance of unbound probe molecule and hence the generation of tissue contrast. Of course this is not a problem if the imaging target is presented in the vasculature [43]. An application where SPIO nanoparticles have proved to be very useful is for cell labelling and cell tracking in vivo [41]. Many cells will readily endocytose SPIO nanoparticles (and also micron sized particles which are even more sensitive to detection [44]) and accumulate these in endocytic vesicles, where they distort the magnetic field way beyond the cell's plasma membrane. Thus, even though MR image resolution in the clinic (1–2 mm) is not at a cellular level, the fact that the field distortion extends beyond the cell, and thus water molecules moving in the vicinity of the cell are affected, means that effectively single cells can be detected using this technique [44]. The technique has already been used in the clinic to track implanted dendritic cells in melanoma patients [45].

The simplest molecular imaging probes used in MRI are the non-targeted Gd^{3+}-chelates that have been used in the clinic to image tumour perfusion and vascular permeability. The agent is injected intravenously and then a series of rapidly acquired T_1-weighted images are collected and used to estimate changes in tumour contrast agent concentration as the agent extravasates into the tumour interstitium (so called dynamic contrast agent enhanced (DCE) MRI). By fitting these data to appropriate kinetic models estimates can be made of the vascular volume and permeability [46], although the relatively small size of these agents (500–1,000 Da) makes estimates of permeability problematic and this is perhaps better achieved using macromolecular agents, which cross the vessel walls more slowly [47]. Macromolecular contrast agents suited to this task, and which could be used clinically, are in development [48]. The increased permeability of tumour vasculature, which is often the result of tumour angiogenesis and increased endothelial cell proliferation [49], means that these agents also allow ready visualisation of tumours (Fig. 10.1).

One of their main applications in clinical oncology has been to assess the efficacy of drugs targeted at the tumour vasculature; anti-vascular drugs that selectively disrupt tumour vasculature and anti-angiogenic drugs that inhibit the growth of new blood vessels [49–52]. Since these drugs often do not produce tumour regression their effects cannot be assessed using the standard RECIST criteria [1], which are based on tumour size. Drug-induced changes in tumour vascular function, however, can readily be detected using DCE MRI. For example, in patients that showed a positive response to treatment with an anti-angiogenic agent there were significantly greater reductions in a pharmacokinetic parameter related to vessel permeability than in those patients with progressive disease [53]. DCE-MRI was used to evaluate the efficacy of the anti-vascular drug, combretastatin A4 phosphate, in a phase-I clinical trial, where tumour perfusion was shown to be decreased in eight out of ten patients with advanced solid malignancies [54].

The Gd^{3+}-chelates can be engineered so that accessibility of water to the paramagnetic metal is a function of some aspect of the tumour microenvironment; perhaps the most interesting of these from the perspective of tumour biology are the pH-sensitive agents [55]. The low extracellular pH in tumours, which is due to a number of factors, including increased lactic acid production, reduced interstitial fluid buffering and reduced perfusion, has been correlated with both prognosis and response to treatment [56]. However, determination of tissue pH using these agents is challenging since an independent estimate of contrast agent concentration in the tissue is required in order to calculate the pH from the change in water signal intensity [57]. Various approaches are being tried to address this issue, although none of these agents has yet progressed to the clinic. Another class of agents in this group assess pH in a different way, by exploiting the fact that the chemical shift of water bound to some lanthanides is very different from free water and is pH dependent. This bound water is then detected by measuring exchange of magnetization between the free and bound water, due to chemical exchange, and which is manifest as a decrease in intensity of the free water resonance when the bound water resonance is selectively saturated [58].

SPIO nanoparticles and Gd^{3+}-chelates can be attached to various ligands and used as targeted imaging probes. An antibody against the Her2/neu receptor, which is up-regulated on some breast cancer cells, was labelled with SPIO nanoparticles and with Gd^{3+}-chelates and used to image these cells in vitro and in a tumour xenograft in vivo [59, 60]. In the latter case the antibody was biotinylated and then linked to avidin, to which Gd^{3+}-chelates had been attached covalently. The integrin $\alpha_v\beta_3$, which is up-regulated on proliferating endothelial cells and is thus a marker of tumour angiogenesis, was imaged in an animal tumour model using an antibody labelled with liposome-encapsulated Gd^{3+}-chelates [61]. The attachment of multiple paramagnetic ions in the liposome increased the sensitivity of detection. This integrin has also been imaged in animal tumour models using integrin-binding peptides, containing the arginine–glycine–aspartic acid (RGD) motif, that had been labelled with paramagnetic nanoparticles [62]. Tumour cell death post-treatment has been imaged using paramagnetically-labelled proteins that bind the phosphatidylserine that is exposed on the surface of apoptotic cells and on the interior of necrotic cells [63–65]. An example is shown in Fig. 10.5.

Targeted MRI probes have the advantage over radionuclide-labelled probes that they do not involve the use of ionizing radiation, which makes them easy to handle, and image resolution is much better, which is a particular advantage for small animal imaging. However, the large size of some of these agents can make tissue penetration

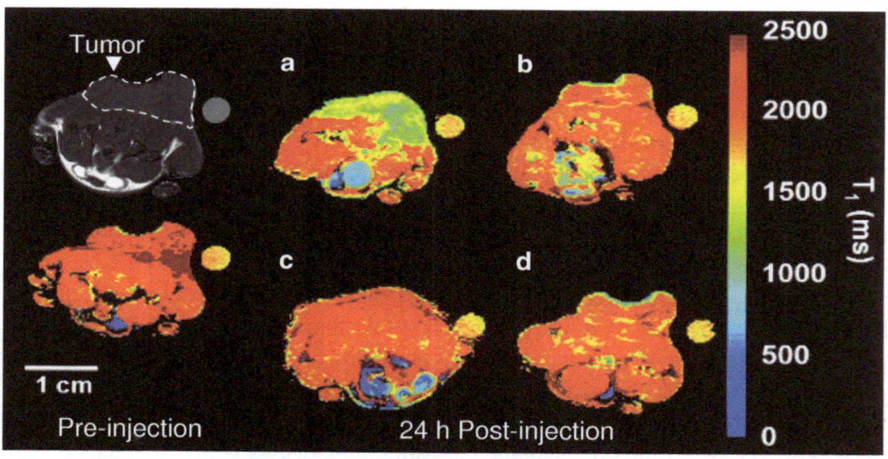

Fig. 10.5 Detection of treatment-induced tumour cell death using a targeted MRI contrast agent that binds phosphatidylserine. The *top left image* shows a conventional gray scale image of tissue water. The tumour margin is outlined. The false colour images show the concentration of the targeted contrast agent; the "colder" the colour the higher the concentration of the agent. The *bottom left image* was acquired prior to injection of the contrast agent. Image (**a**) shows accumulation of the contrast agent in a drug-treated tumour 24 h after injection of the agent. There was very little accumulation in non-treated tumours (**c**). Images (**b**) and (**d**) were acquired from drug-treated and non drug treated animals respectively, which had been injected with a site-directed mutant of the targeted agent that no longer bound phosphatidylserine. Reproduced, with permission, from [65]

and clearance more difficult and while they avoid the use of ionizing radiation there may be a toxicity hazard. The recent toxicity problems encountered with a low molecular weight Gd^{3+}-chelate used in the clinic, in patients with renal insufficiency, signals a potential problem for any targeted Gd^{3+}-based MR contrast agent. The toxicity in these patients was thought to be due to the long lifetime of the agent in the body, which can simply be avoided by not giving these agents to such patients [66]. However, it seems inevitable that most targeted agents will have a long half-life in the body and therefore for this reason it would seem prudent to be cautious about their possible future use in the clinic. Another potential problem with transferring these agents to the clinic is simply the amount of material that is required, which is a reflection of their relative insensitivity when compared to radionuclide-labelled agents. While this is not a problem for a 25 g mouse the amount required for a 70 kg man could be prohibitively expensive. As far as we are aware there are currently no targeted MR imaging agents that have been approved for clinical use.

Magnetic resonance spectroscopy is unique amongst the molecular imaging techniques in terms of the wealth of chemical information that it can provide, being capable, in principle, of providing a profile of tissue metabolites in a non-invasive manner. However, these metabolites are present in only mM concentrations, about $10^4\times$ less than the water protons used for imaging, and in practice the limited sensitivity of the technique means that data acquisition times are long and resolution is relatively poor, with single voxels in localised spectroscopy of 1–8 cm^3, or with spectroscopic imaging resolutions of 0.25–1 cm^3 [67, 68]. Even then only a handful of metabolites can be detected. Nevertheless, this limited set of detectable tumour metabolites can be used to give useful information in the clinic on tumour grade and treatment response.

The early ^{31}P MRS studies showed that tumours were often characterised by relatively high levels of choline-containing metabolites and, in general, elevated levels of phosphocholine (PC) were associated with tumour cell proliferation and decreases with a positive response to treatment [28]. The level of choline kinase, the first enzyme in the pathway of phosphatidylcholine biosynthesis and which is responsible for the synthesis of PC from choline and ATP, was shown to be increased in biopsy material from animal and human tumours. Ras oncogene transformation was shown to stimulate choline kinase activity, leading to increased levels of PC. However, the relatively low sensitivity of ^{31}P compared to ^{1}H MRS (6.6 relative to proton at 100) and the fact that these metabolites often give resolved resonances in the ^{1}H as well as the ^{31}P MR spectrum, has meant that, in the clinic, the tumour levels of these phospholipid metabolites have tended to be investigated using ^{1}H spectroscopy.

The choline metabolite profile is being used increasingly as an adjunct for diagnosis of primary malignant tumours in the breast, prostate and brain and decreases in the levels of choline-containing compounds in these tumours following treatment have been shown to be predictive of treatment response [69, 70]. Prostate epithelial cells synthesize and secrete large quantities of citrate and so the ^{1}H spectra of healthy prostate tissue are characterized by resonances from citrate, whereas in spectra taken from regions of prostate cancer, citrate and polyamines are reduced or absent, while choline is elevated. The ratio of the resonances: Citrate/(Choline+Creatine) is commonly employed to distinguish between prostate cancer, benign prostatic hyperplasia and normal tissue, and to grade malignancy [71], where a linear correlation has been demonstrated between the decrease in citrate and elevation of choline with the pathologic Gleason score [20]. The use of ^{1}H spectroscopic imaging, in addition to conventional MRI in the initial diagnosis of prostate cancer, has also been shown to improve the localization of the disease [72, 73]. In the brain the Choline/N-acetyl aspartate (NAA) ratio has been demonstrated as a prognostic marker to distinguish low- and high-grade disease in astrocytomas [74, 75] and the Choline/Creatine ratio can differentiate high- from low-grade oligodendroglial tumors [76]. In meningioma, a mostly benign disease, decreased NAA [77] or elevated levels of alanine and glutamate [78] are markers of the disease. Multivariate statistical analysis has been applied to these tumour-type specific changes in metabolite profiles and used to develop pattern recognition techniques that can classify brain tumours with 89% accuracy [79]. The hope is that imaging alone could be used to provide a diagnosis, avoiding the requirement for biopsy with its associated morbidity.

^{1}H spectra can provide a measure of the steady state concentrations of some tumour metabolites, however they tell us little of the dynamics of tumour cell metabolism. For this we either need to acquire a series of spectra following some form of perturbation or to introduce an isotopically labelled cell substrate whose metabolites can be detected in the tumour. The ^{13}C nucleus is NMR-active and only 1.1% naturally abundant, which means isotope labelling studies can be performed with ^{13}C-enriched cell substrates. However, ^{13}C is even less sensitive to NMR detection than the ^{31}P nucleus (1.6 relative to the ^{1}H at 100), and so kinetic and imaging studies in the clinic are challenging. Nevertheless, measurements have been made of muscle and liver glycogenesis using ^{13}C-enriched glucose [80]. Recently a technique has been described, which can increase sensitivity in the ^{13}C NMR experiment by more than 10^{4}-fold [81]. In this technique, which has been termed dissolution dynamic nuclear polarization (DNP), the ^{13}C-labelled cell substrate of interest is mixed with a stable free radical and rapidly frozen to form a glass. The sample is then cooled in a bath of liquid helium under vacuum to ~1.2 K and placed in a magnetic field. At this temperature the electron spins on the radical become almost completely polarized. This polarization is then transferred, by microwave irradiation, to the ^{13}C spins and polarizations in excess of 50% can be achieved in the solid state. The sample is then rapidly warmed to room temperature, with little loss of polarization, using pressurized superheated buffer (~180°C at ~10 bar) and injected into the biological system of interest, for example into the tail vein of a tumour-bearing mouse (Fig. 10.6). The huge gain in sensitivity means that we can now image the hyperpolarized ^{13}C-labelled molecule (the expected spatial resolution in the clinic is of the order of 2 mm) and, more importantly, the kinetics of its metabolic conversion into other cell metabolites. The technique promises new insights into the dynamics of tissue metabolism in vivo, both in the laboratory and in the clinic [82]. A drawback of the technique, however, is that the polarization, which is determined by the spin lattice relaxation time (T_1) of the hyperpolarized spin, is relatively short-lived. If the ^{13}C label is placed in a COOH group, where

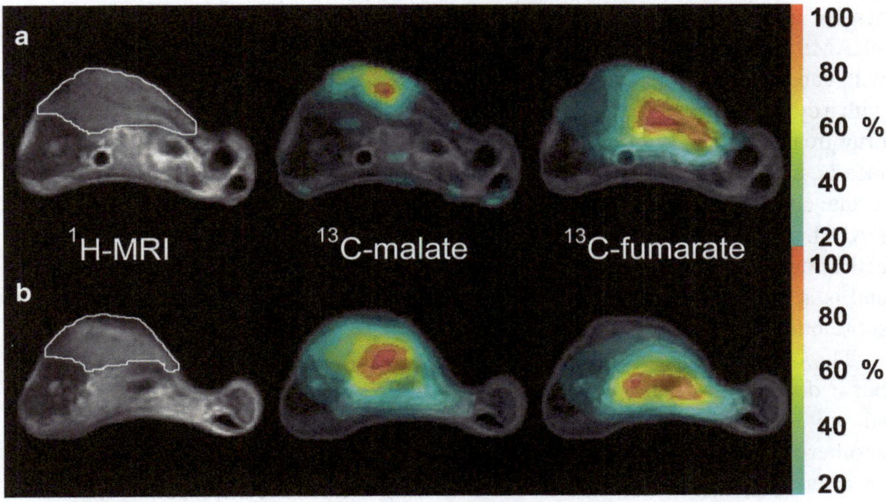

Fig. 10.6 The images on the *left* are conventional ^{1}H images of an implanted murine lymphoma tumour before (**a**) and after drug treatment (**b**). The tumour margins are indicated. The images on the *right* are false colour images of signal from hyperpolarised [1,4-^{13}C]malate and fumarate following intravenous injection of hyperpolarized [1,4-^{13}C]fumarate. The increased malate signal in the drug-treated tumour is thought to be due to tumour cell necrosis. Images adapted, with permission, from [87]

there are no directly bonded protons, the T_1 can be as long as 30–40 s in vivo. However, this still means that the material must be injected and any imaging experiments accomplished within the 2–2.5 min before the polarization has decayed. Moreover, the imaging experiment must make very efficient use of the spin polarization since each excitation pulse inevitably destroys some of the polarization [82]. Another fundamental requirement is that the labelled hyperpolarized molecule must rapidly gain access to the tissue of interest, be rapidly transported into the cell and its subsequent metabolism must be fast, such that there is significant metabolism of the molecule within the life time of the polarization. Despite these limitations numerous studies have now been published in mice and in larger animals, which have demonstrated the potential of the technique and a clinical trial with hyperpolarized ^{13}C-labelled pyruvate in prostate cancer is expected to begin soon.

Most of the studies to date have used hyperpolarized [1-^{13}C]pyruvate. The label can exchange with alanine or lactate, in the reactions catalysed by alanine aminotransferase or lactate dehydrogenase respectively, or lost as CO_2, in the irreversible reaction catalysed by mitochondrial pyruvate dehydrogenase. The exchange reactions are readily observable in tumours, however there appears to be insufficient PDH activity in tumours to give significant hyperpolarized $^{13}CO_2$ production, although this reaction has been observed in heart muscle [83]. There is good evidence that the flux of label between pyruvate and lactate in tumours is due mainly to exchange between the labelled pyruvate and an endogenous lactate pool rather than net conversion of pyruvate to lactate [84]. The high levels of tumour lactate are a well-known consequence of the high levels of aerobic glycolysis that characterise many tumours (the "Warburg effect") [85]. In the TRAMP model of prostate cancer the degree of lactate labelling was shown to correlate with cancer development and progression [86]. In a murine lymphoma model treated with a cytotoxic agent, the degree of lactate labelling was markedly reduced at 24 h after drug treatment [84]. This decrease in labelling was thought to be due to a number of factors, including loss of LDH activity, loss of tumour cellularity, a decrease in tumour lactate concentration and a decrease in the concentration of the coenzymes NAD+ and NADH. The latter was shown to be due to drug-induced DNA damage and consequent activation of poly-ADP ribose polymerase (PARP), which uses NAD+ as a substrate and is activated as part of the DNA damage response. Remarkably, PARP activation substantially depletes the cells of NAD(H).

The labelled pyruvate experiment indicates that the drug has damaged the cells but it doesn't necessarily mean that the cells have actually died. In a subsequent study it was shown that drug-induced tumour cell necrosis could be detected using another hyperpolarized ^{13}C-labelled cell substrate, [1,4-^{13}C]fumarate. Fumarate is an intermediate in the Krebs cycle and is converted into malate in the reaction catalysed by intramitochondrial fumarase. In viable cells transport of fumarate across the cell and/or mitochondrial membrane is too slow for there to be significant conversion of hyperpolarized [1,4-^{13}C]fumarate to malate within the lifetime of the polarization. However, when this permeability barrier is removed by the onset of cellular necrosis there was a marked increase in the rate of malate production and hyperpolarized [1,4-^{13}C]malate was observed in the drug-treated tumour [87] (see Fig. 10.6).

Another interesting substrate from the perspective of tumour cell metabolism is glutamine. As well as providing nitrogen for amino acid and nucleotide biosynthesis it also an important respiratory substrate in tumour cells. Glutaminase, an intramitochondrial enzyme, converts glutamine to glutamate, which undergoes transamination to form α-ketoglutarate, which can then be oxidised in the Krebs cycle, providing reduced coenzymes for oxidative phosphorylation and ATP synthesis. [5-^{13}C]glutamine has been hyperpolarised and its uptake and conversion to glutamate in a human heptoma cell line (HepG2) was sufficiently rapid to allow detection within the lifetime of the polarisation (the T_1 is this case was only ~16 s).

Since glutamine utilisation has been correlated with cell proliferation this may be used in vivo to detect the effects of cytostatic drugs, in much the same way as ^{18}FLT has been used in PET [88]. However, the levels of polarisation obtained were relatively modest (~5%) and these would need to be improved before this experiment could be used to image tumour responses to cytostatic drugs in vivo. Moreover, it is not yet clear whether all tumour cell types have sufficient glutamine transport rates and glutaminase activity to make this technique applicable generally.

The low extracellular pH in tumours has been imaged by intravenous injection of hyperpolarised ^{13}C-labelled bicarbonate into tumour-bearing mice [89]. The labelled bicarbonate is rapidly converted into carbon dioxide in a pH-dependent reaction that is near-to-equilibrium in the body. The reaction is catalysed by carbonic anhydrase, although the non-catalysed reaction is also extremely rapid. Thus the ratio of the ^{13}C signal intensities from bicarbonate and carbon dioxide can be used to estimate the pH using the Henderson Haselbalch equation:

$$pH = pKa + \log_{10}\left[\frac{HCO_3^-}{CO_2}\right]$$

A ratio image, obtained by dividing the CO_2 image by the bicarbonate image, can be used to calculate a map of tumour pH (Fig. 10.7). Since a low tissue pH is a characteristic of various disease states, including cancer, this is potentially a very powerful measurement that could be used in the clinic to detect the presence of disease and its response to treatment. Currently there are no practicab le methods for imaging tissue pH in the clinic.

Since these hyperpolarised ^{13}C-labelled cell substrates are endogenous molecules, that have already been safely infused into humans at relatively high concentrations, there is a reasonable expectation that these will translate into clinical application in the future.

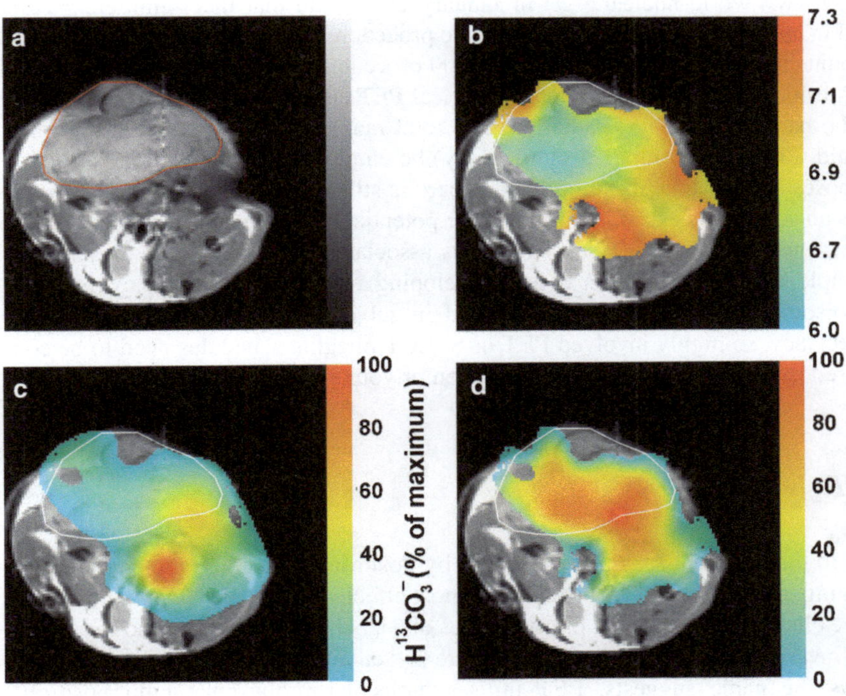

Fig. 10.7 Image (**a**) shows a ^1H image of an implanted murine lymphoma. The tumour margin is indicated. Image (**c**) is a ^{13}C image of hyperpolarized $H^{13}CO_3^-$ obtained immediately following intravenous injection of hyperpolarized $H^{13}CO_3^-$. Note the high levels of signal in an underlying blood vessel. Image (**d**) shows the corresponding ^{13}C image of hyperpolarized $^{13}CO_2$. The ratio of these two images can be used to calculate a pH image (**b**). Note the relatively low extracellular pH in the tumour. Images adapted, with permission, from [89]

Radionuclide-Based Imaging Techniques

Positron Emission Tomography (PET) and Single Photon Emission Computed Tomography (SPECT) are non-invasive molecular imaging techniques that rely upon the detection of radio-labelled molecules. Both techniques possess excellent sensitivity when compared to other imaging techniques, such as MRI (e.g. PET $\leq 10^{-12}$ mol/L, SPECT $\leq 10^{-11}$ mol/L and MRI $\leq 10^{-5}$ mol/L [90]). Overlying tissue does not significantly attenuate signal, so trace quantities of probe can be visualised and accurately quantified from deep tissue locations in the body. However, the resolution of both techniques is relatively low (≥5 mm for PET and SPECT in the clinic, ~1 mm for PET and ≤1 mm for SPECT in the laboratory) and images typically comprise a map of signal intensity without providing anatomic detail.

SPECT imaging is performed in the clinic more often than PET, largely because the hardware and running costs are lower and the necessary infrastructure is much more widespread. Indeed, figures released by the World Nuclear Association (http://www.world-nuclear.org/) in January 2010 state that the γ-emitter ^{99m}Tc is used in about 80% of all nuclear medicine procedures performed worldwide, which amounts to an approximate total of 70,000 procedures per day.

A critical issue when considering clinical PET and SPECT is the total exposure of the patient to ionising radiation. The total radiation dose will increase further should CT (X-ray computed tomography) be employed for attenuation correction purposes at each imaging time point. There is still some debate over what constitutes an acceptable exposure limit and the potential benefits resulting from multiple scans must be balanced against the risks associated with radiation exposure. For example, the risk of a cancer patient developing a secondary malignancy related to radioisotope exposure will be increased in subjects with a predicted long life-expectancy, so highly involved PET or SPECT imaging schedules need to be considered carefully prior to imaging children or young adults [91].

PET

Due to the excellent sensitivity afforded by Positron Emission Tomography (PET) imaging, this technique is currently the most effective molecular imaging modality in the clinic. PET can detect pM quantities of a labelled molecule and so can detect, non-invasively, targets in the body that are present at very low concentrations.

As the name suggests, PET utilises molecular probes that emit positrons, although the positron itself is not detected directly. Once emitted, the positron passes through tissue until it encounters an electron. This results in an annihilation event which produces two 511 keV gamma rays that travel in opposite directions relative to one another. The PET scanner comprises a ring of scintillation detectors that encircle the subject and this arrangement allows for the detection of coincident gamma rays produced from a single annihilation event (see Fig. 10.8). The origin of positron annihilation is then computed by analysing thousands of independent coincidence events.

The resolution of PET is relatively low and is affected by the energy of the emitted positron (i.e. higher energy positrons tend to travel further from source prior to annihilation) but is typically ~5–8 mm in the clinic and ~1 mm with small animal preclinical scanners.

As the annihilation of a positron results in the generation of two gamma rays, which always have an energy of 511 keV, it is not possible to differentiate the signal produced by multiple labelled probes simultaneously. Any given PET probe must therefore be cleared by the body or decay prior to the imaging of a second probe. Although the energies of the γ-rays emitted from a positron annihilation event are relatively high and can readily pass through tissue, there are greater levels of attenuation when passing through bone than soft-tissue and this can affect the determination of probe concentration. The introduction of clinical PET/CT scanners has largely alleviated this problem as they allow a CT scan to be taken prior to the PET scan to generate a map of γ-ray transmission throughout the body. This CT image subsequently enables attenuation correction of the final PET image and more accurate localisation and quantification of signal [92]. Another technique, termed time of flight PET (TOF PET), has also been used to further improve the localisation of the annihilation event within the body. The method relies upon very fast detectors to measure the very small time difference (currently limited to 600 ps) between

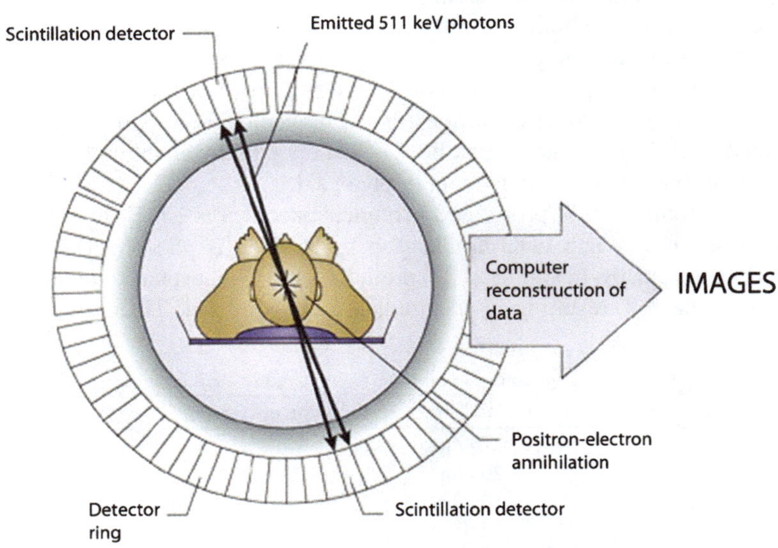

Fig. 10.8 The detector arrangement in a PET scanner. This enables the detection of coincident 511 keV γ-rays that result from the annihilation of a positron with an electron. Image reproduced with permission from [12]

coincident detection events that arise from a single annihilation event, thus enabling the mapping of the annihilation event along the line of response [93].

Various positron emitting isotopes (see Table 10.1) can be used to label a PET probe and these possess different properties in terms of their emission energies, half-life ($t_{1/2}$) and the chemistry associated with probe incorporation. As many positron-emitting isotopes possess a relatively short $t_{1/2}$, an efficient and rapid protocol for probe synthesis is a prequisite for PET. An advantage of PET is that it allows for true isotopic labelling of endogenous cell substrates, for example substitution of naturally abundant ^{12}C with the positron emitting isotope of carbon, ^{11}C. Thus the incorporation of ^{11}C as a positron source will not affect the molecule's chemistry. A major consideration with ^{11}C however is the associated short $t_{1/2}$ (20 min). Its use therefore necessitates that the imaging facility is in close proximity to a cyclotron, in which PET isotopes are generated. Several examples of useful ^{11}C-labelled PET probes include ^{11}C-labelled methionine, which has shown promise for staging glioma in the clinic [94]. Also ^{11}C-labelled acetate, which has shown utility for imaging tumour cell metabolism in a broad variety of tumour types, but in particular may prove most useful for imaging the metabolism of tumours that are not glucose avid (e.g. the prostate) [95].

Another positron-emitting isotope, which is of both preclinical and clinical interest, is ^{64}Cu. Compared to many of the commonly employed positron-emitting isotopes, ^{64}Cu has a relatively long half-life, which means that it can be synthesised in bulk from a centralised facility and shipped to distant imaging facilities. The long half-life is also favourable for labelling probes that have a long life-time in the circulation, for example antibodies, and which are therefore cleared slowly. Further, because ^{64}Cu decays by both positron and gamma emission, this could prove a useful isotope for therapeutic purposes as well as for PET imaging. A novel copper-chelator, called SarAr [96], has been described recently that can very stably retain copper under physiological conditions and a monoclonal antibody labelled with this chelate has demonstrated the utility of ^{64}Cu imaging by enabling PET imaging of both neuroblastoma and melanoma in vivo [97].

The most common PET probe used in clinical oncology is 2-[^{18}F]fluoro-2-deoxy-D-glucose (FDG). When FDG is taken up by a cell it is phosphorylated, in the reaction catalysed by hexokinase, to produce FDG 6-phosphate, which is then retained by the cell, resulting in accumulation of radiolabel. There are two main

Table 10.1 Positron emitting isotopes commonly employed in PET imaging

Positron (β+) emitting isotope	Half-life	Emission energy (keV)	Decay product
^{18}F	110 min	633	^{18}O
^{11}C	20 min	960	^{11}B
^{13}N	10 min	1,199	^{13}C
^{15}O	2 min	1,732	^{15}N
^{124}I	100 h	1,535	^{124}Te
^{68}Ga	68 min	1,899	^{68}Zn
^{64}Cu	12.7 h	653 – β+ (17.9%)	^{64}Ni
		579 – β– (39%)	^{64}Zn

reasons why this probe is so successful at detecting a variety of tumours and their response to therapy. Many tumour types are glucose avid and take up glucose at higher rates than normal tissue. It is also well established that many tumour cells exhibit significantly higher rates of aerobic glycolysis compared to normal cells (the Warburg effect) [85]. Effective tumour treatment perturbs both glucose uptake and cellular metabolism. FDG-PET scans taken before and after treatment can therefore provide the clinician with an early indicator of drug efficacy. If little or no effect is detected, non-responding patients can be identified rapidly and alternative tumour management strategies can be considered [10].

However, several tumour types are difficult to image with FDG PET, in particular brain and prostate tumours. Normal brain tissue is also highly glucose avid whereas prostate tumours tend to have relatively low rates of glucose metabolism and non-metabolised FDG is excreted in the urine [98]. In both cases, high levels of background compared to signal compromise the ability to detect tumours residing close to these locations.

Several other PET probes have been developed to image various aspects of tumour biology and have the potential to influence clinical management of the disease.

A good example is [^{18}F]-Galacto-RGD, which has been used to image tumour angiogenesis and exploits the high affinity between the arginine-glycine-aspartate (RGD) peptide motif and the $\alpha_v\beta_3$-integrin receptor. Studies have shown that [^{18}F]-Galacto-RGD uptake correlates well with $\alpha_v\beta_3$-integrin expression levels and not with overall tumour size across a broad range of human tumour types [99]. The exceptions to this correlation arose largely from tumour types that also express $\alpha_v\beta_3$-integrin on their cell surface (e.g. melanoma cells in lymph node metastases). Expression of the $\alpha_v\beta_3$-integrin has been suggested to be a marker of metastatic potential and so this probe could also prove useful as a prognostic indicator and for non-invasive tumour staging. Sequential PET scans of metastatic lesions with [^{18}F]-FDG and [^{18}F]-Galacto-RGD look different, which adds support to the notion that [^{18}F]-Galacto-RGD PET imaging enables the measurement of a qualitatively different aspect of tumour biology in vivo (i.e. angiogenesis) that cannot be measured by imaging glucose metabolism [100].

Another PET probe, ^{18}F-fluoroestradiol ([^{18}F]-FES), has been used to image the estrogen receptor status of human breast tumours [101, 102]. A high level of the receptor on the surface of breast cancer cells has been associated with a positive outcome to hormone therapy and so it is useful to be able to measure the receptor status of patients non-invasively prior to treatment. Other studies have shown that sequential imaging regimens with [^{18}F]-FES and [^{18}F]-FDG provide complimentary read-outs for predicting and assessing breast tumour treatment response to Tamoxifen. [^{18}F]-FES PET uptake was shown to correlate well with predicted outcome to treatment. In treatment responders, [^{18}F]-FDG uptake was seen to increase (termed a metabolic flare) 7–10 days after treatment, whereas the levels of [^{18}F]-FDG uptake remained unaffected in non-responders [103].

Several PET probes have also been developed to image apoptosis, a common mechanism that underlies the effects of many effective cancer treatments in the clinic. The development of imaging methods that enable the sensitive detection of apoptosis would therefore offer a very powerful means to rapidly evaluate the efficacy of clinical intervention.

An early biomarker of apoptosis is the appearance of phophatidylserine (PS) on the outer surface of the plasma membrane. Annexin V, a 35 kDa protein that has a high affinity for PS, has been used as an imaging probe for apoptosis. A ^{18}F-labelled derivative of annexin V has been used in preclinical PET studies to detect apoptosis in tumours following drug treatment [104] and a ^{99m}Tc-labelled derivative of annexin V is currently undergoing clinical trials as a SPECT imaging probe (see next section). Another apoptosis-specific PET probe currently in development is [^{18}F]-ML-10 or ApoSense [105]. This is a much smaller molecule (206 Da) than annexin V, which should improve tissue bioavailability and also clearance of unbound material and hence the generation of tissue contrast. It is believed that this molecule gives an apoptosis-specific readout by being able to cross the plasma membrane of early stage apoptotic cells in a caspase-dependent manner. Interestingly, ML-10 does not accumulate in cells with disrupted membranes and so does not detect necrotic cell death. Another probe described recently, [^{18}F]ICMT-11, which is based on istatin sulphonamide, detects apoptosis by binding to the activated forms of caspase 3 and 7 (two of the effector proteins of apoptosis) [106]. In a preclinical study this molecule showed increased cellular uptake and retention in apoptotic tumour cells within 24 h of drug treatment in vivo, although a high background was observed in the liver and intestine, which may limit future clinical applications in the abdomen.

Labelled fluoromisonidazole or [^{18}F]FMISO has proven useful for imaging tumour hypoxia. Low levels of oxygen are often present within tumours because of high cellular demand and poor supply and this can affect the outcome of treatment, especially radiotherapy. Techniques to measure non-invasively the levels of tumour hypoxia in vivo would therefore be useful for the clinical management of the disease. In normoxic conditions, [^{18}F]FMISO can diffuse freely through tissue. In low oxygen conditions however, [^{18}F]FMISO is reduced and retained in hypoxic cells.

FMISO-PET imaging has been shown to be useful in predicting treatment response of patients with non-small cell lung carcinoma, head and neck cancer and glioblastoma multiforme [107, 108]. The relationship between hypoxia, as determined by FMISO-PET, and treatment outcome may be context-dependent. For example, a recent study found no clear correlation between hypoxia (as determined by FMISO-PET) and treatment outcome for a cohort of patients with head and neck cancer receiving cisplatin and radiotherapy treatment [109]. Another recent preclinical study found a poor correlation between HIF1α levels and activity (a biomarker of hypoxia) and the accumulation of FMISO [110]. This discrepancy can potentially be explained if intratumoural hypoxia is a transient and dynamic process, as FMISO labelling only offers a "snap-shot" view of tissue hypoxia upon administration. Alternatively, it could be that the levels of hypoxia detected by imidazole-containing compounds are less physiologically relevant than HIF1α biomarker readouts.

The relative abundance of somatostatin receptors have also been imaged with PET using a molecule called Dotatoc [111], however, this topic will be discussed further in Sect. 3.2 (see SPECT).

Several PET reporter transgenes have been developed, including a virally derived thymidine kinase (HSV1-*tk*) and a sodium iodide symporter (NIS). HSV1-*tk* can phosphorylate a range of synthetic nucleoside analogues (based upon pyrimidine or acycloguanosine structures) that are poor substrates for the endogenous mammalian thymidine kinase. These nucleosides are retained by the cell upon phosphorylation, thus HSV1-*tk* labelled cells accumulate radiolabel over time relative to non-labelled cells. Various nucleoside-based probes can be used in conjunction with HSV1-*tk* to image labelled cells by PET including [^{18}F]FIAU, [^{18}F]FMAU, [^{18}F]FEAU and [^{18}F] FHGB [112–114]. Further, HSV1-*tk* can also be used as a therapeutic transgene since it can activate the pro-drug gancyclovir into a cytotoxic form [115, 116]. An engineered mutant transgene called HSV1-sr39tk has been reported that confers greater imaging sensitivity relative to HSV1-*tk* since it exhibits preferential kinase activity with synthetic nucleosides over activity with thymidine [117]. The sodium iodide symporter (NIS), which is expressed naturally by the human thyroid gland, where it transports iodine, can also be used as a gene reporter. Radiolabelled isotopes (^{123}I, ^{124}I or ^{99m}TcO4-pertechnetate) have been shown to be actively pumped into NIS-expressing tumour cells in the laboratory, thus conferring a specific imaging readout for PET or SPECT. Expression of NIS may also confer a potential radiotherapeutic benefit (with ^{131}I) [118–122].

Reporter transgene based PET imaging approaches have to date proven most useful as a means of assessing the efficiency of therapeutic gene delivery and persistence of therapeutic gene expression in gene therapy studies or for tracking the progress of cell based therapies, both in the lab and in the clinic [120, 123–126]. As discussed in Sect. 4.1, reporter transgene-based imaging methods can also confer a high degree of versatility in terms of imaging readout. This is true also for PET reporter transgenes and tumour related PET imaging readouts for p53 response, hypoxia and HSP70 response have all been described in preclinical studies [127–129].

Combined PET/CT scanners can provide functional information (PET) with anatomical context (CT), as well as enabling attenuation correction of clinical PET scans. Significant effort is now also being made in the development of combined PET/MRI scanners. As outlined in Sect. 2, many MRI-based techniques have been developed that enable the clinician or researcher far greater insight into the biology of cancer than simply anatomy alone. For example, [^{18}F]-FDG PET is regularly used to measure the efficacy of cancer treatments in the clinic, however, a drop in signal post-treatment could be explained by either a decrease in tumour cell viability or a down-regulation of glucose transporter expression. The ability to simultaneously perform diffusion-weighted MRI on such a subject to assess viable cell density [39] would therefore be very informative in this regard. Further, unlike MRI, the use of CT involves exposing the patient to an additional amount of ionising radiation.

The combination of MRI and PET presents a significant technical challenge as the PET detectors must be functional in a high magnetic field and the MRI scan must be functional in the presence of γ-ray detection hardware. Significant progress has been made however, and combined scanners have been demonstrated recently in both the laboratory and the clinic [130, 131]. Efforts have also been made to develop MRI-based attenuation correction algorithms for PET scans [132, 133].

SPECT

SPECT relies upon the detection of molecular probes labelled with γ-emitting isotopes. Unlike PET, in which co-incident γ-rays striking the detector ring aid computation of the position of the signal, SPECT probes emit single γ-rays that travel in random directions through the subject. Consequently, to deduce the origin of γ-emission, collimators are needed to restrict the γ-rays that reach the detector to a defined angle. This in turn means that, with a conventional parallel-hole collimator, only a small percentage (~0.02%) of emitted γ-rays reach the detector, which reduces the sensitivity of SPECT relative to PET. However, as the γ-rays are emitted directly from the SPECT probe, unlike the γ-rays generated by positron emission, the resolution of SPECT is theoretically greater than that of PET.

The development of multi-pinhole collimators has dramatically improved the resolution and sensitivity of small animal SPECT in the laboratory (see Fig. 10.9). Because emitted γ-rays travel in a straight line, pinhole collimation has a magnification effect on the image (reviewed in [134]), in a manner similar to the pinhole cameras and projectors from the Victorian era. Upon de-magnification, the resultant image has significantly better resolution than an equivalent image taken with parallel collimation. Further, if the subject is placed close to the pinhole, significant sensitivity gains can also be achieved. Following acquisition, sophisticated software algorithms are used to reconstruct an image from the multiple projections produced by the multi-pinhole collimators, the result being sub-millimetre resolution and approximately a tenfold gain in sensitivity [134]. This collimation approach is less well suited to imaging human-sized subjects but can still be effective if the field of view is substantially reduced.

The isotopes routinely employed in SPECT imaging (see Table 10.2) are not usually found in biologically relevant molecules. This means that the γ-emitter cannot be incorporated into a probe via the substitution of a native atom, but requires attachment, for example in the case of the metals, via a chelating group (e.g. DOTA) [135]. This can be viewed as advantageous in one respect, as the labelling of a molecule with a chelate can greatly simplify the radio-chemistry of probe synthesis. This can also be viewed as a disadvantage, however, as the addition of a chelate group to a molecular probe will alter the overall size, shape and charge of the molecule, which in turn may give rise to differences in biodistribution in vivo and biological activity relative to the native molecule. Another useful feature of SPECT isotopes, such as ^{111}In, is that the radiochemistry required to label a probe is very similar to that of ^{68}Ga, thus a PET probe counterpart can be rapidly developed from a validated SPECT probe [135]. Since the energy of γ-ray emission from the commonly used SPECT isotopes are also very different, the simultaneous detection of multiple SPECT probes in a patient is possible [136–138], although not performed routinely in the clinic.

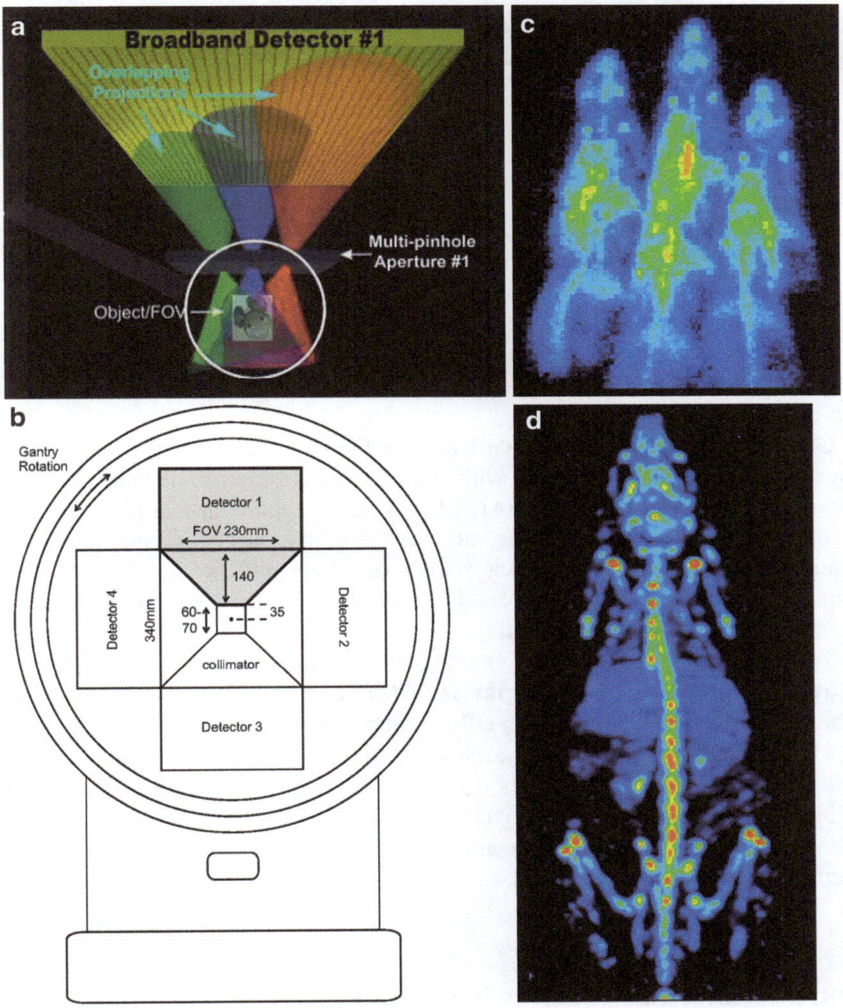

Fig. 10.9 The principles of multi-pinhole SPECT. Image (**a**) illustrates how multiple pinholes result in the projection of magnified and overlapping images onto a single γ-detector. Image (**b**) illustrates how four of the detectors depicted in (**a**) are organised around the bore of a multi-pinhole SPECT system. Image (**c**) depicts what an overlapping multi-pinhole SPECT projection looks like prior to image processing. Image (**d**) shows the processed image from (**c**). Images kindly provided by Dr Christian Lackas and Dr Staf Van Cauter, Bioscan Inc

Many of the imaging probes mentioned in the previous section on PET have also been labelled with γ emitters and used in SPECT imaging studies. For example, a ^{99m}Tc-labelled version of annexin V, ^{99m}Tc-HYNIC annexin V [139], has shown promise as a generic marker of tumour cell death in the clinic [140].

Table 10.2 Radio-isotopes commonly used in preclinical and clinical SPECT imaging

γ (β−) emitting isotope	Half-life	Energy (keV)	Decay product
^{99m}Tc	6 h	140	^{99}Tc
^{123}I	13 h	159	^{123}Te
^{111}In	67 h	245 172	^{111}Cd
^{67}Ga	78 h	70–80	^{67}Zn
^{125}I	60 days	35[a]	^{125}Te

[a]Energy too low for effective clinical imaging

Other notable and clinically applicable SPECT probes that have tumour-specific targets, which have not yet been addressed in this review, include probes that target the somatostatin receptor and probes that measure multi-drug resistant p-glycoprotein expression levels.

Octreoscan (Mallinkrodt Medical), an ^{111}In-DPTA labelled form of octreotide, is a synthetic somatostatin analogue with high binding affinity for the family of somatostatin receptors (sst1 to sst5) [141, 142]. These receptors and in particular sst2, are abundantly expressed, relative to normal tissue, in a variety of malignant human tumours, including neuroendocrine, small cell lung and breast tumours. Once bound, the receptor-ligand complex is internalised by the cell, which results in tumour-specific retention of signal.

^{99m}Tc-MIBI (^{99m}Tc-methoxyisobutylisonitrile) has been used as a means of assessing the relative expression levels of MDR1 and MRP1 in tumours. These genes encode transmembrane drug efflux pumps and confer a drug-resistant phenotype to tumours when overexpressed. Poor uptake of ^{99m}Tc-MIBI correlates strongly with MDR1 and MRP1 overexpression and so enables prediction of which tumours will respond well to chemotherapy [143]. ^{99m}Tc-MIBI has also been used clinically as a means to differentiate malignant and benign lesions since it shows preferential retention in malignant cells [144].

Optical Molecular Imaging Techniques

Optical techniques rely upon the detection of visible or near-visible light to image tumour biology non-invasively. There are primarily two distinct modalities that are used for this purpose; bioluminescence and fluorescence imaging. The former is at present used solely for preclinical research and relies upon the detection of chemiluminescence resulting from the oxidation of a substrate catalyzed by a reporter protein. The latter technique, from a molecular imaging standpoint, has also been used primarily in a preclinical context. In a fashion similar to the radionuclide imaging techniques described in Sect. 3, a molecule can be converted into a fluorescent imaging probe by attaching a fluorescent moiety prior to administration in vivo. Alternatively, target cells may be labelled with a reporter gene that expresses a fluorescent protein, and a broad range of colours are available [145].

Fluorescence imaging techniques are now also being applied in the clinic to aid surgeons determine tumour resection boundaries and to map sentinel lymph nodes in cancer patients in real time [146, 147]. Wavelengths in the near-infrared (NIR) region of the spectrum (between 700 and 1,000 nm) transmit most efficiently through tissue, with longer and shorter wavelengths being absorbed by water and haemoglobin respectively. This so-called tissue "window" is being exploited by fluorescence-based molecular imaging techniques through the use of labels that excite and emit in this wavelength range [148].

Bioluminescence Imaging

Bioluminescence Imaging (BLI) is a sensitive, versatile, low cost and relatively high-throughput technique for preclinical cancer research. BLI relies upon the expression of a luciferase transgene to generate signal from a target population of cells. This can be achieved simply by labelling cells ex vivo for xenograft based models, or via the generation of a transgenic mouse for imaging spontaneous tumour models [149]. There are multiple bioluminescent reporter transgenes available that can be used for BLI in vivo, the most commonly employed being firefly luciferase (FLuc, *Photinus pyralis*), but importantly also Renilla luciferase (RLuc, *Renilla reniformis*) and the secreted Gaussia luciferase (GLuc, *Gaussia princeps*). To image luciferase transgene expression in vivo, a substrate is first administered, typically i.p. or alternatively i.v. D-Luciferin (in the presence of ATP and O_2) is used to image FLuc and coelenterazine (in the presence of O_2) to image RLuc and GLuc. These substrates do not cross-react and so in principal dual labelling strategies may be employed to monitor an additional biological feature within the same subject. The spectrum of emitted light is broad for these enzymes (>100 nm), with an emission maximum of 560 nm for FLuc, 480 nm for RLuc [150] and 480 nm for GLuc [151]. The suboptimal colour of emitted light from GLuc is compensated for by being >1,000-fold brighter than native RLuc. GLuc bioluminescence in vivo appears approximately as bright as FLuc, even though FLuc has a more favourable emission spectrum for light transmission through tissue. Several RLuc mutants have recently been described that are both relatively brighter and red-shifted in terms of their emission spectra than native RLuc (RLuc7-521 and Rluc8.6-535 with emission maxima of 521 and 535 nm respectively [152, 153]).

The amount of light produced in a typical BLI experiment in vivo is very low and requires a highly sensitive detector to be measured. These are available commercially and typically comprise a super-cooled (<–90°C) CCD chip housed in a light-tight box (see Fig. 10.10). Light is typically detected from a single aspect and results in a 2-D bioluminescent intensity map across the field of view. This image is then superimposed on a regular digital photograph of the subject to provide anatomic context. Regular BLI acquisitions are short, ranging from 1 to 300 s depending upon the extent of luciferase expression and the size and depth of the target cell population. This coupled with the fact that up to five subjects may be imaged simultaneously makes BLI the molecular imaging modality with the highest throughput.

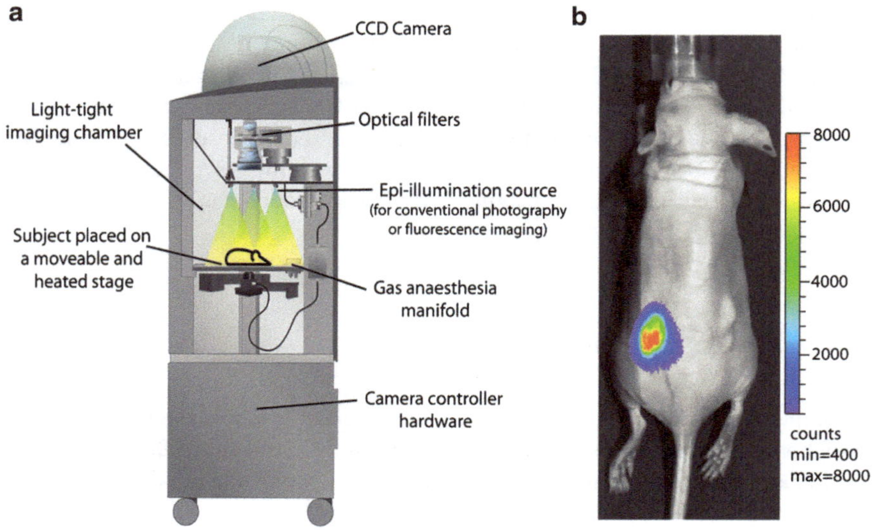

Fig. 10.10 A camera system for detecting bioluminescence in vivo. The schematic depicted in (**a**) shows a side-projection cut-away of a commercially available optical in vivo imaging system, capable of both BLI and fluorescence imaging, with key features annotated. (Image kindly provided by David Panzarella and Stephen Oldfield, Caliper LifeSciences Inc.) The image in (**b**) shows a typical in vivo bioluminescence image. In this image, the mouse has a <100 mm^3 luciferase-labelled LL2 (Lewis Lung) tumour developing subcutaneously on its left flank (5 s acquisition, small binning, fstop 2; Dr Scott Lyons, unpublished data)

Despite the fact that overall light output is low and prone to attenuation and scatter from overlying tissue, background light emission from non-labelled tissue is essentially absent so BLI is a very sensitive technique. It has been reported that as few as three labelled cells implanted subcutaneously can be detected in vivo [154] and another study, which employed multi-modal reporters, recommended BLI over PET as the method of choice to detect the smallest tumours in vivo [155]. Such sensitivity limits are highly dependent upon experimental context, however, and are affected by levels of reporter expression, depth of signal and optical noise arising from other distinct populations of labelled cells in the proximity of the tumour.

In most cases, the analysis of 2-D images provides sufficient information to interpret experimental results. Even though the light emitted from populations of cells located at deep body locations is prone to greater levels of attenuation and scattering than an equivalent cell population located more superficially, the quantification of light emission provides a relative measure of that feature of the tumour's biology which is being probed. When multiple images of a subject are acquired over time (e.g. before and after treatment), the relative changes in tumour biology can be readily visualised irrespective of signal depth and the absolute amount of light detected. If required, the depth of signal can be computed by analysing a series of planar bioluminescent images acquired with a range of defined bandwidth filters. Red wavelengths pass through tissue more efficiently than green, so the ratio of red to green light on the surface of the subject is indicative of relative tissue depth [156].

Luciferase transgene expression may be regulated at the transcriptional or post-translational level and this confers a great degree of versatility in terms of imaging read-out. Transcriptional regulation can be modified by varying the promoter used. For example, a constitutive promoter (e.g. CMV or CAGGS) will result in robust steady-state expression of luciferase. In such circumstances the extent of bioluminescence detected in vivo from a population of labelled cells will be proportional to viable cell number. This strategy has been employed extensively with firefly luciferase to evaluate tumour cell kill following treatment as only viable cells bioluminesce (n.b. FLuc requires ATP and O_2 to generate light [157–159]). A reduction in tumour cell viability can be identified, therefore, by BLI at early time points when typically there has been little evident change in tumour volume or anatomic structure.

Tissue or cell-type specific promoters can also be employed to restrict luciferase expression to a specific organ or to a cell type within an organ. This has been particularly useful in the development of luciferase expressing transgenic mice for imaging spontaneous tumour models as background bioluminescence arising from other body locations, which can severely impact signal-to-noise and overall image sensitivity, is minimised [149, 160, 161]. Context specific promoters have also been used to restrict reporter expression to populations of cells in a defined physiological state. For example, certain promoters may be employed to restrict transgene expression to a specific phase of the cell cycle [162] or in response to a stimulus such as DNA damage [163]. Such reporters have the potential to provide a deeper mechanistic understanding of tumour response to therapy than could be garnered by imaging anatomy alone.

Regulation of luciferase function at the post-translational level has also provided an opportunity to measure key aspects of tumour biology non-invasively in real-time. For example, several apoptosis specific reporters have been developed whereby the firefly luciferase protein has been fused to inhibitory peptides at both N- and C-terminal ends [164], with all three domains separated by the canonical caspase-3 cleavage motif DEVD. Consequently, upon the induction of apoptosis, this non-functional luciferase fusion protein is cleaved, resulting in restoration of function and an overall increase in bioluminescence [165]. A further example of post-translational control of luciferase function is a modified reporter allele that assumes a non-functional conformation until phosphorylated by Akt [166]. This experiment serves as an important paradigm, showing that the relative activity of key cellular signalling pathways can be measured with BLI.

Intracellular protein–protein interactions have also been measured by BLI via the application of a split luciferase allele strategy. The coding sequences of both RLuc and FLuc have been split into two independently non-functional domains [167, 168]. When either half is fused to two other independent proteins, bioluminescence is conditionally restored only when those proteins bind to each other and the two luciferase halves come into close proximity. This has proven to be a highly effective means of screening the effectiveness of chemicals that modulate tumour related protein–protein interactions. For example, molecules that affect homo- and hetero-dimerisation of the CXCR4 and CXCR7 chemokine receptors [169], tumour-related Hsp90/p23 interaction [170], and that promote or antagonise folding of the human estrogen receptor ligand binding domain [171] have all been screened in this way.

Collectively these examples serve to illustrate the versatility of preclinical BLI applications. Several major issues currently prevent the translation of BLI to the clinic however. It is currently not possible to efficiently and safely deliver luciferase transgene expression to target populations of cells in the clinic. Further, it is likely that the increased tissue-depths associated with clinical imaging will give rise to problematic levels of signal attenuation. Given today's imaging technology this would limit any potential clinical BLI applications to relatively superficial locations in the body.

Fluorescence Imaging

Fluorescence imaging has proven to be an effective and highly versatile molecular imaging modality. Although not as sensitive as PET, SPECT or BLI, this approach is still very useful for whole body imaging in vivo and has the added advantage that certain applications can uniquely facilitate microscopic detection of labelled cells in vivo. Further, promising fluorescently-labelled probes developed in the laboratory can in principal be translated directly to clinical application, which cannot yet be said for the other optical imaging approach, BLI.

When a fluorophore absorbs a photon of a defined wavelength it briefly enters an excited electronic state. One way that this energy can be lost is by emitting a photon with a lower energy and hence longer wavelength. It is this red-shifted light that is detected as signal in a fluorescence imaging experiment. Although fluorescence imaging requires and generates substantially more light than a typical in vivo bioluminescence experiment, the sensitivity of whole body imaging, especially when employing labels that excite in the visible range of the spectrum, is relatively poor for several reasons. Both the excitation and the emission wavelengths of probes that fluoresce in the visible region of the spectrum do not pass efficiently through tissue. Furthermore, much of the visible spectrum, especially green light, generates appreciable amounts of autofluorescence from non-labelled tissue and from some food-types in the digestive tract [172]. Taken together this means that many of the fluorophores that have proven so successful in the field of microscopy are poorly suited for non-invasive whole-body fluorescence imaging in vivo. Fluorophores that excite and emit in the far-red and near-infrared portion of the spectrum are better suited, however, as the tissue penetrance of both the exciting and emitted light is improved and background autofluorescence is markedly reduced [148].

Several imaging techniques have been developed for fluorescence imaging in vivo. These include reflectance imaging, where the top surface of the subject or tissue is both illuminated by the excitation light (epi-illumination) and the resultant fluorescence signal is collected. In transmission imaging, the excitation light shines through the subject (trans-illumination) and the resulting fluorescence emission is collected on the opposite side. Reflectance imaging appears to be best suited for fluorescent targets that are located relatively superficially in the subject or tissue whereas transmission imaging is better for targets in deeper body locations. In both cases the use of appropriate and defined optical band-pass filters ensure that only the light emitted from the fluorescent source reaches the detector. Autofluorescence background can also be largely subtracted from these images by acquiring and subtracting a second image that employs an excitation wavelength close to the absorption maximum of the fluorophore, but which is incapable of exciting it.

The signals from several fluorescent labels may also be acquired simultaneously in vivo and differentiated on the basis of their emitted wavelengths using advanced image analysis techniques such as spectral unmixing [173]. In addition to enabling more accurate quantification of multiplex analyses, this analysis method also provides a useful means of reducing tissue autofluorescence.

Another important whole-body fluorescence imaging technique, termed FMT (fluorescence mediated tomography) involves restraining the subject in a tight-fitting chamber prior to the acquisition of two optical measurements. The first comprises a raster scan of the entire subject to model light transmission through the subject at thousands of co-ordinate points. A second raster scan of the whole subject is then taken with light that excites the fluorescent label. These data sets are then paired and processed to accurately quantify the relative amounts of fluorescence at deep-tissue locations, correcting for artefacts arising from differential signal transmission through heterogeneous surrounding tissue. The resolution of this technique has been markedly improved by using custom-built hardware that specifically detects only the very first emitted photons that transmit through the tissue [174]. These early-detected photons reach the detector first because they have undergone less scattering and so the resolution of the technique is correspondingly improved.

Several other important invasive techniques have also been developed to detect fluorescence in vivo. These include both preclinical and clinical fluorescence endoscopy [175–178] and a technique termed intravital microscopy [179]. A key advantage of these techniques over the non-invasive approaches already mentioned is that the target population of labelled cells can be imaged directly without overlying tissue impeding light transmission. This enables a significant gain in sensitivity and resolution, albeit with a substantial reduction in the field of view, and small lesions that would not have been detected via non-invasive whole-body imaging are now visible. Moreover, magnification of the field of view is also possible and intravital microscopy can image tumour biology with single cell resolution. This technique has proven particularly powerful for real-time visualisation of tumour angiogenic processes [180], of cellular mobility and escape from a primary tumour [181] and of cell fate in the establishment of brain metastases [182]. Models of this type involve the engraftment of a glass window into tissue to facilitate the direct detection of labelled cells, so it should not be discounted that this local perturbation of tissue may in some way influence tumour biology. Non-invasive multiphoton fluorescence microscopy is also possible in vivo, however, tissue penetration depth is shallow (<1 mm [183]), effectively limiting this approach to studies of the skin.

A molecule that is not natively fluorescent can be converted into a fluorescent probe by attaching a fluorescent moiety such as a dye or quantum dot. Such simple constitutively fluorescent molecular conjugates can be used to study molecular pharmacokinetics [184] or to image vascular volume following in vivo administration [185]. Should the labelled probe have affinity for a molecular target in the body, such labelling approaches, although not as sensitive as PET or SPECT, can be used to measure the relative location and abundance of a target molecule. In the context of cancer biology, those targets have been markers presented by primary tumours [186, 187] or tumour-associated vasculature [188, 189] and metastatic lesions [190].

However an important advantage that fluorescent imaging has over PET and SPECT has been the development of activatable probes. These are molecules that are non-fluorescent when administered, but become fluorescent upon encountering their target. Such probes have proven very useful in measuring the relative activity of several tumour related classes of proteolytic enzyme such as the caspases, matrix-metalloproteinases and papains [191–195]. This has, in general, been achieved by positioning a light absorbing moiety (or quencher) adjacent to the fluorophore such that no light is emitted by the intact probe upon excitation. A protease-specific cleavage motif is also incorporated into the molecule so that both fluorescent and quenching domains become spatially separated following the specific proteolytic processing of the probe, resulting in a gain of fluorescence.

A new class of pH-activatable fluorescent probes has also been reported recently, whereby a conjugated fluorophore is inactive until endocytosed by the cell and exposed to the low pH conditions present within the lysosome. This breaks down the conjugate, freeing the fluorophore and establishing fluorescence. In this way it was possible to image the binding of a labelled therapeutic antibody to the Her2 receptor on the surface of tumour cells and serves as a new method to image receptor-mediated endocytosis in vivo [196, 197]. Moreover, as the acidic conditions within the lysosome are energy dependent, only viable cells are visualised by this approach, so this may also serve as a useful tool to image tumour response to treatment in the future.

Cells have also been labelled with fluorescent reporter transgenes and imaged in vivo in the laboratory. Non-invasive whole-body imaging of tumours labelled with fluorescent reporter transgene expression has been demonstrated [198, 199], however, the signal-to-noise ratio is relatively low and the lack of sensitivity at deep-tissue locations can be problematic when trying to image small lesions. Reporter transgenes have, however, proven particularly useful when imaged with intravital microscopy as light transmission is not impeded by overlying tissue and labelled cells can be detected without any of the complications associated with probe-based imaging, such as bioavailability, half-life in serum, clearance etc. For example, tumour and stromal/vascular cells have been constitutively and differentially labelled with two colours of fluorescent reporter transgene to facilitate the study of tumour angiogenesis in vivo [200]. Another recent study has reported the development of a fluorescence reporter transgene method to identify replicating cells in vivo. Both GFP and RFP transgenes were fused to two independent peptide domains derived from proteins that are normally tightly regulated at the posttranslational level at different phases of the cell cycle. This labelling strategy resulted in red cells at G1 and green cells at S/G2/M stages of the cell cycle [201]. Cycling cells could clearly be seen in tumours in vivo using intravital microscopy. The relative ease with which fluorescence can be detected at the microscopic level ex vivo has also made these reporter transgenes useful for co-labelling purposes (e.g. for facilitating the assessment of transgene delivery from a therapeutic vector [202, 203]). Several triple modality reporter constructs have also been validated in recent years that can confer fluorescence, bioluminescence and PET imaging capabilities to labelled cells [204, 205].

An entirely new class of fluorescent protein has been described recently based upon a phytochrome molecule from the radiation resistant bacterium *Deinococcus radiodurans [*206]. This new fluorescent protein excites and emits in the infrared region of the spectrum (684 and 708 nm respectively), which is very promising from a whole-body imaging perspective as these wavelengths will pass efficiently through tissue. This new class of proteins is currently not very bright (they possess a low quantum yield), however, future research will undoubtedly improve this and open up new possibilities for molecular imaging with fluorescence reporter transgenes.

Conclusions

Remarkable progress has been made in the field of molecular imaging within the past decade and this has ultimately resulted in a deeper understanding of the cellular biology of tumours and in the clinic has opened up new ways of detecting tumours, of grading and staging them and detecting their response to treatment. This progress has been partly driven by hardware development, with the advent of new preclinical imaging techniques such as hyperpolarised MRI, micro-PET, multi-pinhole SPECT and BLI offering new and innovative imaging possibilities. Some of these new approaches are starting to be evaluated in the clinic and have the potential to further impact clinical practice in the near future.

Novel imaging technologies continue to be developed and several are well positioned for evaluation in tumour-related imaging applications. For example, a new intravital microscopy approach, called optical frequency domain imaging [207], images tissue with light between 1,250 and 1,350 nm and can produce images of tumour vasculature and tissue viability without the use of any contrast agents. Another promising approach has been termed photoacoustic or optoacoustic imaging [208, 209]. This approach uses pulses of light to cause transitory temperature increases in tissue, which in turn give rise to the generation of acoustic waves that are detected in a similar fashion to ultrasound. The technique combines a strength of optical imaging, high contrast, with a strength of acoustic-based imaging, high resolution. New forms of targeted contrast media are also being evaluated, using materials that efficiently absorb light and convert that energy into heat (e.g. gold-plated carbon nanotubules [210]).

As the more established techniques mentioned in this chapter continue to be refined and exciting new modalities continue to be developed, it is clear that molecular imaging could transform the way that cancer is managed in the clinic including in some instances earlier detection of cancers at the pre-invasive stage.

References

1. Eisenhauer E, Therasse P, Bogaerts J et al (2009) New response evaluation criteria in solid tumours: Revised RECIST guideline (version 1.1). Eur J Cancer 45:228–247
2. Weissleder R (1999) Molecular imaging: exploring the next frontier. Radiology 212:609–614
3. Weissleder R, Mahmood U (2001) Molecular imaging. Radiology 219:316–333
4. Weissleder R, Pittet M (2008) Imaging in the era of molecular oncology. Nature 452:580–589
5. Gambhir SS (2002) Molecular imaging of cancer with positron emisson tomography. Nat Rev Cancer 2:683–693
6. Margolis D, Hoffman J, Herfkens R, Jeffrey R, Quon A, Gambhir S (2007) Molecular imaging techniques in body imaging. Radiology 245:333–356
7. Sullivan D, Kelloff G (2005) Seeing into cells – The promise of in vivo molecular imaging in oncology. EMBO Rep 6:292–296
8. Weber W (2005) Use of PET for monitoring cancer therapy and for predicting outcome. J Nucl Med 46:983–995
9. Czernin J, Weber WA, Herschman HR (2006) Molecular imaging in the development of cancer therapeutics. Annu Rev Med 57:99–118
10. Weber WA (2006) Positron emission tomography as an imaging biomarker. J Clin Oncol 24:3282–3292
11. Neves AA, Brindle KM (2006) Assessing responses to cancer therapy using molecular imaging. Biochim Biophys Acta 1766:242–261
12. Brindle K (2008) New approaches for imaging tumour responses to treatment. Nat Rev Cancer 8:1–14
13. Juweid M, Cheson B (2006) Positron-emission tomography and assessment of cancer therapy. N Engl J Med 354:496–507
14. Weissleder R (2001) Scaling down imaging: molecular mapping of cancer in mice. Nat Rev Cancer 2:1–8
15. Frese KK, Tuveson DA (2007) Maximizing mouse cancer models. Nat Rev Cancer 7:654–658
16. Testoni PA, Mangiavillano B (2008) Optical coherence tomography in detection of dysplasia and cancer of the gastrointestinal tract and bilio-pancreatic ductal system. World J Gastroenterol 14:6444–6452
17. Kara MA, Bergman JJ (2006) Autofluorescence imaging and narrow-band imaging for the detection of early neoplasia in patients with Barrett's esophagus. Endoscopy 38:627–631
18. Moghissi K, Dixon K, Stringer MR (2008) Current indications and future perspective of fluorescence bronchoscopy: a review study. Photodiagnosis Photodyn Ther 5:238–246
19. Hsiung PL, Hardy J, Friedland S et al (2008) Detection of colonic dysplasia in vivo using a targeted heptapeptide and confocal microendoscopy. Nat Med 14:454–458
20. Kurhanewicz J, Swanson MG, Nelson SJ, Vigneron DB (2002) Combined magnetic resonance imaging and spectroscopic imaging approach to molecular imaging of prostate cancer. J Magn Reson Imaging 16:451–463
21. Sawyers C (2008) The cancer biomarker problem. Nature 452:548–552
22. Hanash SM, Pitteri SJ, Faca VM (2008) Mining the plasma proteome for cancer biomarkers. Nature 452:571–579
23. Jana S, Blaufox MD (2006) Nuclear medicine studies of the prostate, testes, and bladder. Semin Nucl Med 36:51–72
24. Lauterbur PC (1973) Image formation by induced local interactions: examples employing nuclear magnetic resonance. Nature 242:190–191
25. Hoult D, Busby S, Gadian D, Radda G, Richards R, Seeley P (1974) Observation of tissue metabolites using ^{31}P nuclear magnetic resonance. Nature 252:285–287
26. Gadian DG, Radda GK (1981) NMR studies of tissue metabolism. Ann Rev Biochem 50:69–83
27. Negendank W (1992) Studies of human tumours by MRS: a review. NMR Biomed 5:303–324
28. Glunde K, Jacobs MA, Bhujwalla ZM (2006) Choline metabolism in cancer: implications for diagnosis and therapy. Expert Rev Mol Diagn 6:821–829

29. Gadian DG (1995) NMR and its applications to living systems, 2nd edn. Oxford University Press, Oxford
30. McRobbie DW, Moore EA, Graves MJ, Prince MR (2006) MRI from picture to proton, 2nd edn. Cambridge University Press, Cambridge
31. Wuthrich K (1986) NMR of Proteins and Nucleic Acids. Wiley-Interscience, New York
32. Lindon JC, Nicholson JK, Wilson ID (1996) Direct coupling of chromatographic separations to NMR spectroscopy. Prog Nucl Magn Reson Spectrosc 29:1–49
33. Raichle ME (2001) Bold insights. Nature 412:128–130
34. Logothetis NK (2008) What we can do and what we cannot do with fMRI. Nature 453:869–878
35. Robinson SP, Howe FA, Griffiths JR (1995) Noninvasive monitoring of carbogen-induced changes in tumor blood-flow and oxygenation by functional magnetic-resonance-imaging. Int J Radiat Oncol Biol Phys 33:855–859
36. van Zijl PCM, Moonen CTW, Faustino P, Pekar J, Kaplan O, Cohen JS (1991) Complete separation of intracellular and extracellular information in NMR spectra of perfused cells by diffusion-weighted spectroscopy. Proc Natl Acad Sci USA 88:3228–3232
37. Zhao M, Pipe JG, Bonnett J, Evelhoch JL (1996) Early detection of treatment response by diffusion-weighted 1H-NMR spectroscopy in a murine tumour in vivo. Br J Cancer 73:61–64
38. Chenevert TL, Stegman LD, Taylor JMG et al (2000) Diffusion magnetic resonance imaging: an early surrogate marker of therapeutic efficacy in brain tumors. J Natl Cancer Inst 92:2029–2036
39. Moffat BA, Chenevert TL, Lawrence TS et al (2005) Functional diffusion map: a noninvasive MRI biomarker for early stratification of clinical brain tumor response. Proc Natl Acad Sci USA 102:5524–5529
40. Aime S, Cabella C, Colombatto S, GeninattiCrich S, Gianollio E, Maggioni F (2002) Insights into the use of paramagnetic Gd(III) complexes in MR-molecular imaging investigations. J Magn Reson Imaging 16:394–406
41. Bulte JWM, Kraitchman DL (2004) Iron oxide MR contrast agents for molecular and cellular imaging. NMR Biomed 17:484–499
42. Stuber M, Gilson WD, Schar M et al (2007) Positive contrast visualization of iron oxide-labeled stem cells using inversion-recovery with ON-Resonant water suppression (IRON). Magn Reson Med 58:1072–1077
43. Wickline SA, Neubauer AM, Winter PM, Caruthers SD, Lanza GM (2007) Molecular imaging and therapy of atherosclerosis with targeted nanoparticles. J Magn Reson Imaging 25:667–680
44. Shapiro EM, Skrtic S, Sharer K, Hill JM, Dunbar CE, Koretsky AP (2004) MRI detection of single particles for cellular imaging. Proc Natl Acad Sci USA 101:10901–10906
45. de Vries I, Lesterhuis W, Barentsz J et al (2005) Magnetic resonance tracking of dendritic cells in melanoma patients for monitoring of cellular therapy. Nat Biotechnol 23:1407–1413
46. Leach MO, Brindle KM, Evelhoch JL et al (2005) The assessment of antiangiogenic and antivascular therapies in early-stage clinical trials using magnetic resonance imaging: issues and recommendations. Br J Cancer 92:1599–1610
47. Brasch R, Pham C, Shames D et al (1997) Assessing tumor angiogenesis using macromolecular MR imaging contrast media. J Magn Reson Imaging 7:68–74
48. Barrett T, Kobayashi H, Brechbiel M, Choyke PL (2006) Macromolecular MRI contrast agents for imaging tumor angiogenesis. Eur J Radiol 60:353–366
49. McDonald DM, Choyke PL (2003) Imaging of angiogenesis: from microscope to clinic. Nat Med 9:713–725
50. Hylton N (2006) Dynamic contrast-enhanced magnetic resonance imaging as an imaging biomarker. J Clin Oncol 24:3293–3298
51. Tozer GM, Kanthou C, Baguley BC (2005) Disrupting tumour blood vessels. Nat Rev Cancer 5:423–435
52. Miller JC, Pien HH, Sahani D, Sorensen AG, Thrall JH (2005) Imaging angiogenesis: applications and potential for drug development. J Natl Cancer Inst 97:172–187

53. Morgan B, Thomas AL, Drevs J et al (2003) Dynamic contrast-enhanced magnetic resonance imaging as a biomarker for the pharmacological response of PTK787/ZK 222584, an inhibitor of the vascular endothelial growth factor receptor tyrosine kinases, in patients with advanced colorectal cancer and liver metastases: results from two phase I studies. J Clin Oncol 21:3955–3964
54. Stevenson JP, Rosen M, Sun WJ et al (2003) Phase I trial of the antivascular agent combretastatin A4 phosphate on a 5-day schedule to patients with cancer: magnetic resonance imaging evidence for altered tumor blood flow. J Clin Oncol 21:4428–4438
55. Aime S, Castelli D, Terreno E (2002) Novel pH-reporter MRI contrast agents. Angew Chem Int Ed 41:4334–4336
56. Gillies RJ, Raghunand N, Garcia-Martin ML, Gatenby RA (2004) pH imaging. A review of pH measurement methods and applications in cancers. IEEE Eng Med Biol Mag 23:57–64
57. Aime S, Fedeli F, Sanino A, Terreno E (2006) A R-2/R-1 ratiometric procedure for a concentration-independent, pH-responsive, Gd(III)-based MRI agent. J Am Chem Soc 128: 11326–11327
58. Aime S, Barge A, Castelli DD et al (2002) Paramagnetic lanthanide(III) complexes as pH-sensitive chemical exchange saturation transfer (CEST) contrast agents for MRI applications. Magn Reson Med 47:639–648
59. Artemov D, Mori N, Ravi R, Bhujwalla ZM (2003) Magnetic resonance molecular imaging of the HER-2/neu receptor. Cancer Res 63:2723–2727
60. Artemov D, Mori N, Okollie B, Bhujwalla ZM (2003) MR molecular imaging of the Her-2/neu receptor in breast cancer cells using targeted iron oxide nanoparticles. Magn Reson Med 49:403–408
61. Sipkins DA, Cheresh DA, Kazemi MR, Nevin LM, Bednarski MD, Li KCP (1998) Detection of tumour angiogenesis in vivo by $\alpha_v\beta_3$-targeted magnetic resonance imaging. Nat Med 4:623–626
62. Winter PM, Caruthers SD, Kassner A et al (2003) Molecular Imaging of angiogenesis in nascent vx-2 rabbit tumors using a novel alpha(v)beta(3)-targeted nanoparticle and 1.5 tesla magnetic resonance imaging. Cancer Res 63:5838–5843
63. Zhao M, Beauregard DA, Loizou L, Davletov B, Brindle KM (2001) Non-invasive detection of apoptosis using magnetic resonance imaging and a targeted contrast agent. Nat Med 7:1241–1244
64. van Tilborg GAF, Mulder WJM, Deckers N et al (2006) Annexin A5-functionalized bimodal lipid-based contrast agents for the detection of apoptosis. Bioconjug Chem 17:741–749
65. Krishnan AS, Neves AA, de Backer MM et al (2008) Detection of cell death in tumors using MRI and a gadolinium-based targeted contrast agent. Radiology 246:854–862
66. Lauenstein T, Salman K, Morreira R et al (2007) Nephrogenic systemic fibrosis: center case review. J Magn Reson Imaging 26:1198–1203
67. Podo F, Sardanelli F, Iorio E et al (2007) Abnormal choline phospholipid metabolism in breast and ovary cancer: molecular bases for noninvasive imaging approaches. Curr Med Imaging Rev 3:123–137
68. Hu JN, Feng WZ, Hua J et al (2009) A high spatial resolution in vivo 1H magnetic resonance spectroscopic imaging technique for the human breast at 3 T. Med Phys 36:4870–4877
69. Kurhanewicz J, Vigneron DB, Nelson SJ (2000) Three-dimensional magnetic resonance spectroscopic imaging of brain and prostate cancer. Neoplasia 2:166–189
70. Meisamy S, Bolan PJ, Baker EH et al (2004) Neoadjuvant chemotherapy of locally advanced breast cancer: predicting response with in vivo H-1 MR spectroscopy - A pilot study. Radiology 233:424–431
71. Kumar R, Kumar M, Jagannathan NR, Gupta NP, Hemal AK (2004) Proton magnetic resonance spectroscopy with a body coil in the diagnosis of carcinoma prostate. Urol Res 32:36–40
72. Mueller-Lisse UG, Scherr MK (2007) Proton MR spectroscopy of the prostate. Eur J Radiol 63:351–360
73. Futterer JJ, Heijmink S, Scheenen TWJ et al (2006) Prostate cancer localization with dynamic contrast-enhanced MR imaging and proton MR spectroscopic imaging. Radiology 241:449–458

74. Magalhaes A, Godfrey W, Shen YM, Hu JN, Smith W (2005) Proton magnetic resonance spectroscopy of brain tumors correlated with pathology. Acad Radiol 12:51–57
75. Chen J, Huang SL, Li T, Chen XL (2006) In vivo research in astrocytoma cell proliferation with H-1-magnetic resonance spectroscopy: correlation with histopathology and immunohistochemistry. Neuroradiology 48:312–318
76. Spampinato MV, Smith JK, Kwock L et al (2007) Cerebral blood volume measurements and proton MR spectroscopy in grading of oligodendroglial tumors. AJR Am J Roentgenol 188:204–212
77. Chernov MF, Nakaya K, Kasuya H et al (2009) Metabolic alterations in the peritumoral brain in cases of meningiomas: H-1-MRS study. J Neurol Sci 284:168–174
78. Hazany S, Hesselink JR, Healy JF, Imbesi SG (2007) Utilization of glutamate/creatine ratios for proton spectroscopic diagnosis of meningiomas. Neuroradiology 49:121–127
79. Tate A, Underwood J, Acosta D et al (2006) Development of a decision support system for diagnosis and grading of brain tumours using in vivo magnetic resonance single voxel spectra. NMR Biomed 19:411–434
80. Roden M, Shulman GI (1999) Applications of NMR spectroscopy to study muscle glycogen metabolism in man. Annu Rev Med 50:277–290
81. Ardenkjaer-Larsen JH, Fridlund B, Gram A et al (2003) Increase in signal-to-noise ratio of >10, 000 times in liquid-state NMR. Proc Natl Acad Sci USA 100:10158–10163
82. Gallagher F, Kettunen M, Brindle K (2009) Biomedical applications of hyperpolarized ^{13}C magnetic resonance imaging. Prog NMR Spec 55:285–295
83. Golman K, Petersson JS, Magnusson P et al (2008) Cardiac metabolism measured noninvasively by hyperpolarized ^{13}C MRI. Magn Reson Med 59:1005–1013
84. Day SE, Kettunen MI, Gallagher FA et al (2007) Detecting tumor response to treatment using hyperpolarized ^{13}C magnetic resonance imaging and spectroscopy. Nat Med 13:1382–1387
85. Gatenby RA, Gillies RJ (2004) Why do cancers have high aerobic glycolysis? Nat Rev Cancer 4:891–899
86. Albers M, Bok R, Chen A et al (2008) Hyperpolarized C-13 lactate, pyruvate, and alanine: noninvasive biomarkers for prostate cancer detection and grading. Cancer Res 68:8607–8615
87. Gallagher FA, Kettunen MI, Hu DE et al (2009) Production of hyperpolarized [1, 4-C-13(2)] malate from [1, 4-C-13(2)]fumarate is a marker of cell necrosis and treatment response in tumors. Proc Natl Acad Sci USA 106:19801–19806
88. Gallagher F, Kettunen M, Day S, Lerche M, Brindle K (2008) ^{13}C Magnetic resonance spectroscopy measurements of glutaminase activity in human hepatocellular carcinoma cells using hyperpolarized ^{13}C-labeled glutamine. Magn Reson Med 60:253–257
89. Gallagher F, Kettunen M, Day S et al (2008) Magnetic resonance imaging of pH in vivo using hyperpolarized ^{13}C-labeled bicarbonate. Nature 453:940–943
90. Massoud TF, Gambhir SS (2003) Molecular imaging in living subjects: seeing fundamental biological processes in a new light. Genes Dev 17:545–580
91. Robbins E (2008) Radiation risks from imaging studies in children with cancer. Pediatr Blood Cancer 51:453–457
92. Carney JP, Townsend DW, Rappoport V, Bendriem B (2006) Method for transforming CT images for attenuation correction in PET/CT imaging. Med Phys 33:976–983
93. Moses WW (2007) Recent advances and future advances in time-of-flight PET. Nucl Instrum Methods Phys Res A 580:919–924
94. Ullrich RT, Kracht L, Brunn A et al (2009) Methyl-L-11C-methionine PET as a diagnostic marker for malignant progression in patients with glioma. J Nucl Med 50:1962–1968
95. Soloviev D, Fini A, Chierichetti F, Al-Nahhas A, Rubello D (2008) PET imaging with 11C-acetate in prostate cancer: a biochemical, radiochemical and clinical perspective. Eur J Nucl Med Mol Imaging 35:942–949
96. Di Bartolo N, Sargeson AM, Smith SV (2006) New 64Cu PET imaging agents for personalised medicine and drug development using the hexa-aza cage, SarAr. Org Biomol Chem 4:3350–3357

97. Voss SD, Smith SV, DiBartolo N et al (2007) Positron emission tomography (PET) imaging of neuroblastoma and melanoma with 64Cu-SarAr immunoconjugates. Proc Natl Acad Sci USA 104:17489–17493
98. Emonds KM, Swinnen JV, Mortelmans L, Mottaghy FM (2009) Molecular imaging of prostate cancer. Methods 48:193–199
99. Beer AJ, Haubner R, Sarbia M et al (2006) Positron emission tomography using [18F] Galacto-RGD identifies the level of integrin alpha(v)beta3 expression in man. Clin Cancer Res 12:3942–3949
100. Beer AJ, Lorenzen S, Metz S et al (2008) Comparison of integrin alphaVbeta3 expression and glucose metabolism in primary and metastatic lesions in cancer patients: a PET study using 18F-galacto-RGD and 18F-FDG. J Nucl Med 49:22–29
101. Mortimer JE, Dehdashti F, Siegel BA, Katzenellenbogen JA, Fracasso P, Welch MJ (1996) Positron emission tomography with 2-[18F]Fluoro-2-deoxy-D-glucose and 16alpha-[18F] fluoro-17beta-estradiol in breast cancer: correlation with estrogen receptor status and response to systemic therapy. Clin Cancer Res 2:933–939
102. Peterson LM, Mankoff DA, Lawton T et al (2008) Quantitative imaging of estrogen receptor expression in breast cancer with PET and 18F-fluoroestradiol. J Nucl Med 49: 367–374
103. Mortimer JE, Dehdashti F, Siegel BA, Trinkaus K, Katzenellenbogen JA, Welch MJ (2001) Metabolic flare: indicator of hormone responsiveness in advanced breast cancer. J Clin Oncol 19:2797–2803
104. Shah C, Miller TW, Wyatt SK et al (2009) Imaging biomarkers predict response to anti-HER2 (ErbB2) therapy in preclinical models of breast cancer. Clin Cancer Res 15: 4712–4721
105. Cohen A, Shirvan A, Levin G, Grimberg H, Reshef A, Ziv I (2009) From the Gla domain to a novel small-molecule detector of apoptosis. Cell Res 19:625–637
106. Nguyen QD, Smith G, Glaser M, Perumal M, Arstad E, Aboagye EO (2009) Positron emission tomography imaging of drug-induced tumor apoptosis with a caspase-3/7 specific [18F]-labeled isatin sulfonamide. Proc Natl Acad Sci USA 106:16375–16380
107. Eschmann SM, Paulsen F, Reimold M et al (2005) Prognostic impact of hypoxia imaging with 18F-misonidazole PET in non-small cell lung cancer and head and neck cancer before radiotherapy. J Nucl Med 46:253–260
108. Spence AM, Muzi M, Swanson KR et al (2008) Regional hypoxia in glioblastoma multiforme quantified with [18F]fluoromisonidazole positron emission tomography before radiotherapy: correlation with time to progression and survival. Clin Cancer Res 14:2623–2630
109. Lee N, Nehmeh S, Schoder H et al (2009) Prospective trial incorporating pre-/mid-treatment [18F]-misonidazole positron emission tomography for head-and-neck cancer patients undergoing concurrent chemoradiotherapy. Int J Radiat Oncol Biol Phys 75:101–108
110. Lehmann S, Stiehl DP, Honer M et al (2009) Longitudinal and multimodal in vivo imaging of tumor hypoxia and its downstream molecular events. Proc Natl Acad Sci USA 106:14004–14009
111. Buchmann I, Henze M, Engelbrecht S et al (2007) Comparison of 68Ga-DOTATOC PET and 111In-DTPAOC (Octreoscan) SPECT in patients with neuroendocrine tumours. Eur J Nucl Med Mol Imaging 34:1617–1626
112. Miyagawa T, Gogiberidze G, Serganova I et al (2008) Imaging of HSV-tk Reporter gene expression: comparison between [18F]FEAU, [18F]FFEAU, and other imaging probes. J Nucl Med 49:637–648
113. Kang KW, Min JJ, Chen X, Gambhir SS (2005) Comparison of [14C]FMAU, [3H]FEAU, [14C]FIAU, and [3H]PCV for monitoring reporter gene expression of wild type and mutant herpes simplex virus type 1 thymidine kinase in cell culture. Mol Imaging Biol 7:296–303
114. Yaghoubi SS, Gambhir SS (2006) PET imaging of herpes simplex virus type 1 thymidine kinase (HSV1-tk) or mutant HSV1-sr39tk reporter gene expression in mice and humans using [18F]FHBG. Nat Protoc 1:3069–3075
115. Deng WP, Wu CC, Lee CC et al (2006) Serial in vivo imaging of the lung metastases model and gene therapy using HSV1-tk and ganciclovir. J Nucl Med 47:877–884

116. Maatta AM, Samaranayake H, Pikkarainen J, Wirth T, Yla-Herttuala S (2009) Adenovirus mediated herpes simplex virus-thymidine kinase/ganciclovir gene therapy for resectable malignant glioma. Curr Gene Ther 9:356–367
117. Gambhir SS, Bauer E, Black ME et al (2000) A mutant herpes simplex virus type 1 thymidine kinase reporter gene shows improved sensitivity for imaging reporter gene expression with positron emission tomography. Proc Natl Acad Sci USA 97:2785–2790
118. Dingli D, Kemp BJ, O'Connor MK, Morris JC, Russell SJ, Lowe VJ (2006) Combined I-124 positron emission tomography/computed tomography imaging of NIS gene expression in animal models of stably transfected and intravenously transfected tumor. Mol Imaging Biol 8:16–23
119. Che J, Doubrovin M, Serganova I, Ageyeva L, Zanzonico P, Blasberg R (2005) hNIS-IRES-eGFP dual reporter gene imaging. Mol Imaging 4:128–136
120. Niu G, Gaut AW, Ponto LL et al (2004) Multimodality noninvasive imaging of gene transfer using the human sodium iodide symporter. J Nucl Med 45:445–449
121. Scholz IV, Cengic N, Baker CH et al (2005) Radioiodine therapy of colon cancer following tissue-specific sodium iodide symporter gene transfer. Gene Ther 12:272–280
122. Park SY, Kwak W, Thapa N et al (2008) Combination therapy and noninvasive imaging with a dual therapeutic vector expressing MDR1 short hairpin RNA and a sodium iodide symporter. J Nucl Med 49:1480–1488
123. Kim YJ, Dubey P, Ray P, Gambhir SS, Witte ON (2004) Multimodality imaging of lymphocytic migration using lentiviral-based transduction of a tri-fusion reporter gene. Mol Imaging Biol 6:331–340
124. Penuelas I, Haberkorn U, Yaghoubi S, Gambhir SS (2005) Gene therapy imaging in patients for oncological applications. Eur J Nucl Med Mol Imaging 32(Suppl 2):S384–S403
125. Dubey P, Su H, Adonai N et al (2003) Quantitative imaging of the T cell antitumor response by positron-emission tomography. Proc Natl Acad Sci USA 100:1232–1237
126. Koehne G, Doubrovin M, Doubrovina E et al (2003) Serial in vivo imaging of the targeted migration of human HSV-TK-transduced antigen-specific lymphocytes. Nat Biotechnol 21:405–413
127. Doubrovin M, Ponomarev V, Beresten T et al (2001) Imaging transcriptional regulation of p53-dependent genes with positron emission tomography in vivo. Proc Natl Acad Sci USA 98:9300–9305
128. Serganova I, Doubrovin M, Vider J et al (2004) Molecular imaging of temporal dynamics and spatial heterogeneity of hypoxia-inducible factor-1 signal transduction activity in tumors in living mice. Cancer Res 64:6101–6108
129. Che J, Doubrovin M, Serganova I et al (2007) HSP70-inducible hNIS-IRES-eGFP reporter imaging: response to heat shock. Mol Imaging 6:404–416
130. Catana C, Procissi D, Wu Y et al (2008) Simultaneous in vivo positron emission tomography and magnetic resonance imaging. Proc Natl Acad Sci USA 105:3705–3710
131. Schlemmer HP, Pichler BJ, Schmand M et al (2008) Simultaneous MR/PET imaging of the human brain: feasibility study. Radiology 248:1028–1035
132. Hofmann M, Steinke F, Scheel V et al (2008) MRI-based attenuation correction for PET/MRI: a novel approach combining pattern recognition and atlas registration. J Nucl Med 49:1875–1883
133. Martinez-Moller A, Souvatzoglou M, Delso G et al (2009) Tissue classification as a potential approach for attenuation correction in whole-body PET/MRI: evaluation with PET/CT data. J Nucl Med 50:520–526
134. Beekman F, van der Have F (2007) The pinhole: gateway to ultra-high-resolution three-dimensional radionuclide imaging. Eur J Nucl Med Mol Imaging 34:151–161
135. Sosabowski JK, Mather SJ (2006) Conjugation of DOTA-like chelating agents to peptides and radiolabeling with trivalent metallic isotopes. Nat Protoc 1:972–976
136. Tomura N, Watanabe O, Takahashi S et al (2006) Comparison of 201Tl-chloride SPECT with 99mtc-MIBI SPECT in the depiction of malignant head and neck tumors. Ann Nucl Med 20:107–114

137. Nishiyama Y, Yamamoto Y, Yokoe K et al (2004) Superimposed dual-isotope SPECT using 99mTc-hydroxymethylene diphosphonate and 201Tl-chloride to assess cartilage invasion in laryngohypopharyngeal cancer. Ann Nucl Med 18:527–532
138. Suzuki A, Togawa T, Kuyama J et al (2004) Evaluation of mandibular invasion by head and neck cancers using 99mTc-methylene diphosphonate or 99mTc-hydroxymethylene diphosphonate and 201Tl chloride dual isotope single photon emission computed tomography. Ann Nucl Med 18:399–408
139. van de Wiele C, Lahorte C, Vermeersch H et al (2003) Quantitative tumor apoptosis imaging using technetium-99m-HYNIC annexin V single photon emission computed tomography. J Clin Oncol 21:3483–3487
140. Kartachova M, van Zandwijk N, Burgers S, van Tinteren H, Verheij M, Valdes Olmos RA (2007) Prognostic significance of 99mTc Hynic-rh-annexin V scintigraphy during platinum-based chemotherapy in advanced lung cancer. J Clin Oncol 25:2534–2539
141. Balon HR, Goldsmith SJ, Siegel BA et al (2001) Procedure guideline for somatostatin receptor scintigraphy with (111)In-pentetreotide. J Nucl Med 42:1134–1138
142. Perri M, Erba P, Volterrani D et al (2008) Octreo-SPECT/CT imaging for accurate detection and localization of suspected neuroendocrine tumors. Q J Nucl Med Mol Imaging 52:323–333
143. Akgun A, Cok G, Karapolat I, Goksel T, Burak Z (2006) Tc-99m MIBI SPECT in prediction of prognosis in patients with small cell lung cancer. Ann Nucl Med 20:269–275
144. Saggiorato E, Angusti T, Rosas R et al (2009) 99mTc-MIBI Imaging in the presurgical characterization of thyroid follicular neoplasms: relationship to multidrug resistance protein expression. J Nucl Med 50:1785–1793
145. Shaner NC, Campbell RE, Steinbach PA, Giepmans BN, Palmer AE, Tsien RY (2004) Improved monomeric red, orange and yellow fluorescent proteins derived from Discosoma sp. red fluorescent protein. Nat Biotechnol 22:1567–1572
146. Troyan SL, Kianzad V, Gibbs-Strauss SL et al (2009) The FLARE intraoperative near-infrared fluorescence imaging system: a first-in-human clinical trial in breast cancer sentinel lymph node mapping. Ann Surg Oncol 16:2943–2952
147. Winer JH, Choi HS, Gibbs-Strauss SL, Ashitate Y, Colson YL, Frangioni JV (2010) Intraoperative localization of insulinoma and normal pancreas using invisible near-infrared fluorescent light. Ann Surg Oncol 17:1094–1100
148. Rao J, Dragulescu-Andrasi A, Yao H (2007) Fluorescence imaging in vivo: recent advances. Curr Opin Biotechnol 18:17–25
149. Lyons SK, Lim E, Clermont AO et al (2006) Noninvasive bioluminescence imaging of normal and spontaneously transformed prostate tissue in mice. Cancer Res 66:4701–4707
150. Fan F, Wood KV (2007) Bioluminescent assays for high-throughput screening. Assay Drug Dev Technol 5:127–136
151. Tannous BA, Kim DE, Fernandez JL, Weissleder R, Breakefield XO (2005) Codon-optimized Gaussia luciferase cDNA for mammalian gene expression in culture and in vivo. Mol Ther 11:435–443
152. Loening AM, Wu AM, Gambhir SS (2007) Red-shifted Renilla reniformis luciferase variants for imaging in living subjects. Nat Meth 4:641–643
153. Loening AM, Dragulescu-Andrasi A, Gambhir SS (2010) A red-shifted Renilla luciferase for transient reporter-gene expression. Nat Meth 7:5–6
154. Rabinovich BA, Ye Y, Etto T et al (2008) Visualizing fewer than 10 mouse T cells with an enhanced firefly luciferase in immunocompetent mouse models of cancer. Proc Natl Acad Sci U S A 105:14342–14346
155. Deroose CM, De A, Loening AM et al (2007) Multimodality imaging of tumor xenografts and metastases in mice with combined small-animal PET, small-animal CT, and bioluminescence imaging. J Nucl Med 48:295–303
156. Kuo C, Coquoz O, Troy TL, Xu H, Rice BW (2007) Three-dimensional reconstruction of in vivo bioluminescent sources based on multispectral imaging. J Biomed Opt 12:024007

157. Jenkins DE, Yu SF, Hornig YS, Purchio T, Contag PR (2003) In vivo monitoring of tumor relapse and metastasis using bioluminescent PC-3M-luc-C6 cells in murine models of human prostate cancer. Clin Exp Metastasis 20:745–756
158. Edinger M, Cao YA, Verneris MR, Bachmann MH, Contag CH, Negrin RS (2003) Revealing lymphoma growth and the efficacy of immune cell therapies using in vivo bioluminescence imaging. Blood 101:640–648
159. Zhang C, Yan Z, Arango ME, Painter CL, Anderes K (2009) Advancing bioluminescence imaging technology for the evaluation of anticancer agents in the MDA-MB-435-HAL-Luc mammary fat pad and subrenal capsule tumor models. Clin Cancer Res 15:238–246
160. Vooijs M, Jonkers J, Lyons S, Berns A (2002) Noninvasive imaging of spontaneous retinoblastoma pathway-dependent tumors in mice. Cancer Res 62:1862–1867
161. Zhang N, Lyons S, Lim E, Lassota P (2009) A spontaneous acinar cell carcinoma model for monitoring progression of pancreatic lesions and response to treatment through noninvasive bioluminescence imaging. Clin Cancer Res 15:4915–4924
162. Uhrbom L, Nerio E, Holland EC (2004) Dissecting tumor maintenance requirements using bioluminescence imaging of cell proliferation in a mouse glioma model. Nat Med 10:1257–1260
163. Hamstra DA, Bhojani MS, Griffin LB, Laxman B, Ross BD, Rehemtulla A (2006) Real-time evaluation of p53 oscillatory behavior in vivo using bioluminescent imaging. Cancer Res 66:7482–7489
164. Laxman B, Hall DE, Bhojani MS et al (2002) Noninvasive real-time imaging of apoptosis. Proc Natl Acad Sci USA 99:16551–16555
165. Lee KC, Hamstra DA, Bhojani MS, Khan AP, Ross BD, Rehemtulla A (2007) Noninvasive molecular imaging sheds light on the synergy between 5-fluorouracil and TRAIL/Apo2L for cancer therapy. Clin Cancer Res 13:1839–1846
166. Zhang L, Lee KC, Bhojani MS et al (2007) Molecular imaging of Akt kinase activity. Nat Med 13:1114–1119
167. Paulmurugan R, Gambhir SS (2003) Monitoring protein-protein interactions using split synthetic renilla luciferase protein-fragment-assisted complementation. Anal Chem 75: 1584–1589
168. Luker GD, Sharma V, Pica CM et al (2002) Noninvasive imaging of protein-protein interactions in living animals. Proc Natl Acad Sci USA 99:6961–6966
169. Luker KE, Gupta M, Luker GD (2009) Imaging chemokine receptor dimerization with firefly luciferase complementation. FASEB J 23:823–834
170. Chan CT, Paulmurugan R, Gheysens OS, Kim J, Chiosis G, Gambhir SS (2008) Molecular imaging of the efficacy of heat shock protein 90 inhibitors in living subjects. Cancer Res 68:216–226
171. Paulmurugan R, Gambhir SS (2006) An intramolecular folding sensor for imaging estrogen receptor-ligand interactions. Proc Natl Acad Sci USA 103:15883–15888
172. Inoue Y, Izawa K, Kiryu S, Tojo A, Ohtomo K (2008) Diet and abdominal autofluorescence detected by in vivo fluorescence imaging of living mice. Mol Imaging 7:21–27
173. Xu H, Rice BW (2009) In-vivo fluorescence imaging with a multivariate curve resolution spectral unmixing technique. J Biomed Opt 14:064011
174. Niedre MJ, de Kleine RH, Aikawa E, Kirsch DG, Weissleder R, Ntziachristos V (2008) Early photon tomography allows fluorescence detection of lung carcinomas and disease progression in mice in vivo. Proc Natl Acad Sci USA 105:19126–19131
175. Mayinger B, Neumann F, Kastner C, Haider T, Schwab D (2010) Hexaminolevulinate-induced fluorescence colonoscopy versus white light endoscopy for diagnosis of neoplastic lesions in the colon. Endoscopy 42:28–33
176. Kimura T, Muguruma N, Ito S et al (2007) Infrared fluorescence endoscopy for the diagnosis of superficial gastric tumors. Gastrointest Endosc 66:37–43
177. Upadhyay R, Sheth RA, Weissleder R, Mahmood U (2007) Quantitative real-time catheter-based fluorescence molecular imaging in mice. Radiology 245:523–531

178. Zhong W, Celli JP, Rizvi I et al (2009) In vivo high-resolution fluorescence microendoscopy for ovarian cancer detection and treatment monitoring. Br J Cancer 101:2015–2022
179. Winkler F, Kozin SV, Tong RT et al (2004) Kinetics of vascular normalization by VEGFR2 blockade governs brain tumor response to radiation: role of oxygenation, angiopoietin-1, and matrix metalloproteinases. Cancer Cell 6:553–563
180. Fukumura D, Jain RK (2008) Imaging angiogenesis and the microenvironment. APMIS 116:695–715
181. Giampieri S, Manning C, Hooper S, Jones L, Hill CS, Sahai E (2009) Localized and reversible TGFbeta signalling switches breast cancer cells from cohesive to single cell motility. Nat Cell Biol 11:1287–1296
182. Kienast Y, von Baumgarten L, Fuhrmann M et al (2010) Real-time imaging reveals the single steps of brain metastasis formation. Nat Med 16:116–122
183. Helmchen F, Denk W (2005) Deep tissue two-photon microscopy. Nat Meth 2:932–940
184. Citrin D, Lee AK, Scott T et al (2004) In vivo tumor imaging in mice with near-infrared labeled endostatin. Mol Cancer Ther 3:481–488
185. Montet X, Figueiredo JL, Alencar H, Ntziachristos V, Mahmood U, Weissleder R (2007) Tomographic fluorescence imaging of tumor vascular volume in mice. Radiology 242:751–758
186. Ke S, Wen X, Gurfinkel M et al (2003) Near-infrared optical imaging of epidermal growth factor receptor in breast cancer xenografts. Cancer Res 63:7870–7875
187. Moore A, Medarova Z, Potthast A, Dai G (2004) In vivo targeting of underglycosylated MUC-1 tumor antigen using a multimodal imaging probe. Cancer Res 64:1821–1827
188. Wu Y, Cai W, Chen X (2006) Near-infrared fluorescence imaging of tumor integrin alpha v beta 3 expression with Cy7-labeled RGD multimers. Mol Imaging Biol 8:226–236
189. Mulder WJ, Castermans K, van Beijnum JR et al (2009) Molecular imaging of tumor angiogenesis using alphavbeta3-integrin targeted multimodal quantum dots. Angiogenesis 12:17–24
190. Koyama Y, Hama Y, Urano Y, Nguyen DM, Choyke PL, Kobayashi H (2007) Spectral fluorescence molecular imaging of lung metastases targeting HER2/neu. Clin Cancer Res 13:2936–2945
191. Edgington LE, Berger AB, Blum G et al (2009) Noninvasive optical imaging of apoptosis by caspase-targeted activity-based probes. Nat Med 15:967–973
192. Blum G, Mullins SR, Keren K et al (2005) Dynamic imaging of protease activity with fluorescently quenched activity-based probes. Nat Chem Biol 1:203–209
193. Blum G, von Degenfeld G, Merchant MJ, Blau HM, Bogyo M (2007) Noninvasive optical imaging of cysteine protease activity using fluorescently quenched activity-based probes. Nat Chem Biol 3:668–677
194. Grimm J, Kirsch DG, Windsor SD et al (2005) Use of gene expression profiling to direct in vivo molecular imaging of lung cancer. Proc Natl Acad Sci USA 102:14404–14409
195. McIntyre JO, Matrisian LM (2009) Optical proteolytic beacons for in vivo detection of matrix metalloproteinase activity. Meth Mol Biol 539:155–174
196. Ogawa M, Kosaka N, Choyke PL, Kobayashi H (2009) In vivo molecular imaging of cancer with a quenching near-infrared fluorescent probe using conjugates of monoclonal antibodies and indocyanine green. Cancer Res 69:1268–1272
197. Urano Y, Asanuma D, Hama Y et al (2009) Selective molecular imaging of viable cancer cells with pH-activatable fluorescence probes. Nat Med 15:104–109
198. Katz MH, Takimoto S, Spivack D, Moossa AR, Hoffman RM, Bouvet M (2003) A novel red fluorescent protein orthotopic pancreatic cancer model for the preclinical evaluation of chemotherapeutics. J Surg Res 113:151–160
199. Yang M, Li L, Jiang P, Moossa AR, Penman S, Hoffman RM (2003) Dual-color fluorescence imaging distinguishes tumor cells from induced host angiogenic vessels and stromal cells. Proc Natl Acad Sci USA 100:14259–14262
200. Amoh Y, Katsuoka K, Hoffman RM (2008) Color-coded fluorescent protein imaging of angiogenesis: the AngioMouse models. Curr Pharm Des 14:3810–3819
201. Sakaue-Sawano A, Kurokawa H, Morimura T et al (2008) Visualizing spatiotemporal dynamics of multicellular cell-cycle progression. Cell 132:487–498

202. Mocanu JD, Moriyama EH, Chia MC et al (2004) Combined in vivo bioluminescence and fluorescence imaging for cancer gene therapy. Mol Imaging 3:352–355
203. Kimball KJ, Rivera AA, Zinn KR et al (2009) Novel infectivity-enhanced oncolytic adenovirus with a capsid-incorporated dual-imaging moiety for monitoring virotherapy in ovarian cancer. Mol Imaging 8:264–277
204. Kesarwala AH, Prior JL, Sun J, Harpstrite SE, Sharma V, Piwnica-Worms D (2006) Second-generation triple reporter for bioluminescence, micro-positron emission tomography, and fluorescence imaging. Mol Imaging 5:465–474
205. Ray P, Tsien R, Gambhir SS (2007) Construction and validation of improved triple fusion reporter gene vectors for molecular imaging of living subjects. Cancer Res 67:3085–3093
206. Shu X, Royant A, Lin MZ et al (2009) Mammalian expression of infrared fluorescent proteins engineered from a bacterial phytochrome. Science 324:804–807
207. Vakoc BJ, Lanning RM, Tyrrell JA et al (2009) Three-dimensional microscopy of the tumor microenvironment in vivo using optical frequency domain imaging. Nat Med 15: 1219–1223
208. De la Zerda A, Zavaleta C, Keren S et al (2008) Carbon nanotubes as photoacoustic molecular imaging agents in living mice. Nat Nanotechnol 3:557–562
209. Razansky D, Baeten J, Ntziachristos V (2009) Sensitivity of molecular target detection by multispectral optoacoustic tomography (MSOT). Med Phys 36:939–945
210. Kim JW, Galanzha EI, Shashkov EV, Moon HM, Zharov VP (2009) Golden carbon nanotubes as multimodal photoacoustic and photothermal high-contrast molecular agents. Nat Nanotechnol 4:688–694

Chapter 11
Chemoprevention

Richard A. Hubner

Introduction

In the developed world mortality from major chronic diseases such as cardiovascular and cerebrovascular disease has decreased substantially in the past half century, whilst cancer mortality has only recently shown a modest decline [1]. Despite novel chemotherapeutic and biological agents for cancer treatment, prognosis for the large majority of patients diagnosed with advanced cancer remains poor, and cancer is now the most frequent cause of death in men and women under 85 years in the United States [2]. A promising alternative approach is to prevent the development of invasive disease by treating carcinogenesis rather than cancer itself. Cancer chemoprevention is classically defined as the use of natural, synthetic, or biological chemical agents to interfere with the process of carcinogenesis by either preventing the development of a pre-invasive lesion, inhibiting the progression of a pre-invasive lesion into an invasive cancer, or causing a reversal of a pre-invasive lesion towards the normal state [3]. Although there is a large body of pre-clinical data supporting the concept of cancer chemoprevention, a relatively small number of clinical chemoprevention trials have reported significant benefits, and the use of chemopreventive agents in routine clinical practice is currently limited to high-risk cancer predisposition syndromes.

This chapter describes how pre-invasive disease is embedded in the key principles of chemoprevention, has provided a platform for clinical trials of chemopreventive agents, and will be instrumental in achieving personalised chemoprevention.

R.A. Hubner (✉)
Department of Medicine, Royal Marsden Hospital, London, UK
e-mail: richard.hubner@icr.ac.uk

R.C. Fitzgerald (ed.), *Pre-Invasive Disease: Pathogenesis and Clinical Management*,
DOI 10.1007/978-1-4419-6694-0_11, © Springer Science+Business Media, LLC 2011

Principles of Chemoprevention and Influence of Pre-invasive Disease

Population-Based and Individualised Cancer Prevention Strategies

Data from observational studies indicating differential cancer risk in population subgroups defined by lifestyle or dietary factors implies that cancer prevention may be possible through modification of such risk factors. For example, the recent World Cancer Research Fund/American Institute for Cancer Research report into food, nutrition, physical activity and the prevention of cancer judged regular physical exercise, foods containing dietary fibre, garlic, and milk to be protective against colorectal cancer (CRC), whilst alcohol, abdominal obesity, and processed or red meats confer increased CRC risk [4]. Lifestyle and dietary interventions are generally population-based prevention strategies designed to reduce risk factor prevalence in the whole population and target cancer risk broadly, with a less predictable impact on any one person's cancer risk. In contrast, chemoprevention is more suited to individualised prevention strategies where agents are targeted to subgroups of the population who are at high cancer risk. Population-based chemoprevention is unlikely to be acceptable since large numbers of subjects at low risk of cancer would be exposed to potential adverse effects. A diagnosis of pre-invasive disease, identified either through screening programmes or direct referral pathways on development of symptoms, usually confers a substantially increased risk of invasive disease. Thus, pre-invasive disease provides an opportunity for individualised cancer prevention by identifying subjects at greater risk of cancer compared to the background population and thus likely to gain differential benefit from chemopreventive agents.

The majority of CRC, for example, are thought to develop from colorectal adenoma (CRA) via the adenoma-carcinoma sequence, and development of CRA is one of the most relevant risk factors for CRC, conferring a two- to fourfold increased risk depending on size and histological features [5]. Observational data indicates that endoscopic resection of CRA reduces risk of subsequent invasive disease by 75–90%, although no confirmatory randomised data are available [6]. Thus CRA resection is a form of surgical or local cancer prevention, a further example being colposcopy and excision of cervical pre-invasive lesions identified though cervical smear-test screening. One-off colonoscopy and resection of CRA alone, however, may not convert an individual's CRC risk back to the population risk, since pre-invasive disease confers an increased risk of further pre-invasive lesions. The "field cancerisation" concept of carcinogenesis proposed by Slaughter and colleagues in 1953 [7], postulated that insult from a carcinogen occurs across an entire epithelial field, giving rise to multiple, independent sites of carcinogenesis. Subsequent molecular findings of field-wide genetically altered cells have supported this hypothesis, which explains in part why successful local control of neoplasia frequently does not prevent second, genetically distinct pre-invasive and invasive lesions occurring in the same epithelial field. Repeated endoscopic examinations do not necessarily solve this problem due to the development of interval lesions. By acting systemically, chemoprevention has the potential to impact the whole field, complementing local preventive strategies when used simultaneously.

Cancer Risk Prediction Models

Accurate prediction of cancer risk is a cornerstone of chemoprevention. The population lifetime risk of developing even common cancers is low, for example ~12% for breast cancer and ~5% for CRC, thus most individuals will remain cancer free over considerable periods of time. Individualised prevention strategies such as chemoprevention rely on cancer risk prediction models to identify high risk individuals to maximize efficacy and favourably shift the risk-benefit ratio where even minimal potential side-effects exist. However, unless the relative risks conferred by single or combinations of risk factors are high, perhaps as high as 20-fold or more, the probability that a person with a particular risk factor profile will develop cancer (positive predictive value) will be low due to the low baseline risk [8]. Without cancer risk prediction models with high discriminatory power, population prevention strategies aimed at reducing risk factor prevalence in the whole population will yield greater benefits, since targeting high risk individuals based on inaccurate risk factor profiles may miss a substantial number of individuals who will ultimately develop disease. Overall, the more predictable the cancer risk, the greater the rationale for focusing prevention strategies on high risk individuals.

An important step in cancer risk modelling is accurate estimation of the relative and attributable risks for aetiologic factors, including age, gender, ethnicity, reproductive factors, lifestyle factors (such as smoking and physical exercise), dietary patterns, medication use, genetic factors (including family history and polymorphic variants), and clinical markers (such as serum cancer marker levels, enzyme levels, and histopathologic factors). An understanding of how these factors interact to influence cancer risk is also important. These risk estimates can be obtained from a number of different study designs including case-control, cohort, and clinical studies, national databases, and cross-sectional population surveys. The changing nature and effect magnitude of individual risk factors over time may also need to be considered, and different risk models will be required for cancer-specific subtypes such as oestrogen receptor positive and negative breast cancer.

A diagnosis of pre-invasive disease has the potential to be a powerful predictive factor for development of invasive cancer. An example of a cancer risk prediction model that includes pre-invasive disease as a risk factor is the Gail Breast Cancer Risk Assessment Model [9]. This model was adapted to design the Breast Cancer Prevention Trial (BCPT), which investigated tamoxifen chemoprevention in women at elevated risk of breast cancer, and includes atypical hyperplasia in biopsy specimens as a risk factor for subsequent invasive disease [10]. Pre-invasive disease may also interact with other factors to determine cancer risk. For example, studies in animal models of colon cancer indicate that folic acid supplementation initiated prior to the development of pre-invasive lesions has a protective effect against development of malignancy, whilst supplementation started after pre-invasive lesions have been initiated has a detrimental effect [11, 12]. Current understanding of the risk implications of pre-invasive disease is incomplete, even for well-studied lesions such as CRA. Recent data, for example, indicates that removal of CRA does not impact significantly on subsequent risk of proximal colon cancers [13]. Furthermore, all pre-invasive lesions are not equal in terms of impact on cancer risk; it is estimated that only 2–5% of sporadic CRA have the potential to progress to malignancy, thus the majority of CRA identified at screening and subsequent surveillance are clinically insignificant lesions [14].

Cancer risk prediction has been recognised as an area of extraordinary research opportunity [8]. Further studies investigating the relationships between pre-invasive and invasive disease are required, and should include an assessment of the impact of molecular heterogeneity of pre-invasive lesions, and interactions with other potential risk factors, in particular polymorphic genetic variants.

Toxicity Avoidance

Adverse events represent a major obstacle to the routine use of chemopreventive agents. The low absolute population risk of common cancers means that a large proportion of individuals will remain cancer free, even in subgroups defined by risk factors conferring high relative risk, thus all subjects receiving chemoprevention are exposed to toxicity whilst only a proportion will experience potential benefit. In the setting of chemoprevention trials, evaluating adverse events is as important as preventive efficacy.

Early chemoprevention studies investigated natural agents assumed to be virtually free of toxicity, however supplement doses were selected that raised levels 10- to 20-fold greater than physiologic levels, and unexpected adverse events were encountered [15]. Lung cancer prevention trials of β-carotene in combination with α-tocopherol or retinol reported significantly increased incidences of lung cancer and cardiovascular disease [16, 17], a meta-analysis of trials of antioxidant supplements indicated increased mortality with supplement use [18], whilst high dose folic acid supplements (1,000 mcg daily) increased recurrence of advanced CRA [19]. Vitamin supplementation does not appear to confer cancer reduction when administered to a non-deficient population, and at supraphysiologic doses may increase cancer incidence and cause other adverse effects. Long-term administration of drugs in randomised chemoprevention studies can also reveal unexpected adverse effects of drugs already in routine use in other clinical scenarios. The increased incidence of cardiovascular events and mortality associated with cyclo-oxygenase-2 (COX-2) inhibitors was discovered in CRA recurrence prevention trials, but had not been encountered in shorter trials in arthritis and familial adenomatous polyposis [20].

The risk of adverse events will not be uniform across a population receiving chemoprevention. For example, although the BCPT demonstrated that tamoxifen reduced invasive breast cancer in women at increased disease risk, adverse events such as stroke, pulmonary embolism, and endometrial cancer occurred more often in women taking tamoxifen, and the risk increased with advancing age [21]. Hence the level of risk needed to justify the use of tamoxifen for breast cancer prevention was much higher in older women who had higher risks of adverse events. Similarly, the risk of gastric or duodenal ulceration and serious gastrointestinal bleeding in subjects taking regular aspirin or NSAID increases with advancing age [22].

Pre-invasive disease may beneficially influence the risk-benefit ratio of chemopreventive agents in two different ways. Firstly, it informs risk prediction models allowing more accurate delineation of high-risk individuals as discussed above. Secondly, examining the somatic genetic alterations and molecular aberrations present in the pre-invasive lesion will potentially allow rational selection of the chemopreventive agent most likely to provide maximal preventive efficacy. Such molecular targeting of chemoprevention has already being examined in clinical chemopreventive trials with favourable outcomes when compared with non-targeted chemoprevention, and examples are discussed below.

The more tangible nature of pre-malignant lesions compared to other risk factors may result in an inappropriate acceptance of potential adverse effects, particularly if pre-malignancy occurs in the setting of other emotive risk factors such as a positive family history. It is the responsibility of chemoprevention trialists to ensure that careful evaluation of side effects is undertaken, even when studying agents with an established adverse effect profile. Consideration of the expected frequency of toxicity is also required when designing chemoprevention trials since most studies will be underpowered to detect significant differences in rarely occurring but clinically significant side effects. In the context of chemoprevention even subtle adverse effects such as increases in mean blood sugar or blood pressure are important when treating a healthy population, and may have a major influence on clinical utility.

Molecular-Targeted Chemoprevention

The proof of principle of chemoprevention was demonstrated by Hong and coworkers [23] in a trial initiated in 1983 which showed that adjuvant high dose 13-*cis*-retinoic acid prevented second primary tumours in patients with curatively treated stage I–IV head and neck cancer. Subsequent nutritional supplement cancer chemoprevention trials were largely negative or even harmful as discussed above, and culminated in the negative Selenium and Vitamin E prostate Cancer Prevention Trial (SELECT) in over 35,000 men [24]. Chemoprevention trials designed on the basis of an understanding of molecular mechanisms involved in carcinogenesis have been more successful, and three examples are discussed below.

Selective Oestrogen Receptor Modulators (SERMs) and Breast Cancer Prevention

The reduced risk of contralateral breast cancers in women taking tamoxifen compared to those randomised to placebo in adjuvant endocrine therapy trials, led to the initiation of randomised, placebo-controlled tamoxifen chemoprevention trials. The BCPT (National Surgical Adjuvant Breast and Bowel Project Protocol-1, NSABP P-1 trial) [21] was the largest of these studies, and randomised 13,888 women at high risk for breast cancer on the basis of age ≥60 years, a Gail model 5-year predicted breast cancer risk of ≥1.66%, or history of lobular carcinoma in situ, to either tamoxifen 20 mg daily or placebo for 5 years. At a median follow-up of 55 months, tamoxifen significantly reduced the risk of invasive breast cancer by 49% and non-invasive breast lesions by 50%. The protective effect was limited to oestrogen-receptor (ER) positive tumours, and a recent update after 7 years of follow-up indicated a continuing significant breast cancer risk reduction [25]. Tamoxifen reduced hip fractures, consistent with oestrogen agonist effects in bone, however the incidence of endometrial cancer in women over 50 years was also significantly increased, as was the incidence of thromboembolic events. A meta-analysis of the BCPT and three other tamoxifen chemoprevention trials reported a 48% reduction in ER-positive breast cancer (95% confidence interval (CI); 36–58%) [26], and tamoxifen was approved by the US Food and Drug Administration (FDA) for breast cancer risk reduction in 1998.

Despite the proven cancer prevention efficacy of tamoxifen, only a small proportion of eligible high-risk women are offered and accept tamoxifen for primary breast cancer prevention, largely due to concerns over potential side effects, illustrating the difficulties of implementing chemopreventive strategies in a healthy population. The Study of Tamoxifen and Raloxifene trial (STAR) aimed to address these concerns by testing the hypothesis that raloxifene would have equivalent breast cancer preventive efficacy with fewer side effects [27]. Raloxifene is a SERM with oestrogen antagonist effects on breast and endometrium, and oestrogen agonist effects on bone, lipid metabolism and coagulation. Studies with raloxifene in individuals with osteoporosis or coronary heart disease had indicated a breast cancer preventive effect [28, 29]. In the STAR trial 19,747 post-menopausal women at increased breast cancer risk were randomised to tamoxifen (20 mg daily) or raloxifene (60 mg daily) for 5 years. After a median follow-up of 3.9 years both tamoxifen and raloxifene reduced invasive breast cancer incidence by 50%, however raloxifene did not provide protection against non-invasive breast cancer whereas tamoxifen decreased the incidence by half. Rates of endometrial cancer and thromboembolic events were significantly lower in raloxifene treated individuals. These data support the hypothesis that raloxifene is a safer chemopreventive agent and raloxifene is FDA approved for breast cancer chemoprevention in post-menopausal women with osteoporosis or post-menopausal women with high risk for breast cancer. Currently over half a million post-menopausal women in the US take raloxifene, although the large majority is prescribed for osteoporosis.

5α-Reductase Inhibition and Prostate Cancer Prevention

The enzyme 5α-reductase catalyses the conversion of testosterone to the more potent androgen dihydrotestosterone. The Prostate Cancer Prevention Trial (PCPT) tested the hypothesis that the 5α-reductase inhibitor finasteride would prevent androgen driven prostate cancer development [30]. This study randomly assigned 18,882 men with normal digital rectal examination (DRE) and a prostate specific antigen ≤3.0 ng/mL to placebo or finasteride 5 mg daily. Subjects were followed up with annual DRE, and prostate biopsies were performed for abnormal DRE or elevated PSA ≥4.0 ng/mL, and at the end of the 7-year study period. The prevalence of prostate cancer was significantly reduced in the finasteride group (18.4% compared to 24.4% in the placebo group). However, initial results also indicated an increased prevalence of high-grade (Gleason grade 7–10) prostate cancer (6.4% compared to 5.1%), which led to a lack of enthusiasm for recommending finasteride as a preventive agent. As expected, there were improved urinary symptoms but increased sexual dysfunction in the finasteride group. Subsequent analyses have found that the elevated prevalence of high-grade cancers in the finasteride treated group was an artefact secondary to enhanced detection. Finasteride increases the sensitivity of both PSA and DRE for cancer detection, and improves the diagnostic accuracy of prostate biopsy due to the ~25% reduction in prostate size with finasteride [31]. Analyses accounting for these factors indicated that participants taking finasteride were at significantly reduced risk of both tumours with Gleason grade ≤6 and those with grade 7–10.

Finasteride is currently the only agent to have proven prostate cancer chemopreventive efficacy and modelling analyses have calculated an overall population survival benefit of ~1.7 months [32]. Remaining questions include the optimal age to initiate chemoprevention, and optimal duration.

Cyclooxygenase-2 (COX-2) Inhibition and Colorectal Cancer Prevention

Aspirin and non-steriodal anti-inflammatory drugs (NSAIDs) inhibit the cyclooxygenase activity of prostaglandin G/H synthase (PTGS or COX), thereby blocking prostaglandin synthesis [33]. There are two isoforms of the COX enzyme; COX-1 inhibition results in the adverse effect of promoting gastric ulceration, whilst COX-2 inhibition mediates the beneficial anti-inflammatory effects of NSAIDs. Low dose aspirin is a relatively selective inhibitor of COX-1 in platelets but at higher doses inhibits both COX-1 and COX-2, whilst sulindac, ibuprofen and most other NSAIDs inhibit both isoforms to the same extent [34]. COX-2 selective inhibitors, such as celecoxib and refecoxib, take advantage of structural differences at the active sites of the two enzymes to selectively inhibit only the COX-2 isoform, leading to a significantly improved gastrointestinal side effect profile [35].

Aspirin and non-aspirin NSAIDs are known to stimulate apoptosis and inhibit angiogenesis, and as a consequence there has been much interest in their potential as anticancer drugs [36]. Many epidemiological, in vitro, animal-model, and human interventional studies have been performed investigating the effects of NSAIDs in a variety of tumour types, with the most substantial evidence for benefit being shown in colorectal carcinogenesis [34]. At least 36 epidemiologic studies have investigated the relationship between regular aspirin or other NSAID use and risk of CRC or CRA in different populations and using various study designs, and all but one have found an approximately 30–50% reduced risk in regular users [34, 37]. Data also suggest that the protective effect of aspirin in preventing CRC is dependent on dose and duration of treatment, with a benefit only being observed with higher doses (>150 mg daily) and after more than 5 years of regular use [38, 39].

A randomised trial of sulindac in 77 patients with Familial Adenomatous Polyposis (FAP), a hereditary condition characterised by the development of 100–1,000s of adenomatous polyps and CRC by the third or fourth decade, provided proof of principle that COX-inhibition could influence colorectal carcinogenesis [40]. Celecoxib caused regression of existing polyps and reduced new polyp formation, and was approved for use as an adjunct to standard care in FAP patients. In contrast, two randomised primary prevention trials using aspirin in the general US population reported no significant effect on CRC incidence for either males or females [41, 42]. The first trial, the Physicians' Health Study, was designed to investigate the effects of aspirin on primary prevention of cardiovascular disease, and randomised to intervention for only 5 years [41]. This relatively short duration of aspirin use, combined with a relatively low dose (325 mg every other day), and the lack of systematic screening for either CRA or CRC at either trial entry or termination makes interpretation of the data on CRC incidence difficult. The second study, the Women's Health Study, also used a dose of aspirin, 100 mg daily, that was probably too low to demonstrate protective effects against CRC development [42]. More recently, a combined analysis of the long-term effects of aspirin use in two UK based randomised trials, the British Doctors Aspirin Trial and the UK-TIA Aspirin Trial, which randomised to 5 years of 500 mg daily use and 1–7 years of 1,200 mg daily use respectively, reported a 26% reduction in CRC risk in those allocated to aspirin, which was greatest in those who received aspirin for 5 or more years, and was only seen after a latency of 10 years [43].

Four randomised trials have investigated the influence of various doses of aspirin (81–325 mg daily) in the setting of CRA recurrence [44–47]. These trials aimed to maximize the likelihood of observing a protective effect of aspirin intervention by enrolling subjects who had already been diagnosed with either CRA [44, 45, 47] or CRC [46], and who were therefore at high risk of recurrent CRA. The use of CRA recurrence as a surrogate endpoint for CRC development also allowed the intervention period to be shortened to 3–6 years, rather than the 10–15 years that would likely be required to demonstrate primary preventive effects. All four studies reported a reduction in CRA recurrence in subjects receiving aspirin, and in a pooled analysis (including 2,698 patients, 1,542 of whom received aspirin, with a median follow-up of 33 months), the pooled risk ratio was 0.83 (95%CI, 0.72–0.96) for any adenoma recurrence, and 0.72 (95%CI, 0.57–0.90) for adenoma deemed "advanced" on the basis of size or adverse histological features [48]. Collectively the results of these randomised trials indicate that aspirin has a modest beneficial effect in secondary prevention of CRA recurrence, although the optimal dose is unclear.

The use of COX-2 selective inhibitors appeared to have the potential to achieve the benefits of unselective inhibitors such as aspirin in terms of colorectal neoplasia prevention, without the side-effects of gastric irritation and bleeding associated with COX-1 inhibition. Randomised trials of rofexocib and celecoxib confirmed their efficacy in preventing CRA recurrence, but unfortunately also reported an increased incidence of serious cardiovascular events, precluding their use in primary or secondary prevention [20, 49]. However, recent analyses of data from phase III trials of celecoxib for non-arthritic conditions indicate that celecoxib did not increase cardiovascular adverse events in individuals with low baseline cardiovascular risk, which may provide an opportunity for selective use in such patients with high CRA/CRC risk [50].

The proven benefits of aspirin for cardiovascular disease give it an advantage over other NSAIDs for further study in cancer chemoprevention, although other NSAIDs such as sulindac warrant investigation. Aspirin or NSAIDs may be effective for secondary chemoprevention of colorectal and other gastrointestinal cancers in individuals with no prior history of gastrointestinal bleeding. An alternative approach is combination therapy with a proton-pump inhibitor, and this is currently being studied in the AspECT study of omeprazole and aspirin in patients with Barrett's oesophagus [51].

Combination Chemoprevention

Chemotherapy agents are often used in combination to treat invasive cancer with the aim of preventing the emergence of drug resistant clones by combining agents with different mechanisms of action. Combination chemoprevention may lead to a similar gain in efficacy with the additional benefit of potentially allowing reduced toxicities by lowered doses of individual agents. Pre-clinical data linking increased polyamine synthesis and inflammation with colon carcinogenesis led to a clinical trial in patients with resected CRA combining the NSAID sulindac with difluoromethylornithine (DMFO), an irreversible inhibitor of ornithine decarboxylase

(ODC) [52]. Polyamines affect many processes in carcinogenesis, and ODC is the rate-limiting enzyme in the polyamine synthesis pathway. Inhibition of polyamine synthesis is associated with reduced cell proliferation, increased apoptosis, and suppression of angiogenesis, whilst ODC activity and polyamine levels are increased in many human epithelial tumours including colon cancer [53]. NSAIDs influence polyamine levels by induction of polyamine catabolism, and this may account in part for their chemopreventive effects on colorectal neoplasia [53]. Hence NSAIDs and DMFO act independently at different stages of polyamine metabolism to reduce tissue polyamine levels (Fig. 11.1). In the clinical trial

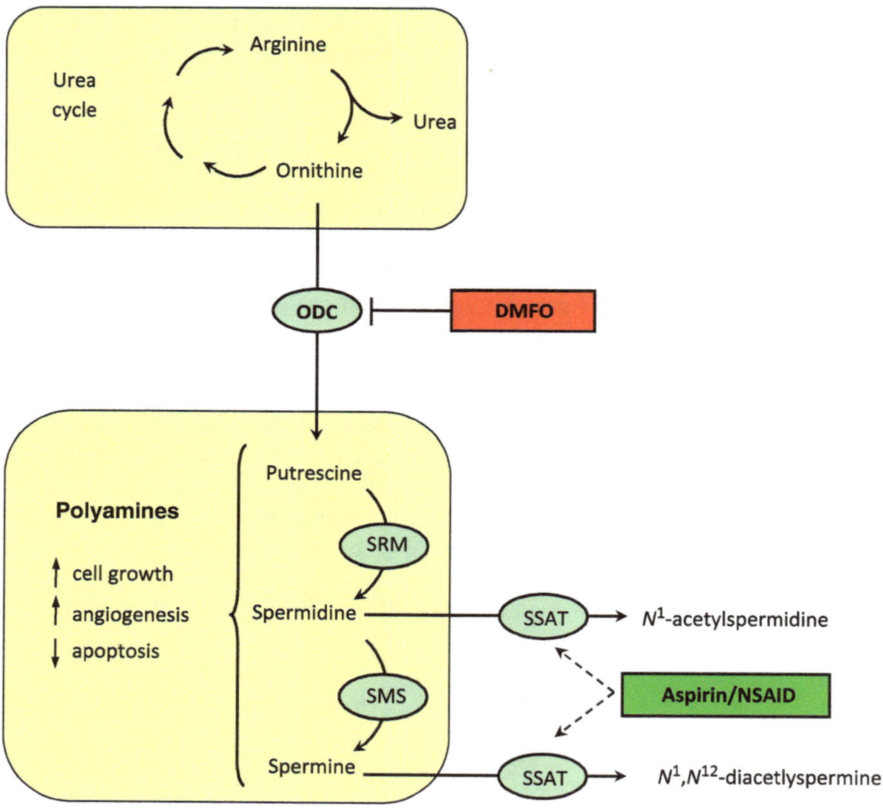

Fig. 11.1 Schematic representation of polyamine metabolism. The metabolism of arginine in the urea cycle results in ornithine production. Ornithine decarboxylase (ODC) catalyses the first step in polyamine synthesis in which ornithine is decarboxylated to produce putrescine. Spermidine synthase (SRM) converts putrescine to spermidine which is subsequently converted to spermine by spermine synthase (SMS). Spermidine/spermine N1-acetyltransferase (SSAT) acetylates spermidine and spermine which are then either converted back to putrescine or exported from the cell and excreted in urine. ODC is inhibited by difluoromethylornithine (DMFO), reducing polyamine synthesis. Aspirin and other non-steroidal anti-inflammatory drugs (NSAID) induce SSAT transcription, promoting polyamine metabolism

patients received either both chemopreventive agents or placebo for 36 months [52]. CRA recurrence rates were 12% in the combination group vs. 41% in the placebo group, and advanced adenoma rates were 0.7 and 8.5% respectively – a highly significant relative risk reduction of over 90%, whilst rates of serious adverse events were similar between the study arms. The drugs for this combination chemoprevention trial were selected on the basis of extensive animal testing [54, 55], and the doses chosen following careful dose de-escalation studies with assessment of polyamine levels in target tissue [56]. This landmark study has validated the concept of combination chemoprevention, with favourable efficacy compared to previous adenoma recurrence prevention trials with single agent aspirin or COX-2 inhibitors. Furthermore, the doses of each agent were lower than that previously shown to be ineffective in advanced colorectal cancer, indicating that drugs with little or no activity in advanced disease may still possess preventive activity at earlier stages of carcinogenesis.

Incorporating Biomarker Data in Chemoprevention Strategies

The identification of predictive markers of response to established and emerging anti-cancer agents is widely recognised as a research priority, with the aim of improving clinical outcomes and cost-efficiency, whilst avoiding toxicity [57]. This is particularly relevant to chemoprevention where treatment of individuals who may be at high-risk but are currently unaffected by cancer broadens the acceptable therapeutic window. Research into the molecular genetic features of pre-invasive disease may identify predictive markers for chemopreventive agents, and a promising example is COX-2 expression level in colorectal neoplasia and response to aspirin chemoprevention. Aspirin has proven efficacy in secondary prevention of CRA, but the balance of risk and benefit is not considered sufficient to routinely recommend aspirin use in individuals diagnosed with CRA or CRC. COX-2 is over-expressed in ~80% of CRC and ~50% of CRA [58], and the likelihood of COX-2 over-expression varies in different CRC subgroups defined by molecular characteristics such as microsatellite instability [59], and increases with increasing CRA size and degree of epithelial dysplasia [60].

Two provocative studies by Chan and coworkers suggest that COX-2 expression levels in colorectal tumour tissue are a predictor of aspirin efficacy in both primary and secondary prevention of CRC [61, 62]. Both studies were retrospective analyses of two large independent cohorts of US women, the Nurses' Health Study (NHS), and US men, the Health Professionals Follow-up Study (HPFS). In the first study [61] the influence of regular aspirin use on CRC risk was evaluated according to over-expression of COX-2 in the tumour. For the analysis, participants taking two or more standard (325 mg) aspirin tablets per week, or aspirin on two or more occasions per week were considered to be regular aspirin users. Out of 1,994 CRCs that were recorded in the follow-up period, COX-2 expression was assessed using immunohistochemistry in 636 (32%), and over-expression was present in 67% of tumours. As had been previously noted in these cohorts, the overall risk of CRC was significantly reduced by regular aspirin use. However, the benefit of aspirin appeared to be confined to cancers with COX-2 over-expression (RR 0.64; 95%CI, 0.52–0.78), with no significant association observed in CRCs with weak or absent COX-2 expression (RR 0.96; 95%CI, 0.73–1.26). Furthermore, significant dose-response and duration-response effects were noted in the influence of regular aspirin use on risk of only COX-2 over-expressing CRC. Remarkably similar results were observed in the two independent cohorts when analysed separately, and these results were consistent with an earlier case-control study in which the association of NSAID use with a reduced risk of CRA was most apparent in cases with high expression of COX-2 mRNA [63].

The second study extended these observations to the effect of tumour COX-2 expression on the associations between regular aspirin use and CRC-specific and overall survival following a diagnosis of stage I–III CRC [62]. The same patient cohorts, definitions of regular aspirin use, and immunohistochemical methods for assessment of COX-2 expression were used, and the influence of aspirin use pre- and post-diagnosis were analysed both together and separately. Overall, regular aspirin use prior to diagnosis had no significant influence on either CRC-specific or overall mortality, whereas aspirin use after diagnosis was associated with significant risk reductions of 29 and 21%, respectively. Further analyses of the effect of post-diagnosis aspirin use indicated that the beneficial effects were confined to those individuals who initiated aspirin use following diagnosis rather than those who continued existing pre-diagnosis aspirin use. COX-2 expression status impacted significantly on the association, with the benefit of post-diagnosis aspirin use being confined to individuals with COX-2 over-expressing tumours, particularly in those initiating aspirin use post-diagnosis who benefited from a 78% (95%CI, 26–93%) reduction in risk of CRC-specific mortality. Receipt of adjuvant chemotherapy did not influence these associations, and aspirin use did not affect the likelihood of receiving adjuvant chemotherapy. These findings corroborated results from a prior analysis of participants in a study of adjuvant therapy in resected stage III colon cancer [64], in whom regular aspirin use conferred a significant prolongation of disease free survival. Together, these studies suggest that aspirin may have a specific effect on the prevention of micrometastases among individuals with invasive disease, that this effect will be absent in tumours which develop in the presence of aspirin, and that COX-2 expression in the tumour is a marker of aspirin efficacy.

Although both studies by Chan and coworkers were retrospective, assessed the influence of non-randomised aspirin administration, and did not consider non-aspirin NSAID or COX-2 selective inhibitor use, the predictive influence of COX-2 over-expression in determining benefit from aspirin use is compelling. Randomised studies of aspirin in patients diagnosed with CRA or CRC stratified by intra-lesion COX-2 expression are warranted.

Influence of Polymorphic Variation on Chemoprevention Efficacy and Toxicity

Recent genome wide association studies in common cancers and other common chronic diseases have confirmed that germline genetic variants with high population frequency can confer small but highly significant influences on disease risk, which when combined with other similar variants can have a clinically relevant impact on individual risk [65]. Polymorphic variation has also been shown to influence drug bioavailability, activity, and toxicity in the treatment of invasive cancer, and it is very probable that similar polymorphic influences exist for chemopreventive agents.

Although pharmacogenomics in the setting of chemoprevention is still in its infancy, important associations have already been identified. Expression of ODC, the rate limiting enzyme in polyamine synthesis, is altered by a functional polymorphism, *ODC* G316A, which lies between two promoter-region transcription factor binding sites, with the minor A allele conferring reduced enzyme expression [66]. Genotyping of participants in a CRA recurrence prevention study investigating the effect of a wheat bran fiber intervention initially reported a 50% reduction in CRA recurrence in individuals with homozygous *ODC* 316AA genotype compared to wild-type individuals [66]. Aspirin impacts on the same metabolic pathway by inducing polyamine catabolism, and *ODC* 316AA genotype participants who reported aspirin use had a 90% reduction in recurrence risk compared to wild-type non-aspirin users. These findings were corroborated in a UK-based trial of aspirin for CRA recurrence prevention, in which *ODC* 316AA genotype participants were at similar significantly decreased risk of recurrence compared to those with *ODC* 316GG or *ODC* 316GA genotypes combined (relative risk 0.43), with a more pronounced effect in those taking aspirin [67]. Finally, a third study by Barry and coworkers, who genotyped participants in an independent randomised trial of aspirin for CRA recurrence prevention, found that *ODC* 316AA genotype did not have an independent prognostic effect, but was a significant predictor of response to aspirin [68]. Pooling the results of all three studies provides compelling evidence of a predictive influence of *ODC* 316AA genotype on the response to aspirin in preventing CRA recurrence (Fig. 11.2) [67]. Although only ~5% of Caucasians carry the *ODC* 316AA genotype, this group appear to gain differential benefit from aspirin in preventing colorectal neoplasia, offering the potential for targeted chemoprevention.

Conclusion

Diagnosis of a pre-invasive lesion significantly influences cancer risk and provides an opportunity to intervene with chemopreventive agents prior to the development of invasive disease. The challenge to researchers is to individualise

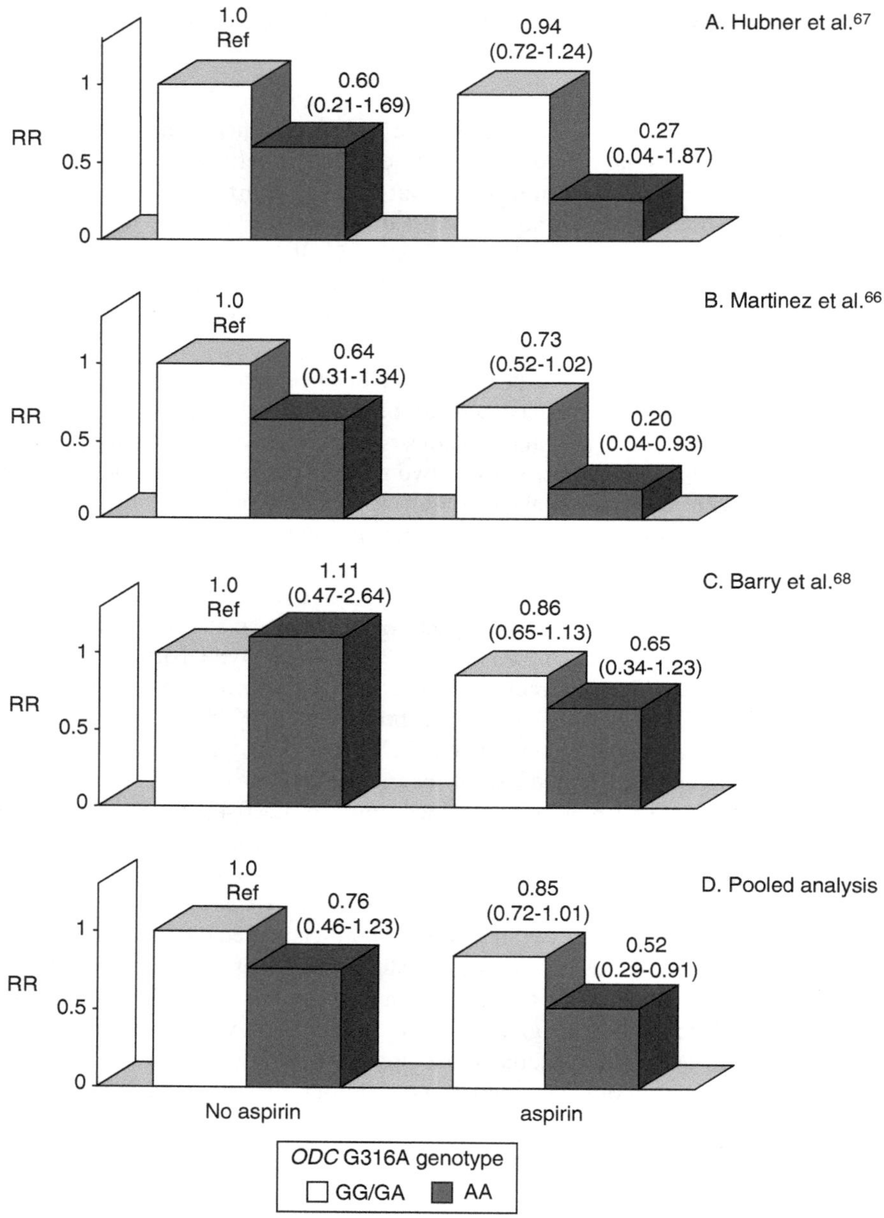

Fig. 11.2 Relative risks (RRs) and 95% confidence intervals (CIs) for adenoma recurrence stratified by *ODC* G316A genotype and aspirin exposure in Hubner et al. [67] (**a**), Martinez et al. [66] (**b**), Barry et al. [68] (**c**), and pooled analysis (**d**). In each panel the reference group is individuals with either *ODC* 316GG or 316GA genotypes who were not exposed to aspirin. For panels B and C RRs and 95%CIs were calculated from published raw data without adjustment

chemopreventive therapy by determining which agent or combination of agents should be used, at what dose, and for what duration to achieve maximal preventive efficacy and minimal toxicity. Factors that will impact on the optimal choice of chemopreventive agent include individual level of cancer risk, molecular features of the pre-invasive lesion, host genotype, and the availability of other pharmacological and non-pharmacological alternatives for cancer prevention. Such personalised chemoprevention strategies will maximize the likelihood of an individual avoiding cancer.

References

1. Ford ES, Ajani UA, Croft JB et al (2007) Explaining the decrease in U.S. deaths from coronary disease, 1980–2000. N Engl J Med 356:2388–2398
2. Jemal A, Siegel R, Ward E et al (2007) Cancer statistics, 2007. CA Cancer J Clin 57:43–66
3. Sporn MB, Dunlop NM, Newton DL et al (1976) Prevention of chemical carcinogenesis by vitamin A and its synthetic analogs (retinoids). Fed Proc 35:1332–1338
4. World Cancer Research Fund/American Institute for Cancer Research: Food, nutrition, physical activity, and the prevention of cancer: a global perspective. Washington DC, 2007
5. Atkin WS, Morson BC, Cuzick J (1992) Long-term risk of colorectal cancer after excision of rectosigmoid adenomas. N Engl J Med 326:658–662
6. Winawer SJ, Zauber AG, Ho MN et al (1993) Prevention of colorectal cancer by colonoscopic polypectomy. The National Polyp Study Workgroup. N Engl J Med 329:1977–1981
7. Slaughter DP, Southwick HW, Smejkal W (1953) Field cancerization in oral stratified squamous epithelium; clinical implications of multicentric origin. Cancer 6:963–968
8. Freedman AN, Seminara D, Gail MH et al (2005) Cancer risk prediction models: a workshop on development, evaluation, and application. J Natl Cancer Inst 97:715–723
9. Gail MH, Brinton LA, Byar DP et al (1989) Projecting individualized probabilities of developing breast cancer for white females who are being examined annually. J Natl Cancer Inst 81:1879–1886
10. Costantino JP, Gail MH, Pee D et al (1999) Validation studies for models projecting the risk of invasive and total breast cancer incidence. J Natl Cancer Inst 91:1541–1548
11. Song J, Sohn KJ, Medline A et al (2000) Chemopreventive effects of dietary folate on intestinal polyps in Apc+/–Msh2–/– mice. Cancer Res 60:3191–3199
12. Song J, Medline A, Mason JB et al (2000) Effects of dietary folate on intestinal tumorigenesis in the apcMin mouse. Cancer Res 60:5434–5440
13. Baxter NN, Goldwasser MA, Paszat LF et al (2009) Association of colonoscopy and death from colorectal cancer. Ann Intern Med 150:1–8
14. Labianca R, Beretta GD, Mosconi S et al (2005) Colorectal cancer: screening. Ann Oncol 16(Suppl 2):ii127–ii132
15. Goodman GE (2008) Assessing toxicity in cancer chemoprevention trials: the other side of the coin. Cancer Prev Res (Phila Pa) 1:499–502
16. The Alpha-Tocopherol, Beta Carotene Cancer Prevention Study Group (1994) The effect of vitamin E and beta carotene on the incidence of lung cancer and other cancers in male smokers. N Engl J Med 330:1029–1035
17. Omenn GS, Goodman GE, Thornquist MD et al (1996) Effects of a combination of beta carotene and vitamin A on lung cancer and cardiovascular disease. N Engl J Med 334: 1150–1155
18. Bjelakovic G, Nikolova D, Gluud LL et al (2007) Mortality in randomized trials of antioxidant supplements for primary and secondary prevention: systematic review and meta-analysis. JAMA 297:842–857

19. Cole BF, Baron JA, Sandler RS et al (2007) Folic acid for the prevention of colorectal adenomas: a randomized clinical trial. JAMA 297:2351–2359
20. Solomon SD, McMurray JJ, Pfeffer MA et al (2005) Cardiovascular risk associated with celecoxib in a clinical trial for colorectal adenoma prevention. N Engl J Med 352:1071–1080
21. Fisher B, Costantino JP, Wickerham DL et al (1998) Tamoxifen for prevention of breast cancer: report of the National Surgical Adjuvant Breast and Bowel Project P-1 Study. J Natl Cancer Inst 90:1371–1388
22. Kune GA, Kune S, Watson LF (1988) Colorectal cancer risk, chronic illnesses, operations, and medications: case control results from the Melbourne Colorectal Cancer Study. Cancer Res 48:4399–4404
23. Hong WK, Lippman SM, Itri LM et al (1990) Prevention of second primary tumors with isotretinoin in squamous-cell carcinoma of the head and neck. N Engl J Med 323:795–801
24. Lippman SM, Klein EA, Goodman PJ et al (2009) Effect of selenium and vitamin E on risk of prostate cancer and other cancers: the Selenium and Vitamin E Cancer Prevention Trial (SELECT). JAMA 301:39–51
25. Fisher B, Costantino JP, Wickerham DL et al (2005) Tamoxifen for the prevention of breast cancer: current status of the National Surgical Adjuvant Breast and Bowel Project P-1 study. J Natl Cancer Inst 97:1652–1662
26. Cuzick J, Powles T, Veronesi U et al (2003) Overview of the main outcomes in breast-cancer prevention trials. Lancet 361:296–300
27. Vogel VG, Costantino JP, Wickerham DL et al (2006) Effects of tamoxifen vs raloxifene on the risk of developing invasive breast cancer and other disease outcomes: the NSABP Study of Tamoxifen and Raloxifene (STAR) P-2 trial. JAMA 295:2727–2741
28. Cummings SR, Eckert S, Krueger KA et al (1999) The effect of raloxifene on risk of breast cancer in postmenopausal women: results from the MORE randomized trial. Multiple outcomes of raloxifene evaluation. JAMA 281:2189–2197
29. Barrett-Connor E, Mosca L, Collins P et al (2006) Effects of raloxifene on cardiovascular events and breast cancer in postmenopausal women. N Engl J Med 355:125–137
30. Thompson IM, Goodman PJ, Tangen CM et al (2003) The influence of finasteride on the development of prostate cancer. N Engl J Med 349:215–224
31. Goodman PJ, Thompson IM Jr, Tangen CM et al (2006) The prostate cancer prevention trial: design, biases and interpretation of study results. J Urol 175:2234–2242
32. Unger JM, Thompson IM Jr, LeBlanc M et al (2005) Estimated impact of the Prostate Cancer Prevention Trial on population mortality. Cancer 103:1375–1380
33. Brown JR, DuBois RN (2005) COX-2: a molecular target for colorectal cancer prevention. J Clin Oncol 23:2840–2855
34. Thun MJ, Henley SJ, Patrono C (2002) Nonsteroidal anti-inflammatory drugs as anticancer agents: mechanistic, pharmacologic, and clinical issues. J Natl Cancer Inst 94:252–266
35. Mamdani M, Rochon PA, Juurlink DN et al (2002) Observational study of upper gastrointestinal haemorrhage in elderly patients given selective cyclo-oxygenase-2 inhibitors or conventional non-steroidal anti-inflammatory drugs. BMJ 325:624
36. Chan TA (2002) Nonsteroidal anti-inflammatory drugs, apoptosis, and colon-cancer chemoprevention. Lancet Oncol 3:166–174
37. Paganini-Hill A, Chao A, Ross RK et al (1989) Aspirin use and chronic diseases: a cohort study of the elderly. BMJ 299:1247–1250
38. Garcia-Rodriguez LA, Huerta-Alvarez C (2001) Reduced risk of colorectal cancer among long-term users of aspirin and nonaspirin nonsteroidal antiinflammatory drugs. Epidemiology 12:88–93
39. Chan AT, Giovannucci EL, Meyerhardt JA et al (2005) Long-term use of aspirin and nonsteroidal anti-inflammatory drugs and risk of colorectal cancer. JAMA 294:914–923
40. Steinbach G, Lynch PM, Phillips RK et al (2000) The effect of celecoxib, a cyclooxygenase-2 inhibitor, in familial adenomatous polyposis. N Engl J Med 342:1946–1952
41. Gann PH, Manson JE, Glynn RJ et al (1993) Low-dose aspirin and incidence of colorectal tumors in a randomized trial. J Natl Cancer Inst 85:1220–1224

42. Cook NR, Lee IM, Gaziano JM et al (2005) Low-dose aspirin in the primary prevention of cancer: the Women's Health Study: a randomized controlled trial. JAMA 294:47–55
43. Flossmann E, Rothwell PM (2007) Effect of aspirin on long-term risk of colorectal cancer: consistent evidence from randomised and observational studies. Lancet 369:1603–1613
44. Baron JA, Cole BF, Sandler RS et al (2003) A randomized trial of aspirin to prevent colorectal adenomas. N Engl J Med 348:891–899
45. Benamouzig R, Deyra J, Martin A et al (2003) Daily soluble aspirin and prevention of colorectal adenoma recurrence: one-year results of the APACC trial. Gastroenterology 125:328–336
46. Sandler RS, Halabi S, Baron JA et al (2003) A randomized trial of aspirin to prevent colorectal adenomas in patients with previous colorectal cancer. N Engl J Med 348:883–890
47. Logan RFA, Muir KR, Grainge MJ, on behalf of the UKCAP Trial Group et al (2006) Aspirin for the prevention of recurrent colorectal adenomas – results of the UKCAP trial. Gut 55(Suppl 2):A90
48. Cole BF, Logan RF, Halabi S et al (2009) Aspirin for the chemoprevention of colorectal adenomas: meta-analysis of the randomized trials. J Natl Cancer Inst 101:256–266
49. Bresalier RS, Sandler RS, Quan H et al (2005) Cardiovascular events associated with rofecoxib in a colorectal adenoma chemoprevention trial. N Engl J Med 352:1092–1102
50. Solomon SD, Wittes J, Finn PV et al (2008) Cardiovascular risk of celecoxib in 6 randomized placebo-controlled trials: the cross trial safety analysis. Circulation 117:2104–2113
51. Das D, Chilton AP, Jankowski JA (2009) Chemoprevention of oesophageal cancer and the AspECT trial. Recent Results Cancer Res 181:161–169
52. Meyskens FL Jr, McLaren CE, Pelot D, et al. (2008) Difluoromethylornithine plus sulindac for the prevention of sporadic colorectal adenomas: a randomized placebo-controlled, double-blind trial. Cancer Prev Res (Phila Pa) 1:32–38
53. Babbar N, Ignatenko NA, Casero RA Jr et al (2003) Cyclooxygenase-independent induction of apoptosis by sulindac sulfone is mediated by polyamines in colon cancer. J Biol Chem 278:47762–47775
54. Rao CV, Tokumo K, Rigotty J et al (1991) Chemoprevention of colon carcinogenesis by dietary administration of piroxicam, alpha-difluoromethylornithine, 16 alpha-fluoro-5-androsten-17-one, and ellagic acid individually and in combination. Cancer Res 51: 4528–4534
55. Piazza GA, Alberts DS, Hixson LJ et al (1997) Sulindac sulfone inhibits azoxymethane-induced colon carcinogenesis in rats without reducing prostaglandin levels. Cancer Res 57:2909–2915
56. Meyskens FL Jr, Emerson SS, Pelot D et al (1994) Dose de-escalation chemoprevention trial of alpha-difluoromethylornithine in patients with colon polyps. J Natl Cancer Inst 86:1122–1130
57. Walther A, Johnstone E, Swanton C et al (2009) Genetic prognostic and predictive markers in colorectal cancer. Nat Rev Cancer 9:489–499
58. Eberhart CE, Coffey RJ, Radhika A et al (1994) Up-regulation of cyclooxygenase 2 gene expression in human colorectal adenomas and adenocarcinomas. Gastroenterology 107:1183–1188
59. Castells A, Paya A, Alenda C et al (2006) Cyclooxygenase 2 expression in colorectal cancer with DNA mismatch repair deficiency. Clin Cancer Res 12:1686–1692
60. McLean MH, Murray GI, Fyfe N et al (2008) COX-2 expression in sporadic colorectal adenomatous polyps is linked to adenoma characteristics. Histopathology 52:806–815
61. Chan AT, Ogino S, Fuchs CS (2007) Aspirin and the risk of colorectal cancer in relation to the expression of COX-2. N Engl J Med 356:2131–2142
62. Chan AT, Ogino S, Fuchs CS (2009) Aspirin use and survival after diagnosis of colorectal cancer. JAMA 302:649–658
63. Haile RW, Yochim JM, Cortessis VK et al (2005) A molecular/epidemiologic analysis of expression of cyclooxygenases 1 and 2, use of nonsteroidal antiinflammatory drugs, and risk of colorectal adenoma. Clin Colorectal Cancer 4:390–395

64. Fuchs CS, Meyerhardt JA, Heseltine DL et al (2005) Influence of regular aspirin use on survival for patients with stage III colon cancer: Findings from Intergroup trial CALGB 89803. J Clin Oncol 23:3530
65. Houlston RS, Webb E, Broderick P et al (2008) Meta-analysis of genome-wide association data identifies four new susceptibility loci for colorectal cancer. Nat Genet 40:1426–1435
66. Martinez ME, O'Brien TG, Fultz KE et al (2003) Pronounced reduction in adenoma recurrence associated with aspirin use and a polymorphism in the ornithine decarboxylase gene. Proc Natl Acad Sci U S A 100:7859–7864
67. Hubner RA, Muir KR, Liu JF et al (2008) Ornithine decarboxylase G316A genotype is prognostic for colorectal adenoma recurrence and predicts efficacy of aspirin chemoprevention. Clin Cancer Res 14:2303–2309
68. Barry EL, Baron JA, Bhat S et al (2006) Ornithine decarboxylase polymorphism modification of response to aspirin treatment for colorectal adenoma prevention. J Natl Cancer Inst 98:1494–1500

Chapter 12
Endoscopic Management of Pre-invasive Esophageal Adenocarcinoma

Namasivayam Vikneswaran and Kenneth K. Wang

Clinical Vignette

A 50-year old white male presents for surveillance endoscopy for Barrett's esophagus. He was diagnosed with Barrett's esophagus 3 years ago after he underwent upper endoscopy for longstanding heartburn. Biopsies from the esophagus then showed intestinal metaplasia with no dysplasia. Currently, upper endoscopy reveals columnar mucosa in the distal 6 cm of the esophagus with no discernible mucosal nodularity. Biopsies show high grade dysplasia. He has no other complaints or comorbidities and physical examination is unremarkable.

How should his condition be managed?

Basic Principles for the Treatment of Pre-invasive Disease

There are two major issues for treatment of pre-invasive cancer. The first is the determination that the lesion truly is pre-invasive. Although the appearance of the lesion can give some information regarding the depth of invasive, for instance, a patient with dysphagia and a long concentric stenotic esophageal cancer almost always has a T3 cancer that is deeply invasive [1]. It is usually necessary to establish lack of invasion through either careful ultrasonography or through actual resection of any lesion. Endoscopic ultrasonography is fairly specific for deep invasion but not very sensitive. One of the problems is that ultrasound usually must see full thickness invasion to establish an invasive tumor. In addition, endoscopic ultrasound in the luminal GI tract is difficult to perform without compressing the lesion

K.K. Wang (✉)
Division of Gastroenterology and Hepatology, Mayo Clinic, 200 2nd Street SW, Rochester, MN, 55905, USA
e-mail: wang.kenneth@mayo.edu

N. Vikneswaran
Division of Gastroenterology and Hepatology, Mayo Clinic, Rochester, Minnesota

R.C. Fitzgerald (ed.), *Pre-Invasive Disease: Pathogenesis and Clinical Management*,
DOI 10.1007/978-1-4419-6694-0_12,

in question since an acoustical interface must be established. In order to truly visualize the lesion, the area must be water filled and the patient rotated so that the pool of water encompasses the lesion. This is not readily doable in areas such as the pulmonary tree or even areas outside of the esophagus [2].

Once the lesion is removed and invasion is excluded, the other problem is to decide whether or not field carcinogenesis has occurred. Most epithelial cancers form because of chronic inflammation and there is a reasonable chance that histological normal appearing mucosa harbor genetic mutations that will generate metachronous cancers. This is not always simple to identify since these changes are so small, that there is no easy method to detect them without performing tests for chromosomal instability or methylation arrays that characterize the pheotype of this tissue [3]. The treatment of some of these epithelial lesions is difficult since these changes are not visible, they may also involve large areas of epithelium.

Chemoprevention with non-steroidal anti-inflammatories that interferes with COX-2 production of PGE2 which produces epithelial proliferation would be reasonable although this effect may depend on whether or not the oncogenic pathways are still susceptible to this manipulation [4–6]. Agents with less side effect profiles are also being investigated since this strategy could decrease cancer formation and decrease the need for further endoscopic procedures.

There is also ablation of the residual tissue which is done particularly in Barrett's esophagus due ot the high rate of metachronous lesions [7]. Squamous cell cancer is more difficult to assess if abnormal tissue is present usually chronic surveillance will need to be done in this high risk subset. In the colon, if there is a hereditary component that satisfies Amsterdam criteria, then surveillance colonscopy is recommended for the life of the patient. Pulmonary tissue is also surveyed periodically since most of the risk factors affect both lungs.

Gastrointestinal Pre-invasive Diseases

Barrett's esophagus is a condition characterized by the replacement of normal esophageal squamous epithelium with metaplastic columnar epithelium [1] resulting in the proximal migration of the squamocolumnar junction. This occurs in response to chronic gastroesophageal reflux. Its significance stems from the 30- to 50-fold increase in the risk of esophageal adenocarcinoma [2]. The incidence of esophageal cancer has increased by over 500% in the past 3 decades in the West [3] and confers a dismal 5-year survival of 13% despite the advances in diagnosis and treatment [4]. Although Barrett's esophagus confers a substantial relative risk of developing cancer, the absolute risk of neoplastic progression in an individual patient with Barrett's esophagus is small at less than 0.5% per year [5]. Hence interventions aimed at preventing the development of invasive adenocarcinoma have focused on identifying high-risk subgroups amongst patients with Barrett's esophagus.

The risk of neoplastic progression in Barrett's esophagus is stratified based on the degree of dysplasia detected on biopsy. This continues to be the main determinant of the need for treatment despite several limitations which include interobserver variability in interpretation of dysplasia, misdiagnosis of regenerative changes as dysplasia and sampling errors in biopsy. All of these issues compromise the therapy of this disorder and has led to redundancy in the evaluation. In the clinical vignette presented, the biopsies need to be examined by an experienced pathologist to determine if the diagnosis can be substantiated to decrease the variation in interpretation. Patients with non-dysplastic Barrett's esophagus and low grade dysplasia have 0.5–0.6% [6] risk of developing cancer per year respectively. While a recent meta-analysis suggests possible benefit from endoscopic ablation in these patients [7], the risks from presently available treatment modalities often outweigh the potential risk of neoplastic progression to justify treatment in these patients. Furthermore eradication of the columnar mucosa does not obviate the need for continued endoscopic surveillance as intestinal metaplasia and dysplasia can recur after endoscopic eradication. The recurrence rates and potential cancer risk reduction of ablative therapies is not well defined and the randomized controlled trials have not obtained important endpoints such as survival and cancer related survival. These endpoints are often impractical given the longevity of these patients and the limitations of conducting clinical trials. It is recommended that patients undergo periodic endoscopic surveillance to detect high grade dysplasia. The presence of high grade dysplasia is associated with a 30% risk of progression to invasive adenocarcinoma and represents the currently accepted threshold for intervention. The current guidelines recommend that one of the following options may be considered in patients with high grade dysplasia – esophagectomy, endoscopic therapy or intensive surveillance to detect esophageal adenocarcinoma [1].

Esophagectomy has traditionally been the treatment of choice for high grade dysplasia. Patients with high grade dysplasia harbor carcinoma in adjacent segments of the Barrett's mucosa in as many as 40% [8] though more recent studies suggest a much lower rate of synchronous lesions [9]. Esophagectomy may completely removes at risk mucosa and may reduce the need for subsequent surveillance although intestinal metaplasia has been reported in the residual esophagus even after surgical resection. However the procedure is associated with significant morbidity and mortality risks even in experienced hands. The morbidity rates are 30–50% [10] and mortality rates of 1–2% in high-volume centres and 10–18% in lower volume centres have been reported [11]. Vagal sparing esophagectomies have been reported that reduce the gastric emptying problems after esophagectomy but the procedure is still associated with significant morbidity despite reporting better outcomes than transhiatal esophagectomy [12]. Minimally invasive esophagectomy has been proposed with the gastric resection performed using laparoscopic techniques with the cervical esophagus anastomosis performed with thoracoscopic methods. Though incisions as much smaller than traditional trans-thoracic and trans-hiatal esophagectomy the overall complications and time in hospital is not reduced. The advanced age and concurrent comorbidities in a typical patient in their sixth decade of life with Barrett's neoplasia often preclude surgery as a treatment option.

Continued endoscopic surveillance has been recommended in patients with high grade dysplasia. This used to be an option in patients who were deemed to be unfit or unwilling to undergo esophagectomy as progression to invasive cancer was not invariable.

However, this incurs the risk of progression to inoperable cancer in between surveillance endoscopies which would preclude curative treatment. The advent of endoscopic therapy and the accumulating evidence of its efficacy and safety may render "watchful waiting" an less tenable option in the near future except for patients with limited life expectancy. The ability to intervene should a cancer develop using endoscopic therapies may be viable in those patients with severe co-morbidities.

Endoscopic Therapy

Endoscopic therapy is based on the principle that injury to metaplastic epithelium followed by healing and acid suppression could lead to re-epithelialization with a neosquamous lining of the esophagus [13, 14]. Endoscopic therapy is directed at high grade dysplasia and intramucosal adenocarcinoma as these lesions generally have a less than 5% risk of nodal metastases [15] which is comparable to the operative mortality of esophagectomies [11, 16, 17]. The presence of submucosal invasion and nodal metastases generally precludes endoscopic therapy as a curative option although the combination of endoscopic therapy with adjuvant chemoradiation therapy has been performed. The basic tenants of endoscopic therapy are to begin by removing the most neoplastic appearing lesions such as nodules or areas of mucosal irregularly detected with either white light or advanced imaging techniques such as narrow band imaging, laser confocal endoscopy, or chromoendoscopy. After clearance of visible lesions which have the highest potential for neoplasia, the second goal of endoscopic therapy is to eradicate the residual columnar mucosa that harbors the potential for malignant change. This endpoint has served as a surrogate measure of endoscopic efficacy in clinical trials despite its limitations due to the large number of patients and the long periods of follow-up required to demonstrate an actual survival benefit in a prospective study. The eradication of columnar mucosa can be achieved either by endoscopic resection or ablation of columnar mucosa with ablation being the most commonly applied method since there is less morbidity associated with these techniques. There are several methods of endoscopic ablation of which radiofrequency ablation, photodynamic therapy and cryotherapy show the most promise. Endoscopic therapy is always combined with acid suppression to facilitate mucosal healing though the optimal dose of acid suppressive medication has not been ascertained. In practice, endoscopic mucosal resection and ablative techniques are often combined to achieve complete eradication of dysplastic mucosa.

Endoscopic Mucosal Resection

Endoscopic Mucosal Resection (EMR) is a technique which involves the removal of a localized segment of mucosa with a modified snare for diagnostic or therapeutic purposes. The basic principle underlying EMR is the mucosa and the muscle layer of the gastrointestinal wall may be separated by the injection of saline into the submucosa thereby facilitating mucosal resection while mitigating the risk of perforation. Developed over 25 years ago in Japan for the treatment of early gastric cancer [18], there are several techniques currently used for performing EMR. The most commonly used technique is the suck-and-cut technique. This involves the creation of a polyp by aspiration of the mucosa into a device followed by resection using snare and electrocautery. This may be performed by two techniques. The cap (EMR-C) technique [19] employs a transparent cap affixed to the distal end of the endoscope. The cap contains a groove on which a specially designed small-diameter crescent-shaped snare is placed. Following injection of diluted epinephrine, the mucosa is retracted into the cap by suction and resected by closure of the snare and electrocautery (Fig. 12.1). Alternatively, the ligation (EMR-L) technique employs a method similar to variceal band ligation. A band ligation device is placed over the mucosal lesion. The mucosa is aspirated into the cap and a band is deployed. The captured mucosa is then resected with electrocautery with the aid of a snare deployed either above or below the band. The development of multiband mucosectomy devices allows for multiple sequential ligations and resections to be performed in a single intubation. The cap and ligation methods have largely replaced the original strip biopsy method of EMR and its variants as they are easier to perform, provide larger specimens and are associated with lower rates of bleeding [20]. EMR is applied focally to resect visible lesions although more recent studies have described circumferential EMR which entails the removal of the entire Barrett's segment [21].

The main advantage of EMR over the ablative techniques is that it provides tissue for histological analysis. The resected specimens are superior to biopsy

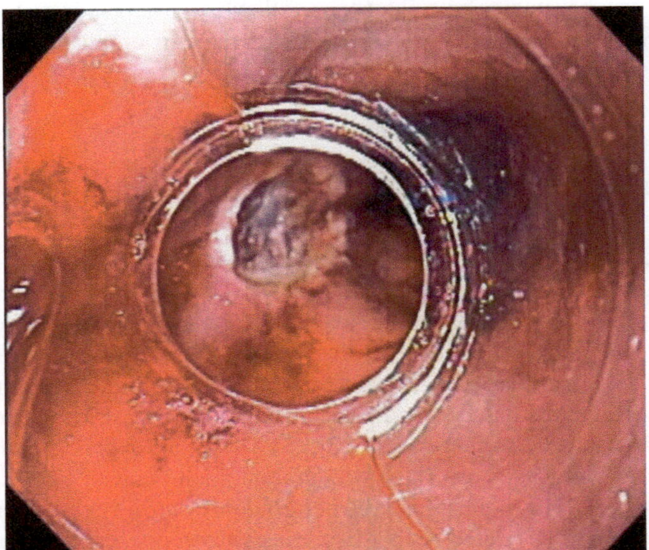

Fig. 12.1 Esophageal ulceration following cap assisted EMR

specimens in assessing the depth of tumour invasion and demonstrate better diagnostic reproducibility as the specimens are larger and mucosal landmarks are preserved [22]. This influences management by altering the assessment of the degree of dysplasia and tumour invasion that was seen on biopsy specimens.

EMR is presently the most reliable investigation for assessing the T stage of esophageal cancer [23].

Several single centre studies have demonstrated the efficacy of EMR in combination with endoscopic ablation in the treatment of high grade dysplasia and intramucosal adenocarcinoma. Endoscopic remission of dysplasia has been reported in over 95% of patients with high grade dysplasia and intramucosal adenocarcinoma [24, 25]. The overall survival in patients with mucosal carcinoma treated endoscopically is comparable to patients undergoing esophagectomy (17 vs. 20%, $p=0.75$) [26]. Complications have been reported in 13–16.6% of patients. These are mainly esophageal strictures which are amenable to dilatations and minor bleeding [25, 26].

Recurrence of high grade dysplasia may occur in 12–21.5% of patients. The risk of recurrence is higher in patients with long-segment Barrett's esophagus, those who had piecemeal resection and/or multifocal neoplasia [25]. The size of specimens that may be resected with EMR is less than 20 mm. Larger lesions require piecemeal resection which creates uncertainties in the assessment of involvement of the lateral margins of the resected specimens by tumour and this in turn is associated with an increased rate of tumour recurrence [27, 28]. Recurrent lesions are usually amenable to endoscopic treatment. The risk of recurrence mandates continued endoscopic surveillance after resection.

Circumferential resection of the entire Barrett's segment (Circumferential EMR) has been described in an attempt to completely remove at risk mucosa to reduce recurrence. Several studies with short term follow-up have demonstrated the feasibility of circumferential EMR but the reported rates of esophageal stenoses are much higher at 12–56% of patients [21, 29, 30].

Endoscopic Submucosal Dissection

Endoscopic submucosal dissection (ESD) was developed in Japan to achieve en bloc resection of larger early gastric cancers. This differs from EMR in its use of an endoscopic knife to incise the margins of the tumour prior to its dissection. The advantage over mucosal resection is the preservation of the tissue margins in lesions that are larger than 1.5–2.0 cm in diameter. Though the feasibility and efficacy of this technique has been well documented in the gastric cancers [31] and esophageal squamous cell cancers [32, 33], there is limited experience in the setting of Barrett's related neoplasia. The procedural duration is much longer than EMR and is associated with higher rates of perforation even in high volume centres. Dissection of Barrett's related neoplasia in the gastroesophageal junction would be technically challenging and the presence of fibrosis and reflux-induced inflammation would conceivably increase the level of difficulty.

Ablation Techniques

Radiofrequency Ablation

Radiofrequency Ablation (RFA) delivers radiofrequency energy to ablate columnar mucosa in the esophagus. The energy is delivered by a 3-cm long ablation balloon catheter that contains multiple electrodes that transmit RF energy in a circumferential manner. The balloon-based delivery system allows for the uniform delivery of RF energy to large segments of the esophagus. Close apposition of the balloon to the mucosa is essential in order to achieve optimal ablation. The ablation balloon catheter comes in different sizes. A sizing balloon catheter is used to ascertain the appropriate size of the balloon catheter required to deliver the RF energy. The sizing balloon is inserted into the esophagus and inflated to an appropriate pressure by a foot pedal. The balloon inflation machine recommends the appropriate size of balloon for ablation. The ablation balloon catheter is then inserted to ablate the mucosa in 3-cm segments under direct endoscopic vision (Fig. 12.2). The mucosa is ablated twice in each treatment session. Following each ablation, the catheter is removed and the sloughed mucosa (Fig. 12.3) is scraped off with a cap affixed to the endoscope before ablation is repeated over the same region. This ensures optimal contact between the balloon and the mucosa during the second ablation.

Alternatively, an endoscopically mounted catheter may deliver RF energy to focal segments of columnar mucosa. This is typically used to ablate residual tongues of columnar mucosa following circumferential ablation with the

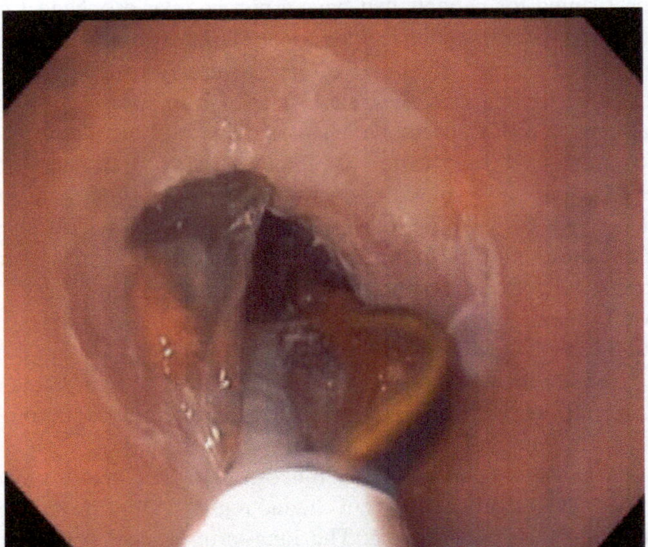

Fig. 12.2 RFA Balloon in situ

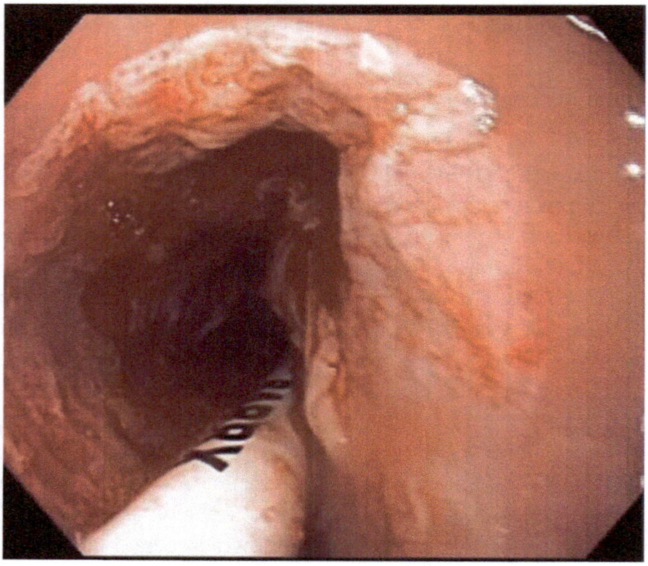

Fig. 12.3 Mucosal slough following balloon RFA

balloon-based delivery system. Several sessions of ablation is usually required to eradicate dysplastic mucosa. The treatment sessions are usually performed at 2–3 monthly intervals to allow for healing of mucosal ulceration prior to repeat ablation.

RFA is best suited for patients that have a non-nodular esophageal mucosa in a relatively straight tubular esophagus with no strictures or tortuosity. This facilitates optimal contact between the ablation balloon and the esophageal mucosa – a pre-requisite for effective ablation. Nodules should be endoscopically resected for optimal treatment as well as definitive characterization of histology.

A recently published multi-centre randomised sham-controlled study reported eradication of high grade dysplasia in over 80% of patients and reduced neoplastic progression over a short-term period [34]. However, long-term results are needed to demonstrate the durability of treatment response as intestinal metaplasia and dysplasia may recur following treatment.

RFA is well tolerated with chest pain being the commonest adverse effect. The reported rate of esophageal strictures with RFA (6%) is lower than other ablative modalities. This is probably a consequence of the effects of RFA being confined to the mucosa. The strictures are usually amenable to endoscopic dilatation. Significant bleeding and perforation are uncommon.

RFA results in the ablated columnar mucosa being replaced by neosquamous epithelium which effectively results in a caudad regression of the squamocolumnar junction often into the gastric cardia. The long-term clinical consequence of this reversal of an essentially adaptive response in a patient predisposed to chronic acid reflux is not known.

Photodynamic Therapy

Photodynamic Therapy (PDT) ablates esophageal mucosa by using light of a specific wavelength (630 nm) on mucosa sensitized by the prior administration of a systemic photosensitizing agent to generate reactive oxygen molecules. These reactive oxygen species mediate tissue ablation in the esophageal mucosa by inducing apoptosis, vascular injury and an immune response [35]. Intravenous porfirmer and oral 5 aminolevulinic acid (ALA) are the two photosensitisers commonly used in PDT. These photosensitisers have a propensity to bind to neoplastic tissue and induce cell death under light of the appropriate wavelength.

Porfimer is administered intravenously 48 h before the procedure and 5 aminolevulinic acid is taken orally 4 h before. Photoradiation is then applied using either a bare cylindrical diffusing fiber or centering balloons. The cylindrical diffusing fiber is passed through the accessory channel of the endoscope and placed in the center of the esophageal lumen. The light is delivered from a laser (Figs. 12.4 and 12.5). Alternatively, the centering balloon is passed into the esophagus over a guide wire, endoscopically positioned adjacent to the targeted area of Barrett's mucosa, and then inflated.

PDT with porfirmer is effective in ablating high grade dysplasia (77 vs. 39% $p<0.0001$) and reducing the incidence of adenocarcinoma in patients with high grade dysplasia (13 vs. 28% $p<0.006$) compared to acid suppression alone [36]. Follow-up studies demonstrate a sustained benefit 5 years after treatment [37]. A retrospective cohort study reports similar survival outcomes between PDT either alone or in combination with EMR and esophagectomy [38] in patients with high grade dysplasia.

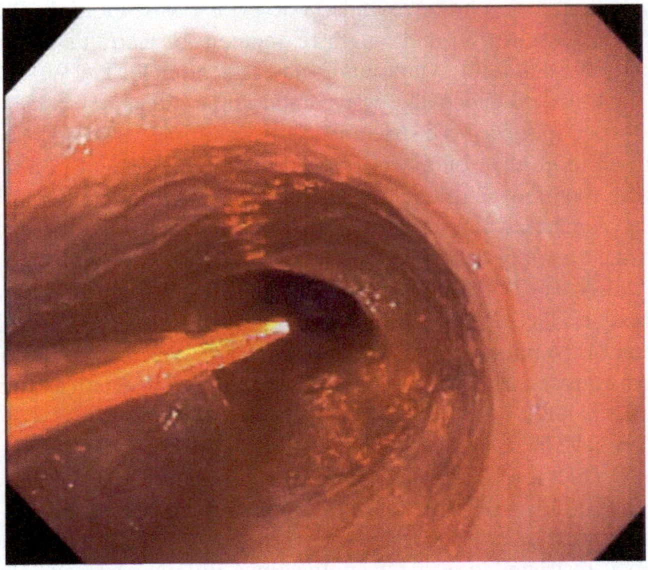

Fig. 12.4 Photodynamic therapy

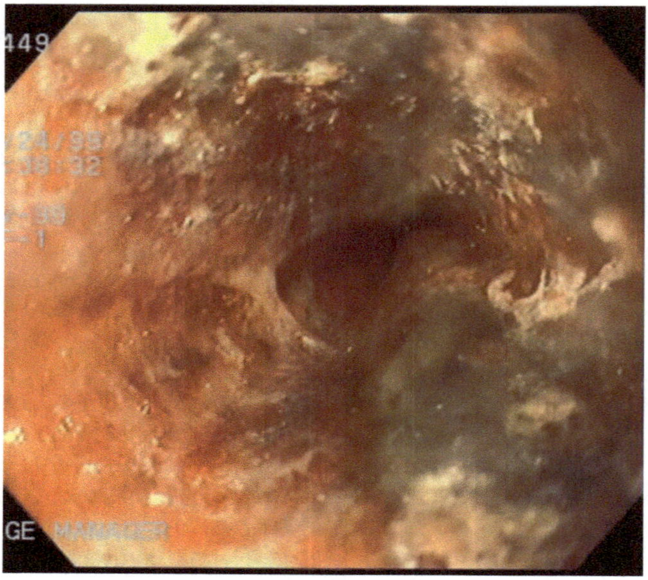

Fig. 12.5 Necrotic mucosa following PDT

However, adverse effects may occur in as many as 94% of patients. Esophageal strictures may occur in 20–36% of patients undergoing PDT, more frequent than other ablative modalities. These are more likely to occur in patients who have pre-existing strictures, those who have undergone prior EMR, multiple PDT applications in a single session [39] and length of segment of Barrett's esophagus [40]. These typically present with symptoms 3–4 weeks after PDT [39]. The strictures are usually thick-walled hence aggressive endoscopic dilatations causing a significant tear is needed to treat these strictures. Often multiple serial endoscopic dilatations performed more than once weekly is needed. One patient in a study by the authors' centre required 42 dilatations and continued self dilatation at home [39]. These adverse events has limited the application of this technique to patients who have an unusual anatomy that is not amendable to other therapies.

PDT may also cause cutaneous phototoxicity that usually manifests as sunburn in exposed body surface. Patients need to avoid bright light for at least 30 days after administration of the photosensitizer. This may not be feasible in patients living in sunny, tropical climates. PDT with ALA seems to be associated with a lower incidence of adverse effects but it is less efficacious [41, 42].

Biomarkers have been studied to predict patients' response to PDT in an attempt to individualise therapy. The loss of p16 allele is associated with a diminished response to PDT [43] while persistence of biomarkers following PDT is associated with increased risk of neoplastic recurrence following PDT [44]. Currently, the use of biomarkers is restricted to research applications. Biomarkers may help determine the best therapy for an individual patient.

Cryotherapy

Cryotherapy is a non-contact method of ablation that employs an endoscopically delivered cryogen – either liquid nitrogen or carbon dioxide. Tissue injury with cryotherapy occur via two main mechanisms – an immediate phase of direct cell injury caused by formation of ice crystals in the tissue and a delayed phase characterized by tissue ischemia from endothelial damage and microthrombi formation. Repetitive cycles of rapid freezing and slow thawing are the basic features of cryotherapy [45].

Though freezing techniques have been used in the palliation of esophageal cancers with modest efficacy in the past, the use of cryotherapy in the ablation of Barrett's dysplasia has only recently gained prominence [46]. Earlier devices which relied on direct contact between a cryoprobe and the esophagus to achieve cryoablation were unable to achieve uniform tissue ablation and were associated with perforation as direct contact with the mucosa resulted in the probe binding to the esophagus [47].

Current devices administer cryogens as a low pressure spray via a catheter passed through the working channel of the endoscope [47]. The spray method of delivery allows for a more uniform application of cryogen to the mucosal surface without the need for direct mucosal contact. There are two commercially available systems. The Polar Wand cryotherapy device (GI Supply, Camp Hill, PA, USA) uses carbon dioxide while the CryoSpray Ablation system (CSA Medical, Inc., Baltimore, MD, USA) uses low pressure liquid nitrogen which achieves a significantly lower temperature. The liquid nitrogen is stored in a console which regulates the dose with a timer. A decompression tube is inserted endoscopically prior to the administration of the cryogen to prevent gaseous distension of the stomach which may lead to perforation [47].

Uncontrolled studies have reported promising safety and efficacy with cryotherapy [48, 49] but long term data is lacking. Cryotherapy facilitates treatment of uneven mucosal surfaces unlike RFA as mucosal contact is not required. However, the presence of frosting on the tip of endoscope often obscures vision during the procedure. The presence of a tight stricture may preclude its use if both the endoscope and the suction catheter cannot be accommodated within the esophageal lumen. The dosimetry needs to be clarified as studies thus far have reported varying freeze times.

Multipolar Electrocoagulation and Argon Plasma Coagulation

Multipolar electrocoagulation (MPEC) utilizes thermal energy to cause tissue injury by passing a current between electrodes that are in contact with tissue. Studies on the utility of MPEC have mainly focused on patients with non-dysplastic Barrett's esophagus [50] and have relatively small cohorts with short periods of follow-up. A randomized control trial comparing MPEC with argon plasma coagulation in patients with mainly non dysplastic Barrett's esophagus showed a statistically insignificant superiority of MPEC in the eradication of Barrett's esophagus (75 vs. 63% $p=0.49$) [51].

Argon plasma coagulation (APC) uses ionised argon gas to deliver a monopolar current to coagulate tissue. Several prospective studies which primarily studied patients with non dysplastic Barrett's esophagus have reported variable efficacy (65–100%) [52, 53] and high rates of recurrence of intestinal metaplasia of up to 66% and subsquamous Barrett's esophagus [54, 55] possibly due to the superficial depth of injury. Complications of perforation and pneumomediastinum have been reported [53, 56]. With the advent of superior ablative modalities, MPEC and APC have been relegated to ablating residual tongues of columnar mucosa in the occasional patient who had been ablated with another modality. Fundamentally, these techniques were developed for treating very small regions of mucosa.

Clinical Evaluation and Management

Successful outcome with endoscopic therapy for Barrett's neoplasia is contingent on careful patient selection. Indiscriminate application of endoscopic therapy may result in progression to incurable cancer in a patient who might otherwise have benefited from a curative esophagectomy. What would be the principal considerations governing therapy in patients with Barrett's neoplasia?

Confirmation of Dysplasia

The degree of dysplasia seen on biopsy specimens should be confirmed with an expert GI pathologist as there may be interobserver variability in interpretation of dysplasia and concomitant inflammation may result in a misdiagnosis of dysplasia. Endoscopic biopsies should be repeated in patients with erosive esophagitis after a course of acid suppression. There is an increased risk of neoplastic progression when the presence of dysplasia is confirmed by two or more pathologists [57]. The confirmation of high grade dysplasia should prompt more thorough surveillance biopsies taken from the four quadrants every one centimeter.

Assessment for Nodal Metastases

The risk of nodal metastases in esophageal adenocarcinoma is related to the depth of tumor invasion. The risk of nodal metastases in esophageal cancer increases from less than 1% for tumors confined to the lamina propria to 35–50% with submucosal invasion. Careful staging of the disease is crucial as the presence of disseminated disease precludes endoscopic resection as a curative treatment. Patients with high grade dysplasia or intramucosal adenocarcinoma confined to the mucosa may undergo curative endoscopic resection. TNM staging is performed with computerized tomography (CT) chest and abdomen to detect disseminated metastases (M) and endoscopic ultrasound (EUS) to detect nodal metastases (N). EUS, however, only has modest accuracy [23] in ascertaining the depth of tumour invasion (T) as the findings may be confounded by the presence of inflammation or the inability to traverse a stricture with an echoendoscope. Presently, EMR offers the most reliable means of T staging. Patients with no evidence of metastases on CT and EUS may be considered for EMR.

Esophagectomy or Endoscopic Therapy?

The choice of treatment modality would be governed by several factors. The availability of local surgical and endoscopic expertise would influence the choice of therapy. Outcomes with esophagectomy are superior in centres with high volume [11]. Conversely, most of the outcomes for endoscopic therapy have been reported by centres of excellence with dedicated endoscopists experienced in the detection of subtle lesions and resection and GI pathologists experienced in the recognition and grading of dysplasia. The reported results probably represent the best outcomes one may expect from endoscopic therapy. It remains to be seen if these can be replicated in a community practice.

There is limited evidence on the durability of treatment response for ablation and resection beyond 5 years. The length of the segment has also been implicated has a factor that may predict response to endoscopic therapy [58]. A younger patient with a ten centimeter segment of Barrett's esophagus and multifocal dysplasia might conceivably benefit more from surgery than an elderly patient with comorbidities that preclude surgery.

Furthermore patients undergoing endoscopic therapy require several sessions of treatment which may require a year to completely eradicate dysplasia. This is followed by intensive endoscopic surveillance every 3–6 months to detect metachronous lesions. The impact of a protracted course of treatment for cancer on the patient's quality of life has not been ascertained. Clearly, a patient who has difficulty adhering to a rigorous treatment and surveillance regimen may be better suited to undergo surgery.

There are no prospective randomized trials comparing outcomes with esophagectomy and endoscopic therapy and it is unlikely one will ever be performed as patients are unlikely to agree to undergo randomization to two radically different treatment arms. Indeed anecdotal evidence suggests that the choice of therapy is often influenced by patients' values and concerns – the fear of missing invasive cancer versus the fear of morbid surgery. Patients undergoing endoscopic therapy need to be informed of the risk of failure of endoscopic treatment, albeit remote which may necessitate surgical resection. This may be related to difficult resections from scarring, undetected submucosal cancers and mucosal non-healing which may preclude further endoscopic therapy [25]. The authors believe a discussion of the risks and benefits in consultation with the thoracic surgeon should be carried out for each patient.

Resection, Ablation or Both?

Patient's undergoing endoscopic therapy should undergo meticulous surveillance of the columnar mucosa for mucosal abnormalities. Narrow band imaging which utilizes light of short wavelength (blue light) to achieve more superficial tissue penetration to highlight mucosal surface patterns and details of microvasculature is used in conjunction with white light endoscopy to visualize the mucosal landscape and identify mucosal abnormalities and nodularities. Any focal lesion especially mucosal nodularities should be targeted for resection as they are associated with coexistent carcinoma [59]. Mucosal resection, unlike ablation, allows for definitive histological assessment of grade and the presence of lymphovascular invasion which are associated with an increased risk of metastatic lymphadenopathy.

The remaining columnar mucosa may be targeted for circumferential resection which involves the complete resection of the entire columnar segment but it is associated with a much higher rate of symptomatic esophageal stenoses. Alternatively, endoscopic resection of focal abnormalities is combined with ablation of the residual columnar mucosa by either RFA or PDT. Ablation is usually performed at least 4 weeks after resection to allow for healing of mucosal ulceration acid suppressive therapy prior to ablation. RFA is preferred in patients with a non-nodular mucosa in a relatively straight tubular esophagus with no strictures or tortuosity. Cryotherapy may be performed in patients with uneven mucosal surfaces which precludes optimal tissue contact with the RFA balloon. Mapping biopsies are obtained during each endoscopy and treatment is continued until there is no evidence of dysplasia. Patients continue to undergo 3–6 monthly endoscopic surveillance with progressively increasing intervals depending on the biopsy findings. Endoscopic ultrasound is performed annually at the authors' unit to detect lymph node metastases.

Conclusion

The patient presented in the clinical vignette has high grade dysplasia in the setting of Barrett's esophagus. This would be confirmed by a repeat endoscopy with thorough biopsies taken from every centimeter each quadrant. The specimens should be reviewed by an expert GI pathologist to confirm the findings.

Once high grade dysplasia is confirmed, the patient should be advised on his treatment options preferably in conjunction with a thoracic surgical consult. CT chest and abdomen and EUS should be performed to exclude disseminated disease. Endoscopic resection of any mucosal abnormalities seen on white light endoscopy or NBI is performed to stage the lesions. The residual dysplastic mucosa is then resected or ablated every 3 months until biopsies no longer show any dysplasia. The patient should continue to undergo periodic surveillance endoscopy to assess for recurrence. The precise interval has not been established but in the authors experience, should be based on the degree of dysplasia prior ablation with more intensive surveillance for early cancer and less intensive for low grade dysplasia.

References

1. Wang KK, Sampliner RE (2008) Updated guidelines 2008 for the diagnosis, surveillance and therapy of Barrett's esophagus. Am J Gastroenterol 103:788–797
2. Sharma P, McQuaid K, Dent J, Fennerty MB, Sampliner R, Spechler S, Cameron A, Corley D, Falk G, Goldblum J, Hunter J, Jankowski J, Lundell L, Reid B, Shaheen NJ, Sonnenberg A, Wang K, Weinstein W (2004) A critical review of the diagnosis and management of Barrett's esophagus: the AGA Chicago Workshop. Gastroenterology 127:310–330
3. Pohl H, Welch HG (2005) The role of overdiagnosis and reclassification in the marked increase of esophageal adenocarcinoma incidence. J Natl Cancer Inst 97:142–146
4. Eloubeidi MA, Mason AC, Desmond RA, El-Serag HB (2003) Temporal trends (1973–1997) in survival of patients with esophageal adenocarcinoma in the United States: a glimmer of hope? Am J Gastroenterol 98:1627–1633
5. Shaheen NJ, Crosby MA, Bozymski EM, Sandler RS (2000) Is there publication bias in the reporting of cancer risk in Barrett's esophagus? Gastroenterology 119:333–338
6. Sharma P, Falk GW, Weston AP, Reker D, Johnston M, Sampliner RE (2006) Dysplasia and cancer in a large multicenter cohort of patients with Barrett's esophagus. Clin Gastroenterol Hepatol 4:566–572
7. Wani S, Puli SR, Shaheen NJ, Westhoff B, Slehria S, Bansal A, Rastogi A, Sayana H, Sharma P (2009) Esophageal adenocarcinoma in Barrett's esophagus after endoscopic ablative therapy: a meta-analysis and systematic review. Am J Gastroenterol 104:502–513
8. Tschanz ER (2005) Do 40% of patients resected for barrett esophagus with high-grade dysplasia have unsuspected adenocarcinoma? Arch Pathol Lab Med 129:177–180
9. Wang VS, Hornick JL, Sepulveda JA, Mauer R, Poneros JM (2009) Low prevalence of submucosal invasive carcinoma at esophagectomy for high-grade dysplasia or intramucosal adenocarcinoma in Barrett's esophagus: a 20-year experience. Gastrointest Endosc 69:777–783
10. Chang AC, Ji H, Birkmeyer NJ, Orringer MB, Birkmeyer JD (2008) Outcomes after transhiatal and transthoracic esophagectomy for cancer. Ann Thorac Surg 85:424–429
11. Birkmeyer JD, Siewers AE, Finlayson EV, Stukel TA, Lucas FL, Batista I, Welch HG, Wennberg DE (2002) Hospital volume and surgical mortality in the United States. N Engl J Med 346:1128–1137
12. Peyre CG, DeMeester SR, Rizzetto C, Bansal N, Tang AL, Ayazi S, Leers JM, Lipham JC, Hagen JA, DeMeester TR (2007) Vagal-sparing esophagectomy: the ideal operation for intramucosal adenocarcinoma and barrett with high-grade dysplasia. Ann Surg 246:665–671, discussion 671–674
13. Berenson MM, Johnson TD, Markowitz NR, Buchi KN, Samowitz WS (1993) Restoration of squamous mucosa after ablation of Barrett's esophageal epithelium. Gastroenterology 104:1686–1691
14. Sampliner RE, Hixson LJ, Fennerty MB, Garewal HS (1993) Regression of Barrett's esophagus by laser ablation in an anacid environment. Dig Dis Sci 38:365–368
15. Buskens CJ, Westerterp M, Lagarde SM, Bergman JJ, ten Kate FJ, van Lanschot JJ (2004) Prediction of appropriateness of local endoscopic treatment for high-grade dysplasia and early adenocarcinoma by EUS and histopathologic features. Gastrointest Endosc 60: 703–710
16. Ancona E, Rampado S, Cassaro M, Battaglia G, Ruol A, Castoro C, Portale G, Cavallin F, Rugge M (2008) Prediction of lymph node status in superficial esophageal carcinoma. Ann Surg Oncol 15:3278–3288
17. Migliore M, Choong CK, Lim E, Goldsmith KA, Ritchie A, Wells FC (2007) A surgeon's case volume of oesophagectomy for cancer strongly influences the operative mortality rate. Eur J Cardiothorac Surg 32:375–380
18. Tada M, Murata M, Tamekoto T (1984) The development of "strip-off" biopsy. Gastroenterol Endosc 26:883–889

19. Inoue H, Takeshita K, Hori H, Muraoka Y, Yoneshima H, Endo M (1993) Endoscopic mucosal resection with a cap-fitted panendoscope for esophagus, stomach, and colon mucosal lesions. Gastrointest Endosc 39:58–62
20. Tanabe S, Koizumi W, Kokutou M, Imaizumi H, Ishii K, Kida M, Yokoyama Y, Ohida M, Saigenji K, Shimao H, Mitomi H (1999) Usefulness of endoscopic aspiration mucosectomy as compared with strip biopsy for the treatment of gastric mucosal cancer. Gastrointest Endosc 50:819–822
21. Seewald S, Akaraviputh T, Seitz U, Brand B, Groth S, Mendoza G, He X, Thonke F, Stolte M, Schroeder S, Soehendra N (2003) Circumferential EMR and complete removal of Barrett's epithelium: a new approach to management of Barrett's esophagus containing high-grade intraepithelial neoplasia and intramucosal carcinoma. Gastrointest Endosc 57:854–859
22. Mino-Kenudson M, Hull MJ, Brown I, Muzikansky A, Srivastava A, Glickman J, Park DY, Zuckerberg L, Misdraji J, Odze RD, Lauwers GY (2007) EMR for Barrett's esophagus-related superficial neoplasms offers better diagnostic reproducibility than mucosal biopsy. Gastrointest Endosc 66:660–666, quiz 767, 769
23. Larghi A, Lightdale CJ, Memeo L, Bhagat G, Okpara N, Rotterdam H (2005) EUS followed by EMR for staging of high-grade dysplasia and early cancer in Barrett's esophagus. Gastrointest Endosc 62:16–23
24. Ell C, May A, Gossner L, Pech O, Gunter E, Mayer G, Henrich R, Vieth M, Muller H, Seitz G, Stolte M (2000) Endoscopic mucosal resection of early cancer and high-grade dysplasia in Barrett's esophagus. Gastroenterology 118:670–677
25. Pech O, Behrens A, May A, Nachbar L, Gossner L, Rabenstein T, Manner H, Guenter E, Huijsmans J, Vieth M, Stolte M, Ell C (2008) Long-term results and risk factor analysis for recurrence after curative endoscopic therapy in 349 patients with high-grade intraepithelial neoplasia and mucosal adenocarcinoma in Barrett's oesophagus. Gut 57:1200–1206
26. Prasad GA, Wu TT, Wigle DA, Buttar NS, Wongkeesong LM, Dunagan KT, Lutzke LS, Borkenhagen LS, Wang KK (2009) Endoscopic and surgical treatment of mucosal (T1a) esophageal adenocarcinoma in Barrett's esophagus. Gastroenterology 137(3):815–823
27. Ishihara R, Iishi H, Takeuchi Y, Kato M, Yamamoto S, Yamamoto S, Masuda E, Tatsumi K, Higashino K, Uedo N, Tatsuta M (2008) Local recurrence of large squamous-cell carcinoma of the esophagus after endoscopic resection. Gastrointest Endosc 67:799–804
28. Esaki M, Matsumoto T, Hirakawa K, Nakamura S, Umeno J, Koga H, Yao T, Iida M (2007) Risk factors for local recurrence of superficial esophageal cancer after treatment by endoscopic mucosal resection. Endoscopy 39:41–45
29. Pouw RE, Peters FP, Sempoux C, Piessevaux H, Deprez PH (2008) Stepwise radical endoscopic resection for Barrett's esophagus with early neoplasia: report on a Brussels' cohort. Endoscopy 40:892–898
30. Peters FP, Kara MA, Rosmolen WD, ten Kate FJ, Krishnadath KK, van Lanschot JJ, Fockens P, Bergman JJ (2006) Stepwise radical endoscopic resection is effective for complete removal of Barrett's esophagus with early neoplasia: a prospective study. Am J Gastroenterol 101:1449–1457
31. Gotoda T (2007) Endoscopic resection of early gastric cancer. Gastric Cancer 10:1–11
32. Ishihara R, Iishi H, Uedo N, Takeuchi Y, Yamamoto S, Yamada T, Masuda E, Higashino K, Kato M, Narahara H, Tatsuta M (2008) Comparison of EMR and endoscopic submucosal dissection for en bloc resection of early esophageal cancers in Japan. Gastrointest Endosc 68:1066–1072
33. Ono S, Fujishiro M, Niimi K, Goto O, Kodashima S, Yamamichi N, Omata M (2009) Long-term outcomes of endoscopic submucosal dissection for superficial esophageal squamous cell neoplasms. Gastrointest Endosc 70(5):860–866
34. Shaheen NJ, Sharma P, Overholt BF, Wolfsen HC, Sampliner RE, Wang KK, Galanko JA, Bronner MP, Goldblum JR, Bennett AE, Jobe BA, Eisen GM, Fennerty MB, Hunter JG, Fleischer DE, Sharma VK, Hawes RH, Hoffman BJ, Rothstein RI, Gordon SR, Mashimo H, Chang KJ, Muthusamy VR, Edmundowicz SA, Spechler SJ, Siddiqui AA, Souza RF, Infantolino

A, Falk GW, Kimmey MB, Madanick RD, Chak A, Lightdale CJ (2009) Radiofrequency ablation in Barrett's esophagus with dysplasia. N Engl J Med 360:2277–2288
35. Dougherty TJ, Gomer CJ, Henderson BW, Jori G, Kessel D, Korbelik M, Moan J, Peng Q (1998) Photodynamic therapy. J Natl Cancer Inst 90:889–905
36. Overholt BF, Lightdale CJ, Wang KK, Canto MI, Burdick S, Haggitt RC, Bronner MP, Taylor SL, Grace MG, Depot M (2005) Photodynamic therapy with porfimer sodium for ablation of high-grade dysplasia in Barrett's esophagus: international, partially blinded, randomized phase III trial. Gastrointest Endosc 62:488–498
37. Overholt BF, Wang KK, Burdick JS, Lightdale CJ, Kimmey M, Nava HR, Sivak MV Jr, Nishioka N, Barr H, Marcon N, Pedrosa M, Bronner MP, Grace M, Depot M (2007) Five-year efficacy and safety of photodynamic therapy with Photofrin in Barrett's high-grade dysplasia. Gastrointest Endosc 66:460–468
38. Prasad GA, Wang KK, Buttar NS, Wongkeesong LM, Krishnadath KK, Nichols FC 3rd, Lutzke LS, Borkenhagen LS (2007) Long-term survival following endoscopic and surgical treatment of high-grade dysplasia in Barrett's esophagus. Gastroenterology 132:1226–1233
39. Prasad GA, Wang KK, Buttar NS, Wongkeesong LM, Lutzke LS, Borkenhagen LS (2007) Predictors of stricture formation after photodynamic therapy for high-grade dysplasia in Barrett's esophagus. Gastrointest Endosc 65:60–66
40. Yachimski P, Puricelli WP, Nishioka NS (2008) Patient predictors of esophageal stricture development after photodynamic therapy. Clin Gastroenterol Hepatol 6:302–308
41. Hage M, Siersema PD, van Dekken H, Steyerberg EW, Haringsma J, van de Vrie W, Grool TE, van Veen RL, Sterenborg HJ, Kuipers EJ (2004) 5-aminolevulinic acid photodynamic therapy versus argon plasma coagulation for ablation of Barrett's oesophagus: a randomised trial. Gut 53:785–790
42. Peters F, Kara M, Rosmolen W, Aalders M, Ten Kate F, Krishnadath K, van Lanschot J, Fockens P, Bergman J (2005) Poor results of 5-aminolevulinic acid-photodynamic therapy for residual high-grade dysplasia and early cancer in barrett esophagus after endoscopic resection. Endoscopy 37:418–424
43. Prasad GA, Wang KK, Halling KC, Buttar NS, Wongkeesong LM, Zinsmeister AR, Brankley SM, Fritcher EG, Westra WM, Krishnadath KK, Lutzke LS, Borkenhagen LS (2008) Utility of biomarkers in prediction of response to ablative therapy in Barrett's esophagus. Gastroenterology 135:370–379
44. Prasad GA, Wang KK, Halling KC, Buttar NS, Wongkeesong LM, Zinsmeister AR, Brankley SM, Westra WM, Lutzke LS, Borkenhagen LS, Dunagan K (2008) Correlation of histology with biomarker status after photodynamic therapy in Barrett esophagus. Cancer 113:470–476
45. Gage AA, Baust J (1998) Mechanisms of tissue injury in cryosurgery. Cryobiology 37: 171–186
46. Pasricha PJ, Hill S, Wadwa KS, Gislason GT, Okolo PI 3rd, Magee CA, Canto MI, Kuo WH, Baust JG, Kalloo AN (1999) Endoscopic cryotherapy: experimental results and first clinical use. Gastrointest Endosc 49:627–631
47. Johnston CM, Schoenfeld LP, Mysore JV, Dubois A (1999) Endoscopic spray cryotherapy: a new technique for mucosal ablation in the esophagus. Gastrointest Endosc 50:86–92
48. Greenwald BD, Dumot JA, Horwhat JD, Lightdale CJ, Abrams JA (2010) Safety, tolerability, and efficacy of endoscopic low-pressure liquid nitrogen spray cryotherapy in the esophagus. Dis Esophagus 23(1):13–19
49. Dumot JA, Vargo JJ 2nd, Falk GW, Frey L, Lopez R, Rice TW (2009) An open-label, prospective trial of cryospray ablation for Barrett's esophagus high-grade dysplasia and early esophageal cancer in high-risk patients. Gastrointest Endosc 70(4):634–644
50. Sampliner RE, Faigel D, Fennerty MB, Lieberman D, Ippoliti A, Lewin K, Weinstein WM (2001) Effective and safe endoscopic reversal of nondysplastic Barrett's esophagus with thermal electrocoagulation combined with high-dose acid inhibition: a multicenter study. Gastrointest Endosc 53:554–558
51. Sharma P, Wani S, Weston AP, Bansal A, Hall M, Mathur S, Prasad A, Sampliner RE (2006) A randomised controlled trial of ablation of Barrett's oesophagus with multipolar electroco-

agulation versus argon plasma coagulation in combination with acid suppression: long term results. Gut 55:1233–1239
52. Dulai GS, Jensen DM, Cortina G, Fontana L, Ippoliti A (2005) Randomized trial of argon plasma coagulation vs. multipolar electrocoagulation for ablation of Barrett's esophagus. Gastrointest Endosc 61:232–240
53. Pereira-Lima JC, Busnello JV, Saul C, Toneloto EB, Lopes CV, Rynkowski CB, Blaya C (2000) High power setting argon plasma coagulation for the eradication of Barrett's esophagus. Am J Gastroenterol 95:1661–1668
54. Mork H, Al-Taie O, Berlin F, Kraus MR, Scheurlen M (2007) High recurrence rate of Barrett's epithelium during long-term follow-up after argon plasma coagulation. Scand J Gastroenterol 42:23–27
55. Kahaleh M, Van Laethem JL, Nagy N, Cremer M, Deviere J (2002) Long-term follow-up and factors predictive of recurrence in Barrett's esophagus treated by argon plasma coagulation and acid suppression. Endoscopy 34:950–955
56. Attwood SE, Lewis CJ, Caplin S, Hemming K, Armstrong G (2003) Argon beam plasma coagulation as therapy for high-grade dysplasia in Barrett's esophagus. Clin Gastroenterol Hepatol 1:258–263
57. Skacel M, Petras RE, Gramlich TL, Sigel JE, Richter JE, Goldblum JR (2000) The diagnosis of low-grade dysplasia in Barrett's esophagus and its implications for disease progression. Am J Gastroenterol 95:3383–3387
58. Yachimski P, Puricelli WP, Nishioka NS (2009) Patient predictors of histopathologic response after photodynamic therapy of Barrett's esophagus with high-grade dysplasia or intramucosal carcinoma. Gastrointest Endosc 69:205–212
59. Buttar NS, Wang KK, Sebo TJ, Riehle DM, Krishnadath KK, Lutzke LS, Anderson MA, Petterson TM, Burgart LJ (2001) Extent of high-grade dysplasia in Barrett's esophagus correlates with risk of adenocarcinoma. Gastroenterology 120:1630–1639

Chapter 13
Psychosocial Outcomes of Screening for Cancer and Pre-invasive Disease

Robert N. Whistance, Shelley Potter, Mark Eveleigh, and Jane M. Blazeby

Introduction

Screening is an important strategy for reducing cancer-related mortality in developed countries. Programmes for breast and cervical cancer screening are well established, while protocols for prostate, colorectal and ovarian cancer are still being developed [1–7]. Population screening programmes help to detect both invasive cancers and pre-malignant disease. Prompt treatment of those identified with cancer can reduce mortality, although screening trials do not consistently improve survival [8–12]. Diagnosing cancer early may mean that less invasive treatments with better clinical outcomes can be offered to patients [13, 14]. The detection of pre-malignant disease through screening also allows sufferers to be offered lifestyle modification advice, entry into surveillance programmes and prophylactic therapy [15–18]. This may help to reduce the incidence of invasive cancers amongst some high-risk populations [17, 19, 20]. In recent years, genetic screening has also helped to predict those at risk of developing cancer in the future, permitting counselling of mutation carriers and their offspring [21–23].

Decisions on the efficacy, acceptability and timing of population screening tests are complex. In 1968, Wilson and Junger published ten criteria on behalf of the World Health Organisation to guide the development of screening programmes (Table 13.1) [24]. These stipulated that the disease being screened for must be an important health problem with a recognised and efficacious treatment. In addition, the disease should be detectable at an early stage with a screening test that is sensitive, specific and easy to perform. In order to ensure that adequate screening uptake is achieved, the test and its subsequent treatment should be acceptable to patients. The vast majority of people who participate in cancer screening programmes will

J.M. Blazeby (✉)
Department of Social Medicine, University of Bristol, Bristol, UK
and
Division of Surgery, Head & Neck, University Hospitals Bristol NHS Foundation Trust, Bristol BS2 8HW, UK
e-mail: J.M.Blazeby@bristol.ac.uk

R.C. Fitzgerald (ed.), *Pre-Invasive Disease: Pathogenesis and Clinical Management*, DOI 10.1007/978-1-4419-6694-0_13, © Springer Science+Business Media, LLC 2011

Table 13.1 Wilson's and Junger criteria for establishing screening programs [168]

Wilson's criteria [24]
The condition being screened for should be an important health problem
The natural history of the condition should be well understood
There should be a detectable early stage
Treatment at an early stage should be of more benefit than at a later stage
A suitable test should be devised for the early stage
The test should be acceptable
Intervals for repeating the test should be determined
Adequate health service provision should be made for the extra clinical workload resulting from screening
The risks, both physical and psychological, should be less than the benefits
The costs should be balanced against the benefits

not be diagnosed with cancer. Healthy participants are, therefore, exposed to physical and psychological risks that may be detrimental to them. The morbidity and mortality associated with screening should be balanced against the sum benefit to the entire at-risk population. The long-term cost-effectiveness of any screening programme should also be taken into consideration, including adequate financial and manpower provision for both diagnosis and treatment.

Individual emotional, social and psychological reactions to cancer screening vary markedly. Some patients may experience anxiety or distress when initially contacted for screening [25–27]. This may be related to the fear of undergoing an invasive test or of being diagnosed with cancer [28, 29]. In certain cases, pre-test distress may present a barrier to screening [30–32]. There is also evidence that pre-test anxiety is associated with persistently elevated levels of anxiety after screening [33, 34]. Cancer worry, anxiety, and fear can conversely motivate patients to enter cancer screening programmes [35, 36]. A negative screening test may provide reassurance, alleviate cancer worry and reduce distress [37–39]. A positive test, by contrast, may cause short or medium-term distress, which often improves with time [38, 40]. The sensitivity and specificity of the screening test is also important. False-positive screening tests may mean that patients are required to undergo unnecessary additional procedures, which may cause further discomfort and distress. False-negative screening tests give disease sufferers false reassurance. The impact of cancer screening therefore on emotional, social and psychological outcomes is variable and depends on the test result, the disease site and the population studied [40–42].

Understanding the psychosocial impact of screening for cancer will provide information that can be useful to inform attendees of possible experiences and outcomes. The information can also be used to inform policy makers regarding decisions to implement screening. It may be possible that psychosocial outcomes associated with particular screening tests may also be used decide between two screening modalities when there is clinical equipoise, for instance, when two screening tests have similar clinical outcomes and cost-effectiveness. This chapter will consider the measures and methods for assessing psycho-social outcomes in cancer screening trials. It will review the published literature related to these issues in breast, cervix, prostate, ovary and gastrointestinal cancer. There will be final sections considering the psycho-social implications of screening for genetic disorders and future research.

Measuring Psycho-social Outcomes of Screening

Assessing psychosocial outcomes of screening has been undertaken using a combination of quantitative and qualitative methodologies. In some early work observer assessment of anxiety caused by screening tests was performed, but more recently it has been recognised that it is necessary to gain information from patients themselves to avoid potential problems with observer bias. Many trials therefore initially incorporated a measure of health-related quality of life (HRQL) into the protocol. Measures of HRQL, however, may not be suitable for this purpose because the majority of them were developed to assess cancer related symptoms and treatment side effects (rather than issues related to the impact of screening itself in a healthy population). More recently screening trials have incorporated questionnaires developed for assessing anxiety and specific psychosocial issues related to screening. The past decade has seen a change in the nomenclature of tools assessing self-reported health and these are now collectively referred to as patient reported outcomes measures (PROMs). The definition of a PROM is that the instrument assesses any aspect of health reported by the patient themselves and it is not a measure of health interpreted by an observer [43]. In screening trials, this is a key feature and using observers' impressions of the impact of screening on psychosocial issues is likely to be inaccurate (leading to both over rating and underscoring the true value). Qualitative research has also been used to understand how screening impacts on participants' experiences and perceptions. Qualitative data may supplement information from questionnaire studies and be used to understand responses from participants (and carers). The following sections will review the literature regarding psychosocial outcomes of screening for specific cancers including published studies that have included validated PROMs.

Quantitative Methods

A wide range of PROMs have been used to assess the psychosocial impact of screening for pre-invasive disease and cancer. Many have been designed specifically for the study being undertaken and it is not uncommon for such questionnaires to lack full psychometric evaluation [44–46]. Studies using this ad hoc approach will provide data that may be unreliable. Others have used more well validated and rigorously designed questionnaires, such as the Spielberger State-trait Anxiety Inventory (S-STAI), the Centre for Epidemiological Studies Depression

Scale (CES-D), the Hospital Anxiety and Depression Scale (HADS), and the EuroQol 5D (EQ-5D) questionnaire [47–50]. Some of these, including the S-STAI and CES-D, assess affective symptoms such as anxiety and depression related to screening, while others including the EuroQol-5D and the Short Form-36 (SF-36) have been used to measure the impact of screening on HRQL [51–53]. In addition, many cancer screening studies have developed and used PROMs that assess the level of cancer worry and distress in participants. This section will consider the different types of PROM that have been used in cancer screening trials and their relative merits and flaws.

Health-Related Quality of Life

Questionnaires assessing health-related quality of life (HRQL) were the first PROMs to be used in cancer screening trials. Most generic HRQL measures assess physical, social, emotional, role and cognitive function, and common symptoms. Examples include the SF-36, the EQ-5D, the European Organisation for Research and Treatment of Cancer (EORTC) QLQ-C30 and the Functional Assessment of Cancer Therapy General (FACT-G) [50, 52, 54, 55]. None of these tools were specifically developed to assess issues related to screening, although the SF-36 was designed to assess the population health but it is unlikely to be sensitive enough to act as a measure of anxiety related to screening. The EORTC and FACT systems were developed in patients with cancer and therefore they focus on the presence of symptoms related to the disease and side effects of specific treatments. Some of these items and domains may not be relevant in cancer screening studies, where the majority of participants are healthy and asymptomatic.

Anxiety and Depression

Other cancer screening studies have used PROMs that assess the presence of affective symptoms such as anxiety and depression in patients prior to and following screening. These are perhaps the most widely used PROMs in cancer screening trials and their use is based on the assumption that screening can cause clinically detectable levels of anxiety and depression. The S-STAI is a 40-item questionnaire divided into two 20-item sections to assess state and trait anxiety [47]. State anxiety pertains to the emotional response one feels when placed in a situation which appropriately generates anxiety which then subsequently subsides once the stimulus has been removed, for instance when undergoing a stressful event such as cancer screening. Trait anxiety refers to the background level of anxiety that each individual experiences throughout their adult lives. Reliability and validity data for the S-STAI have been widely published, although only rarely in cancer screening studies [47, 56–59]. Internal consistency estimates of both the state and trait anxiety scales are on the whole very high (Cronbach's $\alpha > 0.90$), while the S-STAI has also demonstrated good reliability [58]. State anxiety is an appropriate psychosocial outcome in cancer screening studies, as both the anticipation and performance of invasive screening procedures, such as colonoscopy or colposcopy, may induce temporary anxiety. In addition, the S-STAI can distinguish between the anxiety related to a particular event and that which is part of the patient's pre-screening baseline level. However, the S-STAI does not address other issues that may be important to patients undergoing cancer screening, such as the presence of unwanted physical side effects related to the screening test, and it may also miss sub-clinical levels of cancer-worry. Supplementing the S-STAI with a screening specific tool may address this deficit.

The CES-D is another commonly used PROM in cancer screening trials, consisting of 20-items that assess mood, somatic complaints, interactions with others and motor functioning. It was originally developed from Beck's Depression Inventory and Zung's Depression Scale [48, 60–63]. Responses are on a 4-point Likert scale aimed at quantifying the prevalence of depressive symptoms over the preceding week. In this questionnaire, high scores indicate a greater incidence of negative mood symptoms. Since the CES-D was introduced a voluminous amount of psychometric data have been published, and it has generally demonstrated good internal consistency and reliability [63, 64]. The CES-D has also been widely used in studies of patients diagnosed with cancer although its reliability and validity in healthy screening participants is uncertain [65, 66]. The measurement of depressive symptoms in patients undergoing cancer screening may be inappropriate, however, as the tests are unlikely cause clinically detectable levels of depression and are much more likely to cause temporary worry, anxiety and distress which will usually resolve in the short-term. Distinguishing between pre-morbid depression, coincidental post-procedure depression and depressive symptoms directly attributable to the screening process is highly problematic and confounds results.

The Hospital Anxiety and Depression Scale (HADS) has similar limitations as other PROMs that assess affective symptoms [49]. It was originally designed for use in hospital inpatients and consists of two 7-item scales which are concerned with different aspects anxiety and depression. A review of the psychometric data on the HADS found that internal consistency estimates were repeatedly high (Cronbach's α 0.7–0.9) for both the anxiety and depression scales [67]. In addition, the HADS has been used in screening trials of colorectal, prostate, breast and cervical cancer, making it one of the most widely used PROMs in cancer screening [38, 42, 67–72]. However, its use makes the assumption that cancer screening programmes will induce clinically detectable levels of anxiety and depression, which may be unrealistic. It may not, therefore, be sensitive enough to detect minor changes in psychosocial well-being which may be important in the acceptance of and adherence to screening programmes. The HADS alone also does not provide sufficient information on the psychosocial impact of screening, and neglects the impact of physical side effects of screening, such as embarrassment or pain.

Cancer Worry and Distress

Many studies of cancer screening incorporate either a generic or disease-specific assessment of cancer-related worry in patients undergoing screening [73, 74]. Worry is a symptom related to anxiety, but is less serious and could be conceived as a normal reaction to a stressful situation, whereas anxiety may be considered as the excessive manifestation of extreme worry. Patients are more likely to be worried by undergoing cancer screening than to develop frank anxiety as a consequence. Therefore, the assessment of cancer worry is perhaps more appropriate and even more sensitive than using measures of clinical anxiety, which may miss a large proportion of frankly worried but non-anxious participants. Nonetheless it is still important to identify those patients in whom screening-associated anxiety is an issue and, therefore, the use of cancer-worry scales or questions alone is not advocated.

The Impact of Events Scale (IES) was first published in 1979 as a subjective tool to assess distress for any given life event [75]. It is composed of 15-items, eight of which assess avoidance of distressing thoughts and seven of which assess the presence of intrusive thoughts. The scale has demonstrated good internal consistency, reliability and validity in a range of disease states [75–77]. The IES is perhaps the most appropriate tool to use to assess the impact of cancer screening tests on psychosocial well-being. Indeed, the IES measures the incidence of distressing thoughts related to a specific experience, such undergoing a screening test. By contrast, other measures either lack formal psychometric testing or assess affective symptoms or HRQL, which although potentially related to screening, may also be pre-morbid or insensitive.

Qualitative Methods

Qualitative studies embedded within well-designed screening trials provide rich data that can be used to supplement quantitative information collected in self report health questionnaires. The role of qualitative research, however, is important to understand because the samples studied are deliberately small and because many researchers are unfamiliar with these processes. Qualitative research aims to examine people's subjective experiences and understandings of what has happened to them and to interpret social phenomena in terms of the meanings people bring to them; because of this it may be referred to as *interpretative* research. It also studies people in their natural settings rather than in artificial or experimental ones, a phenomenon known as *naturalism.* Standard qualitative methods include talking with people (interviews, focus groups and informal chatting) and observing them (as a participant or non-participant of the situation). Analyses of the data from these processes require considerable time and energy. Interviews or natural settings are audio and/or video-recorded and the outputs transcribed verbatim for analysis. It is then necessary to develop themes from the data (using Grounded theory) and check for reliability and validity by an iterative process of triangulating information.

Accurately interpreting this information (which is often contradictory), to a plausible finding that is relevant to practice is the final and most challenging part. Qualitative interviews enable the perspective of the patient to be brought to the fore, narrowing the gap between the assumptions of health-care professionals and the patient's experience of decisions-making in relation to screening attendance and whether test results are pursued with further investigations.

Psycho-social Outcomes of Cancer Screening Trials

Breast Cancer

The transient anxiety associated with mammographic screening for breast cancer has been well-established [27, 34, 78]. This experience may influence some women's intentions to re-attend for future screening [27, 34] and efforts to reduce this distress have been unsuccessful [79, 80]. Nine studies, (one randomised trial [81], five prospective [27, 74, 82–84] and three cross-sectional studies [85–87]) have demonstrated adverse psychosocial outcomes, most notably high rates of anxiety [27, 82, 83, 87], depression [85, 86], and cancer specific concerns [74, 81] associated with abnormal mammographic findings. The extent to which the requirement for additional diagnostic interventions contributes to these outcomes, however, is inconsistent. Whilst two studies suggested the intensity of follow up and particularly the need for a diagnostic biopsy was related to the amount of anxiety [87] and distress [81] that women experienced, another study suggested that the type of intervention required, whether biopsy or increased mammographic surveillance had little impact on psychosocial distress [84]. Some evidence suggests that responses to mammographic abnormalities may be mediated by individuals' coping strategies [82], and that factors such as reduced waiting periods, consistency in healthcare professionals, giving results in person and good information may also be important in reducing psychosocial distress in these women [87].

Interventions aimed at reducing these adverse experiences such as improved information provision [88], counselling [89], teaching coping skills [81] and immediate reading of mammography [81] may ameliorate the negative psychological effects of an abnormal mammogram. The success of these interventions, however, has been variable. No differences in psychological or behavioural measures were seen in response to additional information provision [88] or as a result of teaching patients additional coping skills [81]. Counselling, however, did appear to decrease dysfunction at follow-up [89] and immediate reading of mammograms significantly decreased anxiety in the abnormal result group [81].

There has also been work studying how chemoprevention of breast cancer affects psychological health in women. Tamoxifen reduces the occurrence of breast cancer [90–92], but its rare and life threatening adverse effects, particularly endometrial cancer and thromboembolic disease have restricted its prophylactic use in all but the highest risk groups [93]. Alternative chemopreventative agents such as raloxifene and aromatase inhibitors have therefore been investigated [94]. Two large randomised clinical trials, IBIS II [95] and the NSABP STAR P-2 [96] have evaluated clinical and psychosocial outcomes of these drugs. Anastrozole (an aromatase inhibitor) does not cause problems with cognitive impairment [95] and there do not seem to be adverse health-related quality of life effects of gonadotrophic-releasing hormone agonists [97] used in a chemopreventative setting. The STAR-P2 [96] study compared tamoxifen with raloxifene and although side effect profiles differed for these treatments, the study demonstrated no significant differences between the drugs in terms of key aspects of health-related quality of life. An additional large RCT, the NCIC CTG MAP.3 study evaluating the clinical effectiveness and health-related quality of life impact of the steroidal aromatase inhibitor exemestane versus placebo for prevention of breast cancer in post-menopausal women is currently ongoing [98]. With such significant potential benefits associated with the use of chemoprevention, two further studies have explored whether psychosocial factors, particularly distress and satisfaction with information influence treatment uptake. One study found that high risk women may wish to take prophylactic tamoxifen, but they may be dissatisfied with this [99]. There is therefore a need for more research into understanding how women perceive and experience chemoprevention to inform this debate. It is also necessary to develop interventions to allow women to make fully informed decisions.

Cervical Cancer

There has been routine screening for cervical carcinoma in the UK since the 1980s and estimates suggest that this has reduced mortality by around 80% [100]. Cervical papaninicolaou (Pap) smears are the mainstay of cervical screening but are hampered by low sensitivity and the need for colposcopy and/or invasive cone biopsy in screening-positive individuals [101]. Pre-test worry is high amongst women contacted for colposcopy, with up to 50% of women admitting to avoiding or delaying Pap smears due to worries or anxieties about the invasiveness or consequences of screening [32, 102]. This is perhaps compounded by the widespread knowledge that equivocal results are commonplace with the need for regular follow-up. Indeed, there is evidence to suggest that anxiety prior to colposcopy is directly associated with ongoing post-test anxiety, indicative of dissatisfaction with the embarrassing nature of the test and concern over the possibility of positive or equivocal test results [33]. Despite this, it has also been shown that most women report a favourable attitude to future colposcopy perhaps because of the reassurance that a negative screening test provides [103].

On the whole negative cytological and Human Papilloma Virus (HPV) screening have been shown to reduce anxiety and induce relief amongst those screened [104, 105]. Another study has, however, shown women not to be reassured by a negative HPV test [106]. Positive screening results, by contrast, are marred by the low specificity of cervical smears making the interpretation of psychosocial responses to screening complicated by the high incidence of false positive test results. Equivocal or inadequate smears are associated with a higher level of concern at 3 months even in women who later return a normal smear [45]. State anxiety was initially raised in these women, but subsequently reduced to baseline at 3 months indicating that the negative psychosocial effects of colposcopy are short-lived. Interestingly, women with initially inadequate smears who then had normal smears experienced relief at the result, but still had higher levels of concern and lower satisfaction than those who initially tested normal [45].

Women who receive abnormal smear results feel frustrated, unprepared, disempowered, anxious and distressed [107–110]. Sexual promiscuity is often perceived as a cause of an abnormal smear result and those women who identified promiscuity with their abnormal result felt ashamed and were embarrassed by the result [110]. A perceived increased risk of cancer and concerns over future fertility have also been associated with negative feelings following an abnormal cytology result [109, 110]. As previously mentioned, test-induced anxiety may be short-lived with reassurance being gained from future screening [108, 109, 111]. Despite this, a subset of women report lasting negative effects from screening especially on their sexual health [109].

Prostate Cancer

The clinical role of screening for prostate cancer with PSA (prostate specific antigen) testing remains controversial. In the past few years major randomised trials from the US (PLC, Prostate, Lung, Colorectal and Ovarian Cancer Screening Trial) and continental Europe (ERSPC, European Randomised Study of Screening for Prostate Cancer) have published some inconclusive evidence testing [11, 112]. These both included validated PROMs although it appears that these were assessed within subgroups. In the ERSPC trial, the short term effects of screening for prostate cancer were measured with the SF-36, EQ-5D and the State-Trait Anxiety Inventory [113] before and immediately prior to testing and after receiving the PSA results. Results showed that participants reported few problems related to screening except that men with a predisposition for anxiety experienced high anxiety levels throughout the process. Data from the Swedish part of the ERSPC trial including 1,781 screen detected men who also showed that anxiety levels were moderate to low during the screening process although there is a subset of men who had severe anxiety [114]. In the US PLCO trial using the mental health component of the SF12 and four items from the IES (assessing intrusion specific to cancer distress) a small sample of 149 men and women being screened for lung, prostate, ovarian and colorectal cancer showed higher levels of intrusive thoughts about cancer than those with all normal results in the short term, but these reduced by the intermediate term follow up (where abnormal screening results had been verified) [40]. In the UK, a screening trial including a comprehensive assessment of PROMs is underway [115] (ISRCTN92187251). Some of the early prospective longitudinal data nested within the study reports results from the HADS and SF-12 questionnaires and a validated measure of lower urinary tract symptoms [116]. Results from men before PSA testing and in those with raised PSA levels prior to biopsy show similar scores, implying very little impact of the process on anxiety and depression [71]. Another report from the same study in men responding or not responding to invitations for PSA testing and from men with raised PSA levels undergoing or refusing a biopsy [69] found similar PROM scores between men accepting or non-responding to invitations for a PSA test, but men subsequently accepting biopsy were more likely to report more lower urinary tract symptoms than those declining this test. These results are important because they suggest that men do not understand the association between lower urinary tract symptoms and the risk of prostate cancer. A qualitative study integrated with this trial explored men's views and perceptions of these processes and confirmed this hypothesis [117]. In addition to these trials, there have been several prospective cohorts and cross sectional studies examining these issues, however, it is necessary to wait for the full results from the three randomised trials to be able to inform men of the overall impact of screening on psycho-social health.

Ovarian Cancer

Some of Wilson's and Junger's criteria for screening are met for ovarian cancer because it is a fatal illness that can be effectively treated with early intervention. There are problems, however, with this disease as the natural history and development and risk factors are uncertain. Other issues are that the screening and diagnostic tests for ovarian cancer require high sensitivity and specificity because currently the only certain way to confirm the diagnosis is surgery and excision of the fallopian tube. Because of these challenging issues there is no regular screening program in existence for ovarian cancer in the developed world although these issues are the focus of several large RCTs that are expected to report in the next few years [7, 11].

Colorectal Cancer

There is a lack of published data regarding the impact of screening in healthy populations for colorectal cancer on PROMs, although several studies have considered these issues within high risk populations (e.g. HPNCC with a genetic tendency for polyp formation). Investigations used for colorectal cancer screening including faecal occult blood testing and endoscopic examination of the gastrointestinal tract are associated with physical side effects, embarrassment and fear. These tests also require fairly extensive preparation by the patient (to empty and clear the bowel) [118–120]. The invasive nature of these tests and associated embarrassment is likely to be implicated in the lower overall attendance rate for screening for colorectal cancer than for breast cancer (data for colorectal in US/UK versus breast).

The impact of undergoing screening was initially thought to have little effect on anxiety and depression when participants were compared with controls using the HADS [121]. In a multi-centre prospective study with a baseline assessment of anxiety and a comprehensive battery of tests designed to measure the psychological consequences of screening in 3,535 participants, it was found that bowel cancer worry decreased significantly following flexible sigmoidoscopic screening, although participants with high health anxiety were less likely to be reassured by screening than those with health anxiety levels within normal limits [26]. Patients with a high health anxiety, however, showed the greatest reduction in state and trait anxiety (measured with the S-STAI) after screening and were more likely to report positive emotional responses to screening [26]. In another large prospective study of 1,951 patients undergoing flexible sigmoidoscopic screening, state anxiety was shown to drop after screening [39]. In addition, bowel cancer worry reduced most dramatically after screening in those participants who had a high level of anxiety at baseline [39]. Other authors have shown an improvement in certain HRQL domains including vitality and role function after colonoscopic screening [41]. Taken as a whole screening for colorectal cancer seems to alleviate anxiety and cancer worry and provide reassurance to those who have been screened.

Oesophago-gastric Cancer

The increasing incidence of adeno-carcinoma of the oesophagus and gastric cardia in Western parts of the world and the knowledge that early disease is often asymptomatic raises the important role of screening in this area. Early work evaluating endoscopic screening and surveillance for Barrett's oesophagus has shown inconclusive evidence of the impact on mortality and efforts to evaluate the psycho-social impact are limited [122]. In some parts of the world efforts to screen for gastric cancer with endoscopy may be more acceptable because of the high incidence of the disease, however, few studies have comprehensively evaluated how testing impacts on patient-reported outcomes. In the UK current efforts to evaluate chemoprevention and the incidence of upper GI cancers are underway with integrated assessment of psycho-social health [123]. It is necessary however, to link these studies with trials evaluating treatment of upper GI cancer because of the current risks and negative impact of surgical approaches on HRQL. Until minimal access endoscopic techniques can successfully treat early lesions it is unlikely that screening or surveillance will be shown to be cost effective. Encouraging results using radiofrequency ablation [124] have just been published.

Lung Cancer

Lung cancer is the most common cancer worldwide and since the widespread use of computerised tomography (CT), the role of screening for this malignancy has increased. A Cochrane review summarised the trials addressing the role of chest

X ray (CXR) and found six randomised studies addressing this issue, although there were no studies with an unscreened control group [125]. There was some reduction in mortality associated with CXR screening, although many trials were methodologically weak and none assessed HRQL. The impact of using CT for lung cancer screening is awaited [126–128]. Some of the results from the NELSON trial, a Dutch-Belgian CT screening trial in high risk subjects using the IES before and 6 months after CT have been published [129]. They showed that a subset of participants with a high risk perception remained more anxious 6 months after the CT than participants with low risk perception. This shows that within the screening populations there is a subset of anxious participants who need attention whilst undergoing investigations. Whether population based testing for lung cancer becomes established remains a subject of debate.

Impact of Genetic Screening on Psychosocial Health

The advent of modern molecular genetics has lead to an upsurge in the identification of mutations that predispose to common forms of cancer. Testing for these mutations has become commonplace in families with a disproportionately high incidence of certain malignancies at younger ages. Testing positive to a specific mutation means sufferers are at a greater risk of developing cancer and this carries with it a significant psychological burden. Consequently, genetic counselling is routinely offered prior to testing to help to address and limit some of the psychosocial impact of genetic screening. Much of the current literature has focussed on the BRCA1 and BRCA2 mutations in breast cancer, although there is a growing volume of research looking at the effect of screening for Familial Adenomatous Polyposis (FAP) and Hereditary Non-polyposis Colorectal Cancer (HNPCC). This section will summarise the current literature in this area.

Hereditary Breast Cancer

Identifying hereditary breast cancer genes (BRCA1/2) in high-risk women allows affected individuals the opportunity to take part in appropriate risk reduction strategies. The process of genetic counselling, testing and the subsequent knowledge of BRCA status, however, may dramatically affect the well-being of both the individual and their family and the impact of genetic testing on psychosocial outcomes has become the subject of intensive research in recent years. Genetic counselling primarily aims to meet the psychosocial need of those being screened by providing information and support, allowing individuals to form more accurate assessments of their genetic risk and thus make informed decisions about genetic testing. High risk women seeking testing for BRCA1/2 have been shown to experience high levels of anxiety and distress [130]. Although counselling appears to address women's psychosocial concerns, decreasing anxiety, depression and cancer related distress [131–134], it has little or no impact on improving the accuracy of their cancer risk assessments. Women in all studies consistently overestimated their breast cancer risk [131–133, 135, 136]. Low satisfaction with the genetic counselling process has also been associated with high levels of general and cancer specific distress [137], a prevalent outcome in women awaiting genetic counselling [138] and of particular relevance given the high rates of depressive symptoms reported in this population [139]. Additionally, high levels of cancer specific distress and low levels of social support may act as barriers to participation in counselling interventions [140, 141].

Despite the explosion in the number of publications in this area, there remains a lack of consensus regarding the psychosocial impact of testing for BRCA1/2. Although a number of well-designed prospective studies suggest that genetic testing has no adverse long-term psychological sequalae [42, 142–146], the short-term effects on both individuals and their families [147–150] are more controversial and may be influenced by a number of factors, most notably carrier status. Receiving a negative screening test has consistently been shown to reduce anxiety as well as general and cancer-specific distress [151–156]. A positive BRCA1/2 test, by contrast, increases general and cancer-specific distress in the weeks following disclosure of carrier status and although the levels of distress decrease over time, they remain higher than in non-carriers [155, 157]. The positive impact of genetic testing is mediated at least in part through the elimination of uncertainty. The disclosure of an inconclusive finding or "variant of uncertain clinical significance" (VUCS) has therefore been the subject of increasing interest as these women are not provided with a definitive result. Some studies [152, 153, 156] suggest that compared with true negatives, women with inconclusive test results report more cancer worry, higher perceived cancer risks and impaired quality of life as a consequence of undergoing genetic testing [153]. By contrast, it has also been suggested that the receipt of an inconclusive result has no adverse effects on psychosocial outcomes [144, 158, 159]. The heterogeneity of the inconclusive group, however, has been highlighted and an individualised approach to each woman recommended [156]. A number of factors other than carrier status may also influence women's responses to genetic testing. Pre-testing levels of cancer worry [68, 142, 160], personality traits [68, 142], passive coping mechanisms [160, 161], inadequate social and family support [162, 163], parental cancer [164], gender [165] and less open communications [160] have all been shown to be predictive of increased psychosocial distress associated with genetic testing.

Hereditary Colon Cancer

In comparison to hereditary breast cancer, few studies have assessed the effect that genetic counselling and testing have on people undergoing screening for FAP and HNPCC. Furthermore, many of the studies that have been undertaken are cross-sectional or have a small sample size, limiting their validity and widespread application [25, 44, 68]. In hereditary colorectal cancer, carrier status is again a strong predictor of the psychological response to genetic testing, with the levels of cancer worry, distress, anxiety and depression being greater amongst carriers than non-carriers [37, 38, 44]. Distress, anxiety and depression generally decreased with time irrespective of carrier status [38, 42, 166, 167], although persistently elevated levels of cancer worry amongst carriers of genetic mutations have been shown even at long-term follow-up [37]. Patients from high-risk families but without a proven mutation also had more anxiety and depression than sufferers with a proven mutation [68].

Summary

Population screening programmes are being increasingly utilised in the Western world for the early detection of cancer and pre-invasive disease. The screening tests themselves are often invasive and embarrassing and can have temporary or lasting effects on the psychological health of participants. The tests also carry physical risks and occasionally lack sensitivity and specificity meaning that participants are exposed to the possibility of missed diagnoses or unnecessary additional procedures. The measurement of PROs is, therefore, warranted in all studies of cancer screening to ensure that the full scale of the psychological burden placed on participants is well understood and catered for. Improving patient satisfaction with the screening process is likely to increase compliance, which it is hoped will have an ensuing effect on cancer-related deaths and survival.

Psychosocial responses to screening vary significantly between individuals, and while it is expected that embarrassing screening tests will induce anxiety and distress and reduce HRQL, this is not always the case. Indeed, some studies have shown that psychosocial outcomes improve after screening, and this is likely to be the consequence of the reassurance that the participant receives. Any negative psychological impact of screening is, on the whole, short-lived and many studies have shown that anxiety, depression and distress levels return to baseline by a year, even in participants who have a positive screening result. These results are encouraging and suggest that although screening can impact negatively on psychological well-being in the short-term, there is little evidence for a long-term detrimental effect. The main exception to this, however, is in participants who have high levels of pre-test anxiety or depression, who have been shown to have enduring psychological symptoms following screening. Improving counselling services and patient information, offering prompt test results and addressing pre-test psychological problems in susceptible individuals may help to alleviate these sequelae. The psychological response to screening is also highly dependent upon whether a positive, negative or inconclusive result is obtained, with screening-positive individuals often showing worse psychosocial function that those who test negative, although this is not a universal finding. At present, there is a paucity of research into the effect on psychosocial outcomes of false positive, false negative and inconclusive test results and further work is warranted in this area, as these participants are likely to be subjected to unique psychological sequelae not experienced by others undergoing screening.

A wide range of PROMs have been used in clinical trials of cancer screening, however, most of these were initially developed to measure affective symptoms, distress and HRQL in other disease settings. Their use may thus be inappropriate and the data collected may be unreliable or invalid. In addition, many studies use questionnaires designed specifically for the study being undertaken meaning that the results are often heterogeneous and non-comparable between studies, hindering meta-analyses of data. At present no PROM exists that has been specifically designed and validated for use in cancer screening trials and this is an area for future work. A proportion of studies assessing the psychosocial impact of cancer screening have lacked power and longevity of follow-up, meaning that there is a need for further well-designed longitudinal trials with appropriate PROMs, especially in colorectal, ovarian and prostate cancer. Breast cancer is a notable exception, where significant research resources have already been invested. Cancer screening is also a growing phenomenon and with the introduction of full-body computed tomography or magnetic resonance scanning, patients will be able to opt for comprehensive periodic screening at their discretion. In addition, genetic profiling will become available in future years, allowing the prediction of patients likely to develop certain forms of cancer in later life. These two new-forms of cancer screening raise important ethical issues with potentially profound effects on the way cancer screening is conducted, and consequently will need to be addressed in future psychosocial studies.

This chapter has reviewed the impact that screening for cancer and pre-invasive disease has on psychosocial well-being. The PROMs most commonly used in these assessments have been discussed and their weaknesses and appropriateness for use in cancer screening trials evaluated. The literature for each of the major forms of cancer that are routinely screened for has also been critically reviewed and areas for future research identified. As screening programmes are continuously improved attention to these details will enhance participant understanding of the benefits and risks (including psychosocial impact) of screening.

Conclusions

Understanding how screening for cancer and pre-invasive disease impacts of psycho-social health is important to inform participants and to identify high risk individuals with higher anxiety levels to assist them during the process. Well designed trials including valid relevant PROMs are needed to answer these questions and integrating qualitative research can yield useful information to understand health behaviours related to screening. Valid measures of anxiety most suited to screening trials include the Impact of Events Scale and the SF12 and STAI/TRAIT measures. The timing of assessments needs to be chosen carefully to avoid missing transient changes. Many screening programmes have been introduced without these issues being fully evaluated and it is recommended that new methods (e.g. whole body PET) are evaluated comprehensively from the outset. There is also a lack of data about the long term impact for screening on psycho-social health. Finally methods are needed to develop a comprehensive communication system to ensure that participants appreciate the short and long term risks and benefits on anxiety of screening and that they receive information about the potential impact of experiencing false negative and positive results.

References

1. Gøtzsche P, Nielsen M (2006) Screening for breast cancer with mammography. Cochrane Database Syst Rev (4):CD001877
2. Bergstrom R, Sparen P, Adami H (1999) Trends in cancer of the cervix uteri in Sweden following cytological screening. Br J Cancer 81(159):166
3. Naucler P, Ryd W, Tornberg S, Strand A, Wadell G, Elfgren K et al (2007) Human papillomavirus and Papanicolaou tests to screen for cervical cancer. N Engl J Med 357(16): 1589–1597
4. Benson V, Patnick J, Davies A, Nadel M, Smith R, Atkin W et al (2008) Colorectal screening: a comparison of 35 initiatives in 17 countries. Int J Cancer 122:1357–1367
5. Hewitson P, Glasziou P, Irwig L, Towler B, Watson E (2007) Screening for colorectal cancer using the faecal occult blood test, Haemoccult. Cochrane Database Syst Rev 1(CD001216)
6. Ilic D, O'Connor D, Green S, Wilt T (2009) Screening for prostate cancer. Cochrane Database Syst Rev 3(CD004720)
7. Menon U, Gentry-Maharaj A, Hallett R, Ryan A, Burnell M, Sharma A et al (2009) Sensitivity and specificity of multimodal and ultrasound screening for ovarian cancer, and stage distribution of detected cancers: results of the prevalence screen of the UK Collaborative Trial of Ovarian Cancer Screening (UKCTOCS). Lancet Oncol 10(4):327–340
8. Andersson I, Aspegren K, Janzon L, Landberg T, Lindholm K, Linell F et al (1988) Mammographic screening and mortality from breast cancer: the Malmo mammographic screening trial. BMJ 297(6654):943–948
9. Adami H, Ponten J, Sparen P, Bergstrom R, Gustafsson L, Friberg L (1994) Survival trend after invasice cervical cancer diagnosis in Sweden before anf after cytologic screening. Cancer 73(1):140–147
10. Mandel JS, Bond JH, Church TR, Snover DC, Bradley GM, Schuman LM et al (1993) Reducing mortality from colorectal cancer by screening for fecal occult blood. N Engl J Med 328(19):1365–1371
11. Andriole GL, Crawford ED, Grubb RL III, Buys SS, Chia D, Church TR et al (2009) Mortality results from a randomized prostate-cancer screening trial. N Engl J Med 360(13):1310–1319
12. Miller AB, To T, Baines CJ, Wall C (2002) The Canadian National Breast Screening Study-1: breast cancer mortality after 11 to 16 years of follow-up: a randomized screening trial of mammography in women age 40 to 49 years. Ann Intern Med 137:305–312
13. Veronesi U, Cascinelli N, Mariani L, Greco M, Saccozzi R, Luini A et al (2002) Twenty-year follow-up of a randomized study comparing breast-conserving surgery with radical mastectomy for early breast cancer. N Engl J Med 347(16):1227–1232
14. Ganz PA, Kwan L, Stanton AL, Krupnick JL, Rowland JH, Meyerowitz BE et al (2004) Quality of life at the end of primary treatment of breast cancer: first results from the moving beyond cancer randomized trial. J Natl Cancer Inst 96(5):376–387
15. Wang K, Samplinrer R (2008) The Practice Parameters Committee of the American College of Gastroenterology. Updated guidelines 2008 for the diagnosis, surveillance and therapy of Barrett's esophagus. Am J Gastroenterol 103(788):797
16. Playford RJ (2006) New British Society of Gastroenterology (BSG) guidelines for the diagnosis and management of Barrett's oesophagus. Gut 55(4):442

17. Winawer SJ, Zauber AG, Ho MN, O'Brien MJ, Gottlieb LS, Sternberg SS et al (1993) Prevention of colorectal cancer by colonoscopic polypectomy. N Engl J Med 329(27):1977–1981
18. Atkin WS, Saunders BP (2002) Surveillance guidelines after removal of colorectal adenomatous polyps. Gut 51(90005):v6–v9
19. Atkin WS, Morson BC, Cuzick J (1992) Long-term risk of colorectal cancer after excision of rectosigmoid adenomas. N Engl J Med 326(10):658–662
20. Selby JV, Friedman GD, Quesenberry CP, Weiss NS (1992) A case-control study of screening sigmoidoscopy and mortality from colorectal cancer. N Engl J Med 326(10):653–657
21. Lynch HT, Lynch JF (1986) Breast cancer genetics in an oncology clinic: 328 consecutive patients. Cancer Genet Cytogenet 22(4):369–371
22. Kinzler KW, Nilbert MC, Su LK, Vogelstein B, Bryan TM, Levy DB et al (1991) Identification of FAP locus genes from chromosome 5q21. Science 253(5020):661–665
23. Leach FS, Nicolaides NC, Papadopoulos N, Liu B, Jen J, Parsons R et al (1993) Mutations of a mutS homolog in hereditary nonpolyposis colorectal cancer. Cell 75(6):1215–1225
24. Wilson J, Junger G (1968) Principles and practice of screening for disease. WHO Chron 22(11):473
25. Esplen M, Madlensky L, Aronson M, Rothenmund H, Gallinger S, Butler K et al (2007) Colorectal cancer survivors undergoing testing for hereditary non-polyposis colorectal cancer: motivational factors and pyschosocial functioning. Clin Genet 72:394–401
26. Miles A, Wardle J (2006) Adverse psychological outcomes in colorectal cancer screening: does health anxiety play a role? Behav Res Ther 44(8):1117–1127
27. Brown SJ, Lehlbach M (2008) The role of anxiety in a mammography screening program. Psychosomatics 49(1):49–55
28. Janz NK, Wren PA, Schottenfeld D, Guire KE (2003) Colorectal cancer screening attitudes and behavior: a population-based study. Prev Med 37(6):627–634
29. Tessaro I, Mangone C, Parkar I, Pawar V (2006) Knowledge, barriers and predictors of colorectal cancer screening in an Appalachian church population. Prev Chronic Dis 3(4):A123
30. Sun WY, Basch CE, Wolf RL, Li XJ (2004) Factors associated with colorectal cancer screening among Chinese-Americans. Prev Med 39(2):323–329
31. Aro A, de Koning HJ, Absetz P, Schreck M (2001) Two distinct groups of non-attenders in an organised mammography screening program. Breast Cancer Res Treat 70(2):145–153
32. Duffett-Leger L, Letourneau N, Croll J (2008) Cervical cancer screening practices among university women. J Obstet Gynecol Neonatal Nurs 37:572–581
33. Chan YM, Lee PWH, Ng TY, Ngan HYS (2004) Could precolposcopy information and counseling reduce women's anxiety and improve knowledge and compliance to follow-up? Gynecol Oncol 95(2):341–346
34. Brunton M, Jordan C, Campbell I (2005) Anxiety before, during, and after participation in a population-based screening mammography programme in Waikato Province, New Zealand. N Z Med J 118(1209):U1299
35. Lagerlund M, Hedin A, Sparqn P, Thurfjell E, Lambe M (2000) Attitudes, beliefs, and knowledge as predictors of nonattendance in a Swedish population-based mammography screening program. Prev Med 31(4):417–428
36. Consedine NS, Magai C, Neugut AI (2004) The contribution of emotional characteristics to breast cancer screening among women from six ethnic groups. Prev Med 38(1):64–77
37. Gritz ER, Peterson SK, Vernon SW, Marani SK, Baile WF, Watts BG et al (2005) Psychological impact of genetic testing for hereditary nonpolyposis colorectal cancer. J Clin Oncol 23(9):1902–1910
38. Meiser B, Collins V, Warren R, Gaff C, St John D, Young M et al (2004) Psychological impact of genetic testing for hereditary non-polyposis colorectal cancer. Clin Genet 66:502–511
39. Wardle J, Williamson S, Sutton S, Biran A, McCaffery K, Cuzick J et al (2003) Psychological impact of colorectal cancer screening. Health Psychol 22(1):54–59
40. Taylor KL, Shelby R, Gelmann E, McGuire C (2004) Quality of life and trial adherence among participants in the prostate, lung, colorectal, and ovarian cancer screening trial. J Natl Cancer Inst 96(14):1083–1094

41. Taupin D, Chambers S, Corbett M, Shadbolt B (2006) Colonoscopic screening for colorectal cancer improves quality of life measures: a population-based screening study. Health Qual Life Outcomes 4(1):82
42. Arver B, Haegermark A, Platten U, Lindblom A, Brandberg Y (2004) Evaluation of psychosocial effects of pre-symptomatic testing for breast/ovarian and colon cancer pre-disposing genes: a 12-month follow-up. Fam Cancer 3(2):109–116
43. FDA (2009) Guidance for industry patient-reported outcome measures: use in medical product development to support labeling claims. FDA, USA
44. Bleiker EMA, Menko FH, Taal BG, Kluijt I, Wever LDV, Gerritsma MA et al (2003) Experience of discharge from colonoscopy of mutation negative HNPCC family members. J Med Genet 40(5):e55
45. French D, Maissi E, Marteau T (2006) The psychological costs of inadequate cervical smear test results: three-month follow-up. Psychooncology 15(6):498–508
46. Fowler F Jr, Barry M, Walker-Corkery B, Caubet J, Bates D, Lee J et al (2006) The impact of a suspicious prostate biopsy on patients' psychological, socio-behavioral, and medical care outcomes. J Gen Intern Med 21:715–721
47. Spielberger C (1983) Manual for the state/trait anxiety inventory (form Y): (self evaluation questionnaire). Consulting Psychologists Press, Palo Alto, CA
48. Radloff L (1977) The CES-D scale: a self report depression scale for research in the general population. Appl Psychol Meas 1:385–401
49. Zigmond A, Snaith R (1983) The hospital anxiety and depression scale. Acta Psychiatr Scand 67:361–370
50. The Euro-Qol Group (1990) EuroQol – a new facility for the measurement of health-related quality of life. Health Policy 16(3):199–208
51. Gray NM, Sharp L, Cotton SC, Avis M, Philips Z, Russell I et al (2005) Developing a questionnaire to measure the psychosocial impact of an abnormal cervical smear result and its subsequent management: the TOMBOLA (Trial Of Management of Borderline and Other Low-grade Abnormal smears) trial. Qual Life Res 14(6):1553–1562
52. McHorney CA, Ware JE Jr, Raczek AE (1993) The MOS 36-Item Short-Form Health Survey (SF-36): II. Psychometric and clinical tests of validity in measuring physical and mental health constructs. Med Care 31(3):247–263
53. Bloom JR, Stewart SL, Oakley-Girvans I, Banks PJ, Chang S (2006) Family history, perceived risk, and prostate cancer screening among African American men. Cancer Epidemiol Biomark Prev 15(11):2167–2173
54. Aaronson NK, Ahmedzai S, Bergman B, Bullinger M, Cull A, Duez NJ et al (1993) The European Organization for Research and Treatment of Cancer QLQ-C30: a quality-of-life instrument for use in international clinical trials in oncology. J Natl Cancer Inst 85(5):365–376
55. Cella DF, Tulsky DS, Gray G, Sarafian B, Linn E, Bonomi A et al (1993) The functional assessment of cancer therapy scale: development and validation of the general measure. J Clin Oncol 11(3):570–579
56. Spielberger C (1970) Manual for the stait-trait anxiety inventory. Consulting Psychologists Press, Palo Alto, CA
57. Spielberger C, Reheiser E, Ritterband L, Sydeman S, Unger K (1995) Assessment of emotional states and personality traits: measuring psychological vital signs. In: Butcher J (ed) Clinical personality assessment: practical approaches. Oxford University Press, New York
58. Barnes LLB, Harp D, Jung WS (2002) Reliability generalization of scores on the Spielberger State-Trait Anxiety Inventory. Educ Psychol Meas 62(4):603–618
59. Vernon SW, Gritz ER, Peterson SK, Amos CI, Perz CA, Baile WF et al (1997) Correlates of psychologic distress in colorectal cancer patients undergoing genetic testing for hereditary colon cancer. Health Psychol 16(1):73–86
60. Beck A, Ward C, Mendelson M, Mock J, Brbaugh J (1961) An inventory for measuring depression. Arch Gen Psychiatry 4:561–571
61. Zung W (1965) A self-rating depression scale. Arch Gen Psychiatry 12:63–70

62. Raskin A, Schulterbrandt J, Reatig N, Rice CE (1967) Factors of psychopathology in interview, ward behavior, and self-report ratings of hospitalized depressives. J Consult Psychol 31(3):270–278
63. Devins GM, Orme CM, Costello CG, Binik YM, Frizzell B, Stam HJ et al (1988) Measuring depressive symptoms in illness populations: Psychometric properties of the Center for Epidemiologic Studies Depression (CES-D) Scale. Psychol Health 2(2):139–156
64. Basen-Engquist K, Shinn EH, Warneke C, de Moor C, Le T, Richards-Kortum R et al (2003) Patient distress and satisfaction with optical spectroscopy in cervical dysplasia detection. Am J Obstet Gynecol 189(4):1136–1142
65. van Wilgen C, Dijkstra P, Stewart R, Ranchor A, Roodenburg J (2006) Measuring somatic symptoms with the CES-D to assess depression in cancer patients after treatment: comparison among patients with oral/oropharyngeal, gynaecological, colorectal and breast cancer. Psychosomatics 47:465–470
66. Tiffen J, Sharp L, O'Toole C (2005) Depressive symptoms prescreening and postscreening among returning participants in an ovarian cancer early detection program. Cancer Nurs 28(4):325–330
67. Bjelland I, Dahl AA, Haug TT, Neckelmann D (2002) The validity of the Hospital Anxiety and Depression Scale: an updated literature review. J Psychosom Res 52(2):69–77
68. Geirdal AO, Dahl AA (2008) The relationship between psychological distress and personality in women from families with familial breast/ovarian or hereditary non-polyposis colorectal cancer in the absence of demonstrated mutations. J Genet Couns 17(4):384–393
69. Avery K, Metcalfe C, Blazeby J, Lane J, Neal D, Hamdy F et al (2008) Prostate specific antigen testing and prostate biopsy: are self-reported lower urinary tract symptoms and health-related quality of life associated with the decision to undergo these investigations? BJU Int 102:1629–1633
70. AWsare N, Green J, Aldwinckle B, Boustead G, McNicholas T (2008) The measurement of psychological distress in men being investigated for the presence of prostate cancer. Prostate Cancer Prostatic Dis 11(4):384–389
71. Brindle L, Oliver S, Dedman D, Donovan J, Neal D, Hamdy F et al (2006) Measuring the psychosocial impact of population-based prostate-specific antigen testing for prostate cancer in the UK. BJU Int 98:777–782
72. Whynes D, Woolley C, Philips Z, for the TOMBOLA Group (2008) Management of low-grade cervical abnormalities detected at screening: which method do women prefer? Cytopathology 19(6):355–362
73. Tyndel S, Austoker J, Henderson BJ, Brain K, Bankhead C, Clements A et al (2007) What is the psychological impact of mammographic screening on younger women with a family history of breast cancer? Findings from a prospective cohort study by the PIMMS Management Group. J Clin Oncol 25(25):3823–3830
74. Absetz P, Aro AR, Sutton SR (2003) Experience with breast cancer, pre-screening perceived susceptibility and the psychological impact of screening. Psychooncology 12(4):305–318
75. Horowitz M, Wilner N, Alavarez W (1979) Impact of events scale: a measure of subjective stress. Psychosom Med 41:209–218
76. Sundin E (2002) Impact of events scale: psychometric properties. Br J Psychiatry 180:205–209
77. Thewes B, Meiser B, Hickie I (2001) Psychometrci properties of the impact of events scale among women at increased risk of hereditary breast cancer. Psychooncology 10:459–468
78. Brown W, Pakenham K (2004) Mammography screening distress and pain: changes over time and relations with breast symptoms, implants and cancer detection concerns. Psychol Health Med 9(4):403–410
79. Domar AD, Eyvazzadeh A, Allen S, Roman K, Wolf R, Orav J et al (2005) Relaxation techniques for reducing pain and anxiety during screening mammography. AJR Am J Roentgenol 184(2):445–447
80. Lambertz C, Johnson C, Montgomery P, Maxwell J (2008) Premedication to reduce discomfort during screening mammography. Radiology 248(3):765–772

81. Barton MB, Morley DS, Moore S, Allen JD, Kleinman KP, Emmons KM et al (2004) Decreasing women's anxieties after abnormal mammograms: a controlled trial [see comment]. J Natl Cancer Inst 96(7):529–538
82. Heckman BD, Fisher EB, Monsees B, Merbaum M, Ristvedt S, Bishop C (2004) Coping and anxiety in women recalled for additional diagnostic procedures following an abnormal screening mammogram. Health Psychol 23(1):42–48
83. Lampic C, Thurfjell E, Sjoden PO (2003) The influence of a false-positive mammogram on a woman's subsequent behaviour for detecting breast cancer. Eur J Cancer 39(12):1730–1737
84. Currence BV, Pisano ED, Earp JA, Moore A, Chiu YF, Brown ME et al (2003) Does biopsy, aspiration or six-month follow-up of a false-positive mammogram reduce future screening or have large psychosocial effects? Acad Radiol 10(11):1257–1266
85. Jatoi I, Zhu K, Shah M, Lawrence W (2006) Psychological distress in U.S. women who have experienced false-positive mammograms. Breast Cancer Res Treat 100(2):191–200
86. Alderete E, Juarbe TC, Kaplan CP, Pasick R, Perez-Stable EJ (2006) Depressive symptoms among women with an abnormal mammogram. Psychooncology 15(1):66–78
87. Pineault P (2007) Breast cancer screening: women's experiences of waiting for further testing. Oncol Nurs Forum Online 34(4):847–853
88. Bottorff JL, Ratner PA, Johnson JL, Hislop TG, Buxton JA, Zeisser C et al (2007) Women's responses to information on mammographic breast density. Can J Nurs Res 39(1):38–57
89. Bowland L, Cockburn J, Cawson J, Anderson HC, Moorehead S, Kenny M (2003) Counselling interventions to address the psychological consequences of screening mammography: a randomised trial. Patient Educ Couns 49(2):189–198
90. Powles T, Ashley S, Tidy A, Smith I, Dowsett M (2007) Twenty-year follow up of the Royal Marsden randomised double blinded tamoxifen breast cancer prevention trial. J Natl Cancer Inst 99(4):283–290
91. Cuzick J, Forbes J, Sestak I, Cawthorn S, Hamed H, Holli K et al (2007) Long-term results of tamoxifen prophylaxis for breast cancer – 96 month follow up of the randomised IBIS-I trial. J Natl Cancer Inst 99(4):272–282
92. Fisher B, Costantino J, Wickerham D, Cecchini R, Cronin W, Robidoux A et al (2005) Tamoxifen for the prevention of breast cancer: current status of the National Surgical Adjuvant Breast and Bowel Project P-1 study. J Natl Cancer Inst 97(22):1652–1662
93. Cuzick J, Powles T, Veronesi U, Edwards R, Asheky S, Boyle P (2003) Overview of the main outcomes in breast cancer prevention trials. Lancet 361:296–300
94. Cuzick J (2005) Aromatase inhibitors for breast cancer prevention. J Clin Oncol 23(8):1636–1643
95. Jenkins VA, Ambroisine LM, Atkins L, Cuzick J, Howell A, Fallowfield LJ (2008) Effects of anastrozole on cognitive performance in postmenopausal women: a randomised, double-blind chemoprevention trial (IBIS II) [see comment]. Lancet Oncol 9(10):953–961
96. Land S, Wickerham D, Constantino J, Ritter M, Vogel V, Lee M et al (2006) Patient-reported symptoms and quality of life during treatment with tamoxifen or raloxifene for breast cancer prevention. The NSABP Study of tamoxifen and raloxifene (STAR) P-2 trial. JAMA 295(23):2742–2751
97. Weitzel JN, Buys SS, Sherman WH, Daniels A, Ursin G, Daniels JR et al (2007) Reduced mammographic density with use of a gonadotropin-releasing hormone agonist-based chemoprevention regimen in BRCA1 carriers. Clin Cancer Res 13(2 Pt 1):654–658
98. Goss P, Richardson H, Chlebowski R, Johnston D, Sarto G, Maunsell E et al (2007) National Cancer Institute of Canada Clinical Trials Group MAP.3: evaluation of exemestane to prevent breast cancer in post menopausal women. Clin Breast Cancer 7(11):895–900
99. Bober SL, Hoke LA, Duda RB, Regan MM, Tung NM (2004) Decision-making about tamoxifen in women at high risk for breast cancer: clinical and psychological factors. J Clin Oncol 22(24):4951–4957
100. Peto J, Gilham C, Fletcher O, Matthews F (2004) The cervical cancer epidemic that screening has prevented in the UK. Lancet 364(9430):249–256

101. Nanda K, McCrory DC, Myers ER, Bastian LA, Hasselblad V, Hickey JD et al (2000) Accuracy of the papanicolaou test in screening for and follow-up of cervical cytologic abnormalities. Ann Intern Med 132(10):810–819
102. Tahseen S, Reid P, Tahseen S (2008) Psychological distress associated with colposcopy: patients' perception. Eur J Obstet Gynecol Reprod Biol 139(1):90–94
103. Breitkopf C, Catero J, Jaccard J, Berenson A (2004) Psychological and sociocultural perspectives on follow-up of abnormal Papanicolaou results. Obstet Gynecol 104(6): 1347–1354
104. Pruitt SL, Parker PA, Peterson SK, Le T, Follen M, Basen-Engquist K (2005) Knowledge of cervical dysplasia and human papillomavirus among women seen in a colposcopy clinic. Gynecol Oncol 99(3 Suppl 1):S236–S244
105. Waller J, McCaffery K, Kitchener H, Nazroo J, Wardle J (2007) Women's experiences of repeated HPV testing in the context of cervical cancer screening. A qualitative study. Psychooncology 16:196–204
106. Maissi E, Marteau TM, Hankins M, Moss S, Legood R, Gray A (2004) Psychological impact of human papillomavirus testing in women with borderline or mildly dyskaryotic cervical smear test results: cross sectional questionnaire study. BMJ 328(7451):1293
107. Basen-Engquist K, Fouladi RT, Cantor SB, Shinn E, Sui D, Sharman M et al (2007) Patient assessment of tests to detect cervical cancer. Int J Technol Assess Health Care 23(02):240–247
108. Hounsgaard L, Petersen LK, Pedersen BD (2007) Facing possible illness detected through screening – experiences of healthy women with pathological cervical smears. Eur J Oncol Nurs 11(5):417–423
109. Idestrom M, Milson I, Andersson-Ellstrom A (2003) Women's experience of coping with a positive Pap smear: A register-based study of women with two consecutive Pap smears reported as CIN 1. Acta Obstet Gynecol Scand 82(8):756–761
110. Karasz A, McKee MD, Roybal K (2003) Women's experiences of abnormal cervical cytology: illness representations, care processes, and outcomes. Ann Fam Med 1(4):196–202
111. Walsh JC, Curtis R, Mylotte M (2004) Anxiety levels in women attending a colposcopy clinic: a randomised trial of an educational intervention using video colposcopy. Patient Educ Couns 55(2):247–251
112. Schroder FH, Hugosson J, Roobol MJ, Tammela TLJ, Ciatto S, Nelen V et al (2009) Screening and prostate-cancer mortality in a randomized European study. N Engl J Med 360(13):1320–1328
113. Essink-Bot ML, de Koning HJ, Nijs HG, Kirkels WJ, van der Maas PJ, Schroder FH (1998) Short-term effects of population-based screening for prostate cancer on health-related quality of life. J Natl Cancer Inst 90(12):925–931
114. Carlsson S, Aus G, Wessman C, Hugosson J (2007) Anxiety associated with prostate cancer screening with special reference to men with a positive screening test (elevated PSA) – results from a prospective, population-based, randomised study. Eur J Cancer 43(14):2109–2116
115. Metcalfe C, Martin RM, Noble S, Lane JA, Hamdy FC, Neal DE et al (2008) Low risk research using routinely collected identifiable health information without informed consent: encounters with the Patient Information Advisory Group. J Med Ethics 34(1):37–40
116. Donovan J, Abrams P, Peters T, Kay H, Reynard J, Chapple C et al (1996) The ICS-'BPH' Study: the psychometric validity and reliability of the ICS*male* questionnaire. Br J Urol 77:554–562
117. Avery KNL, Blazeby JM, Lane JA, Neal DE, Hamdy FC, Donovan JL (2008) Decision-making about PSA testing and prostate biopsies: a qualitative study embedded in a primary care randomised trial. Eur Urol 53(6):1186–1193
118. Dominitz J, Provenzale D (1997) Patient preferences and quality of life associated with colorectal cancer screening. Am J Gastroenterol 92(12):2171–2178
119. Winawer SJ, Miller C, Lightdale C, Herbert E, Ephram R, Gordon L et al (1987) Patient response to sigmoidoscopy. A randomised controlled trial of rigid and flexible sigmoidoscopy. Cancer 60:1905–1908

120. Drossman D, Brandt L, Sears C, Li Z, Nat J, Bozymski E (1996) A preliminary study of patients' concerns related to GI endoscopy. Am J Gastroenterol 91:287–291
121. Thiis-Evensen E, Wilhelmsen I, Hoff GS, Blomhoff S, Sauar J (1999) The psychologic effect of attending a screening program for colorectal polyps. Scand J Gastroenterol 34(1):103–109
122. Garside R, Pitt M, Somerville M, Stein K, Price A, Gilbert N (2006) Surveillance of Barrett's oesophagus: exploring the uncertainty through systematic review, expert workshop and economic modelling. Health Technol Assess 10(8):1–142
123. Das D, Chilton AP, Jankowski JA (2009) Chemoprevention of oesophageal cancer and the AspECT trial. Cancer Prevention II. Recent Results Cancer Res 181:161–169
124. Shaheen NJ, Sharma P, Overholt BF, Wolfsen HC, Sampliner RE, Wang KK et al (2009) Radiofrequency ablation in Barrett's esophagus with dysplasia. N Engl J Med 360(22): 2277–2288
125. Manser R, Irving L, Stone C, Byrnes G, Abramson M, Campbell D (2009) Screening for lung cancer. Cochrane Database Syst Rev (4)
126. Bach PB, Jett JR, Pastorino U, Tockman MS, Swensen SJ, Begg CB (2007) Computed tomography screening and lung cancer outcomes. JAMA 297:953–961 [see comment] [erratum appears in JAMA. 2007 Aug 1;298(5):518]
127. Gohagan J, Marcus P, Fagerstrom R, Pinsky P, Kramer B, Prorok P (2004) Baseline findings of a randomized feasibility trial of lung cancer screening with spiral CT scan vs chest radiograph*. Chest 126(1):114–121
128. van Iersel C, de Koning H, Draisam G, Mali P, Scholten E, Nackaerts K et al (2006) Risk-based selection from the general population in a screening trial: selection criteria, recruitment and power for the Dutch-Belgian randomised lung cancer multi-slice CT screening trial. Int J Cancer 120:868–874
129. Bunge EM, van den Bergh KA, Essink-Bot ML, van Klaveren RJ, de Koning HJ (2008) High affective risk perception is associated with more lung cancer-specific distress in CT screening for lung cancer. Lung Cancer 62(3):385–390
130. Dorval M, Bouchard K, Maunsell E, Plante M, Chiquette J, Camden S et al (2008) Health behaviors and psychological distress in women initiating BRCA1/2 genetic testing: comparison with control population. J Genet Couns 17(4):314–326
131. Kelly K, Leventhal H, Andrykowski M, Toppmeyer D, Much J, Dermody J et al (2004) The decision to test in women receiving genetic counseling for BRCA1 and BRCA2 mutations. J Genet Couns 13(3):237–257
132. Rimes KA, Salkovskis PM, Jones L, Lucassen AM (2006) Applying a cognitive behavioral model of health anxiety in a cancer genetics service. Health Psychol 25(2):171–180
133. Bjorvatn C, Eide GE, Hanestad BR, Oyen N, Havik OE, Carlsson A et al (2007) Risk perception, worry and satisfaction related to genetic counseling for hereditary cancer. J Genet Couns 16(2):211–222
134. McInerney-Leo A, Biesecker BB, Hadley DW, Kase RG, Giambarresi TR, Johnson E et al (2004) BRCA1/2 testing in hereditary breast and ovarian cancer families: effectiveness of problem-solving training as a counseling intervention. Am J Med Genet A 130A(3):221–227
135. Matloff ET, Moyer A, Shannon KM, Niendorf KB, Col NF (2006) Healthy women with a family history of breast cancer: impact of a tailored genetic counseling intervention on risk perception, knowledge, and menopausal therapy decision making. J Womens Health 15(7):843–856
136. Gurmankin AD, Domchek S, Stopfer J, Fels C, Armstrong K (2005) Patients' resistance to risk information in genetic counseling for BRCA1/2. Arch Intern Med 165(5):523–529
137. Tercyak KP, Demarco TA, Mars BD, Peshkin BN (2004) Women's satisfaction with genetic counseling for hereditary breast-ovarian cancer: psychological aspects. Am J Med Genet A 131(1):36–41
138. Mikkelsen EM, Sunde L, Johansen C, Johnsen SP (2008) Psychosocial conditions of women awaiting genetic counseling: a population-based study. J Genet Couns 17(3):242–251

139. Kodl MM, Lee JW, Matthews AK, Cummings SA, Olopade OI (2006) Correlates of depressive symptoms among women seeking cancer genetic counseling and risk assessment at a high-risk cancer clinic. J Genet Couns 15(4):267–276
140. Halbert CH, Wenzel L, Lerman C, Peshkin BN, Narod S, Marcus A et al (2004) Predictors of participation in psychosocial telephone counseling following genetic testing for BRCA1 and BRCA2 mutations. Cancer Epidemiol Biomark Prev 13(5):875–881
141. Caruso A, Vigna C, Maggi G, Sega F, Cognetti F, Savarese A (2008) The withdrawal from oncogenic counselling and testing for hereditary and familial breast and ovarian cancer. A descriptive study of an Italian sample. J Exp Clin Cancer Res 27:75
142. Reichelt JG, Moller P, Heimdal K, Dahl AA (2008) Psychological and cancer-specific distress at 18 months post-testing in women with demonstrated BRCA1 mutations for hereditary breast/ovarian cancer. Fam Cancer 7(3):245–254
143. Lynch HT, Snyder C, Lynch JF, Karatoprakli P, Trowonou A, Metcalfe K et al (2006) Patient responses to the disclosure of BRCA mutation tests in hereditary breast-ovarian cancer families. Cancer Genet Cytogenet 165(2):91–97
144. Beran TM, Stanton AL, Kwan L, Seldon J, Bower JE, Vodermaier A et al (2008) The trajectory of psychological impact in BRCA1/2 genetic testing: does time heal? Ann Behav Med 36(2):107–116
145. van Oostrom I, Meijers-Heijboer H, Lodder LN, Duivenvoorden HJ, Van Gool AR, Seynaeve C et al (2003) Long-term psychological impact of carrying a BRCA1/2 mutation and prophylactic surgery: a 5-year follow-up study. J Clin Oncol 21(20):3867–3874
146. Foster C, Watson M, Eeles R, Eccles D, Ashley S, Davidson R et al (2007) Predictive genetic testing for BRCA1/2 in a UK clinical cohort: three-year follow-up. Br J Cancer 96(5):718–724
147. Stroup AM, Smith KR (2007) Familial effects of BRCA1 genetic mutation testing: changes in perceived family functioning. Cancer Epidemiol Biomark Prev 16(1):135–141
148. McInerney-Leo A, Biesecker BB, Hadley DW, Kase RG, Giambarresi TR, Johnson E et al (2005) BRCA1/2 testing in hereditary breast and ovarian cancer families II: impact on relationships. Am J Med Genet A 133A(2):165–169
149. Hamann HA, Smith TW, Smith KR, Croyle RT, Ruiz JM, Kircher JC et al (2008) Interpersonal responses among sibling dyads tested for BRCA1/BRCA2 gene mutations. Health Psychol 27(1):100–109
150. Coyne JC, Kruus L, Racioppo M, Calzone KA, Armstrong K (2003) What do ratings of cancer-specific distress mean among women at high risk of breast and ovarian cancer? Am J Med Genet A 116A(3):222–228
151. Andrews L, Meiser B, Apicella C, Tucker K (2004) Psychological impact of genetic testing for breast cancer susceptibility in women of Ashkenazi Jewish background: a prospective study. Genet Test 8(3):240–247
152. van Dijk S, van Asperen CJ, Jacobi CE, Vink GR, Tibben A, Breuning MH et al (2004) Variants of uncertain clinical significance as a result of BRCA1/2 testing: impact of an ambiguous breast cancer risk message. Genet Test 8(3):235–239
153. Dorval M, Gauthier G, Maunsell E, Dugas MJ, Rouleau I, Chiquette J et al (2005) No evidence of false reassurance among women with an inconclusive BRCA1/2 genetic test result. Cancer Epidemiol Biomark Prev 14(12):2862–2867
154. McInerney-Leo A, Hadley D, Kase RG, Giambarresi TR, Struewing JP, Biesecker BB (2006) BRCA1/2 testing in hereditary breast and ovarian cancer families III: risk perception and screening. Am J Med Genet A 140(20):2198–2206
155. Watson M, Foster C, Eeles R, Eccles D, Ashley S, Davidson R et al (2004) Psychosocial impact of breast/ovarian (BRCA1/2) cancer-predictive genetic testing in a UK multi-centre clinical cohort. Br J Cancer 91(10):1787–1794
156. van Dijk S, Timmermans DR, Meijers-Heijboer H, Tibben A, van Asperen CJ, Otten W (2006) Clinical characteristics affect the impact of an uninformative DNA test result: the course of worry and distress experienced by women who apply for genetic testing for breast cancer. J Clin Oncol 24(22):3672–3677

157. van Roosmalen MS, Stalmeier PF, Verhoef LC, Hoekstra-Weebers JE, Oosterwijk JC, Hoogerbrugge N et al (2004) Impact of BRCA1/2 testing and disclosure of a positive test result on women affected and unaffected with breast or ovarian cancer. Am J Med Genet A 124A(4):346–355
158. Claes E, Evers-Kiebooms G, Boogaerts A, Decruyenaere M, Denayer L, Legius E (2004) Diagnostic genetic testing for hereditary breast and ovarian cancer in cancer patients: women's looking back on the pre-test period and a psychological evaluation. Genet Test 8(1):13–21
159. Low CA, Bower JE, Kwan L, Seldon J (2008) Benefit finding in response to BRCA1/2 testing. Ann Behav Med 35(1):61–69
160. van Oostrom I, Meijers-Heijboer H, Duivenvoorden HJ, Brocker-Vriends AH, van Asperen CJ, Sijmons RH et al (2007) Comparison of individuals opting for BRCA1/2 or HNPCC genetic susceptibility testing with regard to coping, illness perceptions, illness experiences, family system characteristics and hereditary cancer distress. Patient Educ Couns 65(1):58–68
161. van Oostrom I, Meijers-Heijboer H, Duivenvoorden HJ, Brocker-Vriends AH, van Asperen CJ, Sijmons RH et al (2007) The common sense model of self-regulation and psychological adjustment to predictive genetic testing: a prospective study. Psychooncology 16(12):1121–1129
162. Manne S, Audrain J, Schwartz M, Main D, Finch C, Lerman C (2004) Associations between relationship support and psychological reactions of participants and partners to BRCA1 and BRCA2 testing in a clinic-based sample. Ann Behav Med 28(3):211–225
163. van Oostrom I, Meijers-Heijboer H, Duivenvoorden HJ, Brocker-Vriends AH, van Asperen CJ, Sijmons RH et al (2007) Family system characteristics and psychological adjustment to cancer susceptibility genetic testing: a prospective study. Clin Genet 71(1):35–42
164. van Oostrom I, Meijers-Heijboer H, Duivenvoorden HJ, Brocker-Vriends AH, van Asperen CJ, Sijmons RH et al (2006) Experience of parental cancer in childhood is a risk factor for psychological distress during genetic cancer susceptibility testing. Ann Oncol 17(7): 1090–1095
165. Daly PA, Nolan C, Green A, Ormiston W, Cody N, McDevitt T et al (2003) Predictive testing for BRCA1 and 2 mutations: a male contribution. Ann Oncol 14(4):549–553
166. Claes E, Denayer L, Evers-Kiebooms G, Boogaerts A, Phillippe K, Tejpar S et al (2005) Predictive testing for hereditary non polyposis colorectal cancer. Subjective perception regarding colorectal and endometrial cancer, distress and health-related behaviour at one year post-test. Genet Test 9(1):54–65
167. Codori A, Zawacki K, Petersen G, Miglioretti D, Bacon J, Trimbath J et al (2003) Genetic testing for hereditary colorectal cancer in children: Long term psychological effects. Am J Med Genet A 116A(117):128
168. Agency for Healthcare Research and Quality US Preventive Services Task Force (USPSTF) (2009) http://www.ahrq.gov/clinic/uspstfix.htm

Part III
Disease Specific Examples

Chapter 14
Pre-invasive Disease of the Lung

Ornella Belvedere, Anindo K. Banerjee, and Pamela Rabbitts

Abstract Histologically distinct pre-invasive lesions have been identified as precursors, or putative precursors, of lung cancer; the extent to which pre-invasive disease precedes invasive disease is, however, still unknown. In the context of lung cancer screening, understanding the biology behind pre-invasive disease is potentially of importance as it may lead to the identification of specific and selective markers of pre-invasive lesions at high risk to develop into invasive lung cancer, useful for both the development of screening tools and also for the development of effective targeted strategies for chemoprevention and early treatment of such disease. In this chapter we focus on current knowledge and future directions of research on pulmonary pre-invasive lesions.

Abbreviations

AAH	atypical adenomatous hyperplasia
AFB	autofluorescence bronchoscopy
BAC	bronchiolo-alveolar carcinoma
CIS	carcinoma in situ
CT	computed tomography
DIPNECH	diffuse idiopathic pulmonary neuroendocrine hyperplasia
FDG-PET	[^{18}F]fluoro-2-deoxy-d-glucose positron emission tomography
HGL	high grade lesion
LDCT	low dose spiral computed tomography
LGL	low grade lesion
LOH	loss of heterozygosity
Nd-YAG	neodymium:yttrium-aluminum-garnet
OCT	optical coherence tomography

O. Belvedere (✉)
Leeds Institute of Molecular Medicine, University of Leeds, St. James's University Hospital, Beckett Street, LS9 7TF, Leeds, UK
e-mail: ornella.belvedere@gmail.com

R.C. Fitzgerald (ed.), *Pre-Invasive Disease: Pathogenesis and Clinical Management*, DOI 10.1007/978-1-4419-6694-0_14, © Springer Science+Business Media, LLC 2011

PDT	photodynamic therapy
PET	positron emission tomography
SHR-CT	super high-resolution computed tomography
SqCC	squamous cell carcinoma
WHO	World Health Organization
WLB	white light bronchoscopy

Lung cancer is the leading cause of cancer death in Europe, with an estimated 386,000 new cases and 334,800 deaths in 2006, corresponding to 12% of all cancers diagnosed and 20% of total cancer deaths, respectively [27]. Most patients with lung cancer are diagnosed with disease that is at least locally advanced and often incurable [43, 113]; in Western countries the overall survival rate at 5-years from diagnosis is only 5–16% [40, 94, 98].

As first proposed by Doll and Hill in their seminal early epidemiological study [25], smoking is the single most important cause of lung cancer. Major international research efforts are currently focused on screening methods to identify lung cancer at an early and potentially curable stage in cohorts of heavy smokers using low-dose spiral computed tomography (LDCT) [29]. However, even if the ongoing randomized LDCT screening trials demonstrate a reduction in lung cancer mortality, it is likely that the costs and workload of screening millions of smokers will be prohibitive for many health-care services, especially in developing countries where lung cancer incidence rates are increasing more rapidly. There remains therefore a need to develop novel, reliable, quick, cheap and non-invasive screening strategies that can be easily applied to large populations to further identify the subset of smokers at higher risk, in whom the potential of LDCT screening is likely to be greatest. In addition, LDCT is not as sensitive in detecting small central cancers and airway tumours (usually squamous cell carcinomas, more likely to be diagnosed in smokers) as it is for small peripheral cancers (usually adenocarcinomas) [37]. This limitation may be overcome using a screening approach that integrates LDCT and autofluorescence bronchoscopy (AFB). In fact, bronchoscopy allows the direct evaluation of the central airways and the identification of early, centrally located, tumours and pre-invasive lesions; AFB further increases the ability of the bronchoscopist to detect pre-invasive lesions [47]. However, AFB is an invasive procedure requiring highly trained bronchoscopists. Encouraging results have been reported for this bimodality approach [35, 69] but further studies are necessary to address the impact on lung cancer mortality and the cost-effectiveness of this strategy. It will however be impractical and not cost-effective to screen the entire population of at risk smokers; therefore further targeting of the highest risk population is required, hence the value of the novel, cheap, rapid and accurate screening strategies to further risk stratify the at-risk population.

Histologically distinct pre-invasive lesions have been identified as precursors, or putative precursors, of lung cancer; the extent to which pre-invasive disease precedes invasive disease is, however, still unknown. In the context of lung cancer screening, understanding the biology behind pre-invasive disease is potentially of importance as it may lead to the identification of specific and selective markers of pre-invasive lesions at high risk to develop into invasive lung cancer, useful for both the development of screening tools and also for the development of effective targeted strategies for chemoprevention and early treatment of such disease.

In the current World Health Organization (WHO) histological classification of lung cancer (2004), three morphologically distinct pulmonary preneoplastic lesions are listed: bronchial dysplasia and carcinoma in situ (CIS), a precursor for bronchial squamous cell carcinoma (SqCC); atypical adenomatous hyperplasia (AAH), the putative precursor for adenocarcinomas with bronchiolo-alveolar carcinoma (BAC) component; and diffuse idiopathic pulmonary neuroendocrine cell hyperplasia (DIPNECH), which is the proposed precursor for carcinoid tumours (Table 14.1) [117]. No morphological precursor for small cell lung cancer has been identified so far.

In this chapter we focus on current knowledge and future directions of research on pulmonary pre-invasive disease.

Bronchial Dysplasia and Carcinoma In Situ

Definition, General Overview

Pre-invasive bronchial lesions are defined as "a precursor lesion of squamous cell carcinoma arising in the bronchial epithelium. Squamous dysplasia and carcinoma in situ are a continuum of recognizable histologic changes in the large airways. They can occur as single or multifocal lesions throughout the tracheobronchial tree. Dysplasia or carcinoma in situ may exist as an isolated finding or as a bronchial surface lesion accompanying invasive carcinoma" [117]. The model of multistep carcinogenesis from normal bronchial mucosa to invasive SqCC is shown in Fig. 14.1.

The association between pre-invasive bronchial lesions and squamous cell carcinoma was first described in the 1950s by Auerbach and colleagues [6, 7]. Saccomanno et al. subsequently reported that, on serial sputum cytology in a cohort of uranium miners, the presence of abnormal cells with increasingly malignant characteristics preceded the development of lung cancer [96]. It was however only in 1981 that pre-invasive bronchial lesions were added to the WHO classification of lung and pleural tumours [128].

Microscopic parameters for the diagnosis and grading of pre-invasive bronchial lesions include thickness of the bronchial epithelium, cell size, cell maturation and orientation, nuclear/cytoplasmic ratio and other nuclear characteristics [117]. In the grading between normal bronchial epithelium and invasive SqCC, bronchial hyperplasia and metaplasia are viewed as reactive changes rather than pre-invasive lesions. Dysplasia and carcinoma in situ are considered pre-invasive lesions, with mild and moderate dysplasia often grouped together as low-grade lesions (LGL), and severe dysplasia and carcinoma in situ referred to as high-grade lesions (HGL), at higher risk of progression to invasive cancer [35].

The term "angiogenic squamous dysplasia" has been introduced to refer to dysplastic bronchial mucosa associated with intramucosal capillary loops observed

Table 14.1 Main features of pulmonary pre-invasive lesions

	Bronchial dysplasia/CIS	Atypical adenomatous hyperplasia	DIPNECH
Synonyms	Squamous atypia, angiogenic squamous dysplasia, bronchial premalignancy, pre-invasive squamous lesion, early non-invaisve cancer	Atypical alveolar cuboidal cell hyperplasia, alveolar epithelial hyperplasia, atypical alveolar hyperplasia, atypical bronchioloalveolar cell hyperplasia, bronchioloalveolar cell adenoma	Peripheral bronchial adenomas [26]
Precursor of	Bronchial squamous cell carcinoma	Adenocarcinoma, non-mucinous BAC	Carcinoid
Lesion size	Variable from few millimeters to few centimeters	Usually <5 mm [117]	Usually <5 mm
Location	Bronchial epithelium; usually central airway lesions (mainly in lobar or segmental bronchi)	Bronchiolar and alveolar epithelium; usually peripheral airway lesions, close to the pleura; most frequent in the upper lobes	Bronchiolar epithelium; usually peripheral airway lesions
Microscopic features	Increased thickness of bronchial epithelium, cellular atypia with increased cell size, decreased or no progression of maturation from base to luminal surface, increased N/C ratio [117]	Proliferation of minimally atypical cuboidal type II pneumocytes with gaps between cells; usually not associated with interstitial inflammation and fibrosis [117]	Widespread pulmonary neuroendocrine cells proliferation usually in the setting of airway fibrosis and/or inflammation, not breaching the basement membrane [15]
Detection and presentation	Usually asymptomatic; detected in bronchial biopsy, often AF +ve lesions or incidentally discovered in resected lung cancer specimens	Usually asymptomatic; incidental findings in lung specimens resected for lung cancer [15]. Often visible as ground-glass lesions on CT	A years-long history of dry cough and shortness of breath usually precedes the diagnosis

Patient characteristics	Most frequently observed in men than in women. Usually history of smoking or occupational exposure (asbestos, uranium, silica, polycyclic aromatic hydrocarbons, etc.) [89]	Most frequently observed in women than in man; in Caucasian series history of smoking	More frequent in women, typically in their forties or fifties; most common in non-smokers
Differential diagnosis	Inflammatory bronchial mucosal atypia; post-radiation changes	Reactive pneumocyte hyperplasia/atypia associated with scars or organizing alveolar injury, micronodular pneumocyte hyperplasia, bronchiolar metaplasia, non-mucinous BAC	Reactive pulmonary neuroendocrine cell proliferation often associated with chronic inflammatory diseases, such as bronchiectasis and chronic lung abscess

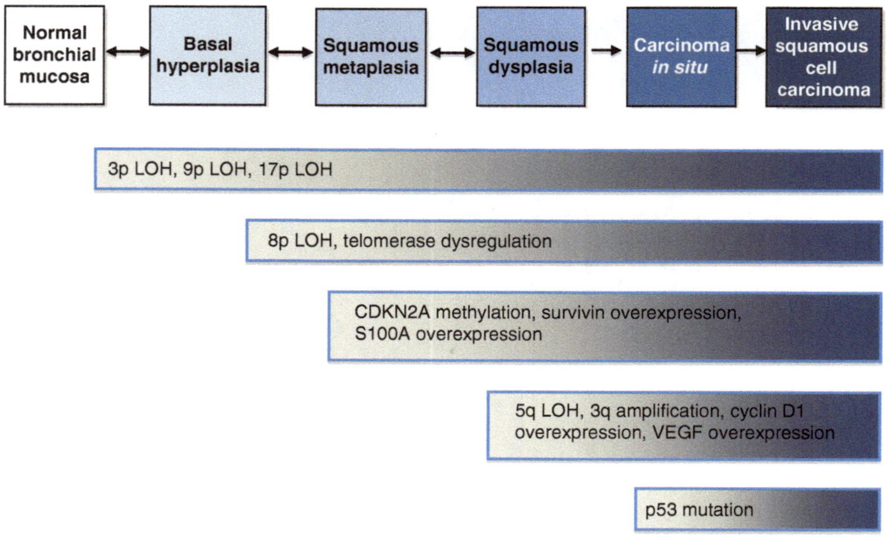

Fig. 14.1 Model of multistep carcinogenesis of lung squamous cell carcinoma

in approximately one-third of subjects at high risk for lung cancer enrolled in autofluorescence bronchoscopy trials at a single North-American institution [46]. To date, only few prevalence data are available for angiogenic squamous dysplasia; prospective surveillance studies will address the natural history of this distinct lesion and whether the presence of neoangiogenesis is a marker for invasive potential in pre-invasive bronchial lesions. This hypothesis is supported by the fact that neoangiogenesis is critical for tumour growth, invasion and metastasis [32]. If longitudinal studies confirm angiogenic squamous dysplasia as a high-risk lesion, a chemoprevention strategy including anti-angiogenic drug(s) is worthy of investigation in patients with these lesions.

Squamous dysplasia and carcinoma in situ are virtually always observed in subjects with a history of smoking, suggesting that cigarette smoking is the main cause of pre-invasive lesions in ever smokers [7, 8, 82].

Genomic Instability and Molecular Abnormalities

Advances in molecular techniques have enabled the study of the molecular genetics and biology of invasive lung cancer, and abnormalities specific for different histological types have been reported [39, 101, 120]. As molecular abnormalities were detected in fully invasive tumours and chromosomal regions or candidate genes were identified, it became possible to interrogate their involvement at the pre-invasive stage. Molecular studies on bronchial pre-invasive lesions are much more challenging: their small size makes detection difficult and severely limits the scope of molecular analysis.

Nevertheless, over the past 20 years, several molecular abnormalities have been described in pre-invasive bronchial lesions, with a direct correlation between the frequency of the specific molecular changes and the severity of the lesion as defined by histology (Fig. 14.1). The most common genetic changes in pre-invasive lesions include gain at 3q [74, 75, 91] and 1p [33], loss/deletion at 3p, 5q, 8p, 9p, 17p [20, 106, 114, 125, 126]. Also, mutations of *K-RAS* [110] and *p53* [92, 99, 111]; overexpression of cyclin D1 [44], survivin [2], VEGF [60, 76], S100A2 [104], heterogeneous nuclear ribonucleoprotein A2/B1 [71]; increased telomerase activity [102]; and a two-step evolution of microRNAs expression levels [73] have been described in the progression towards invasive cancer. Most of the studies above however are not longitudinal studies, i.e. studies that report on molecular changes in the same lesions over time. It should also be noted that different lesions in different locations in a single patient may have different genetic profiles [10, 14]. These same molecular changes have previously been reported for invasive SqCC [100].

Molecular abnormalities in pre-invasive lesions are expected to be fewer than in invasive tumours [114]. The study of pre-invasive disease at a molecular level should therefore be more informative with regards to the relevant genes driving tumour initiation and progression. Nevertheless, a potentially confounding factor to the identification of the relevant molecular abnormalities for lesion progression is the observation of similar genetic changes in histologically normal or metaplastic bronchial biopsies of healthy former or current heavy smokers, including 3p14 LOH, 9p21 LOH and 17p13 LOH [72, 124]. This is consistent with the concept of "field cancerization", first introduced by Danely Slaughter in 1953 to refer to the presence of "multifocal areas of precancerous change" in the oral mucosa of patients with SqCC of the oral cavity [103], and subsequently extended to the entire upper aerodigestive tract [109]. This should be taken into account when developing these molecular changes as biomarkers for early detection as they would not have the specificity required. In fact, there is a need to differentiate cigarette smoke markers from malignant potential markers, and also to determine HGL with malignant potential from HGL with likelihood to regress. Therefore, an ideal marker, or panel of markers, for early detection will be associated with HGL with the greatest malignant potential, and not with normal bronchial mucosa or LGL.

No mouse models corresponding to human squamous bronchial dysplasia have yet been reported through gene targeting to the mouse bronchial epithelium but a potentially useful model has been generated in mice in which the Nkx2.8 gene (a homeodomain transcription factor) was constitutionally inactivated. Although the expectation was that the Nkx2.8$^{-/-}$ mice would show abnormal liver development, fortuitously, these mice were observed to have bronchial hyperplasia from birth and dysplasia in their large airways by 1 year. Mice sacrificed later had occasionally developed fully malignant lung tumours including squamous cell carcinoma [116].

Detection

Pre-invasive bronchial lesions are usually very small, not visible radiologically and easily missed using conventional white light bronchoscopy (WLB) [127]. The detection rate of these lesions has significantly increased since the introduction of autofluorescence bronchoscopy (AFB), developed in the late 1980s at the British Columbia Cancer Agency in Vancouver [42, 53]. AFB is based on the observation that normal bronchial mucosa and pre-invasive lesions/microinvasive SqCC fluoresce differently when exposed to violet-blue light (380–450 nm wavelength) due to differences in tissue architecture and fluorophores present [42, 93]. Specifically, normal bronchial mucosa fluoresces green much greater than red, while pre-invasive lesions and microinvasive SqCC show a decrease in the intensity of green fluorescence but no change in red fluorescence, and usually appear red-brownish. Since its introduction, AFB has become the gold standard for the detection of pre-invasive bronchial lesions. At present, several autofluorescence bronchoscopy systems are commercially available, including the Storz D-light (Karl Storz, Tuttlingen, Germany), SAFE 3000 (Pentax Europe, Hamburg, Germany), EVIS Lucera (Olympus, Tokyo, Japan), and PINPOINT (Novadaq Technologies, Mississauga, Canada). Overall, AFB has a sensitivity of 80% (range 43–100%) compared to 40% (range 0–78%) with WLB, increasing the detection of pre-invasive bronchial lesions by 1.2–6.2-fold [9, 47]. These figures are however obtained against random biopsies rather than a systematic histological assessment of the bronchial mucosa accessible to bronchoscopy. The variability in sensitivity may be explained by differences among series in terms of (1) experience of the bronchoscopist; (2) population studied; (3) indication for bronchoscopy; (4) type of lesions looked for (i.e. all lesions vs. LGL and/or HGL and/or invasive SqCC). The quality of the WL and AF images and inter-observer variability are rarely an issue. Despite a significant improvement in sensitivity, AFB has a lower specificity compared with WLB (60 and 81% respectively) (Kennedy 2007): positive lesions on AFB may include benign lesions such as inflammation, granulomas, benign tumours, areas of traumatized mucosa but also histopathologically normal areas, still harboring chromosomal aberrations [36]. To increase the specificity of AFB, the use of colour fluorescence ratio (red reflectance to green fluorescence ratio) combined with visual score has recently been proposed and prospectively validated, resulting in 80% sensitivity and 88% specificity [63].

In order to improve the accuracy of the detection of pre-invasive lesions and to identify alternative procedures to fiberoptic bronchoscopy when the latter is not feasible, contraindicated or when the patient refuses it, novel technologies have been evaluated, including [^{18}F]fluoro-2-deoxy-d-glucose positron emission tomography, virtual bronchoscopy, super high-resolution computed tomography scan and optical coherence tomography. The role of [^{18}F]fluoro-2-deoxy-d-glucose positron emission tomography (FDG-PET) for the detection and staging of radiologically occult pre-invasive bronchial lesions and early SqCC has been investigated in a small study from a single institution [90]. Eleven of 13 (85%) histologically proven dysplastic bronchial lesions were FDG-PET negative, whereas 8 of 11 microinvasive SqCC were FDG positive. In general, two characteristics of pre-invasive bronchial lesions, namely small size and superficial spread, may limit the usefulness of FDG-PET making the lesion FDG-PET negative even if the abnormal cells may have increased glucose uptake. Based on these limited and preliminary data, pre-invasive bronchial lesions seem to be FDG-PET negative. A larger multicenter and ideally longitudinal study is required to definitely address the role of FDG-PET in the detection and characterization of pre-invasive bronchial lesions or evaluate alternative tracers to detect lesions rather than glucose, although PET positivity might be altered by biopsy.

Only very limited data are available for the evaluation of mucosal abnormalities by virtual bronchoscopy (VB) and super high-resolution computed tomography scan (SHR-CT) [30, 31, 67]. Sensitivity of SHR-CT scans and VB was low (range 0–16%) suggesting that these technologies are currently not reliable for the detection of pre-invasive lesions. Despite the development of inhaled contrast agents that might improve the diagnostic value of CT based imaging in this setting, important limitations to the use of VB for the diagnosis and surveillance of pre-invasive bronchial lesions include inability to visualize and biopsy the lesion, radiation exposure, and cost.

Optical coherence tomography (OCT) is a promising imaging method for the characterization of white-light and AFB detected lesions is. OCT is an interferometric imaging technique that translates depth-wise reflections of near-infrared light from tissues in cross-sectional images [130]. In a recent study, Lam et al. demonstrated that OCT of AFB positive lesions can discriminate invasive carcinoma from CIS, and dysplasia from metaplasia, hyperplasia or normal bronchial mucosa [58]. The main advantage of OCT is that it provides a reliable assessment of pre-invasive lesions without the need for a biopsy. This is most important in the setting of surveillance and chemoprevention studies where conclusions are undermined by the possibility that the diagnostic/surveillance biopsies might be responsible for the frequently observed lesion regression due to complete excision.

Prevalence

Pre-invasive bronchial lesions are almost exclusively observed in ever smokers. In the 1950s, Auerbach et al. were the first to report prevalence data on pre-invasive bronchial lesions (Auerbach 1957); the value of this report is, however, largely historical as (1) all pre-invasive bronchial lesions were labeled as carcinoma in situ, defined as "all bronchial epithelial lesions composed entirely of atypical cells and lacking cilia", with no distinction between lesions that would currently be classified as "dysplasia" and carcinoma in situ; (2) changes in smoking behavior, cigarette design (i.e. the introduction of filter tips) and tobacco preparation (including low tar and nicotine cigarettes) over the past decades have resulted in changes in the histopathology of lung cancer, with an increase in the incidence of adenocarcinoma and a decline of SqCC [115]. It is likely that the prevalence of different lung cancer precursor lesions may have changed as well.

Contemporary prevalence data are available from the chemoprevention studies by Lam et al. where 401 volunteer smokers older than 40 years of age underwent

AFB. The prevalence of carcinoma in situ was 1.8%, severe dysplasia 6.5%, moderate dysplasia 14% and mild dysplasia 40% [54]. Paris et al. investigated the prevalence of high grade bronchial pre-invasive lesions detected by AFB in a population at high risk for lung cancer as defined by the International Association for the Study of Lung Cancer, including 241 patients with a personal history of treated lung or head and neck cancer, a cigarette smoking history of ≥30 pack-years or exposure to occupational respiratory carcinogens for >10 years. In this group of patients at much higher risk than in the chemoprevention studies, the overall prevalence of high grade pre-invasive bronchial lesions was 9%, ranging from 4 to 12% in former and current smokers, respectively.

Natural History

Invasive bronchial SqCC is believed to be the final stage of the multistep process: normal epithelium→hyperplasia/metaplasia→dysplasia→carcinoma in situ→invasive cancer. To date, a small number of studies have investigated the natural history of pre-invasive bronchial lesions [13, 16, 35, 41, 44, 56, 57, 59, 83, 99, 114]. The overall limited number of lesions along with the heterogeneity of patient inclusion criteria, schedule for follow-up, duration of follow-up, criteria for intervention, definition of response and the unavoidable involvement of different pathologists, make it difficult to draw definitive conclusions from these studies [11]. The interpretation of these findings is further complicated by the possibility of surveillance biopsies removing the whole pre-invasive lesion, resulting in apparent complete regression at the following surveillance biopsy [13]. With these limitations, it is however accepted that (1) bronchial pre-invasive lesions may spontaneously regress; (2) the probability of regression decreases with the severity of the pre-invasive lesion; (3) the probability of progression to invasive SqCC increases with the severity of the lesion, being higher for high-grade lesions than low-grade lesions.

Figure 14.2a summarizes the outcome of pre-invasive lesions from 11 studies in the literature [13, 16, 35, 41, 44, 56, 57, 59, 83, 99, 114]. Overall, progression rate for HGL is 22%; this is probably an underestimate as in the study by Bota et al. which includes 59 out of 165 HGL considered, the 49 CIS lesions were followed for only 3 months before endobronchial treatment in case of persistent HGL [13].

At present, the natural history of pre-invasive bronchial lesions remains ill defined: the proportion of CIS that progress to invasive cancer varies widely among studies, ranging from 16 to 67% and there are no validated molecular features predictive of outcome. A well-designed, long-term, large, multicentre, international, prospective surveillance study with well-defined inclusion criteria, follow-up schedule, intervention criteria and centralized pathology review is required in order to (1) determine the natural history of pre-invasive bronchial lesions; (2) provide scientists with sequential biopsies from the same lesion to enable the identification of molecular changes associated with progression to invasive disease.

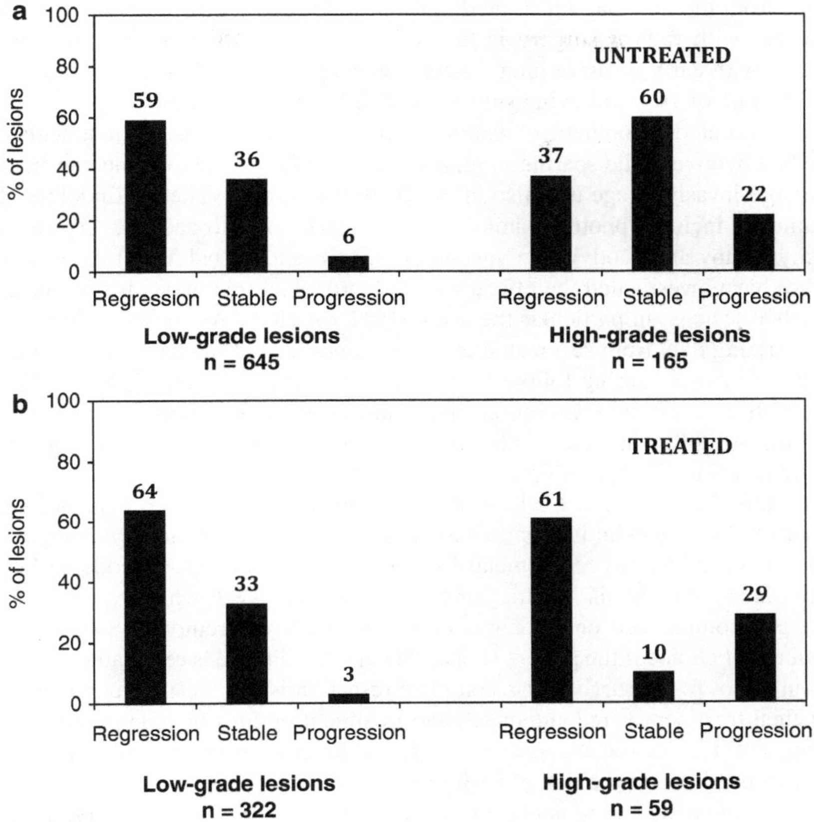

Fig. 14.2 Outcome of untreated and treated pre-invasive bronchial lesions

Management

In the absence of a predictive morphological or molecular marker(s) to identify lesions at higher risk of progression, the management of patients with pre-invasive bronchial disease is challenging and controversial.

The only treatment available and proven to be curative for early invasive lung cancer is surgery. Even when the disease is identified by either sputum cytology or bronchoscopy when still roentgenographically occult, treatment with curative intent requires at least a lobectomy, potentially leaving the patient without the option of further surgery in the event of a second lung primary cancer [22]. In this scenario, the observation that HGL may remain stable, or even regress to LGL or histologically normal mucosa, supports a watchful waiting strategy, with surgical treatment being considered only when there is evidence of microinvasive disease. However, support for a more aggressive approach for HGL and in particular CIS comes from the fact that when the disease is still at a pre-invasive stage (i.e. CIS), cure rate with radical surgery is theoretically 100%, while survival figures for patients with early invasive lung cancer (i.e. stage IA, pT1N0M0) report a 5-year survival rate of 70% following surgery with radical intent [18, 84].

The recent development of endobronchial therapies provides treatments that may be effective while sparing lung, and therefore lung function, and can be used at the pre-invasive stage and also in medically inoperable patients. Endobronchial treatments include photodynamic therapy (PDT), electrocautery, cryotherapy, brachytherapy and neodymium:yttrium-aluminum-garnet (Nd-YAG) laser. Several studies have investigated the efficacy of endobronchial treatments for pre-invasive bronchial lesions, in particular the use of PDT for HGL. As shown in Fig. 14.2b, summarizing data from seven studies, almost one-third of treated HGL progressed to invasive cancer during follow-up after endobronchial treatment [24, 55–57, 83, 107, 119]. Interestingly, endobronchial treatment does not seem to impact on the outcome of LGL, with outcome figures very similar between untreated (Fig. 14.2a) and treated (Fig. 14.2b) lesions.

In 2007 the American College of Chest Physicians published evidence-based guidelines for bronchial intraepithelial neoplasia/early central airways lung cancer [47]. These guidelines recommend bronchoscopic follow-up of moderate/severe dysplasia and carcinoma in situ, using WLB and also AFB, when available; treatment is recommended only for microinvasive/invasive carcinoma. Surgery is the treatment of choice if the patient is operable and the disease is resectable; when the patient is not fit for surgery or a complete resection is not feasible, curative endobronchial treatment is recommended and treatment options include photodynamic therapy (PDT), electrocautery, cryotherapy and brachytherapy. Nd-YAG laser is not recommended due to the risk of perforation.

Finally, smoking cessation may play an important role in patients with pre-invasive bronchial lesions. It is possible that smoking cessation might reduce the likelihood of these lesions progressing towards invasive cancer. So far, published data show that (1) the prevalence of pre-invasive bronchial lesions is higher in current than in former smokers (12 and 4%, respectively) [89]; (2) the severity of pre-invasive bronchial lesions in current smokers correlates with the duration and number of pack year smoking [82]. Therefore, smoking cessation counseling should then be encouraged in patients with pre-invasive bronchial lesions and the diagnostic/surveillance bronchoscopy should be considered a "teachable moment" for smoking cessation.

Chemoprevention

Based on epidemiologic observations and preclinical data, two large randomized trials evaluated the chemopreventive efficacy of vitamin supplementation to reduce lung cancer incidence and mortality in heavy smokers. In the ATBC trial, over 29,000 subjects were randomized to alpha-tocopherol (vitamin E) and/or beta-carotene or placebo [12]; in the CARET trial, over 18,000 subjects were randomized to retinol (vitamin A) and beta-carotene or placebo [88]. Both studies failed to demonstrate a reduction in lung cancer incidence or mortality. Even more disappointing, there was an increased incidence of lung cancer in current smokers randomized to receive beta-carotene, either alone or in combination. Time and effort (of patients and clinicians) as well as cost of these and other large negative trials [12, 68, 88, 118] cannot be underestimated. Therefore, to increase the success rate of randomized phase III chemopreventive trials, there is a need to improve the design of phase II studies, to better select the candidate chemopreventive agents more likely to be effective when tested in subsequent larger studies. Intermediate surrogate endpoints to be used instead of lung cancer are then required. In this context, the evaluation of pre-invasive lesions has been proposed, and several studies have already been conducted using this endpoint [52, 55, 57, 61]. Nevertheless, to date, there is no consensus on the criteria to assess the histological changes of these lesions. There is no way to discriminate between the effects of the chemopreventive agent(s) and the natural history of the lesion under observation, as the natural (i.e. untreated) history of the individual lesion cannot be predicted using any known criteria. Moreover, no validation of surrogate endpoints is however possible in this setting, until there will be an effective chemopreventive strategy.

In general, chemoprevention studies looking at histological endpoints are very difficult to conduct, as the following issues need to be addressed: (1) availability of bronchoscopy facilities and experienced bronchoscopists; (2) high costs due to bronchoscopy facility time, histopathology and bronchoscopy equipment; (3) low patient accrual rate, due to the overall low prevalence of detectable pre-invasive bronchial lesions in the smokers population and also due to the evolving prevalence of the different lung cancer histological types, with a decreasing incidence of SqCC in favor of more peripheral adenocarcinomas; (4) possible high patient drop-out rate due to refusal to undergo repeated bronchoscopies; (5) the influence of biopsy on the natural history and outcome of an individual lesion.

Atypical Adenomatous Hyperplasia

Definition, General Overview

The association between atypical epithelial proliferation and peripheral lung carcinomas was first described by Meyer and Liebow in the 1960s [77]. It was 20 years later that Miller et al. paid renewed interest to this topic, with the observation of localized *foci* of atypical bronchioloalveolar cells proliferation associated with lung adenocarcinoma and proposed the hypothesis of these lesions being precursors for peripherally arising lung adenocarcinoma [78].

Atypical adenomatous hyperplasia (AAH) is the term currently used to refer to these areas of abnormal proliferation, although other terms are being used including atypical alveolar hyperplasia, bronchioloalveolar cell adenoma, atypical cuboidal cell hyperplasia, and alveolar atypical hyperplasia. AAH is defined as "a localized

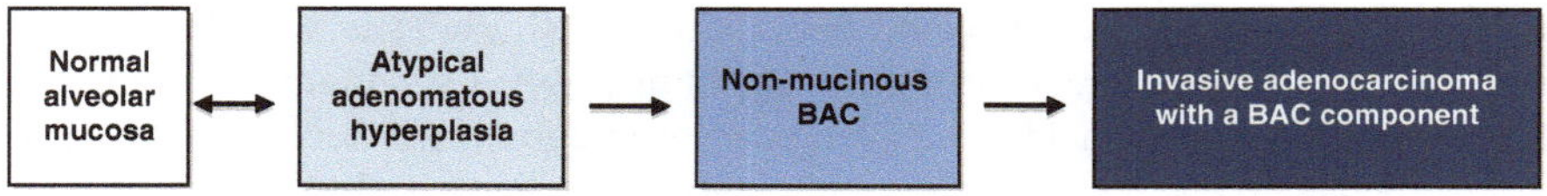

Fig. 14.3 Model of multistep carcinogenesis of lung adenocarcinoma

proliferation of mild to moderately atypical cells lining involved alveoli and, sometimes, respiratory bronchioles, resulting in focal lesions in peripheral alveolated lung, usually less than 5 mm in diameter and generally in the absence of underlying interstitial inflammation and fibrosis" [117]. AAH can present as a single or more frequently as multiple lesions, with up to 161 AAH lesions reported in an individual patient [3]. Typically, AAH is found in conjunction with BAC and/or invasive adenocarcinoma. The model of multistep cancerogenesis from normal alveolar mucosa to adenocarcinoma with BAC component is shown in Fig. 14.3.

In the spectrum of histology towards invasive cancer, AAH is believed to progress to non-mucinous bronchioloalveolar carcinoma (BAC), which is defined as "growth of neoplastic cells along pre-existing alveolar structures (lepidic growth) without evidence of stromal, vascular or pleural invasion" [117]. Two histological variants have been described: mucinous BAC and non-mucinous BAC. The distinction between AAH and a small non-mucinous BAC may be difficult; in general, differential diagnosis between AAH and BAC is based on multiple criteria, including morphological features and lesion diameter, usually ≥10 mm for BAC [117]. The pure localized BAC is an adenocarcinoma in situ, by definition a pre-invasive lesion.

Most of the literature on AAH and BAC until recently has been produced by groups based in Japan and East Asia, where adenocarcinoma has always been the most common histology for lung cancer.

Molecular Abnormalities

Several genetic and molecular changes have been described in AAH, including LOH at 3p (*ROBO1/DUTT1* gene, *FHIT gene, RASSF1A*, *FUS-1*, *BAP-1*), 9p (*CDKN2A*), 17p (*p53*), *K-RAS* mutations (mainly codon 12), p53 mutations, *EGFR* mutations and gene amplification, promoter hypermethylation of genes involved in lung cancer pathogenesis (*p16*, *TIMP3*, *DAPK*, *MGMT*, *RARβ*, *hTERT*, *Wnt* antagonists), increased Ki-67 proliferation index [48, 51, 65, 66, 105, 123].

The observation that *EGFR* and *KRAS* mutations in AAH are mutually exclusive suggests the existence of two distinct AAH subtypes and therefore two pathways for the development of invasive adenocarcinoma from AAH [97, 105, 129]. The study by Sakamoto et al. shows that the frequency of *KRAS* mutations decreases along the putative progression process from AAH (33%) through BAC (12%), then minimally invasive adenocarcinoma (8%), to well differentiated adenocarcinoma

(0%); the frequency of *EGFR* mutations does not show a clear trend being 25, 36, 86 and 67% in AAH, non-mucinous BAC, minimally invasive adenocarcinoma and well differentiated adenocarcinoma, respectively. Based on these observations, a novel theory for lung adenocarcinoma development is proposed, where both *EGFR* and *KRAS* mutations can result in AAH but only *EGFR* mutated AAH may progress to BAC and then invasive adenocarcinoma, while *KRAS* mutated AAH do not progress or do so at a lesser extent [97]. This hypothesis also includes the existence of another distinct pathway for the development of lung adenocarcinoma, to explain the presence of *KRAS* mutations in invasive adenocarcinomas. Larger studies are required to address this hypothesis. The correlation between *KRAS* and *EGFR* mutations and smoking status in AAH remains unclear [97, 129].

Detection

There are no typical clinical signs or symptoms and in most cases AAH is detected as an incidental finding in lung specimens resected for lung cancer [15]. Bronchoscopy is of no use for its detection and surveillance due to the peripheral location in the airways. AAH is usually not visualized on chest X-ray. Computed tomography (CT) may detect AAH, which usually appears as a ground-glass opacity [50, 86, 87]. Pulmonary nodules with ground-glass opacity are a frequent finding of lung cancer screening trials with low-dose CT in asymptomatic smokers [38, 64]. The appearance or increase of a solid component is observed with the progression towards BAC and invasive adenocarcinoma, probably reflecting a decrease in the air content and increase in cellular content [49]. To date, no validated radiological criteria for the differentiation of AAH, BAC and invasive carcinoma with predominant BAC component on CT imaging have been established, although nodular sphericity and internal air bronchograms have been proposed to differentiate between AAH and BAC [87].

Prevalence

The prevalence of AAH in lungs resected for primary lung cancer ranges between 9 and 21% [19, 79, 81, 85, 122]. This rate increases up to 35.5% in patients with lung adenocarcinoma (range 16–35%), while it is lower in SqCC (3–11%) [19, 79, 81, 85, 122]. AAH has also been detected in patients undergoing resection for cancer other than lung (range 4–11%) [19, 81, 122] and in 2% of noncancerous patients at autopsy [108]. The relatively wide variation in prevalence of AAH among series within each population may be partially due to differences in sampling technique: it might also reflect a true prevalence difference between Caucasian and East Asian patients.

Natural History and Management

Longitudinal studies for the understanding of the natural history of AAH are virtually impossible for two reasons: (1) AAH lesions are usually too peripheral to be accessible to bronchoscopy or other direct visualization methods that would allow the repeat biopsies required to characterize and follow the development of these lesions; (2) AAH is usually identified in resected lung specimens when the natural history of the lesion has already been changed by the surgical removal.

Insights on the natural history of AAH however come from the follow-up of patients who underwent curative surgery for lung adenocarcinoma and had incidental finding of AAH in the resected lung specimen. Based on the observation that AAH is usually multifocal [3, 19], the assumption is that these patients still have AAH lesions in the remaining lung tissue. No difference has been observed in terms of postoperative survival between these patients and patients with similar stage adenocarcinoma who also underwent curative surgery but did not have coexisting AAH in the resected lung [19, 70, 95, 112]. Based on this observation, the detection of AAH in resected lung does not affect the decision on postoperative (adjuvant) treatment. Similarly, the detection of AAH in the absence of a known or suspected lung cancer does not prompt treatment. Close follow-up and smoking cessation, if applicable, are warranted; participation in chemoprevention trials should be offered, whenever available.

Diffuse Idiopathic Pulmonary Neuroendocrine Cell Hyperplasia

Definition, General Overview

Diffuse idiopathic pulmonary neuroendocrine cell hyperplasia (DIPNECH) is a very rare pre-invasive lesion first described in the 1950s by Felton and Colleagues in a case report of "peripheral bronchial adenomas" [26]. Other authors reported a few similar cases in the following decades but it was only in 1992 that this histological entity was better characterized and named "diffuse idiopathic pulmonary neuroendocrine cell hyperplasia" by Aguayo et al. [1]. DIPNECH is a putative precursor of peripheral tumourlets and typical and atypical carcinoids. To date, there is no large study on DIPNECH. A PubMed search performed at the time of writing using the search string "Diffuse idiopathic pulmonary neuroendocrine cell hyperplasia" returned only 32 items, mainly case reports.

DIPNECH is defined as "a generalized proliferation of scattered single cells, small nodules (neuroendocrine bodies) or linear proliferations of pulmonary neuroendocrine cells that may be confined to the bronchial and bronchiolar epithelium, include extraluminal proliferation in the form of tumorlets, or extend to the development of carcinoid tumors. It is sometimes accompanied by intra- and extraluminal fibrosis of involved airways, but other pathology that might induce reactive pulmonary neuroendocrine

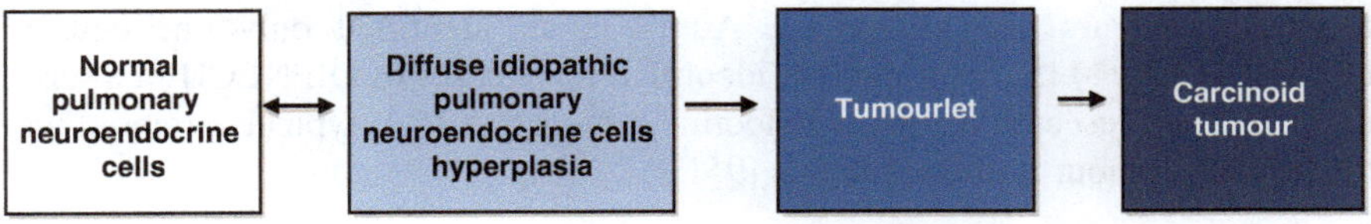

Fig. 14.4 Model of multistep carcinogenesis of carcinoid tumours

cells proliferation is absent" [117]. When the pulmonary neuroendocrine cells breach the basement membrane with local invasion, the lesion is then referred to as "tumourlet" if the lesion diameter is ≤5 mm or carcinoid if the diameter is >5 mm [117]. The proposed model of multistep carcinogenesis from normal pulmonary neuroendocrine cells to carcinoid tumours is shown in Fig. 14.4.

DIPNECH is typically observed in women in their 50s or 60s and long standing dry cough and dyspnoea usually precedes the diagnosis [1, 4, 23, 28, 34, 80, 95].

Molecular Abnormalities

To date, only few, small studies have reported on the molecular features of DIPNECH and most of them have focused on the expression of one or few specific markers by immunohistochemistry rather than providing a molecular profile of the disease [21, 23, 34, 121]. No data are available on genetic abnormalities in this disease.

Detection

DIPNECH is often an incidental finding in patients asymptomatic for the disease undergoing investigations for other diseases [23]. Nonetheless, most of the reports of DIPNECH in the literature describe case histories of years of persistent and often slowly progressive nonproductive cough and dyspnea, typically initially misdiagnosed as asthma.

Standard chest radiography may be within normal limits, whereas chest CT scan usually shows mosaic attenuation pattern suggestive of small airways obstruction [23]. Multiple millimetric nodules can also be present, usually corresponding to tumourlets or carcinoids [1, 4, 17, 23, 62].

Prevalence

Prevalence data for DIPNECH are limited to small series of patients treated with surgery for lung cancer. In a series of 28 patients treated with surgery for multiple carcinoid tumours and tumourlets, Aubry et al. identified only one case of DIPNECH (3.6%) [5]. Ruffini et al. identified three cases of DIPNECH in a series of 55 patients resected for neuroendocrine tumours (5.4%): typical carcinoid was the primary tumour in these patients [95].

Natural History and Management

DIPNECH is listed among the pre-invasive lesions of the lung as precursor of pulmonary tumourlets and carcinoid tumours but very little is known about its biology and natural history. Similar to AAH, longitudinal studies for the understanding of the natural history of DIPNECH are virtually impossible as such lesions are usually too peripheral to be accessible to bronchoscopy or other direct visualization methods that would allow the repeat biopsies required to characterize and follow the development of these lesions.

Based on limited follow-up in the small series reported in the literature, DIPNECH is typically an indolent and slow progressive disease. For most of the patients, clinical and radiologic follow-up is a reasonable strategy; no specific therapy is however available and treatment is usually symptomatic.

References

1. Aguayo SM, Miller YE, Waldron JA, Bogn RM, Sunday ME, Staton GW, Beam WR, King TE (1992) Brief report: idiopathic diffuse hyperplasia of pulmonary neuroendocrine cells and airway disease. N Engl J Med 327:1285–1288
2. Akyurek N, Mamis L, Ekinci O, Kokturk N, Ozturk C (2006) Survivin expression in pre-invasive lesions and non-small cell lung carcinoma. Virchows Arch 449:164–170
3. Anami Y, Matsuno Y, Yamada T, Takeuchi T, Nakayama H, Hirohashi S, Noguchi M (1998) A case of double primary adenocarcinoma of the lung with multiple atypical adenomatous hyperplasia. Pathol Int 48:634–640
4. Armas OA, White DA, Erlandson RA, Rosai J (1995) Diffuse idiopathic pulmonary neuroendocrine cell proliferation presenting as interstitial lung disease. Am J Surg Pathol 19:963–970
5. Aubry MC, Thomas CF, Jett JR, Swensen SJ, Myers JL (2007) Significance of multiple carcinoid tumors and tumorlets in surgical lung specimens. Analysis of 28 patients. Chest 131:1635–1643
6. Auerbach O, Forman JB, Gere JB, Kassouny DY, Muehsam GE, Petrick TG, Smolin HJ, Stout AP (1957) Changes in the bronchial epithelium in relation to smoking and cancer of the lung; a report of progress. N Engl J Med 256:97–104
7. Auerbach O, Stout AP, Hammond EC, Garfinkel L (1961) Changes in the bronchial epithelium in relation to cigarette smoking and in relation to lung cancer. N Engl J Med 265:253–267
8. Auerbach O, Hammond EC, Garfinkel L (1979) Changes in bronchial epithelium in relation to cigarette smoking, 1955–1960 vs. 1970–1977. N Engl J Med 300:381–385
9. Banerjee AK, George PJM (2007) Fluorescence bronchoscopy. In: Rose BD (ed) UpToDate. UpToDate, Waltham
10. Banerjee AK, Read CA, Griffiths MH, George PJ, Rabbitts PH (2007) Clonal divergence in lung cancer development is associated with allelic loss on chromosome 4. Genes Chromosomes Cancer 46:852–860

11. Banerjee AK (2009) Preinvasive lesions of the bronchus. J Thorac Oncol 4:545–551
12. Beta Carotene Cancer prevention Study Group – The Alpha-Tocopherol (1994) The effect of vitamin E and beta carotene on the incidence of lung cancer and other cancers in male smokers. N Engl J Med 330:1029–1035
13. Bota S, Auliac JB, Paris C, Metayer J, Sesboue R, Nouvet G, Thiberville L (2001) Follow-up of bronchial precancerous lesions and carcinoma in situ using fluorescence endoscopy. Am J Respir Crit Care Med 164:1688–1693
14. Boyle JO, Lonardo F, Chang JH, Klimstra D, Rusch V, Dmitrovsky E (2001) Multiple high-grade bronchial dysplasia and squamous cell carcinoma: concordant and discordant mutations. Clin Cancer Res 7:259–266
15. Brambilla E, Travis WD, Colby TV, Corrin B, Shimosato Y (2001) The new World Health Organization classification of lung tumors. Eur Respir J 18:1059–1068
16. Breuer RH, Pasic A, Smit EF, van Vliet E, Vonk Noordegraaf A, Risse EJ, Postmus PE, Sutedja TG (2005) The natural course of preneoplastic lesions in bronchial epithelium. Clin Cancer Res 11:537–543
17. Brown MJ, English J, Muller NL (1997) Bronchiolitis obliterans due to neuroendocrine hyperplasia: high-resolution CT-pathologic correlation. AJR Am J Roentgenol 168: 1561–1562
18. Chansky K, Sculier JP, Crowley JJ, Giroux D, Van Meerbeeck J, Goldstraw P (2009) The international association for the study of lung cancer staging project. J Thorac Oncol 4:792–801
19. Chapman AD, Kerr KM (2000) The association between atypical adenomatous hyperplasia and primary lung cancer. Br J Cancer 83:632–636
20. Chung GT, Sundaresan V, Hasleton P, Rudd R, Taylor R, Rabbitts PH (1995) Sequential molecular genetic changes in lung cancer development. Oncogene 11:2591–2598
21. Cohen AJ, King TE Jr, Gilman LB, Magill-Solc C, Miller YE (1998) High expression of neutral endopeptidase in idiopathic diffuse hyperplasia of pulmonary neuroendocrine cells. Am J Respir Crit Care Med 158:1593–1599
22. Cortese DA, Pairolero PC, Bergstralh EJ, Woolner LB, Uhlenhopp MA, Piehler JM, Sanderson DR, Bernatz PE, Williams DE, Taylor WF, Payne WS, Fontana RS (1983) Roentgenographically occult lung cancer. A ten year experience. J Thorac Cardiovasc Surg 86:373–380
23. Davies SJ, Gosney JR, Hansell DM, Wells AU, du Bois RM, Burke MM, Sheppard MN, Nicholson AG (2007) Diffuse idiopathic pulmonary neuroendocrine cell hyperplasia: an under-recognised spectrum of disease. Thorax 62:248–252
24. Deygas N, Froudarakis M, Ozenne G, Vergnon JM (2001) Cryotherapy in early superficial bronchogenic carcinoma. Chest 120:26–31
25. Doll R, Hill AB (1950) Smoking and carcinoma of the lung. Preliminary report. Br Med J 2:739–748
26. Felton WL, Liebow AA, Lindskog GE (1953) Peripheral and multiple bronchial adenomas. Cancer 6:555–566
27. Ferlay J, Autier P, Boniol M, Heanue M, Colombet M, Boyle P (2007) Estimates of the cancer incidence and mortality in Europe in 2006. Ann Oncol 18:581–592
28. Fessler MB, Cool CD, Miller YE, Schwarz MI, Brown KK (2004) Idiopathic diffuse hyperplasia of pulmonary neuroendocrine cells in a patient with acromegaly. Respirology 9:274–277
29. Field JK, Smith RA, Duffy SW, Berg CD, van Klaveren R, Henschke CI, Carbone D, Postmus PE, Paci E, Hirsch FR, Mulshine JL (2006) The Liverpool statement 2005: priorities for the European Union/United States spiral computed tomography collaborative group. J Thorac Oncol 1:497–498
30. Finkelstein SE, Summers RM, Nguyen DM, Stewart JH, Tretler JA, Schrump DS (2002) Virtual bronchoscopy for evaluation of malignant tumors of the thorax. J Thorac Cardiovasc Surg 123:967–972
31. Finkelstein SE, Schrump DS, Nguyen DM, Hewitt SM, Kunst TF, Summers RM (2003) Comparative evaluation of super high-resolution CT scan and virtual bronchoscopy for the detection of tracheobronchial malignancies. Chest 124:1834–1840
32. Folkman J (1995) Clinical applications of research on angiogenesis. N Engl J Med 333:1757–1763

33. Garnis C, Campbell J, Davies JJ, MacAulay C, Lam S, Lam WL (2005) Involvement of multiple developmental genes on chromosome 1p in lung tumorigenesis. Hum Mol Genet 14:475–482
34. Ge Y, Eltorky MA, Ernst RD, Castro CY (2007) Diffuse idiopathic pulmonary endocrine cell hyperplasia. Ann Diagn Pathol 11:122–126
35. George PJ, Banerjee AK, Read CA, O'Sullivan C, Falzon M, Pezzella F, Nicholson AG, Shaw P, Laurent G, Rabbitts PH (2007) Surveillance for the detection of early lung cancer in patients with bronchial dysplasia. Thorax 62:43–50
36. Helfritzsch H, Junker K, Bartel M, Scheele J (2002) Differentiation of positive autofluorescence bronchoscopy findings by comparative genomic hybridization. Oncol Rep 9: 697–701
37. Henschke CI, Naidich DP, Yankelevitz DF, McGuinness G, McCauley DI, Smith JP, Libby D, Pasmantier M, Vazquez M, Koizumi J, Flieder D, Altorki N, Miettinen OS (2001) Early lung cancer action project. Initial findings on repeat screening. Cancer 92:153–159
38. Henschke CI, Yankelevitz DF, Mirtcheva R, McGuinness G, McCauley D, Miettinen OS, ELCAP Group (2002) CT screening for lung cancer: frequency and significance of part-solid and nonsolid nodules. AJR Am J Roentgenol 178:1053–1057
39. Herbst RS, Heymach JV, Lippman SM (2008) Lung cancer. N Engl J Med 359:1367–1380
40. Horner MJ, Ries LAG, Krapcho M, Neyman N, Aminou R, Howlader N, Altekruse SF, Feuer EJ, Huang L, Mariotto A, Miller BA, Lewis DR, Eisner MP, Stinchcomb DG, Edwards BK (eds) SEER cancer statistics review, 1975–2006. National Cancer Institute, Bethesda, MD. Available at: http://www.seer.cancer.gov/csr/1975_2006/. Accessed July 2009
41. Hoshino H, Shibuya K, Chiyo M, Iyoda A, Yoshida S, Sekine Y, Iizasa T, Saitoh Y, Baba M, Hiroshima K, Ohwada H, Fujisawa T (2004) Biological features of bronchial squamous dysplasia followed up by autofluorescence bronchoscopy. Lung Cancer 46:187–196
42. Hung J, Lam S, LeRiche JC, Palcic B (1991) Autofluorescence of normal and malignant bronchial tissue. Lasers Surg Med 11:99–105
43. Imperatori A, Harrison RN, Leitch DN, Rovera F, Lepore G, Dionigi G, Sutton P, Dominioni L (2006) Lung cancer in Teesside (UK) and Varese (Italy): a comparison of management and survival. Thorax 61:232–239
44. Jeanmart M, Lantuejoul S, Fievet F, Moro D, Sturm N, Brambilla C, Brambilla E (2003) Value of immunohistochemical markers in preinvasive bronchial lesions in risk assessment of lung cancer. Clin Cancer Res 9:2195–2203
45. Keith RL, Miller YE, Gemmill RM, Drabkin HA, Dempsey EC, Kennedy TC, Prindiville S, Franklin WA (2000) Angiogenic squamous dysplasia in bronchi of individuals at high risk for lung cancer. Clin Cancer Res 6:1616–1625
46. Kennedy T, McWilliams A, Edell E, Sutedja T, Downie G, Yung R, Gazdar A, Mathur PN (2007) Bronchial intraepithelial neoplasia/early central airways lung cancer. ACCP evidence-based clinical practice guidelines (2nd edition). Chest 132:221S–233S
47. Kerr KM, Carey FA, King G, Lamb D (1994) Atypical alveolar hyperplasia: relationship with pulmonary adenocarcinoma, p53, and c-erbB-2 expression. J Pathol 174:249–256
48. Kim HY, Shim YM, Lee KS, Han J, Yi CA, Kim YK (2007) Persistent pulmonary nodular ground-glass opacity at thin-section CT: histopathologic comparisons. Radiology 245: 267–275
49. Kim TJ, Goo JM, Lee KW, Park CM, Lee HJ (2009) Clinical, pathological and thin-section CT features of persistent multiple ground-glass opacity nodules: comparison with solitary ground glass opacity nodule. Lung Cancer 64:171–178
50. Kitaguchi S, Takeshima Y, Nishisaka T, Inai K (1998) Proliferative activity, p53 expression and loss of heterozygosity on 3p, 9p, 17p in atypical adenomatous hyperplasia of the lung. Hiroshima J Med Sci 47:17–25
51. Kurie J, Lee JS, Khuri FR, Mao L, Morice RC, Lee JJ, Walsh GL, Broxson A, Lippman SM, Ro JY, Kemp BL, Liu D, Fritsche HA, Xu X, Lotan R, Hong WK (2000) *N*-(4-hydroxyphenyl) retinamide in the chemoprevention of squamous metaplasia and dysplasia of the bronchial epithelium. Clin Cancer Res 6:2973–2979

52. Lam S, MacAulay C, LeRiche J, Profio AE, Palcic B (1993) Detection of dysplasia and carcinoma in situ with a lung imaging fluorescence endoscope device. J Thorac Cardiovasc Surg 105:1035–1040
53. Lam S, leRiche JC, Zheng Y, Coldman A, MacAulay C, Hawk E, Kelloff G, Gazdar AF (1999) Sex-related differences in bronchial epithelial changes associated with tobacco smoking. J Natl Cancer Inst 91:691–696
54. Lam S, MacAulay C, LeRiche JC, Dyachkova Y, Coldman A, Guillaud M, Hawk E, Christen MO, Gazdar AF (2002) A randomized phase IIb trial of anethole dithiolethione in smokers with bronchial dysplasia. J Natl Cancer Inst 94:1001–1009
55. Lam S, Xu X, Parker-Klein H, LeRiche JC, Macaulay C, Guillaud M, Coldman A, Gazdar A, Lotan R (2003) Surrogate end-point biomarker analysis in a retinol chemoprevention trial in current and former smokers with bronchial dysplasia. Int J Oncol 23:1607–1613
56. Lam S, leRiche JC, McWilliams A, Macaulay C, Dyachkova Y, Szabo E, Mayo J, Schellenberg R, Coldman A, Hawk E, Gazdar A (2004) A randomized phase IIb trial of pulmicort turbuhaler (budesonide) in people with dysplasia of the bronchial epithelium. Clin Cancer Res 10:6502–6511
57. Lam S, Standish B, Baldwin C, McWilliams A, leRiche J, Gazdar A, Vitkin AI, Yang V, Ikeda N, MacAulay C (2008) In vivo optical coherence tomography imaging of preinvasive bronchial lesions. Clin Cancer Res 14:2006–2011
58. Lamy A, Sesboue R, Bourguignon J, Dautreaux B, Metayer J, Frebourg T, Thiberville L (2002) Aberrant methylation of the CDKN2A/P16INK4A gene promoter region in preinvasive bronchial lesions: a prospective study in high risk patients without invasive cancer. Int J Cancer 100:189–193
59. Lantuejoul S, Costantin B, Drabkin H, Brambilla C, Roche J, Brambilla E (2003) Expression of VEGF, semaphoring SEMA3F, and their common receptors neuropilins NP1 and NP2 in preinvasive bronchial lesions, lung tumours, and cell lines. J Pathol 200:336–347
60. Lee JS, Lippman SM, Benner SE, Lee JJ, Ro JY, Lukeman JM, Morice RC, Peters EJ, Pang AC, Fritsche HA, Hong WK (1994) Randomized placebo-controlled trial of isotretinoin in chemoprevention of bronchial squamous metaplasia. J Clin Oncol 12:937–945
61. Lee JS, Brown KK, Cool C, Lynch DA (2002) Diffuse pulmonary neuroendocrine cell hyperplasia: radiologic and clinical features. J Comput Assist Tomogr 26:180–184
62. Lee P, van den Berg RM, Lam S, Gazdar AF, Grunberg K, McWilliams A, LeRiche J, Postmus PE, Sutedja TG (2009) Color fluorescence ratio for detection of bronchial dysplasia and carcinoma in situ. Clin Cancer Res 15:4700–4705
63. Li F, Sone S, Abe H, MacMahon H, Doi K (2004) Malignant versus benign nodules at CT screening for lung cancer: comparison of thin-section CT findings. Radiology 233:793–798
64. Licchesi JDF, Westra WH, Hooker CM, Herman JG (2008) Promoter hypermethylation of hallmark cancer genes in atypical adenomatous hyperplasia of the lung. Clin Cancer Res 14:2570–2578
65. Licchesi JDF, Westra WH, Hooker CM, Machida EO, Baylin SB, Herman JG (2008) Epigenetic alteration of Wnt pathway antagonists in progressive glandular neoplasia of the lung. Carcinogenesis 29:895–904
66. Liewald F, Lang G, Fleiter TH, Sokiranski R, Halter G, Orend KH (1998) Comparison of virtual and fiberoptic bronchoscopy. Thorac Cardiovasc Surg 46:361–364
67. Lippman SM, Lee JJ, Karp DD, Vokes EE, Benner SE, Goodman GE, Khuri FR, Marks R, Winn RJ, Fry W, Graziano SL, Gandara DR, Okawara G, Woodhouse CL, Williams B, Perez C, Kim HW, Lotan R, Roth JA, Hong WK (2001) Randomized phase III intergroup trial of isotretinoin to prevent second primary tumors in stage I non-small cell lung cancer. J Natl Cancer Inst 93:605–618
68. Loewen G, Natarajan N, Tan D, Nava E, Klippenstein D, Mahoney M, Cummings M, Reid M (2007) Autofluorescence bronchoscopy for lung cancer surveillance based on risk assessment. Thorax 62:335–340
69. Logan M, Miller RR, Evans K, Muller NL (1996) Bronchogenic carcinoma and coexistent bronchioloalveolar cell adenomas. Chest 109:713–717

70. Man YG, Martinez A, Avis IM, Hong SH, Cuttitta F, Venzon DJ (2000) Phenotypically different cells with heterogeneous nuclear ribonucleoprotein A2/B1 overexpression show similar genetic alterations. Am J Respir Cell Mol Biol 23:636–645
71. Mao L, Lee JS, Kurie JM, Fan YH, Lippman SM, Lee JJ, Ro JY, Broxson A, Yu R, Morice RC, Kemp BL, Khuri FR, Walsh GL, Hittelman WN, Hong WK (1997) Clonal genetic alterations in the lungs of current and former smokers. J Natl Cancer Inst 89:857–862
72. Mascaux C, Laes JF, Anthoine G, Haller A, Ninane V, Burny A, Sculier JP (2009) Evolution of microRNA expression during human bronchial squamous carcinogenesis. Eur Respir J 33:352–359
73. Massion PP, Taflan PM, Jamshedur Rahman SM, Yildiz P, Shyr Y, Edgerton ME, Westfall MD, Roberts JR, Pietenpol JA, Carbone DP, Gonzalez AL (2003) Significance of p63 amplification and overexpression in lung cancer development and prognosis. Cancer Res 63:7113–7121
74. Massion PP, Taflan PM, Shyr Y, Jamshedur Rahman SM, Yildiz P, Shakthour B, Edgerton ME, Ninan M, Andersen JJ, Gonzalez AL (2004) Early involvement of the phosphatidylinositol 3-kinase/Akt pathway in lung cancer progression. Am J Respir Crit Care Med 170:1088–1094
75. Merrick DT, Haney J, Petrunich S, Sugita M, Miller YE, Keith RL, Kennedy TC, Franklin WA (2005) Overexpression of vascular endothelial growth factor and its receptors in bronchial dysplasia demonstrated by quantitative RT-PCR analysis. Lung Cancer 48:31–45
76. Meyer EC, Liebow AA (1965) Relationship of interstitial pneumonia honeycombing and atypical epithelial proliferation to cancer of the lung. Cancer 18:322–351
77. Miller RR, Nelems B, Evans KG, Muller NL, Ostrow DN (1988) Glandular neoplasia of the lung: a proposed analogy to colonic tumors. Cancer 61:1009–1014
78. Miller RR (1990) Bronchioloalveolar cell adenomas. Am J Surg Pathol 14:904–912
79. Miller RR, Muller NL (1995) Neuroendocrine cell hyperplasia and obliterative bronchiolitis in patients with peripheral carcinoid tumors. Am J Surg Pathol 19:653–658
80. Morinaga S, Shimosao Y (1987) Pathology of the microadenocarcinoma in the periphery of the lung. Pathol Clin Med Jpn 5:74–80
81. Moro-Sibilot D, Jeanmart M, Lantuejoul S, Arbib F, Laverriere MH, Brambilla E, Brambilla C (2002) Cigarette smoking, preinvasive bronchial lesions, and autofluorescence bronchoscopy. Chest 122:1902–1908
82. Moro-Sibilot D, Fievet F, Jeanmart M, Lantuejoul S, Arbib F, Laverriere MH, Brambilla E, Brambilla C (2004) Clinical prognostic indicators of high-grade pre-invasive bronchial lesions. Eur Respir J 24:24–29
83. Mountain CF (1986) A new international staging system for lung cancer. Chest 89:225S–233S
84. Nakanishi K (1990) Alveolar epithelial hyperplasia and adenocarcinoma of the lung. Arch Pathol Lab Med 114:363–368
85. Nakata M, Saeki H, Takata I, Segawa Y, Mogami H, Mandai K, Eguchi K (2002) Focal ground-glass opacity detected by low-dose helical CT. Chest 121:1464–1467
86. Oda S, Awai K, Liu D, Nakaura T, Yanaga Y, Nomori H, Yamashita Y (2008) Ground-glass opacities on thin-section helical CT: differentiation between bronchioloalveolar carcinoma and atypical adenomatous hyperplasia. AJR Am J Roentgenol 190:1363–1368
87. Omenn GS, Goodman GE, Thornquist MD, Balmes J, Cullen MR, Glass A, Keogh JP, Meyskens FL, Valanis B, Williams JH, Barnhart S, Hammar S (1996) Effects of a combination of beta carotene and vitamin A on lung cancer and cardiovascular disease. N Engl J Med 334:1150–1155
88. Paris C, Benichou J, Bota S, Sagnier S, Metayer J, Eloy S, Auliac J-B, Nouvet G, Thiberville L (2003) Occupational and nonoccupational factors associated with high grade bronchial pre-invasive lesions. Eur Respir J 21:332–341
89. Pasic A, Brokx HA, Comans EF, Herder GJ, Risse EK, Hoekstra OS, Postmus PE, Sutedja TG (2005) Detection and staging of preinvasive lesions and occult lung cancer in the central airways with ^{18}F-fluorodeoxyglucose positron emission tomography: a pilot study. Clin Cancer Res 11:6186–6189

90. Pelosi G, Del Curto B, Trubia M, Nicholson AG, Manzotti M, Veronesi G, Spaggiari L, Maisonneuve P, Pasini F, Terzi A, Iannucci A, Viale G (2007) 3q26 Amplification and polysomy of chromosome 3 in squamous cell lesions of the lung: a fluorescence in situ hybridization study. Clin Cancer Res 13:1995–2004
91. Ponticiello A, Barra E, Giani U, Bocchino M, Sanduzzi A (2000) p53 Immunohistochemistry can identify bronchial dysplastic lesions proceeding to lung cancer: a prospective study. Eur Respir J 15:547–552
92. Qu J, MacAulay C, Lam S, Palcic B (1995) Laser-induced fluorescence spectroscopy at endoscopy: tissue optics, Monte Carlo modeling, and in vivo measurements. Opt Eng 34:3334–3343
93. Rachet B, Quinn MJ, Cooper N, Coleman MP (2008) Survival from cancer of the lung in England and Wales up to 2001. Br J Cancer 99:S40–S42
94. Ruffini E, Bongiovanni M, Cavallo A, Filosso PL, Giobbe R, Mancuso M, Molinatti M, Oliaro A (2004) The significance of associated pre-invasive lesions in patients resected for primary lung neoplasms. Eur J Cardiothorac Surg 26:165–172
95. Saccomanno G, Archer VE, Auerbach O, Saunders RP, Brennan LM (1974) Development of carcinoma of the lung as reflected in exfoliated cells. Cancer 33:256–270
96. Sakamoto H, Shimizu J, Horio Y, Ueda R, Takahashi T, Mitsudomi T, Yatabe Y (2007) Disproportionate representation of *KRAS* gene mutation in atypical adenomatous hyperplasia, but even distribution of *EGFR* gene mutation from preinvasive to invasive adenocarcinomas. J Pathol 212:287–294
97. Sant M, Aareleid T, Berrino F, Bielska Lasota M, Carli PM, Faivre J, Grosclaude P, Hedelin G, Matsuda T, Moller H, Moller T, Verdecchia A, Capocaccia R, Gatta G, Micheli A, Santaquilani M, Roazzi P, Lisi D, EUROCARE Working Group (2003) EUROCARE-3: survival of cancer patients diagnosed 1990–1994 – results and commentary. Ann Oncol 14(Suppl 5):v61–v118
98. Satoh Y, Ishikawa Y, Nakagawa K, Hirano T, Tsuchiya E (1997) A follow-up study of progression from dysplasia to squamous cell carcinoma with immunohistochemical examination of p53 protein overexpression in the bronchi of ex-chromate workers. Br J Cancer 75:678–683
99. Seikido Y, Fong KM, Minna JD (2003) Molecular genetics of lung cancer. Annu Rev Med 54:73–87
100. Shen H, Gao W, Wu Y, Qiu H, Shu Y (2009) Multicolor fluorescence in situ hybridization and comparative genomic hybridization reveal molecular events in lung adenocarcinomas and squamous cell lung carcinomas. Biomed Pharmacother 63:396–403
101. Shibuya K, Fujisawa T, Hoshino H, Baba M, Saitoh Y, Iizasa T, Sekine Y, Suzuki M, Hiroshima K, Ohwada H (2001) Increased telomerase activity and elevated hTERT mRNA expression during multistage carcinogenesis of squamous cell carcinoma of the lung. Cancer 92:849–855
102. Slaughter DP, Southwick HW, Smejkal W (1953) "Field cancerization" in oral stratified squamous epithelium. Clinical implications of multicentric origin. Cancer 6:963–968
103. Smith SL, Gugger M, Hoban P, Ratschiller D, Watson SG, Field JK, Betticher DC, Heighway J (2004) S100A2 is strongly expressed in airway basal cells, preneoplastic bronchial lesions and primary non-small cell lung carcinomas. Br J Cancer 91:1515–1524
104. Soh J, Toyooka S, Ichihara S, Asano H, Kobayashi N, Suehisa H, Otani H, Yamamoto H, Ichimura K, Kiura K, Gazdar AF, Date H (2008) Sequential molecular changes during multistage pathogenesis of small peripheral adenocarcinomas of the lung. J Thorac Oncol 3:340–347
105. Sozzi G, Miozzo M, Donghi R, Pilotti S, Cariani CT, Pastorino U, Della Porta G, Pierotti MA (1992) Deletions of 17p and p53 mutations in preneoplastic lesions of the lung. Cancer Res 52:6079–6082
106. Sozzi G, Oggionni M, Alasio L, Conte D, Tavecchio L, Pilotti S, Spinelli P, Calarco G (2002) Molecular changes track recurrence and progression of bronchial precancerous lesions. Lung Cancer 37:267–270
107. Sterner DJ, Mori M, Roggli VL, Fraire AE (1997) Prevalence of pulmonary atypical alveolar hyperplasia in an autopsy population: a study of 100 cases. Mod Pathol 10:469–473
108. Strong MS, Incze J, Vaughan CW (1984) Field cancerization in the aerodigestive tract – its etiology, manifestation, and significance. J Otolaryngol 13:1–6

109. Sugio K, Kishimoto Y, Virmani AK, Hung JY, Gazdar AF (1994) *K-ras* mutations are a relatively late event in the pathogenesis of lung carcinomas. Cancer Res 54:5811–5815
110. Sundaresan V, Ganly P, Hasleton P, Rudd R, Sinha G, Bleehen NM, Rabbitts P (1992) p53 and chromosome 3 abnormalities, characteristic of malignant lung tumours, are detectable in preinvasive lesions of the bronchus. Oncogene 7:1989–1997
111. Suzuki K, Nagai K, Yoshida J, Yokose T, Kodama T, Takahashi K, Nishimura M, Kawasaki H, Yokozaki M, Nishiwaki Y (1997) The prognosis of resected lung carcinoma associated with atypical adenomatous hyperplasia. A comparison of the prognosis of well-differentiated adenocarcinoma associated with atypical adenomatous hyperplasia and intrapulmonary metastasis. Cancer 79:1521–1526
112. The National Lung Cancer Audit (2007) Information Centre, HQIP, Royal College of Physicians. http://www.ic.nhs.uk/webfiles/Services/NCASP/audits%20and%20reports/7089_Lung_Cancer_V5.pdf. Accessed August 2009
113. Thiberville L, Payne P, Vielkinds J, Leriche J, Horsman D, Nouvet G, Palcic B, Lam S (1995) Evidence of cumulative gene losses with progression of premalignant epithelial lesions to carcinoma of the bronchus. Cancer Res 55:5133–5139
114. Thun MJ, Lally CA, Flannery JT, Calle EE, Flanders WD, Heath CW (1997) Cigarette smoking and changes in the histopathology of lung cancer. J Natl Cancer Inst 89:1580–1586
115. Tian J, Mahmood R, Hnasko R, Locker J (2006) Loss of Nkx2.8 deregulates progenitor cells in the large airways and leads to dysplasia. Cancer Res 66:10399–10407
116. Travis WD, Brambilla E, Muller-Hermelink HK, Harris CC (eds) (2004) WHO classification of tumors. Pathology and genetics of tumours of the lung, pleura, thymus and heart. IARC, Lyon
117. Van Zandwijk N, Dalesio O, Pastorino U, de Vries N, van Tinteren H (2000) EUROSCAN, a randomized trial of vitamin A and *N*-acetylcysteine in patients with head and neck cancer or lung cancer. J Natl Cancer Inst 92:977–986
118. Venmans BJ, van Boxem TJ, Smit EF, Postmus PE, Sutedja TG (2000) Outcome of bronchial carcinoma in situ. Chest 117:1572–1576
119. Virmani AK, Fong KM, Kodagoda D, McIntire D, Hung J, Tonk V, Minna JD, Gazdar AF (1998) Allelotyping demonstrates common and distinct patterns of chromosomal loss in human lung cancer types. Genes Chromosomes Cancer 21:308–319
120. Warth A, Herpel E, Schmahl A, Storz K, Schnabel PA (2008) Diffuse idiopathic pulmonary neuroendocrine cell hyperplasia (DIPNECH) in association with an adenocarcinoma: a case report. J Med Case Reports 2:21
121. Weng SY, Tsuchiya E, Kasuga T, Sugano H (1992) Incidence of atypical bronchioloalveolar cell hyperplasia of the lung: relation to histological subtypes of lung cancer. Virchows Arch A Pathol Anat Histopathol 420:463–471
122. Westra WH, Baas IO, Hruban RH (1996) K-ras oncogene activation in atypical alveolar hyperplasia of the human lung. Cancer Res 56:2224–2228
123. Witsuba II, Lam S, Behrens C, Virmani AK, Fong KM, LeRiche J, Samet JM, Srivastava S, Minna JD, Gazdar AF (1997) Molecular damage in the bronchial epithelium of current and former smokers. J Natl Cancer Inst 89:1366–1373
124. Witsuba II, Behrens C, Virmani AK, Milchgrub S, Syed S, Lam S, McKay B, Minna JD, Gazdar AF (1999) Allelic losses at chromosome 8p21–23 are early and frequent events in the pathogenesis of lung cancer. Cancer Res 59:1973–1979
125. Witsuba II, Behrens C, Virmani AK, Mele G, Milchgrub S, Girard L, Fondon JW, Garner HR, McKay B, Latif F, Lerman MI, Lam S, Gazdar AF, Minna JD (2000) High resolution chromosome 3p allelotyping of human lung cancer and preneoplastic/preinvasive bronchial epithelium reveals multiple, discontinuous sites of 3p allele loss and three regions of frequent breakpoints. Cancer Res 60:1949–1960
126. Woolner LB, Fontana RS, Cortese DA, Sanderson DR, Bernatz PE, Payne WS, Pairolero PC, Piehler JM, Taylor WF (1984) Roentgenographically occult cancer: pathologic findings and frequency of multicentricity during a 10-year period. Mayo Clin Proc 59:453–466
127. World Health Organization (1981) Histological typing of lung tumours, 2nd edn. World Health Organization, Geneva

128. Yoshida Y, Shibata T, Kokubu A, Tsuta K, Matsuno Y, Kanai Y, Asamura H, Tsuchiya R, Hirohashi S (2005) Mutations of the epidermal growth factor receptor gene in atypical adenomatous hyperplasia and bronchioloalveolar carcinoma of the lung. Lung Cancer 50:1–8
129. Zysk AM, Nguyen FT, Oldenburg AL, Marks DL, Boppart SA (2007) Optical coherence tomography: a review of clinical development from bench to bedside. J Biomed Opt 12:051403–051421

Chapter 15
Progress in Early Detection and Management of Oral Dysplasia: Components for a Multifaceted Progression Risk Model

Miriam P. Rosin, Catherine F. Poh, S.Y. Catherine Kang, Calum E. MacAulay, and Lewei Zhang

Abstract A chief barrier to prevention of oral squamous cell carcinoma is our limited ability to differentiate oral premalignant lesions (OPLs) that are likely to progress to cancer from their more benign counterparts. This paper describes some of the newer technologies being used to capture novel information in OPLs of clinical, histological and molecular changes that are associated with progression risk. These approaches include: the use of tissue optics and molecular paints to improve lesion visualization; high resolution computer microscopy to detect subtle histological change; and genomics for tracking high-risk molecular clones across the oral mucosa and for gene-specific targeting of future drug therapies. The integration of information from these different approaches into multifaceted risk models can guide the evolution of new strategies for detecting and managing OPLs.

Introduction

The surge of biological and technological discovery in recent years has begun to shine new light on the myriad of tissue changes accompanying evolution of normal tissue to cancer. The integration of this knowledge into new multifaceted models for oral carcinogenesis is greatly needed if we are to improve oral cancer control.

Oral squamous cell carcinoma (OSCC) is a disease of high public health impact with nearly 300,000 cases identified annually worldwide [13]. It has a poor prognosis with 5-year survival rates of only 30–60%, depending on the global locale. This is

M.P. Rosin (✉)
Department of Cancer Control Research, British Columbia Cancer Agency Research Centre, University of British Columbia, Vancouver, BC, Canada
and
Department of Biomedical Physiology and Kinesiology, Simon Fraser University, Burnaby, BC, Canada
and
BC Oral Cancer Prevention Program, British Columbia Cancer Agency Research Centre, 675 West 10th Avenue, Vancouver, BC, Canada
e-mail: mrosin@bccrc.ca

R.C. Fitzgerald (ed.), *Pre-Invasive Disease: Pathogenesis and Clinical Management*, DOI 10.1007/978-1-4419-6694-0_15,

largely attributed to diagnosis at late-stage when therapies have had only a limited impact [61, 72]. The ability to detect high-risk disease at a premalignant stage, and take action to pre-empt or delay the onset of cancer, is the "grail" that many of us seek.

A chief barrier to such early intervention is our limited ability to detect oral premalignant lesions (OPLs) and to classify them into risk categories. OPLs comprise a wide spectrum of lesions with variable outcome. Rates of malignant transformation for leukoplakia, the most commonly diagnosed OPL, diverge widely and time to progression ranges from months to decades [2, 36, 57–59]. The presence of dysplastic areas in OPLs provides some indication of risk, especially for high-grade dysplasia [36, 58]. However, a lesion can have little or no dysplasia and yet have a significant risk of progression [38, 59, 69]. An intriguing question is whether the recent acceleration in pathway specific discovery in cancer biology can be focused more tightly on the premalignant process, to provide biomarkers that let us better predict behaviour for OPLs (see also Chap. 9 for discussion of biomarkers).

This paper will describe some of the newer technologies being used to capture critical information on OPLs and progression risk. These include: tissue optics, molecular paints, computer-based microscopy and genomics. These technologies are still at an early stage of development; however, they each have the potential of impacting significantly on our understanding of oral mucosal fields. The objective of this paper is to demonstrate that the integration of this technology into clinical settings can be a driving force for change, creating new paradigms and strategies for detecting and managing OPLs.

Evaluating Tissue Change in a Technological Era

One of the goals for new technology in the health field is to feed information on tissue change into a knowledge framework for use in building disease models. From a cancer standpoint, such models are beginning to shift away from a focus centred on microscopically identified premalignant and malignant foci alone to a study that also encompasses the niches in which these cells reside.

Squamous epithelium is maintained throughout adult life by stem cells, with their activity regulated by intercellular crosstalk and cell-stroma interaction [10] (see Fig. 15.1). It is well accepted that genetic and epigenetic alterations in these stem cells are critical to the necessary deregulation of signaling pathways that is required for carcinogenesis [23]. However, there is also growing support for involvement of microenvironment modification in cancer initiation and progression [20]. Evidence suggests that changes in the stem cell niche, abnormal cell-cell interaction and loss of extrinsic control facilitate the initiation and maintain these genetic and epigenetic mutations [70]. Over time there is an outgrowth of molecularly altered cells to abnormal clones or patches that are clinically, histologically and molecularly heterogeneous. They can be discrete or multifocal or can be scattered across the affected epithelium, sometimes clinically and histologically apparent and at other times not. These lesions alter with time, with changes extending over decades.

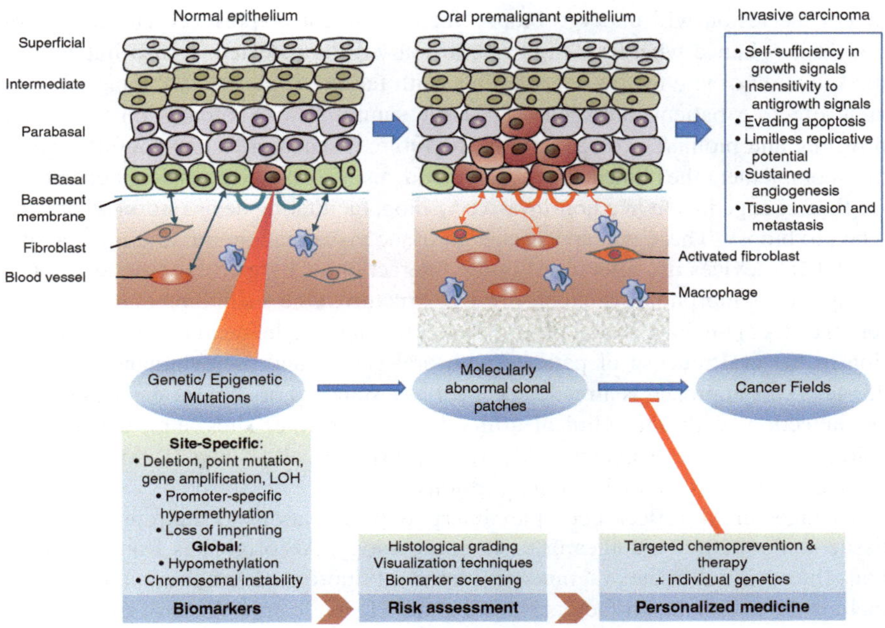

Fig. 15.1 Intrinsic and extrinsic contributions to cancer initiation and progression. Normal tissue is regulated by crosstalk between stem cells (*dark*), their differentiated cells (*light*) and the stromal microenvironment. Genetic and epigenetic in these stem cells, results in inactivation of tumour suppressor genes and activation of oncogenes. Positive selection of cells with such change leads to clonal outgrowth through processes that involve the stem cell niche, cell-cell interactions and microenvironmental modification. The integration of innovative visualization, computer imaging technology and novel biomarkers into the assessment of OPLs can produce risk models that enhance our ability to distinguish high risk OPLs from benign lesions, a process that is essential for effective intervention, and ultimately prevention of oral cancer

From the clinical standpoint, there is a need for discovery of markers for all of these different types of change, clinical, histological and molecular, and for an integration of these different approaches to create new strategies for risk stratification. Given the dynamic nature of the processes involved, ideal biomarkers should reflect the complexity of change occurring within the tissue and the driving forces involved, providing "windows" to ongoing alteration in the individual's clinical condition and enhancing our ability to identify and monitor high-risk subgroups. The following sections describe progress in identifying such biomarkers.

Visualization of Clinical Change

One the critical challenges to risk determination lies in the capacity of clinicians to discriminate sometimes subtle premalignant lesions and cancers from reactive and inflammatory conditions. The decision made at this point determines whether or not the lesion will undergo biopsy for assessment of presence and degree of dysplasia – hence whether a high-risk lesion will be detected. It also impacts on the selection of site for tissue sampling, with failure to biopsy in the highest risk area affecting patient management. Tissue sampling also impacts on molecular profiling and biomarker discovery. In the future, tissue optics and contrast agents may complement the clinical exam and provide us with an ability to better characterize field change in situ in a non-invasive fashion, facilitating decisions on where and when to biopsy. These two approaches to tissue visualization are described below.

Optical devices use alterations in the interaction of light with tissue to identify change in its morphology, chemistry and structure. One such approach, autofluorescence (AF) imaging shows promise for detecting and delineating fields of alteration in the oral mucosa of patients with oral cancer and premalignancy [32, 43, 45–47]. This approach is already accepted as a standard of care for early lung cancer detection, with near clinical utility for several other sites, e.g., the bladder, colon, cervix, skin, esophagus [11, 31, 50, 74], (see also Chap. 10 on molecular imaging as well as Chap. 14 on lung lesions).

Changes in AF reflect a complex interplay of alterations to fluorophores in the tissue and structural changes in tissue morphology. AF originates from endongenous fluorophores in the oral mucosa. Important fluorophores in the epithelial layer include the metabolic co-factors NADH and FAD while cross-links of the collagen are the principle fluorophores of the lamina propria [49, 51]. Alterations to fluorophore distribution include tissue remodeling such as the breakdown of the collagen matrix and elastin composition as well as alterations to metabolism [14]. The interaction between the light source and tissue is also affected by alterations to epithelial thickness, nuclear morphology (dysplastic nuclei) and vascularization, all characteristic changes associated with disease progression.

Several studies have shown that spectroscopy of AF can discriminate between normal and neoplastic mucosa (for review see [43]). However, clinical application of this approach to the oral cavity has occurred only in recent years, beginning with the development of a simple handheld device for real time AF visualization in patients within an ongoing Oral Cancer Prediction Longitudinal (OCPL) Study in British Columbia. That study is following ~400 patients with primary dysplasia, developing and validating markers for progression [53, 54]. This developmental device allowed for rapid direct visualization of alterations to autofluorescence across the oral mucosa, with these changes apparent to the viewer as an alteration from the pale green of normal tissue to dark brown to black regions in abnormal tissue.

Initial reports with this approach described pilot work in a very small number of patients (N = 44). That work was promising with a 98% sensitivity and 100% specificity for discriminating dysplasia and cancers from normals [32]. Since then, interim analysis of a further number of cases as they entered the OCPL study has shown that the approach correctly identifies nearly all cases of invasive OSCC (~95% of 120 examined) and severe dysplasia/carcinoma in situ (82 of 83 cases). In addition, 59 of 76 low-grade (mild/moderate) dysplasias had loss of AF. An intriguing possibility being explored is that low-grade lesions with AF might represent lesions with a greater risk of malignant transformation. Follow-up time for these cases (~24 months) at the interim analysis was too short to make this determination. Although its long term clinical value in screening needs to be determined, a tool using this technology is already commercially available, marketed as VELscope® (LED Med., Inc.).

A further interesting observation made during patient follow-up was that AF was detecting lesions that were clinically occult under white light inspection, yet showed dysplasia and/or cancer at biopsy (example in Fig. 15.2) [46]. This ability is being further monitored in the OCPL study. However, an offshoot of this observation has been the demonstration that AF can provide real-time guidance to surgical tumor margin delineation for invasive and pre-invasive cancer. Local recurrence is a frequent problem for OSCC (occurring in up to 30% of cases) [6, 25, 34, 40, 62, 63] and is thought to be associated with occult residual disease left at the surgery site. A small pilot study of 20 consecutive patients has shown that loss of AF extends beyond clinically apparent tumors in the majority of cases, with the extension varying from 4 to 25 mm. These AF positive, clinically occult margins were high-risk histologically and/or molecularly. Of 36 margins, 17 had OSCC or severe dysplasia/carcinoma in situ, 15 were mild/moderate dysplasia and only four were benign with no dysplasia. Molecular analysis of the margins with low-grade or no dysplasia showed the presence of high-risk molecular patterns (loss of heterozygosity patterns, to be described in Sect. 5.3) in 12 of 19 cases.

Will use of AF to guide margins reduce disease recurrence? We recently reported on data from 60 patients undergoing surgery between 2004 and 2008; 38 had AF-guided surgery (the surgical margin was placed at 10 mm beyond the perimeter of AF loss), the remaining patients (control group) had the surgical margin placed at 10 mm beyond the tumor edge defined by standard white-light examination. Seven of the 60 cases (12%) developed a recurrence of severe dysplasia or worse neoplasia

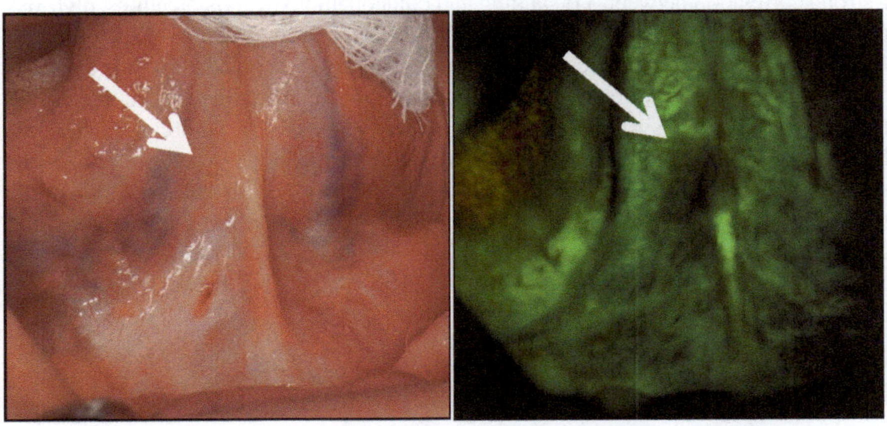

Fig. 15.2 Example of a high-risk occult lesion detected with AF visualization. A 58-year-old male in follow-up 15 months after surgical excision of carcinoma in situ. (**a**) White light image showed a well-healed scar at right floor of mouth close to lingual frenum (*arrow*) with no clinically visible lesion. (**b**) The same area (*arrow*) under FV showing a *dark area* of AF loss. Comparative biopsy of this area showed recurrent carcinoma in situ

at the treated site, all in the control group (P = 0.002) [45]. A large randomized multicentre trial is now being planned to further test this association among patients with T1/T2 OSCC and with preinvasive disease (severe dysplasia/*CIS*).

AF imaging systems are continuing to evolve. Studies to date have been largely restricted to referral settings and to use by oral specialists. They have not addressed the device utility within the typical spectrum of oral pathologies seen in community settings where the more common benign inflammatory conditions are the more prevalent clinical presentation. Several approaches are being taken in an attempt to improve the ability of the device to discriminate such lesions from OPLs in preparation for making this transition. These approaches include alterations to wavelengths illuminations for excitation (the Identifi™ 3000 – Trimera™ system), integration of reflectance imaging [44] and computer manipulation of fluorescence/reflectance image data to generate probability maps [52].

Another approach to lesion visualization that has yet to be explored is to couple the use of AF to use of contrast agents to better define clinical fields. Contrast agents are optically active agents that can be "painted" on the tissue surface to increase our ability to distinguish normal structures from abnormal structures.

There is some precedence for this approach based on use of toluidine blue (TB), a metachromatic vital dye. TB has been used for over 40 years to detect oral mucosal abnormalities, with numerous reports on its utility for screening, although primarily within secondary care settings. There is a general consensus that the dye has a fairly high sensitivity for cancer in such settings [44]; however, specificity can be low and is usually associated with nonspecific binding of the dye to rough areas of the tissue, generated by inflammation and trauma. Of interest is recent work with the dye in patients with OPLs. Data from the OCPL study suggests that TB may preferentially stain lesions with an increased risk of cancer development [75]. An early report showed a strong correlation between TB staining and clinicopathological risk features, high-risk molecular patterns (loss of heterozygosity profiles, described in Sect. 5.3) and outcome. Overall there was a sixfold elevation in cancer risk for OPLs positive for this dye.

The hope for the future will be to engineer markers that link molecular probes to nontoxic delivery systems (e.g., nanoparticles, nano-rods, fluorescent markers, beacons to create paints that can track the spread of high-risk clones across the surface of the oral mucosa). [44]. This will be critical to both risk assessment and treatment, allowing the clinician to directly map tissue with specific molecular change and to assess the impact of drugs on that tissue.

Histology and Risk Assessment: Optimizing Microscopy by Integrating Computer Technology

The classification of dysplasia is built on consensus among pathologists of the association of specific features with the likely progression to cancer. The current WHO criteria is based on 16 features (nine cytological and seven architectural) and a judgment of their severity [3]. However, dysplasia represents a spectrum of change and categorization is challenging.

The strongest association with transformation is for the higher grade severe dysplasia which are often linked with carcinoma in situ (*CIS*) as high-risk OPLs that are characterized by persistence, recurrence, and a high probability of eventual progression to invasive squamous cell carcinoma [9, 15, 24, 60]. Our experience in the OCPL study is consistent with this observation. We determined frequency of progression for 124 such lesions, 68 of which had been treated with conventional surgical excision and 54 left to follow-up (decision to treat had been left to the referring clinician). Progression to cancer occurred in 45% of patients not receiving treatment compared with 22% of the lesions that were treated ($P=0.045$). These high progression rates have resulted in the development of a consensus in British Columbia for treatment of this stage, at this point, by surgery, with recognition of the need to set guidelines for surgical margins for such treatment. To this end, the multi-centre AF surgery trial mentioned above will include severe dysplasia/*CIS* lesions in addition to T1/T2 OSCC to look for impact of AF as a guide to margin delineation at this preinvasive stage.

In contrast to the association of severe dysplasia with outcome, determination of prognosis for lesions with histological changes that are less than severe is more problematic. The majority of OPLs without dysplasia or with low-grade dysplasia (mild and moderate dysplasia) will not progress into cancer [5, 38, 57, 59, 71] and histology alone does not clearly differentiate between those that will progress and those that will not. Unfortunately, as a group, these lesions represent the bulk of leukoplakia and account for the majority of cases that later progress to cancer.

The rapid evolution of computer imaging and processing technology is creating a framework that will in future impact significantly on the way in which we describe and objectively quantify the myriad combinations of subtle alterations to histological and cytological features that associate with outcome prediction. High resolution computer imaging systems have been developed for many tumor sites with some of these commercially available. What has been lacking has been a harnessing of this technology to address specific questions on probability of progression for premalignant lesions. A key barrier to such development has been the access to the critical specimens with known outcome required for training such systems. We have taken advantage of the ongoing OCPL study to develop a Quantitative Tissue Pathology (QTP) imaging system that is targeted toward prediction of progression for OPLs [76]. The system semi-automatically detects and quantifies alteration to ~110 nuclear features in cell nuclei of hundreds of cells in each tissue specimen, looking at not only size and shape of the nuclei but also distribution of DNA within the nuclei (see Fig. 15.3). For example, for hyperchromasia, one of the criteria used in dysplasia assessment, the computer measures multiple features, such as whether the increased DNA is distributed around the edge of the nucleus or clustered in the center; whether the nucleus is dark with light areas or light with dark areas; whether the increased chromatin is evenly distributed (euchromatin) or clumped locally (heterochromatin); what is the distance between the locally clumped chromatin or the fraction of nuclear diameter one can travel before an intensity change is encountered and others. The components of the nuclear phenotypes are broken down into multiple quantifiable units to be studied independently and in combination to obtain diagnostic algorithms. A recent study evaluated the use of this system to judge progression risk of OPLs with no or low-grade (mild/moderate) dysplasias, using five of these system features combined

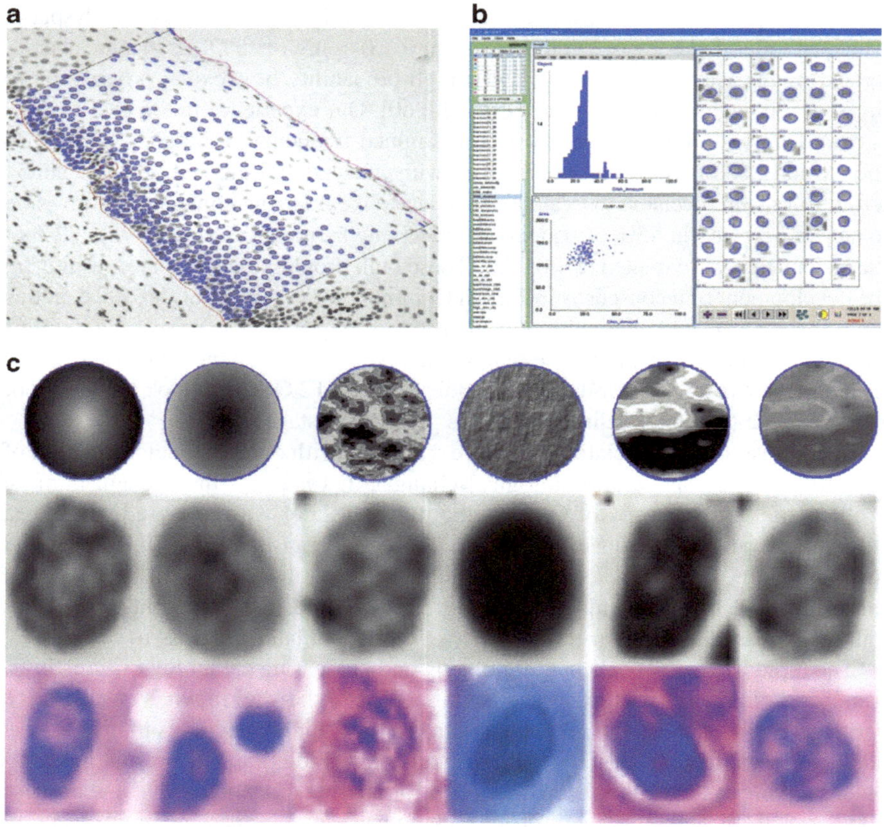

Fig. 15.3 Quantitative tissue phenotype of an oral dysplastic epithelium. (**a**) Delineation of the region of interest manually by the pathologist (area with dark staining nuclei). Nuclei within this region are automatically segmented by the computer and assessed for 100 features. (**b**) Histogram distribution of one of the 110 nuclear features in cell population of region of interest. (**c**) *Top row*, graphic representation of three of the five textural changes chosen for progression risk assessment. *OD-Skewness* measures whether the nucleus is dark with light areas or light with dark areas (first two images on far *left*). *Long90_Run* measures the fraction of nuclear diameter one can travel before an intensity change is encountered (*center* two images). *Fractal_area1* measures heterochromatin versus euchromatin organization, i.e., large intensity contrast between highly condensed chromatin and noncondensed chromatin (images on the far *right*). *Middle and lower rows*, captured images of nuclei showing these features

to derive a nuclear phenotype score (NPS) [21]. Elevated NPS was strongly associated with risk of malignant progression, with a tenfold increase in progression for dysplasia with high NPS. Of further interest, lesions with high NPS also showed an increased presence of high-risk molecular patterns (loss of heterozygosity profiles, to be discussed in the next section). In a multivariate Cox model, LOH and NPS together provided the strongest prediction for cancer development, supporting a fusion of quantitative pathology and molecular analysis as the best judge of progression risk.

These findings are very exciting. From a mechanistic point of view, the results confirm that histomorphological changes are critical for cancer progression, and that there are indeed microscopic differences between OPLs with no/mild/moderate dysplasia that are at high risk of cancer progression and similar lesions that are at low-risk. From a diagnostic point of view, such imaging systems can be easily adopted by any pathologist for use on tissue sections from the routine diagnostic paraffin block. In the future, this approach might provide a quick, reliable method of triaging OPLs with no/mild/moderate dysplasia for further risk assessment by molecular analysis. The combination of multiple biomarkers will improve the accuracy of the risk model.

Molecular Markers of Progression Risk

Building the Multifaceted Risk Model

The above text has shown how visualization and high resolution computer microscopy can facilitate sample collection for molecular analysis, providing critical specimens for biomarker discovery targeted to better prediction of behaviour of OPLs. The challenge is to use molecular analysis of such samples to further drive technological development, for example, to optimize visualization tools and create molecular paints to better target high-risk clinical change and to expand computer imaging systems to allow them to histologically track molecular clones through tissue samples. This will involve the construction of high-risk molecular profiles more tightly focused on the premalignant process, with pathway specific discovery leading to new gene and protein targets for OPL risk stratification. The selection of pathways and gene targets associated with key biological events may further facilitate this process, for example, a focus on altered genes that impact on stem cell regulation and microenvironmental change. In future such information will guide choice of which lesions to treat (through risk stratification), choice of treatment (e.g., surgical excision for tightly confined lesions and drug therapy for more diffuse or multifocal lesions), choice of drugs in chemopreventive therapies (use of drugs that target lesions with specific molecular alterations) and a more precise method of monitoring the success of interventions (e.g., visualization of clones left behind, early identification of disease recurrence, identification of new foci in patients with high-risk disease).

We are still at a very early stage in the molecular analysis of oral premalignant disease. Most molecular profiling has occurred in frank cancers: however an increasing number of publications deal with OPLs. At present, the majority of such studies are cross sectional in nature, with associations to clinical OPLs and dysplasias, sometimes reporting on low-grade versus high-grade disease. A few studies have examined molecular changes in progressing OPLs versus non-progressing lesions. Figure 15.4 presents a summary of such studies and the biomarkers examined. These studies will be discussed briefly below.

Reference	Marker	Effect Size	95% CI
Rosin, 2000	3p LOH	3.74	[1.98, 4.19]
	9p LOH	3.97	[2.29, 5.18]
	3p and/or 9p LOH	24.10	[20.80, 151.9]
	3p and/or 9p LOH + LOH at any other arm	33.40	[28.92, 215.6]
Guillaud, 2008	Nuclear phenotype score	10.30	[7.40, 49.70]
Garnis, 2009	Chromosomal alteration (≥2 regions)	48.00	[43.70, 487.3]
Tsui, 2008	3p segmental deletion	22.75	[20.14, 175.5]
Torres-Rendon, 2009	Aneuploidy	2.63	NR
Lee, 2000	Chromosomal polysomy	1.85	[0.80, 1.40]
	p53 (parabasal layer)	1.53	[0.62, 1.06]
	LOH 3p or 9p	1.94	[1.35, 2.29]
	CP.p53.LOH combined	2.27	[1.13, 1.39]
	CP.p53.LOH & Histology (multicovariate)	2.68	[1.11, 1.91]
Hall, 2009 & Cao, 2009	p16 methylation (pooled)	5.37	[2.40, 4.35]
Cao, 2009	p16 methylation (age adjusted; ≥ 60yr)	12.00	[9.64, 49.05]
Kawaguchi, 2009	Podoplanin	3.09	[1.56, 3.14]
Saintigny, 2009	ΔNp63	3.31	[1.65, 3.27]
	Intraepithelial inflammatory cells (EIC)	2.03	[1.05, 2.18]
	Podoplanin, ΔNp63 and EIC combined	4.37	[2.46, 5.62]
Benchekroun, 2010	EGFR	3.62	[2.18, 5.48]
Yoon, 2009	pChk2	10.50	[5.70, 12.10]
	pChk2 (risk of progression in < 3yr)	5.80	[3.40, 8.00]
	pChk2 (risk of progression in > 3yr)	19.90	[12.60, 35.60]

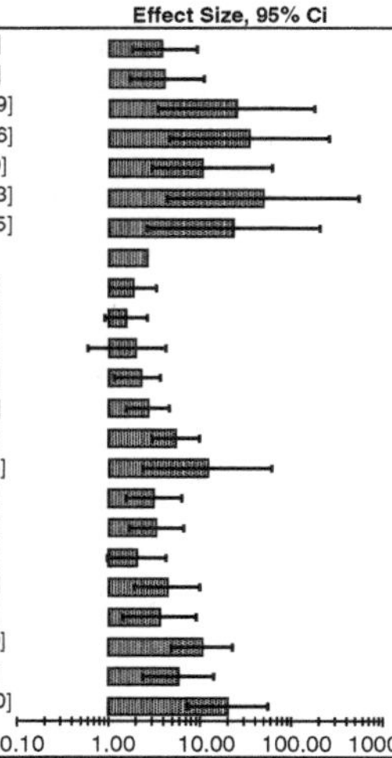

Fig. 15.4 Biomarkers of progression risk for OPLs. HR, RR or OR are shown as presented in the indicated publications. If not given, they were calculated for this article. They are graphed as an estimation of effect size, i.e., the measure of the strength of the relationship between the presence of the markers in OPL and the risk of progression. Ratios greater than one indicate an increased risk for malignant progression. *CI* confidence interval, *LOH* loss of heterozygosity, *CP* chromosomal polysomy, *EGFR* epidermal growth factor, *pChk2* checkpoint kinase 2, *NR* not reported

Molecular Profiling

Molecular profiling of progressing and non-progressing lesions has been limited to only a few studies. A recent article used high resolution genomic analysis with tiling-path array comparative genomic hybridization (CGH) [17, 18] to compare genomic imbalances in low-grade (mild and moderate) dysplastic lesions that progressed to cancer to histologically similar non-progressors. That study showed a significant difference in the number of genomic segmental alterations in progressors compared to non-progressors ($P<10^{-4}$). Non-progressors showed little chromosomal alteration. The probability of a lesion having chromosomal alterations in two or more regions was markedly higher in progressive lesions than in non-progressive counterparts (OR 48; 95% CI, 43.7–487.3), suggesting that overall genetic instability can be a valuable predictive marker for progressive risk of low-grade dysplasia. In a second study, segmental alterations to chromosome 3p were determined using the same genomic profiling technique. Analysis showed six regions of recurrent alteration in high-grade dysplasia as well as OSCC; change in these regions was present at a significantly higher frequency in progressive low-grade dysplasia compared with non-progressive counterparts (OR 22.75; 95% CI, 20.14–175.5) [66]. These alterations to CGH profiles appear to have potential clinical significance. [65] mapped out the regions of recurrent DNA amplifications and homozygous deletions in a set of OPLs and looked for expression changes in these regions using five independent head and neck datasets. Genes showing alteration belonged to several critical signalling pathways, including the canonical ERK/MAPK, FGF, p53, PTEN and P13K/AKT pathways, which share common nodes and interplay as a single network [65]. These changes were present in severe dysplasia and in progressing low-grade dysplasia but were not observed in non-progressing low-grade dysplasia.

LOH as an Example of a Risk Indicator

Virtually all biomarker studies based on known outcome for OPL have come from single institutional analyses. An exception to this has been the use of loss of heterozygosity (LOH) in key chromosomal loci, a finding that has been consistently identified in several laboratories as an independent indicator of risk of progression of OPLs to malignancy [7, 35, 37]. In an early study, Mao and workers showed that patients with OPLs with LOH at 3p14 (location of *FHIT*) and/or 9p21 regions (location of *p16/p15/p14*) had a substantially increased risk of developing OSCC compared to those with retention of these loci. These observations were confirmed in a subsequent study by [55] that assessed LOH at these regions plus loci on an additional five arms (4q, 8p, 11q, 13q, and 17p). That study showed that LOH at 3p14 or 9p21 increased the risk of progression by 3.74 and 3.97-fold respectively and that additional losses on 4q, 8p, 11q, or 17p further contributed to cancer progression by increasing the risk of SCC by 33-fold, with 47% of such cases progressing to cancer within 5 years. This strong association of LOH and risk of progression is currently being validated in an independent prospectively collected set of OPLs from the OCPL study. LOH analysis is already being used to select high-risk patients with OPLs for chemoprevention in two multi-institutional chemoprevention trials: the phase III Erlotinib Prevention of Oral Cancer (EPOC) study [26] and the phase II Cetuximab for treatment of high-risk pre-malignant upper aerodigestive lesions [27]. As mentioned previously, the process of integrating LOH analysis with other technologies is already ongoing, with associations reported among toluidine blue-positive OPLs, LOH status and outcome [75] and among nuclear phenotype score (using quantitative tissue phenotype analysis), LOH status and outcome [21].

p16 Promoter Hypermethylation

CpG hypermethylation of p16 has been shown to correlate with the degree of oral dysplasia in multiple cross-sectional studies [39, 67]. Recently, two case-control studies demonstrated that p16 promoter methylation may also be a novel predictor of risk for progression of OPLs. Cao et al. [8] showed an increased risk of developing OSCC for cases with hypermethylated p16, with 14 of 32 (44%) of such cases progressing to cancer compared with eight of 46 (17.4%) of cases with unmethylated p16 (OR 3.7; 95% CI, 1.31–10.39; $P=0.013$). This association was highest among individuals ≥60 years (age-adjusted OR 12.0, 95% CI, 2.36–61.05; $P = 0.003$), which is consistent with the often reported association of methylation and aging [28]. In a separate study. Hall et al. [22] reported the presence of p16 CpG methylation in 57% (8 of 14) of patients with progressing OPLs compared with only 8% (2 or 24) of non-progressors OPL. In this study, the investigators collected biopsies as well as scrapes of histologically confirmed oral epithelial dysplasia. When methylation status was compared between the two sources of DNA, 80% of the samples showed concordant methylation (61 of 76 samples). Interestingly, among 15 discordant results, p16 promoter methylation was more frequently detected in the scrapes, suggesting that the brushing technique may be a noninvasive alternative to biopsy.

Aneuploidy

Most solid tumor cells are aneuploid [30]; that is, they do not have the normal complement of genetic material. i.e. the cells have 0, 1 or 2+ copies of part or all of some chromosomes. The association between cancer and abnormal chromosome distribution was noted as far back at 1890 by van Hansemann [68].

Aneuploidy has been shown to be related to a high risk of progression at some sites, for example in Barrett's oesophagus [12, 41], (see Chap. 16); however its association with progression risk in OPLs is less well documented. Correlation between the DNA ploidy status and a risk of progression of OPLs was investigated in a recent case-control study using cell suspensions generated from thick tissue sections [64]. The study showed that 14 of 19 aneuploid OPL (74%) progressed to SCC compared with 28 of 67 (42%) diploid lesions. Also, the cancer free survival rate was significantly lower in the aneuploid cases (HR 2.63; log rank, $P = 0.003$).

Lee et al. [33] examined the association of five potential biomarkers in OPL with risk of progression to cancer: chromosomal polysomy, p53 parabasal protein expression, loss of heterozygosity at chromosome 3p or 9p, retinoic acid receptor β and micronuclei. The univariant Cox proportional hazards model showed a significant association with only one of these features, chromosomal polysomy, as an independent predictor of progression risk; however, in the multivariant analysis, the combined biomarker score of chromosomal polysomy, p53 and LOH were each strongly associated with cancer risk (RR 2.27; 95% CI, 1.14–3.66; $P = 0.0008$).

Our data from more than 500 cases suggests that an automated cytological image analysis system, based on targeted brushing of suspect lesions, which uses the frequency of aneuploid cells could be an efficient and effective second step when used in combination with AF in a comprehensive screening program, directing the high risk patient population to appropriate care while not necessitating a large number of biopsies.

Specific Gene Biomarkers of Risk

A few promising gene-specific markers have been reported that are able to differentiate OPL progressors from non-progressors, but these data are restricted to single institutional studies, requiring validation on independent cohorts. These include podoplanin, ΔNp63, pChk2 and EGFR, described below.

Podoplanin, is a member of the type-1 transmembrane sialomucin-like glycoprotein family and has been used previously as a biomarker of lymphatic vessels. Its overexpression is associated with lymph node metastasis and poor survival in OSCC [42, 48]. Kawaguchi et al. reported a strong association between expression level of podoplanin, the presence of dysplasia and risk of progression for OPLs [29]. At 5 years after the sample assessment, less than 8% of the patients with negative podoplanin expression developed oral cancer (95% CI, 0.86–0.98), compared with 37% of those with positive podoplanin expression (95% CI, 0.51–0.77; $P<0.001$) The hazard ratio of cancer progression in podoplanin-positive cases was 3.09 (95% CI, 1.530–6.231; $P=0.002$).

ΔNp63 is a homologue of the *p53* tumour suppressor gene. The first demonstration of ΔNp63 as a potential biomarker for progressive OPL appeared in a cohort study conducted by Saintigny et al [56]. That study showed that ΔNp63 expression in low grade dysplasia is strongly associated with risk of progression to OSCC (HR 3.308; 95% CI, 1.663–6.580; P=0.0007). An increase of immune cell infiltration has been associated with dysplastic progression from hyperkeratosis to dysplasia to OSCC and so this association was examined in that same study [16]. Although association between clusters of intraepithelial inflammatory cells (EIC) in the basal cell layer and progression risk was not statistically significant, ($P=0.057$), a concurrent expression of all three markers, podoplanin, ΔNp63 and EIC, showed the highest risk of malignant transformation (HR 4.37; 95% CI, 1.912–9.992; $P=0.0005$).

pChk2 is a mediator of cell cycle checkpoint in response to DNA damage. The pChk2 isoform has recently been shown to be expressed at exceptionally high levels in premalignant lesions and to persist throughout malignant transformation [1, 19]. Yoon et al. undertook a retrospective case-control study to investigate the value of pChk2 as an early indicator of cancer progression. pChk2-positive OPL lesions showed a 10.5-fold increase in risk of cancer development compared with pChk2-negative OPLs (OR 10.5; 95% CI, 4.8–22.6). The risk of progressing to SCC after 3 years was 19.9 times higher in pChk2-positive group than it was in pChk2-negative OPL (95% CI, 7.3–55.5) [73].

Epidermal Growth Factor Receptor (EGFR) signaling occurs through a multidimensional pathway, of which deregulation plays a profound role in tumor proliferation and patient survival in many cancers. A recent novel report describes EGFR expression and gene copy number in OPLs in a series of longitudinal and prospectively collected samples [4]. It showed that a striking increase in progression to oral squamous cell carcinoma (OSCC) occurred among EGFR overexpressors that also had an increased EGFR gene copy number, as measured by fluorescence in situ hybridization (FISH). Only 40% of patients with lesions expressing high level of EGFR and chromosome 7 remained cancer-free for 5 years while 79% of patients with low expression remained cancer-free for the same period of time (HR 3.620; 95% CI, 1.439–9.104). The significant association between high level of EGFR and the risk of development of oral cancer suggests that EGFR-targeted chemotherapy may enable effective intervention of high risk premalignant lesions and enhance cancer-free survival rates. These data suggest that EGFR copy number change could be a targetable marker, indicating a higher-risk group with a potentially higher likelihood of benefit from EGFR inhibitors.

Conclusion

The harnessing of new technology to explore clinical issues is a powerful way in which to drive the development of new paradigms for disease management. Although the potential of molecular analysis is widely discussed in the literature as a promising approach to gathering information on the critical genetic and epigenetic change underlying cancer development, attention needs to be paid to parallel and complementary devices that will facilitate the collection of molecular information that is better targeted towards direct clinical application. As discussed in this paper, focusing such technology on OPLs has already created useful information about clinical and histological change that would otherwise not be available. The integration of such technology with molecular analysis will drive this process forward more quickly. It is time to begin to build new, more multifaceted risk models that incorporate a broader vision of the dynamic change that is occurring during oral carcinogenesis.

Acknowledgements Supported by grants from the National Institute of Dental and Craniofacial Research R01DE13124 and R01 DE17013R01DE13124.

References

1. Ahn J, Urist M, Prives C (2004) The Chk2 protein kinase. DNA Repair 3:1039–1047
2. Axell T, Pindborg JJ, Smith CJ et al (1996) Oral white lesions with special reference to precancerous and tobacco-related lesions: conclusions of an international symposium held in Uppsala, Sweden, May 18–21, 1994. International Collaborative Group on Oral White Lesions. J Oral Pathol Med 25:49–54
3. Barnes L, Eveson J, Reichart P et al (eds) (2005) World Health Organization classification of tumours: pathology and genetics of head and neck tumours. IARC, Lyon
4. Benchekroun MT, Saintigny P, Thomas SM, et al (2010) Epidermal growth factor receptor expression and gene copy number in the risk of oral cancer. Cancer Prev Res [Epub ahead of print] PMID:20570883
5. Bouquot J (1999) Oral cancers with leukoplakia. Oral Dis 5:183–184
6. Brennan JA, Mao L, Hruban RH et al (1995) Molecular assessment of histopathological staging in squamous-cell carcinoma of the head and neck. N Engl J Med 332:429–435
7. Califano J, van der Riet P, Westra W et al (1996) Genetic progression model for head and neck cancer: implications for field cancerization. Cancer Res 56:2488–2492

8. Cao J, Zhou J, Gao Y et al (2009) Methylation of p16 CpG island associated with malignant progression of oral epithelial dysplasia: a prospective cohort study. Clin Cancer Res 15:5178–5183
9. Crissman JD, Zarbo RJ (1989) Dysplasia, in situ carcinoma, and progression to invasive squamous cell carcinoma of the upper aerodigestive tract. Am J Surg Pathol 13(Suppl 1): 5–16
10. Donjacour AA, Cunha GR (1991) Stromal regulation of epithelial function. Cancer Treat Res 53:335–364
11. Drezek R, Guillaud M, Collier T et al (2003) Light scattering from cervical cells throughout neoplastic progression: influence of nuclear morphology, DNA content, and chromatin texture. J Biomed Opt 8:7–16
12. Fang M, Lew E, Klein M et al (2004) DNA abnormalities as marker of risk for progression of Barrett's esophagus to adenocarcinoma: image cytometric DNA analysis in formalin-fixed tissues. Am J Gastroenterol 99:1887–1894
13. Ferlay J, Bray F, Pisani P, GLOBOCAN et al (2004) Cancer incidence, mortality and prevalence worldwide. IARC cancer base no. 5 version 2.0. IARC, Lyon
14. Follen M, Crain S, MacAulay C et al (2005) Optical technologies for cervical neoplasia: update of an NCI program project grant. Clin Adv Hematol Oncol 3:41–53
15. Fresko D, Lazarus SS (1981) Oral carcinoma in situ. Its progression to squamous, basosquamous, and basal-cell carcinoma. Arch Pathol Lab Med 105:15–19
16. Gannot G, Gannot I, Vered H et al (2002) Increase in immune cell infiltration with progression of oral epithelium from hyperkeratosis to dysplasia and carcinoma. Br J Cancer 86: 1444–1448
17. Garnis C, Campbell J, Zhang L et al (2004) OCGR array: an oral cancer genomic regional array for comparative genomic hybridization analysis. Oral Oncol 40:511–519
18. Garnis C, Chari R, Buys TP et al (2009) Genomic imbalances in precancerous tissues signal oral cancer risk. Mol Cancer 8:50
19. Gorgoulis VG, Vassiliou LV, Karakaidos P et al (2005) Activation of the DNA damage checkpoint and genomic instability in human precancerous lesions. Nature 434:907–913
20. Gudjonsson T, Magnusson MK (2005) Stem cell biology and the cellular pathways of carcinogenesis. APMIS 113:922–929
21. Guillaud M, Zhang L, Poh C et al (2008) Potential use of quantitative tissue phenotype to predict malignant risk for oral premalignant lesions. Cancer Res 68:3099–3107
22. Hall GL, Shaw RJ, Field EA et al (2008) p16 Promoter methylation is a potential predictor of malignant transformation in oral epithelial dysplasia. Cancer Epidemiol Biomarkers Prev 17:2174–2179
23. Hanahan D, Weinberg RA (2000) The hallmarks of cancer. Cell 100:57–70
24. Hayward JR, Regezi JA (1977) Oral dysplasia and in situ carcinoma: clinicopathologic correlations of eight patients. J Oral Surg 35:756–762
25. Hittelman WN, Kim HJ, Lee JS et al (1996) Detection of chromosome instability of tissue fields at risk: in situ hybridization. J Cell Biochem Suppl 25:57–62
26. A Service of the U.S. National Institute of Health (2006) Erlotinib prevention of oral cancer (EPOC). http://www.clinicaltrials.gov/ct2/show/NCT00402779
27. ClinicalTrials.gov – A Service of the U.S. National Institute of Health (2007) Phase II study of single-agent Cetuximab for treatment of high-risk pre-malignant upper aerodigestive lesions. http://www.clinicaltrials.gov/ct2/show/NCT00524017
28. Issa JP, Ottaviano YL, Celano P et al (1994) Methylation of the oestrogen receptor CpG island links ageing and neoplasia in human colon. Nat Genet 7:536–540
29. Kawaguchi H, El-Naggar AK, Papadimitrakopoulou V et al (2008) Podoplanin: a novel marker for oral cancer risk in patients with oral premalignancy. J Clin Oncol 26:354–360
30. Kops GJ, Weaver BA, Cleveland DW (2005) On the road to cancer: aneuploidy and the mitotic checkpoint. Nat Rev Cancer 5:773–785
31. Lam S, MacAulay C, Hung J et al (1993) Detection of dysplasia and carcinoma in situ with a lung imaging fluorescence endoscope device. J Thorac Cardiovasc Surg 105:1035–1040

32. Lane PM, Gilhuly T, Whitehead P et al (2006) Simple device for the direct visualization of oral-cavity tissue fluorescence. J Biomed Opt 11:24006
33. Lee JJ, Hong WK, Hittelman WN et al (2000) Predicting cancer development in oral leukoplakia: ten years of translational research. Clin Cancer Res 6:1702–1710
34. Leemans CR, Tiwari R, Nauta JJ et al (1994) Recurrence at the primary site in head and neck cancer and the significance of neck lymph node metastases as a prognostic factor. Cancer 73:187–190
35. Lippman SM, Hong WK (2001) Molecular markers of the risk of oral cancer. N Engl J Med 344:1323–1326
36. Lumerman H, Freedman P, Kerpel S (1995) Oral epithelial dysplasia and the development of invasive squamous cell carcinoma. Oral Surg Oral Med Oral Pathol Oral Radiol Endod 79:321–329
37. Mao L, Lee JS, Fan YH et al (1996) Frequent microsatellite alterations at chromosomes 9p21 and 3p14 in oral premalignant lesions and their value in cancer risk assessment. Nat Med 2:682–685
38. Mincer HH, Coleman SA, Hopkins KP (1972) Observations on the clinical characteristics of oral lesions showing histologic epithelial dysplasia. Oral Surg Oral Med Oral Pathol 33:389–399
39. Papadimitrakopoulou V, Izzo J, Lippman SM et al (1997) Frequent inactivation of p16INK4a in oral premalignant lesions. Oncogene 14:1799–1803
40. Partridge M, Pateromichelakis S, Phillips E et al (2000) A case-control study confirms that microsatellite assay can identify patients at risk of developing oral squamous cell carcinoma within a field of cancerization. Cancer Res 60:3893–3898
41. Paulson TG, Maley CC, Li X et al (2009) Chromosomal instability and copy number alterations in Barrett's esophagus and esophageal adenocarcinoma. Clin Cancer Res 15(10): 3305–3314
42. Petrova TV, Makinen T, Makela TP et al (2002) Lymphatic endothelial reprogramming of vascular endothelial cells by the Prox-1 homeobox transcription factor. EMBO J 21:4593–4599
43. Poh C, Lane P, MacAulay C et al (2009) The application of tissue autofluorescence in detection and management of oral cancer and premalignant lesions. Springer, New York
44. Poh C, MacAulay C, Laronde D, et al (2010) Squamous cell carcinoma and precursor lesions: diagnosis and screening in a technical era. Periodontology 2000 (in press)
45. Poh CF, MacAulay CE, Zhang L et al (2009) Tracing the "at-risk" oral mucosa field with autofluorescence: steps toward clinical impact. Cancer Prev Res 2:401–404
46. Poh CF, Ng SP, Williams PM et al (2007) Direct fluorescence visualization of clinically occult high-risk oral premalignant disease using a simple hand-held device. Head Neck 29:71–76
47. Poh CF, Zhang L, Anderson DW et al (2006) Fluorescence visualization detection of field alterations in tumor margins of oral cancer patients. Clin Cancer Res 12:6716–6722
48. Raica M, Cimpean AM, Ribatti D (2008) The role of podoplanin in tumor progression and metastasis. Anticancer Res 28:2997–3006
49. Ramanujam N (2000) Fluorescence spectroscopy of neoplastic and non-neoplastic tissues. Neoplasia 2:89–117
50. Ramanujam N, Mitchell MF, Mahadevan A et al (1994) In vivo diagnosis of cervical intraepithelial neoplasia using 337-nm-excited laser-induced fluorescence. Proc Natl Acad Sci U S A 91:10193–10197
51. Richards-Kortum R, Sevick-Muraca E (1996) Quantitative optical spectroscopy for tissue diagnosis. Annu Rev Phys Chem 47:555–606
52. Roblyer D, Kurachi C, Stepanek V et al (2009) Objective detection and delineation of oral neoplasia using autofluorescence imaging. Cancer Prev Res 2:423–431
53. Rosin MP, Poh CF, Elwood JM et al (2008) New hope for an oral cancer solution: together we can make a difference. J Can Dent Assoc 74:261–266
54. Rosin MP, Poh CF, Guillard M et al (2007) Visualization and other emerging technologies as change makers for oral cancer prevention. Ann N Y Acad Sci 1098:167–183

55. Rosin MP, Cheng X, Poh C et al (2000) Use of allelic loss to predict malignant risk for low-grade oral epithelial dysplasia. Clin Cancer Res 6(2):357–362
56. Saintigny P, El-Naggar AK, Papadimitrakopoulou V et al (2009) DeltaNp63 overexpression, alone and in combination with other biomarkers, predicts the development of oral cancer in patients with leukoplakia. Clin Cancer Res 15:6284–6291
57. Schepman KP, van der Meij EH, Smeele LE et al (1998) Malignant transformation of oral leukoplakia: a follow-up study of a hospital-based population of 166 patients with oral leukoplakia from The Netherlands. Oral Oncol 34:270–275
58. Silverman S, Gorsky M, Kaugars GE (1996) Leukoplakia, dysplasia, and malignant transformation. Oral Surg Oral Med Oral Pathol Oral Radiol Endod 82:117
59. Silverman S, Gorsky M, Lozada F (1984) Oral leukoplakia and malignant transformation. A follow-up study of 257 patients. Cancer 53:563–568
60. Summerlin DJ (1996) Precancerous and cancerous lesions of the oral cavity. Dermatol Clin 14:205–223
61. Surveillance Epidemiology and End Results (SEER) Program, National Cancer Institute Surveillance Research Program (2006) Oral cancer 5-year survival rates by race, gender, and stage of diagnosis, vol. 2008
62. Tabor MP, Brakenhoff RH, Ruijter-Schippers HJ et al (2004) Genetically altered fields as origin of locally recurrent head and neck cancer: a retrospective study. Clin Cancer Res 10:3607–3613
63. Tabor MP, Brakenhoff RH, van Houten VM et al (2001) Persistence of genetically altered fields in head and neck cancer patients: biological and clinical implications. Clin Cancer Res 7:1523–1532
64. Torres-Rendon A, Stewart R, Craig GT et al (2009) DNA ploidy analysis by image cytometry helps to identify oral epithelial dysplasias with a high risk of malignant progression. Oral Oncol 45:468–473
65. Tsui IF, Poh CF, Garnis C et al (2009) Multiple pathways in the FGF signaling network are frequently deregulated by gene amplification in oral dysplasias. Int J Cancer 125:2219–2228
66. Tsui IF, Rosin MP, Zhang L et al (2008) Multiple aberrations of chromosome 3p detected in oral premalignant lesions. Cancer Prev Res 1:424–429
67. Vairaktaris E, Yapijakis C, Psyrri A et al (2007) Loss of tumour suppressor p16 expression in initial stages of oral oncogenesis. Anticancer Res 27:979–984
68. von Hansemann D (1890) Ueber asymmetrische zellheilteilung in epithelkrebsen und deren biologische bedeutung. Virschows Arch Pathol Anat 199:299–326
69. Waldron CA, Shafer WG (1975) Leukoplakia revisited. A clinicopathologic study 3256 oral leukoplakias. Cancer 36:1386–1392
70. Walker M, Patel KK, Stappenbeck TS (2009) The stem cell niche. J Pathol 217(2):169–180
71. Wright JM (1998) A review and update of oral precancerous lesions. Tex Dent J 115:15–19
72. Yeole BB, Ramanakumar AV, Sankaranarayanan R (2003) Survival from oral cancer in Mumbai (Bombay), India. Cancer Causes Control 14:945–952
73. Yoon AJ, Shen J, Santella RM et al (2007) Activated checkpoint kinase 2 expression and risk for oral squamous cell carcinoma. Cancer Epidemiol Biomarkers Prev 16:2768–2772
74. Zeng H, McLean DI, MacAulay C, et al (2000) Autofluorescence properties of skin and applications in dermatology. In: Proceedings of the SPIE – the international society for optical engineering biomedical photonics and optoelectronic imaging, vol. 4224, pp. 366–373, 8–10 November 2000
75. Zhang L, Williams M, Poh CF et al (2005) Toluidine blue staining identifies high-risk primary oral premalignant lesions with poor outcome. Cancer Res 65:8017–8021
76. Guillard M, Zhang L, Poh CF et al (2008) Potential use of quantitative tissue phenotyne to predict malignant risk for oral premalignant lesions. Cancer Res 68:1–9

Chapter 16
Barrett's Oesophagus

Rebecca Fitzgerald

Abstract Barrett's oesophagus (or columnar lined epithelium of the oesophagus) is the precursor lesion for oesophageal adenocarcinoma which is a cancer with a very poor prognosis. The clinical accessibility of the Barrett's segment and the opportunity for repeated, longitudinal sampling make it an ideal system in which to study the pathogenesis of metaplasia and the progression to cancer. From a clinical standpoint there has been much controversy over how to manage patients with this condition since it is often clinically silent, only a minority of patients will progress to cancer and until recently the treatment options have been limited and highly invasive. The two key clinical questions are therefore: how to identify patients with Barrett's oesophagus who are at high risk for progression to adenocarcinoma and how to manage those at high risk in order to prevent cancer development. It is also possible that if one had a thorough understanding of the disease pathogenesis then maybe one could prevent individuals with duodeno-gastro-oesophageal reflux developing Barrett's oesophagus in the first place. The explosion in endoscopic technology coupled with molecular biology tools at the –omics level mean that advances are being made which are having an impact on clinical practice although the field remains dogged by a lack of consensus in many areas.

Introduction

Oesophageal adenocarcinoma has been highlighted as a public health concern in the western world due to its increasing incidence and poor prognosis [1]. It is not yet clear whether or not this alarming increase in incidence that has occurred over the last 30 years is waning [2, 3]. There is also the possibility that we are starting

R. Fitzgerald (✉)
MRC Cancer Cell Unit, Hutchison-MRC Research Centre, Hills Road, CB22 0XZ Cambridge, UK
e-mail: rcf@hutchison-mrc.cam.ac.uk

R.C. Fitzgerald (ed.), *Pre-Invasive Disease: Pathogenesis and Clinical Management*, DOI 10.1007/978-1-4419-6694-0_16, © Springer Science+Business Media, LLC 2011

to witness an increase in the incidence of this oesophageal cancer subtype in the east, where traditionally squamous cell carcinoma has predominated [4]. One strategy to reduce the incidence of this disease and to improve outcomes is through early detection at the pre-invasive stage.

Barrett's oesophagus is the precursor lesion for oesophageal adenocarcinoma and hence the race, ethnicity and sex differences are similar in these conditions with a preponderance in white, males with a peak incidence in the sixth decade [5]. Barrett's oesophagus is defined as a metaplastic columnar-lined epithelium which is visible endoscopically with histopathological confirmation of glandular mucosa, (Fig. 16.1). The glandular mucosa is considered to be a result of a metaplastic processs, in which the mature adult squamous epithelium has been replaced by a glandular phenotype. The presence of intestinal cells including mucous producing goblet within the metaplasia has up until recently generally a pre-requisite for diagnosis in order to avoid mis-diagnosis of a hiatus hernia and since this is the subtype with the highest risk of malignant progression [6]. The British Society of Gastroenterology also include the gastric sub-type in their diagnostic classification [7] and this broader definition is currently a subject of debate by other International societies. How these subtypes relate to each other is not clear but it has been suggested that metaplastic gastric epithelium may occur prior to the formation of goblet cells, since non-goblet columnar epithelium has been shown to have expression of intestinal immunohistochemical markers such as MUC2 and villin [8, 9].

The risk of progression to adenocarcinoma is 5.98 per 1,000 patient years in patients with non-dysplastic Barrett's oesophagus increasing to 16.98 and 65.8 per 1,000 patient years for patients with low grade and high grade dysplasia respectively [10]. This is a 30–50 fold increased risk compared to the general population. Hence, although the absolute risk of progression to cancer is small the relative increase is significant.

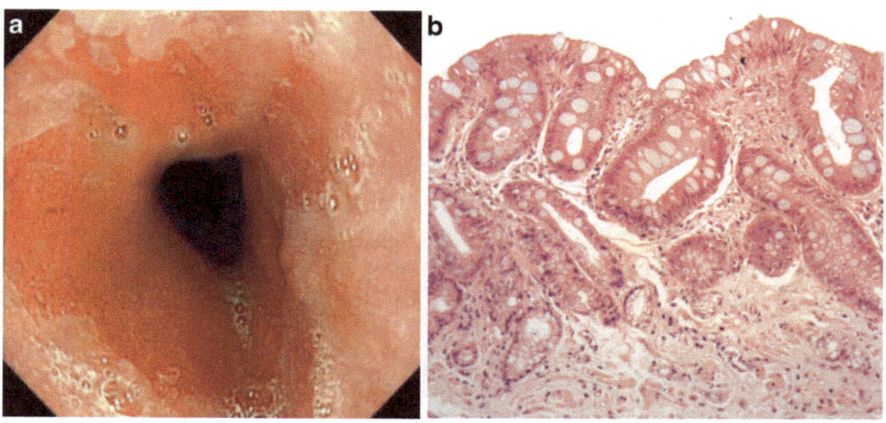

Fig. 16.1 (**a**) Endoscopic appearance of Barrett's oesophagus and (**b**) corresponding light microscopic section with goblet cells characteristic of intestinal metaplasia

The more frequent diagnosis of individuals with Barrett's oesophagus [5] coupled with the poor outcome for invasive oesophageal adenocarcinoma compels us to understand the underlying pathophysiology in order to manage these individuals appropriately.

Molecular Pathophysiology

Remarkably little is understood about the pathogenesis of Barrett's oesophagus at a cell and molecular level. One hypothesis is that Barrett's metaplasia may be considered as a wounding response to injurious factors in the luminal environment (refluxate, dietary factors such as nitric oxide) and in the stroma (inflammatory cells). This chronic injury may result in stem cells undergoing a fundamental switch in their transcriptional regulation with the result that a columnar phenotype is generated. Continued injurious inflammation secondary to reflux exposure may then set the scene for an accumulation and clonal expansion of cancer causing mutations (Fig. 16.2).

Cell of Origin and Stem Cells

Embryologically, the oesophagus starts life as columnar in origin and "transdifferentiates" to a squamous epithelium as a result of altered expression of key transcriptional regulators [11]. This process has been observed in the developing murine oesophagus in which a proportion of cells co-express markers of both squamous (cytokeratin 14) and columnar (cytokeratin 8) differentiation during this

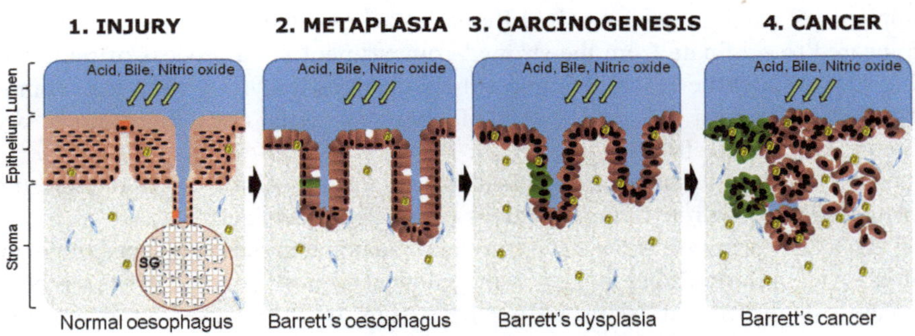

Fig. 16.2 A model for Barrett's pathogenesis. In the normal stratified squamous oesophagus putative stem cells (*red*) reside in both the basal epithelial cell layer and in the submucosal gland (SG) ducts. Injurious factors in the luminal environment (refluxate, dietary nitric oxide) and in the stroma (inflammatory cells: *yellow*, fibroblasts: *blue*) are hypothesized to cause wounding thereby inducing metaplasia. Increasing inflammation and the expansion of mutated epithelial clones (*green*) drive an invasive phenotype

conversion process [12]. This switch is thought to be independent of cell proliferation and apoptosis and to depend on alterations in gene expression.

In contrast to transdifferentiation of fully differentiated cell types another theory is that Barrett's occurs as a change in the commitment of multipotent stem cells (see Chap. 1 on stem cells in intraepithelial neoplasia). Surprisingly the stem cells of the normal human oesophagus have not been clearly identified. It has been suggested that candidate stem cells may be identified on the basis their undergoing asymmetric cell division, (i.e. division to generate one basal and one suprabasal layer daughter cell). A study using conventional 2D histological sectioning suggested that cells which undergo asymmetric division lie in the inter-papillary zone of the human basal layer [13]. However, these cells had several surprising characteristics including low expression of the epidermal stem cell marker β1 integrin [14]. Another possibility is that stem cells could reside within submucosal gland ducts [15], (Fig. 16.2), which are interestingly often seen in continuity with Barrett's epithelium [16] and contain columnar cells in their proximal potion [17]. This hypothesis is based on the ulcer-associated cell lineage [18], in which there is a migration of the glandular cells to the surface adjacent to areas of ulceration in the gastro-intestinal tract. There are several lines of evidence in support of this theory. An immunohistochemical characterization study in pig tissues and cultures indicated similarities between the submucosal glands and BE [19]. A molecular analysis of microdissected areas from the same resection specimen demonstrated a common p16 mutation in a submucosal gland duct and adjacent Barrett's epithelium suggesting a common genetic origin for these cells [15]. In a similar study islands of neo-squamous epithelium were found to be wild type at genetic loci containing mutations within the adjacent Barrett's epithelium. This suggests that the neo-squamous epithelium originates in different cells from those responsible for self-renewal of the Barrett's epithelium and again gland ducts have been suggested as a possible source [20]. (3) In a study in which retinoic acid (RA) was applied as a stimulus for cell differentiation ex vivo, columnar epithelium appeared to originate from the stromal compartment via a process of remodeling [21]. Whilst the cell of origin for these changes was not proven the submucosal glands are a possible source of columnar cells since these are a key component of the stroma.

More work is required to establish for certain the cell of origin of Barrett's metaplasia and the role of the squamous oesophageal stem cells.

As stated earlier metaplasia at a number of anatomical sites is induced by tissue injury, and in Barrett's oesophagus damage induced by reflux components has been widely established as a risk factor (e.g. [22]), (Fig. 16.2). However, reflux is a very common symptom which in the majority of individuals does not lead to Barrett's oesophagus [23, 24]. This therefore calls into question which constellation of risk factors, both environmental and perhaps genetic lead to individual susceptibility to this disease (see Chap. 3). These risk factors may be relevant both for the development of Barrett's metaplasia as well as in the progression to cancer and it is sometimes difficult to tease their precise role apart.

Risk Factors

The chronic exposures to damaging agents required for cancer in general to occur are reflected in the long lag phase from development of a pre-invasive lesion to the development of the invasive stage. Precise data is not available for Barrett's oesophagus, but in colorectal tumorigenesis comparative lesion sequencing suggests that it takes 17 years, and around four clonal expansions with an accumulation of mutations, for a large benign adenoma to evolve into advanced cancer [25]. Similar time frames are likely to be true for mutagens to sensitize the Barrett's epithelium [26].

Whilst for some cancers, such as tobacco smoke and lung cancer, the carcinogens are clearly delineated for Barrett's oesophagus and oesophageal adenocarcinoma the stimulus is less clear. As stated earlier, it has long been known that Barrett's oesophagus occurs on the background of chronic gastro-oesophageal reflux disease [27, 28], and heartburn symptoms are an independent risk factor for oesophageal adenocarcinoma [29]. More recently it has become apparent that these diseases are another casualty of the rising prevalence of obesity and maybe connected with a metabolic syndrome [30–32]. Smoking may play some roel but is not a strong risk factor and modest alcohol consumption may have a protective effect [33–35]. The male preponderance with a lag-phase for the age-related incidence in women has raised questions about whether hormones and iron status are important [36]. Relatively little is understood about dietary factors and the risk of Barrett's oesophagus, although a diet rich in fruit and vegetables appears to be protective [37] and dietary nitrates may increase the local oesophageal concentrations of nitric oxide [38, 39]. There has been no convincing evidence to date for an infective cause for Barrett's in contrast to the link between *H. pylori* infection and intestinal metaplasia of the stomach and thence gastric carcinoma or the link between Human Paplilloma Virus and cervical metaplasia, for example (discussed in Chaps. 17 and 21). Recently a study of the microbiome has suggested a correlation between the microorganisms colonizing the lower oesophagus and the type of oesophageal disease [40].

There is still a gap between our understanding of risk factors and disease causation and how to use this to aid patient management. The questions that arise are whether modification of risk factors could prevent the development of Barrett's oesophagus and cancer or help in the identification of high risk individuals to screen (for example, obese, males with reflux).

Relationship Between Risk Factors and Disease Pathogenesis (Fig. 16.3)

Reflux Components

The acid and bile constituents of reflux have been shown to induce expression of caudal homeobox genes such as *CDX1* and *CDX2* in in vitro experiments using cell

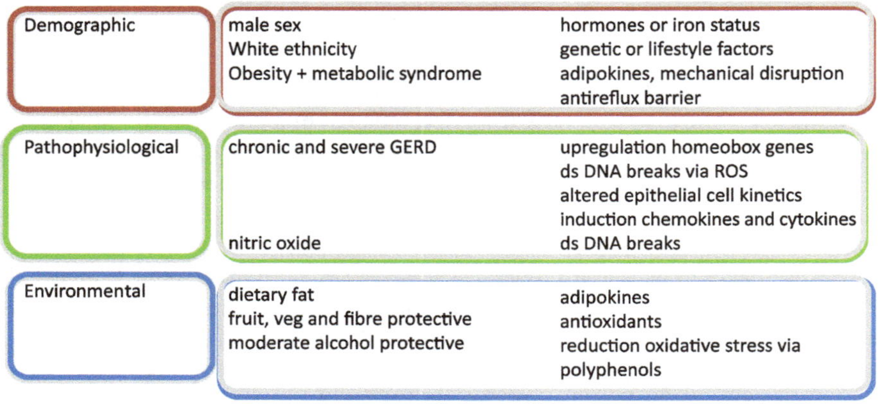

Fig. 16.3 A summary of the main identified demographic, pathophysiological and environmental risk factors for Barrett's oesophagus and progression to cancer. The far *right column* suggests the mechanisms or broad cell processes via which these risk factors might influence cancer risk

lines [41–44]. Cdx genes are transcription factors which are critical determinants of cell fate in embryogenesis and hence their designation "homeobox" from the Greek homeosis meaning a shift in structural development. Aberrant expression of these factors in adulthood can influence cell fate [45, 46]. However, despite attempts by a number of investigators, induction of Cdx2 alone does not appear to be sufficient to generate the metaplastic phenotype [47–49]. This failure could be as a result of problems of using murine models with very different gastro-oesophageal physiology, inability to transfect the appropriate cell of origin, or misguided focus on a single transcription factor when 3 or 4 are likely to be required [50].

Homeobox gene expression is epigenetically regulated via alterations in methylation status [41, 48] as well as via cell signaling pathways including hedgehog, bone morphogenetic proteins (*BMP*s) (belonging to the transforming growth factor beta family) and growth factor signaling pathways such as fibroblast growth factor. *BMP4* expression is increased in Barrett's metaplasia compared with normal squamous oesophagus and in a rat model of GERD induced Barrett's, *BMP4* expression was increased in the stroma underlying the Barrett's epithelium [51]. Furthermore, culture of human oesophageal squamous cells with *BMP4* led to induction of cytokeratins specific for columnar cells [51]. It has also been shown that bile acids alone or in combination with acid, can lead to *CDX2* induction through ligand-dependent transactivation of the epidermal growth factor receptor [52]. It has therefore been suggested that GERD induced *CDX* genes, via *BMP4* and perhaps *EGFR*, might mediate the development of Barrett's oesophagus [46].

With regards to the role of reflux exposure in the progression of Barrett's oesophagus it is not clear whether refluxate can cause tumor initiation. There is a direct cytotoxic effect of H^+ ions, but the main consequence of repeated acid and bile exposure is a chronic inflammatory response which in turn causes epithelial damage. For example, recent data suggests that acid exposure can induce double strand DNA breaks [53] and the bile acid deoxycholic acid can induce DNA damage in a dose-dependent, but non-linear fashion [54, 55]. Both of these effects appear to be mediated by reactive oxygen species raising questions about the potential therapeutic role of antioxidants. Acid and bile have also been shown to lead to altered cell kinetics [56–59] which in the context of sustained DNA damage may enable Barrett's cells to resist apoptosis via activation of the NFkappaB pathway [60]. These findings are in keeping with other evidence suggesting that increased NFkappaB activity [61] and other parts of the inflammatory response are modulated by acid and bile [62–64]. For example, the farnesoid X receptor (FXR), which is involved in regulation of bile acid synthesis, is up-regulated by deoxycholic acid in vitro and is also involved in the induction of the innate immune response [65]. Bile acid can also dysregulate the newly identified inflammation associated pathway tuberous sclerosis complex 1 (SC1) and mammalian target of rapamycin (mTOR) through I kappaB kinases (IKK) beta signaling [66].

The role of specific components of reflux induced inflammation in Barrett's carcinogenesis still needs further analysis but as discussed in Chap. 2, it is well known from other cancer types that inflammation aids proliferation and survival of malignant cells, stimulates angiogenesis and metastasis, subverts adaptive immunity and alters response to hormones and chemotherapy [67]. It would be surprising if this is not the case in this disease.

Obesity, Metabolic Syndrome and Dietary Factors

It is possible that obesity is relevant in Barrett's pathogenesis simply as a consequence of mechanical effects on the usual anatomical anti-reflux barrier. However, in view of the association between Barrett's oesophagus, obesity and inflammation it has been hypothesized that the adipocytokines associated with the metabolic syndrome of central adiposity may also be relevant [68]. In keeping with this there is an increased prevalence of central adiposity associated with hypertension and hyper-insulinaemia in the Barrett's population compared to that expected from the general population [69]. The causal and mechanistic relationship between the metabolic syndrome and Barrett's carcinogenesis remains to be established.

The role of specific dietary factors in Barrett's pathogenesis is largely unknown. As discussed above dietary nitrates in the context of GERD may increase the local oesophageal concentrations of nitric oxide [38, 39] and the resulting nitrosating species are capable of causing ds DNA breaks in vitro probably secondary to stalled replication forks [53]. Reactive oxygen species (ROS) also play important dose dependent roles in the regulation of cell survival and induction of *p53* target genes is a conserved response to oxidative stress [70]. The level of ROS is tightly controlled but there is recent evidence to suggest that the endogenous anti-oxidases may be silenced by hypermethylation in Barrett's adenocarcinoma [71]. It has also been suggested that the protective effect of moderate alcohol consumption might be secondary to the reduction of oxidative stress via polyphenols [33].

Alterations in intracellular iron transport have been linked to cancer and recently this has been demonstrated in the context of Barrett's metaplasia with effects on cell proliferation in vitro [72]. It has been suggested that reduced iron levels in pre-menopausal women may explain the delayed onset for adenocarcinoma in females [36]. It is interesting to note that there is no link between hemochromatosis gene status and Barrett's oesophagus suggesting that any relationship between iron metabolism and disease may not be straightforward [73].

Causal Somatic Genetic Changes

Whatever the causative factors underlying oesophageal carcinogenesis these will lead to pathogenic genetic and epigenetic alterations within the Barrett's tissue. The precise sequence of changes has been difficult to elucidate and the literature appears conflicting and imprecise with lack of a clear sequence. This is in contrast to the linear accumulation of mutations common across the majority of cases for colonic and pancreatic cancer, for example which have led to the concept of a "Vogelgram" (see Chap. 18). This difficulty in defining a precise sequence is likely to be due to the enormous genetic heterogeneity of Barrett's oesophagus and oesophageal adenocarcinoma which is also dominated by alterations in tumor suppressor genes (for review see [74, 75] and Chap. 1). Furthermore, some of these molecular changes are likely to be by-products of the high cell turnover and genetic instability leading to "hitchhiker mutations" rather than being causally related to cancer development and progression [76]. It therefore follows that it is not clear the extent to which the observed genetic changes lead to oncogenic dependence (defined as the situation whereby a particular genetic change is essential for tumor maintenance) which could be exploited for diagnosis and therapy.

Having said this there are some genetic alterations which occur at high frequency in the progression from Barrett's metaplasia to adenocarcinoma and these particularly relate to tumor suppressor genes p16 and TP53 (Fig. 16.4). Loss of one functional p16 (CDKN2A) allele occurs prior to the onset of dysplasia in over 85% of cases (Fig. 16.4 panel b), [77, 78]. This is generally caused by promoter methylation and less frequently by mutation [79]. The mutation spectrum is consistent with that caused by oxidative damage and chronic inflammation [80]. This early clone expands and is associated with the loss of the second p16 allele, commonly by loss of heterozygosity (LOH), thus creating a p16 null clone (Fig. 16.4, panel c), [77, 78, 81]. These changes are initiating events and as such are devoid of alterations in proliferation and the cells remain diploid. As a result no dysplasia is evident histopathologically [80, 82]. Due to the high frequency of p16 loss this is not a useful biomarker for predicting future adenocarcinoma risk [76].

The p16 (CDKN2A) gene shares its exon 2 region with p14ARF (or Alternate Reading Frame, ARF), another tumour suppressor which is estimated to be silenced in 30% of cancers overall. There has therefore been interest in whether this is simultaneously lost early in Barrett's carcinogenesis. Data suggests that in Barrett's

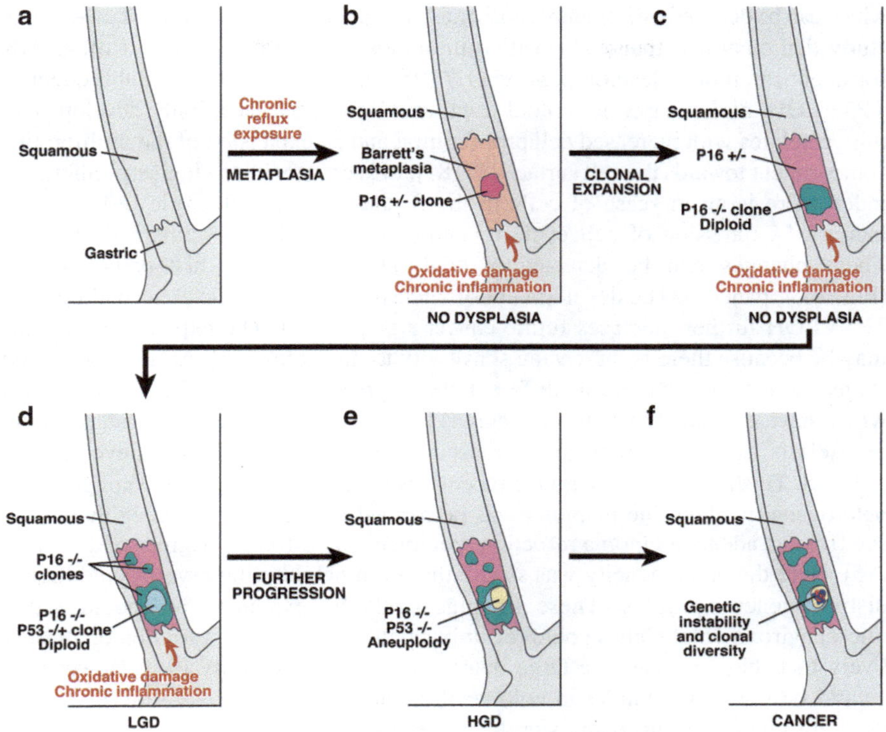

Fig. 16.4 A schematic illustrating the sequential somatic genetic changes in the progression from the squamous esophagus to Barrett's oesophagus to adenocarcinoma. The normal squamous oesophagus (**a**) undergoes a metaplastic transformation with the oxidative damage and chronic inflammation that accompanies chronic gastro-oesophageal reflux. The initial metaplastic change is followed early on by the loss of one p16 allele (**b**); this clone may then expand (*pink* area panel **c**), followed by loss of the second p16 allele and the formation of some p16 null clones (*blue* area, **c**). The subsequent loss of p53 may be associated with morphological changes of low grade dysplasia (LGD), (**d**). Genetic instability may lead to aneuploidy, which is commonly seen with high grade dysplasia (HGD), (panel **e**). Numerous clones may develop, and there may be heterogeneity within clones especially as the degree of genetic instability increases and invasive adenocarcinoma develops (**f**)

p14ARF loss occurs secondary to CpG or histone methylation and is a relatively late event independent of p16 loss [83].

The development of low grade dysplasia (LGD) is commonly seen to coincide with the loss of functional protein expression from one or both TP53 alleles. This occurs by promoter CpG island methylation, mutation or LOH within the p16 null clones (Fig. 16.4, panel d). The timing of TP53 mutation is in keeping with data from other tumors with a pre-invasive stage [25, 84]. When TP53 LOH is present there is an increased progression rate to cancer with a relative risk (RR) of 16 compared to those with no loss [85]. Depending on the precise mechanism for TP53 inactivation there may be a nuclear accumulation of non-functional p53 protein which can be detected by immunohistochemistry. A population based nested case-control study demonstrated that p53 positive immunostaining is associated with an OR for adenocarcinoma development of 11.7 (95% CI 1.93, 71.4) [86]. Subsequent to TP53 LOH, an increased tetraploid fraction followed by aneuploidy develops and this correlates with increased cell proliferation and an expansion of the proliferative compartment towards the cell surface [87–89]. In keeping with the higher proliferative index there is an increase of cells in the S phase of the cell cycle [80, 90] and increased expression of cell cycle related proteins such as cyclins [80, 91, 92]. These changes can be detected as high grade dysplasia histopathologically (Fig. 16.4, panel e). The development of widespread cytogenetic abnormalities and TP53 LOH further increases future cancer risk [93, 94]. The explanation for this may be because there is increasing sensitivity to mutagens [26]. At these advanced stages there are often multiple different clones present within the Barrett's segment which have expanded to differing degrees [95]. A higher degree of clonal diversity in itself is associated with an increased risk of adenocarcinoma development [93, 96]. This is consistent with the recent observation of a large degree of genomic heterogeneity when fine mapping was performed on microdissected epithelial tissue from an adenocarcinoma resection specimen with differing degrees of dysplasia [15]. Here the heterogeneity was so rife that even neighboring crypts could harbor distinct genetic profiles. These findings could be explained by the idea that microenvironmental niches could result in small scale regional variation or alternatively that they are due to a large degree of genetic instability [96]. However, it should be noted that unlike in colorectal carcinogenesis microsatellite instability does not seem to occur to any significant degree in Barrett's carcinogenesis [97].

The presence of aneuploidy is known to have diverse effects on cell metabolism, proliferation and immortalization [98]. Chromosomal copy number changes are not believed to be random events in Barrett's oesophagus. Chromosome 4 and 7 aneuploidy tends to occur early, followed by chromosome 8 and 17 aneuploidy and then loss of the Y chromosome in males [99, 100]. The presence of ploidy abnormalities have been shown to dramatically increase the RR of adenocarcinoma development (4.4 and 11 for tetraploidy and aneuploidy respectively) and this increases to 20 if both abnormalities are present [101].

Genome Wide Approaches to Understanding Molecular Pathogenesis

The rapid advancement in technology over the past 5–10 years has meant that in contrast to the candidate approach, which has largely been responsible for our understanding of disease progression as outlined above, it is now possible to perform genome wide analyses for a number of parameters without an a priori hypotheses (see Chap. 6). These analyses include gene profiling at the level of the chromosome, transcriptome (RNA and small interfering RNAs), epigenome and proteome (Fig. 16.5). Recently large-scale sequencing of the vast majority of protein-coding genes in human tumors has become possible [25]. Furthermore, microdissection and low input amplification protocols has enabled researchers to look at the contribution of individual cell types to the observed changes and to perform fine-mapping across the Barrett's segment [15]. It will take a while before

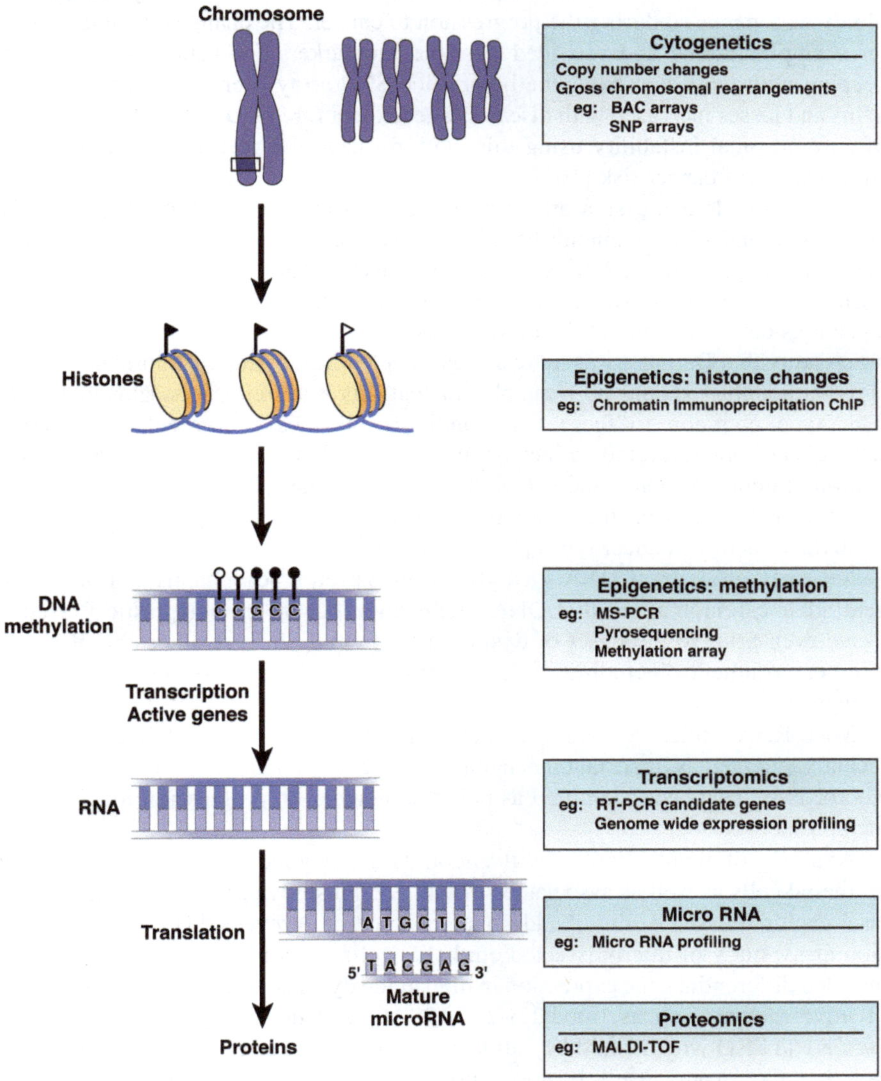

Fig. 16.5 A summary of the –omics technologies (*right hand column*) which have been applied to understanding cancer, and more recently to pre-invasive disease, from the level of the chromosome through to the protein

these technologies are applied to oesophageal datasets with large enough sample sizes to perform robust statistical analyses.

As mentioned above copy number alterations are common in cancer and in contrast to cytogenetic analyses of specific loci of interest, genome wide analyses are possible using chromosome (BAC) array genomic hybridisation [102] and now using high density single nucleotide polymorphism (SNP) technology [103]. The BAC arrays revealed that copy number aberrations correlated highly with aneuploidy and increased during the progression to cancer. The changes included high-level amplifications and provided possible biomarkers for validation [102]. In keeping with work that has gone before, the SNP arrays demonstrated that copy gains and losses increased with disease stage (except for 9pLOH) and that measures of chromosomal instability using this platform have the potential to be used for stratification of cancer risk [103].

Genome wide expression arrays at the level of the transcriptome for Barrett's oesophagus and adenocarcinoma have largely been proof of principle. Several studies have demonstrated that RNA expression profiles were able to distinguish between normal squamous oesophagus, Barrett's, oesophageal adenocarcinoma and squamous cell carcinoma of the oesophagus [104–108]. From such analyses it was noteworthy that Barrett's was more similar to adenocarcinoma that normal oesophagus, although it should be remembered that this may reflect the glandular cell phenotype common to these two conditions. Pathways up-regulated in both Barrett's and adenocarcinoma include those involved in tissue development, proliferation, immune response and extracellular matrix genes [107].

Published studies on methylation so far have focused on genes known to be methylated in other cancer types [109, 110]. These data sets have shown that there is similarity of aberrant DNA methylation in Barrett's oesophagus and oesophageal adenocarcinoma and that DNA methylation occurs in metaplastic Barrett's tissue even prior to the onset of dysplasia [111, 112]. It is also possible that the microenvironment, including reflux exposure, could induce such epigenetic changes (e.g. [71]).

MicroRNAs (miRNAs) are abundant small non-protein coding RNAs that have recently emerged as important mechanisms for gene silencing in cancer [113, 114]. MicroRNAs have been identified as potential markers of progression for Barrett's metaplasia [40, 113].

Analysis of whole tissues will encompass the gene expression of normal epithelial cells as well as associated stroma. A pilot study demonstrated that when laser captured tissue was used additional information is revealed [115]. An expression array study of microdissected epithelial cells without contaminating stroma revealed differential gene expression in high grade dysplasia including up-regulation of novel genes such as lipocalin-2, S100A9, and down-regulation of trefoil factor 1 (TFF1) which could be validated at the protein level [116]. This is not to say that the stroma itself is not important. It is increasingly recognised that stromal-epithelial interactions have profound effects on the pathogenesis of cancer [117–119]. For example, manipulation of TGFβ signaling in the stromal compartment of mice, such as deletion of its receptor or inactivation of a signaling molecule

SMAD in T cells has been shown to induce intraepithelial neoplasia in the prostate and invasive squamous cell carcinoma of the forestomach [120]. In Barrett's oesophagus a gene expression profiling study identified a stromal signature by subtraction of an epithelial cell line signature from that obtained from whole biopsy samples [121]. In order to then more directly examine the contribution of the stroma this compartment was microdissected from samples from each of the different stages of Barrett's oesophagus [122]. Supervised clustering of gene expression profiles from microdissected stroma identified a gene signature which could distinguish between Barrett's metaplasia, dysplasia and adenocarcinoma. Patients with adenocarcinoma over-expressing any of five genes (*TMEPAI*, *JMY*, *TSP1*, *FAPα*, *BCL6*) identified from this stromal signature had a significantly poorer outcome. Gene ontology analysis identified a strong inflammatory component in progression of Barrett's oesophagus and key pathways included cytokine-cytokine receptor interactions and TGFβ. Increased protein levels of inflammatory related genes significantly up-regulated in adenocarcinoma compared with pre-invasive stages were confirmed in the stroma of independent samples and in vitro assays confirmed functional relevance of these genes. This is in keeping with previous data suggesting TGFbeta is dysregulated in Barrett's carcinogenesis [123, 124] and fits with the idea that the inflammatory microenvironment can be considered as the seventh cancer hallmark [125].

High throughput proteomics technologies have been technically more difficult than genomics but mass spectrometry (MALDI TOF MS) has identified candidate novel proteins for further study [126]. Quantitative differential protein expression analysis in oesophageal adenocarcinoma has indentified four cellular stress response proteins (heat-shock protein (HSP) 27, HSP60, glucose-regulated protein (GRP) 94, and GRP78) associated with response to chemotherapy in 34 patients [127]. These findings have not yet been externally validated and it is not yet clear what role, if any they play in the preinvasive state.

Overall, these molecular alterations are in many cases a descriptive catalogue rather than explaining cause and effect. Never the less, whilst many biological questions still need addressing in the meantime this knowledge can be put to use for the identification of clinical biomarkers.

Biomarkers for Screening and Surveillance

Screening to detect Barrett's oesophagus is not yet part of routine clinical practice but merits consideration since it is estimated that only 5% of patients with this condition are currently diagnosed despite the increasing use of endoscopy [128]. Hitherto the utility of screening for BE has been questionable given the lack of treatment options. However, there has been rapid advancement in technologies such as endoscopic mucosal resection and radiofrequency ablation with randomised controlled trial evidence to support their efficacy [129, 130], (see also Chap. 12). In addition, chemoprevention measures are being evaluated in a large CRUK funded trial (AspECT), [131]. Therefore screening-detected cases of Barrett's oesophagus could potentially be coupled to interventions to prevent adenocarcinoma thus avoiding the need for oesophagectomy which has significant mortality and morbidity [132].

As discussed the current diagnosis of Barrett's depends on an endoscopic evaluation which is invasive for the patient and costly for the health care provider. Alternative screening modalities include video capsule endoscopy and ultra-thin transnasal endoscopy [133, 134]. However, the video capsule does not permit tissue sampling and both require expensive technology. The sensitivity and specificity for the diagnosis of Barrett's oesophagus, even for the video capsule, remain relatively low with values of 78 and 88% respectively [135].

We have recently developed a novel immuno-cytological approach (Cytosponge) for screening. This device comprises a spherical sponge which is tethered onto a string and compressed into a capsule. The capsule is swallowed and after entering the proximal stomach it dissolves after 3–5 min allowing the expanded to be pulled back out through the mouth thus collecting cells from along the length of the oesophagus. Use of a biomarker specific for Barrett's oesophageal cells permits one to diagnose Barrett's oesophagus. This approach is proving to be sensitive and specific; overcomes issues of sampling bias; is applicable to primary care; is acceptable to patients and cost effective (International patent filed in UK and Internationally, MHRA approved 2007), (Fig. 16.6). The biomarkers have been selected using a candidate approach [88] as well as from gene expression profiling datasets to select genes significantly up-regulated in Barrett's oesophagus compared with adjacent squamous oesophagus and gastric cardia, which are also sampled by the Cytosponge [136]. In studies comparing Cytosponge specimens from patients with known Barrett's oesophagus compared with healthy volunteers the most promising biomarkers were an antibody raised against the proliferation

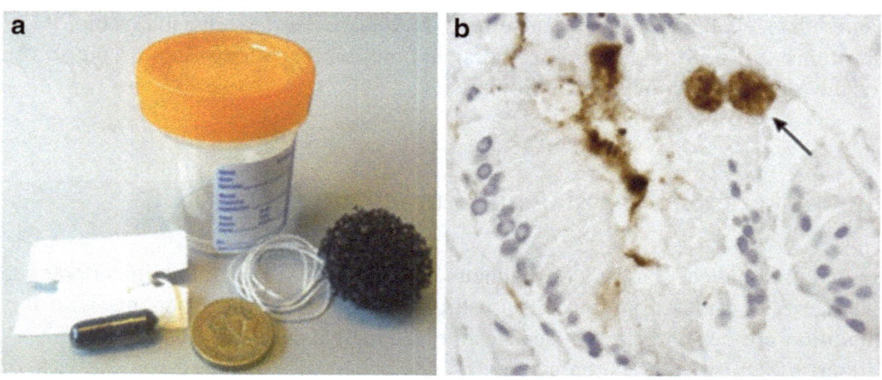

Fig. 16.6 (**a**) Cytosponge within the capsule (*left*) and expanded (*right*) in comparison to a UK£ 1 coin. Once withdrawn the expanded device is placed in a container with preservative and processed for immunohistochemistry. (**b**) A representative picture of positive TFF3 staining in a sample from a patient with Barrett's oesophagus

marker Mcm2; and a mucin characteristic of the intestinal metaplastic phenotype TFF3 [136, 137]. We chose protein based assays on the basis that these are currently the preferred platform for routine clinical diagnostic pathology laboratories. This test has now been piloted in a primary care cohort study of 500 individuals with a history of reflux and the sensitivity and specificity of the TFF3 immuno-test compared with gastroscopy was 73.3 and 93.5% for ≥1 cm circumferential (C1 using the Prague classification, [138]) and 90.0 and 93.5% for ≥C2. The mcm2 biomarker lacked sufficient sensitivity and specificity. Any anxiety returned to low levels by day 7 and Impact of Events Scale suggested that <4.5% displayed significant distress [162]. The Cytosponge test now requires further validation in a larger primary care screening trial.

Once Barrett's oesophagus has been diagnosed the holy grail is to identify those at greatest risk for progression to cancer. As alluded to above there has been much interest in using the information gained about key molecular changes for use as predictive biomarkers. Currently, dysplasia grade is the only biomarker used to risk-stratify patients in clinical practice.

Even when sound scientific data exists to support the use of a biomarker a number of practical hurdles must be overcome before they can be considered for clinical practice. These include clinically reliable assays, biomarkers deemed to be "reasonable and necessary" using a cost-benefit analysis and regulatory approvals. Five conceptual phases of biomarker development have been proposed [139] and out of the many biomarkers which have been proposed in the field only a few describe phase 3 and 4 studies according to Early Detection Research Network (EDRN) criteria.

Much of the biomarker work has focused on the confirmed, common abnormalities of TP53 LOH, p16 LOH and ploidy discussed earlier. These biomarkers are predictive individually but with significantly increased OR when used in combination [140] and when the size of the clone is taken into account [93]. It is now becoming possible to replace the complex flow cytometry based assays previously required to evaluate these biomarkers with single nucleotide polymorphism-based chromosome copy number analyses which may be more amenable to clinical applications [103].

An alternative methodology which is being actively explored is the use of FISH on oesophageal brushings in an attempt to overcome cell sampling bias. This approach has been quite successful [141–143] although there has been concern that FISH will miss LOH without copy number change and that dual probe FISH is required to detect the complex genetic changes associated with a tetraploid intermediate [144]. Phase 3 and 4 studies using FISH assessment of genome specific copy number changes are required to determine the utility of this approach. As an extension of cytological based cell collection methods there has recently been interest in applying biomarkers to non-endoscopic screening tools including the Cytosponge device described above [137].

There is also interest in using epigenetic changes as biomarkers. These molecular readouts can also be usefully combined with clinical characteristics such as age, sex and length of segment and an example of this is a three-tiered risk stratification strategy, based on systematically selected epigenetic and clinical parameters [145]. Further work is required to validate these models on independent datasets and to develop clinically applicable methylation assays. It may also be possible to apply these biomarkers to the cytosponge.

In addition to biomarkers predictive for the future development of cancer, biomarkers may also have a role in the identification of clinically silent advanced pre-invasive lesions (high grade dysplasia) which arise in flat mucosa. For example, in the future it is hoped that molecular biomarkers will also be coupled to endoscopic imaging modalities in order to target biopsies towards dysplastic areas (see Chap. 10 on molecular imaging). Proof of principle studies have been performed for colonic adenomas in which peptides specific for dysplasia determined from a peptide library screen were fluorescently labeled and tested in vivo [146].

Another potential application of biomarkers is as a prognostic tool to determine the likelihood of recurrence following endoscopic treatment (see Chap. 12). Most studies to date have been performed in the context of photodynamic therapy (PDT), but now attention is turning towards patients who have received radiofrequency ablation (RFA). FISH for a panel of biomarkers in a small number of patients demonstrated that patients with persistently positive biomarkers appeared to be at a higher risk of recurrent HGD [147] and patients with p16 allelic loss were more likely to be resistant to therapy [148].

In order to move biomarkers into the clinical arena the current challenge for the academic community is to form consortia which together have large tissue sets to perform appropriately powered validation studies.

Applications of Pathophysiology Knowledge to Therapy

Aside from improving diagnostics it is also hoped that improved knowledge of the pathophysiology of Barrett's carcinogenesis will lead to improved treatment options. Endoscopic therapies have improved significantly over recent years and provide the opportunity to treat those with early lesions confined to the submucosa (see Chap. 12). As mentioned above, longer-term follow-up is required to determine the longevity of response and whether the underlying molecular abnormalities are eradicated or just temporarily stalled.

Prior to the development of high grade dysplasia and cancer, and in contrast to the endoscopic "slash and burn" type of approaches, there has been interest in how one might use our knowledge of disease pathogenesis to prevent cancer from developing in the first place. For example, due to the causal role of refluxate there has been interest in the role of pharmacological and surgical anti-reflux treatments as chemoprevention strategies. Even though anti-reflux treatments may reduce molecular endpoints associated with the cancer phenotype (e.g. [149, 150]), as well as decrease the risk of dysplasia [151–153], these drugs may not reduce the formation of DNA adducts [154]. Overall, although there is some suggestive data with regards cancer incidence [155] the efficacy of these measures in reducing the incidence of cancer is unknown. Additionally, there have been concerns about the sequelae of hypergastrinaema resulting from proton pump inhibitors [161] (Harris 2004). Prospective randomized controlled trials are required in additional to current data from longitudinal follow-up studies.

Similarly, in view of the mounting evidence for a role of chemokines and cytokines in Barrett's progression there is interest in anti-inflammatory agents, aspirin and selective cyclo-oxygenase inhibitors. A meta-analysis of observational human studies demonstrated a 33% reduction in the odds ratio of developing oesophageal adenocarcinoma for patients using aspirin or NSAIDs with a dose dependent effect [156], although the frequency and duration of usage did not have an impact [94]. There are few randomized controlled trials and most of these do not have cancer as the endpoint. In a trial in which patients with Barrett's oesophagus received either celecoxib or placebo there was no difference in the overall area of Barrett's or the grading of dysplasia [157]. In view of the interest in oxidative stress and the development of oesophageal adenocarcinoma there has been an interest in using antioxidants as a chemopreventive measure. To date there is little clinical trial data although a cohort study showed favorable results for individuals who used multivitamins and antioxidant supplements [158].

The advent of therapies targeted against specific molecular abnormalities has led to a new era of cancer therapy. These agents are generally well tolerated and it is possible that they could be used in the chemopreventative setting for intraepithelial neoplasia (HGD), as shown through a number of animal studies [159]. The key alterations described in the biomarker literature for Barrett's, such as TP53, do not lend themselves well to therapy. However, the finding that HER-2 or ErbB2 is overexpressed secondary to genomic amplification in the transition from dysplasia to adenocarcinoma is an example of how these drugs could be applied in the future [160]. However, it is becoming clear that due to the low frequency of such changes a personalised approach or a multidrug regime may be required.

Conclusions

The catalogue of molecular abnormalities in Barrett's has exploded with the advance of high throughput screening for genomic and epigenetic alterations. However, an understanding of the functional relevance of these findings and how to relate them to improved patient management lags behind. Cross disciplinary inputs including the application of concepts from evolutionary biology (see Chap. 7) and bioinformatics (see Chap. 6) should enable progress to be made in understanding causality of molecular genetic changes. There are developments in technologies for: detecting Barrett's oesophagus, for example the Cytosponge linked to a protein phenotypic biomarker; and for treatments of early lesions through radiofrequency ablation and mucosal resection. The advances in diagnostic and therapeutic endoscopy offer an exciting opportunity to revolutionise the diagnostic and treatment algorithms for Barrett's oesophagus but coupling this with our knowledge of molecular pathophysiology will be essential to accurately target our interventions to those individuals at greatest risk.

Acknowledgments Rebecca Fitzgerald is supported by a Medical Research Council programme Grant, as well as from the Cambridge Experimental Cancer Medicine Centre and the NIHR Cambridge Biomedical Research Centre.

References

1. Donaldson SL (2008) Annual report of the Chief Medical Officer: on the state of public health. London, Contract No.: Document Number 1
2. Pohl H, Sirovich B, Welch HG. (2005) Esophageal adenocarcinoma incidence: are we reaching the peak? Cancer Epidemicol Biomarkers Prev19(6):1468–70
3. Lepage C, Rachet B, Jooste V, Faivre J, Coleman MP (2008) Continuing rapid increase in esophageal adenocarcinoma in England and Wales. Am J Gastroenterol 103(11):2694–2699
4. Cheung TK, Wong BC, Lam SK (2008) Gastro-oesophageal reflux disease in Asia: birth of a 'new' disease? Drugs 68(4):399–406
5. Corley DA, Kubo A, Levin TR, Block G, Habel L, Rumore G et al (2009) Race, ethnicity, sex and temporal differences in Barrett's oesophagus diagnosis: a large community-based study, 1994–2006. Gut 58(2):182–188
6. Wang KK, Sampliner RE (2008) Updated guidelines 2008 for the diagnosis, surveillance and therapy of Barrett's esophagus. Am J Gastroenterol 103(3):788–797
7. Watson A, Heading RC, Shepherd NA (2005) Guidelines for the diagnosis and management of Barrett's columnar-lined oesophagus. British Society of Gastroenterology, London, Contract No.: Document Number 1
8. Chandrasoma PT, Der R, Dalton P, Kobayashi G, Ma Y, Peters J et al (2001) Distribution and significance of epithelial types in columnar-lined esophagus. Am J Surg Pathol 25(9):1188–1193
9. Hahn HP, Blount PL, Ayub K, Das KM, Souza R, Spechler S et al (2009) Intestinal differentiation in metaplastic, nongoblet columnar epithelium in the esophagus. Am J Surg Pathol 33(7):1006–1015
10. Wani S, Puli SR, Shaheen NJ, Westhoff B, Slehria S, Bansal A et al (2009) Esophageal adenocarcinoma in Barrett's esophagus after endoscopic ablative therapy: a meta-analysis and systematic review. Am J Gastroenterol 104(2):502–513
11. Montgomery RK, Mulberg AE, Grand RJ (1999) Development of the human gastrointestinal tract: twenty years of progress. Gastroenterology 16(3):702–731
12. Yu WY, Slack JM, Tosh D (2005) Conversion of columnar to stratified squamous epithelium in the developing mouse oesophagus. Dev Biol 284:157–170
13. Seery JP, Watt FM (2000) Asymmetric stem-cell divisions define the architecture of human oesophageal epithelium. Curr Biol 10(22):1447–1450
14. Seery JP (2002) Stem cells of the oesophageal epithelium. J Cell Sci 115(Pt 9):1783–1789
15. Leedham SJ, Preston SL, McDonald SA, Elia G, Bhandari P, Poller D et al (2008) Individual crypt genetic heterogeneity and the origin of metaplastic glandular epithelium in human Barrett's oesophagus. Gut 57(8):1041–1048
16. Coad RA, Woodman AC, Warner PJ, Barr H, Wright NA, Shepherd NA (2005) On the histogenesis of Barrett's oesophagus and its associated squamous islands: a three-dimensional study of their morphological relationship with native oesophageal gland ducts. J Pathol 206:388–394
17. Guillem PG (2005) How to make a Barrett esophagus: pathophysiology of columnar metaplasia of the esophagus. Dig Dis Sci 50(3):415–424
18. Ahnen DJ, Poulsom R, Stamp GW, Elia G, Pike C, Jeffery R, Longcroft J, Rio MC, Chambon P, Wright NA (1994) The ulceration-associated cell lineage (UACL) reiterates the Brunner's gland differentiation programme but acquires the proliferative organization of the gastric gland. J Pathol 173:317–326

19. Abdulnour-Nakhoul S, Nakhoul NL, Wheeler SA, Haque S, Wang P, Brown K et al (2007) Characterization of esophageal submucosal glands in pig tissue and cultures. Dig Dis Sci 52(11):3054–3065
20. Paulson TG, Xu L, Sanchez C, Blount PL, Ayub K, Odze RD et al (2006) Neosquamous epithelium does not typically arise from Barrett's epithelium. Clin Cancer Res 12(6):1701–1706
21. Chang CL, Lao-Sirieix P, Save V, De La Cueva Mendez G, Laskey R, Fitzgerald RC (2007) Retinoic acid-induced glandular differentiation of the oesophagus. Gut 56(7):906–917
22. Vaezi M, Richter J (1996) Role of acid and duodenogastroesophageal reflux in gastro-oesophageal reflux disease. Gastroenterology 111:1192
23. Flameling RD, Numans ME, Ter Linde J, de Wit NJ, Siersema PD (2010) Different characteristics of patients with gastro-oesophageal reflux disease on their path through healthcare: a population follow-up study. Eur J Gastroenterol Hepatol 22(5):578–582
24. Falkenback D, Oberg S, Johnsson F, Johansson J (2009) Is the course of gastroesophageal reflux disease progressive? A 21-year follow-up. Scand J Gastroenterol 44(11):1277–1287
25. Jones S, Chen WD, Parmigiani G, Diehl F, Beerenwinkel N, Antal T et al (2008) Comparative lesion sequencing provides insights into tumor evolution. Proc Natl Acad Sci U S A 105(11): 4283–4288
26. Chao DL, Maley CC, Wu X, Farrow DC, Galipeau PC, Sanchez CA et al (2006) Mutagen sensitivity and neoplastic progression in patients with Barrett's esophagus: a prospective analysis. Cancer Epidemiol Biomarkers Prev 15(10):1935–1940
27. Winters C, Spurling T, Chobanian S, Curtis D, Esposito R, Hacker JF et al (1987) Barrett's esophagus: a prevalent occult complication of gastro-oesophageal reflux disease. Gastroenterology 92:118–124
28. Chiu PW, Ayazi S, Hagen JA, Lipham JC, Zehetner J, Abate E et al (2009) Esophageal pH exposure and epithelial cell differentiation. Dis Esophagus 22(7):596–599
29. Lagergren J, Bergstrom R, Lindgren A, Nyren O (1999) Symptomatic gastroesophageal reflux as a risk factor for oesophageal adenocarcinoma. N Engl J Med 340(11):825–832
30. Cameron A, Kamath P, Carpenter H (1997) Prevalence of Barrett's esophagus and intestinal metaplasia at the esophagogastric junction. Gastroenterology 112:A82
31. Jacobson BC, Chan AT, Giovannucci EL, Fuchs CS (2009) Body mass index and Barrett's oesophagus in women. Gut 58(11):1460–1466
32. Mulholland HG, Cantwell MM, Anderson LA, Johnston BT, Watson RG, Murphy SJ et al (2009) Glycemic index, carbohydrate and fiber intakes and risk of reflux esophagitis, Barrett's esophagus, and esophageal adenocarcinoma. Cancer Causes Control 20(3):279–288
33. El-Serag HB, Lagergren J (2009) Alcohol drinking and the risk of Barrett's esophagus and esophageal adenocarcinoma. Gastroenterology 136(4):1155–1157
34. Anderson LA, Cantwell MM, Watson RG, Johnston BT, Murphy SJ, Ferguson HR et al (2009) The association between alcohol and reflux esophagitis, Barrett's esophagus, and esophageal adenocarcinoma. Gastroenterology 136(3):799–805
35. Kubo A, Levin TR, Block G, Rumore GJ, Quesenberry CP Jr, Buffler P et al (2009) Alcohol types and sociodemographic characteristics as risk factors for Barrett's esophagus. Gastroenterology 136(3):806–815
36. Derakhshan MH, Liptrot S, Paul J, Brown IL, Morrison D, McColl KE (2009) Oesophageal and gastric intestinal-type adenocarcinomas show the same male predominance due to a 17 year delayed development in females. Gut 58(1):16–23
37. Kubo A, Levin TR, Block G, Rumore GJ, Quesenberry CP Jr, Buffler P et al (2008) Dietary patterns and the risk of Barrett's esophagus. Am J Epidemiol 167(7):839–846
38. Iijima K, Henry E, Moriya A, Wirz A, Kelman AW, McColl KE (2002) Dietary nitrate generates potentially mutagenic concentrations of nitric oxide at the gastroesophageal junction. Gastroenterology 122(5):1248–1257
39. Winter JW, Paterson S, Scobie G, Wirz A, Preston T, McColl KE (2007) *N*-nitrosamine generation from ingested nitrate via nitric oxide in subjects with and without gastroesophageal reflux. Gastroenterology 133(1):164–174

40. Kan T, Sato F, Ito T, Matsumura N, David S, Cheng Y et al (2009) The miR-106b-25 polycistron, activated by genomic amplification, functions as an oncogene by suppressing p21 and Bim. Gastroenterology 136(5):1689–1700
41. Wong NA, Wilding J, Bartlett S, Liu Y, Warren BF, Piris J, Maynard N, Marshall R, Bodmer WF (2005) CDX1 is an important molecular mediator of Barrett's metaplasia. Proc Natl Acad Sci U S A 102:7565–7570
42. Kazumori H, Ishihara S, Kinoshita Y (2009) Roles of caudal-related homeobox gene Cdx1 in oesophageal epithelial cells in Barrett's epithelium development. Gut 58(5):620–628
43. Pera M, Pera M, de Bolos C, Brito MJ, Palacin A, Grande L et al (2007) Duodenal-content reflux into the esophagus leads to expression of Cdx2 and Muc2 in areas of squamous epithelium in rats. J Gastrointest Surg 11(7):869–874
44. Hu Y, Williams VA, Gellersen O, Jones C, Watson TJ, Peters JH (2007) The pathogenesis of Barrett's esophagus: secondary bile acids upregulate intestinal differentiation factor CDX2 expression in esophageal cells. J Gastrointest Surg 11(7):827–834
45. Beck F (2004) The role of Cdx genes in the mammalian gut. Gut 53(10):1394–1396
46. Souza RF, Krishnan K, Spechler SJ (2008) Acid, bile, and CDX: the ABCs of making Barrett's metaplasia. Am J Physiol Gastrointest Liver Physiol 295(2):G211–G218
47. Kazumori H, Ishihara S, Rumi MA, Kadowaki Y, Kinoshita Y (2006) Bile acids directly augment caudal related homeobox gene Cdx2 expression in oesophageal keratinocytes in Barrett's epithelium. Gut 55:16–25
48. Liu T, Zhang X, So CK, Wang S, Wang P, Yan L et al (2007) Regulation of Cdx2 expression by promoter methylation, and effects of Cdx2 transfection on morphology and gene expression of human esophageal epithelial cells. Carcinogenesis 28(2):488–496
49. Morrow DJ, Avissar NE, Toia L, Redmond EM, Watson TJ, Jones C et al (2009) Pathogenesis of Barrett's esophagus: bile acids inhibit the Notch signaling pathway with induction of CDX2 gene expression in human esophageal cells. Surgery 146(4):714–721, discussion 21–22
50. Zhou Q, Brown J, Kanarek A, Rajagopal J, Melton DA (2008) In vivo reprogramming of adult pancreatic exocrine cells to beta-cells. Nature 455(7213):627–632
51. Milano F, van Baal JW, Buttar NS, Rygiel AM, de Kort F, DeMars CJ et al (2007) Bone morphogenetic protein 4 expressed in esophagitis induces a columnar phenotype in esophageal squamous cells. Gastroenterology 132(7):2412–2421
52. Avissar NE, Toia L, Hu Y, Watson TJ, Jones C, Raymond DP et al (2009) Bile acid alone, or in combination with acid, induces CDX2 expression through activation of the epidermal growth factor receptor (EGFR). J Gastrointest Surg 13(2):212–222
53. Clemons NJ, McColl KE, Fitzgerald RC (2007) Nitric oxide and acid induce double-strand DNA breaks in Barrett's esophagus carcinogenesis via distinct mechanisms. Gastroenterology 133(4):1198–1209
54. Jenkins GJ, D'Souza FR, Suzen SH, Eltahir ZS, James SA, Parry JM et al (2007) Deoxycholic acid at neutral and acid pH, is genotoxic to oesophageal cells through the induction of ROS: the potential role of anti-oxidants in Barrett's oesophagus. Carcinogenesis 28(1):136–142
55. Jenkins GJ, Cronin J, Alhamdani A, Rawat N, D'Souza F, Thomas T et al (2008) The bile acid deoxycholic acid has a non-linear dose response for DNA damage and possibly NF-kappaB activation in oesophageal cells, with a mechanism of action involving ROS. Mutagenesis 23(5):399–405
56. Fitzgerald RC, Omary MB, Triadafilopoulos G (1996) Dynamic effects of acid on Barrett's esophagus. An ex vivo proliferation and differentiation model. J Clin Invest 98(9): 2120–2128
57. Fitzgerald R, Omary M, Triadafilopoulos G (1998) Altered sodium–hydrogen exchange activity is a mechanism for acid-induced hyperproliferation in Barrett's esophagus. Am J Physiol 275: G47–G55
58. Kaur BS, Triadafilopoulos G (2002) Acid- and bile-induced PGE(2) release and hyperproliferation in Barrett's esophagus are COX-2 and PKC-epsilon dependent. Am J Physiol Gastrointest Liver Physiol 283(2):G327–G334

59. Souza RF, Shewmake K, Pearson S, Sarosi GA Jr, Feagins LA, Ramirez RD et al (2004) Acid increases proliferation via ERK and p38 MAPK-mediated increases in cyclooxygenase-2 in Barrett's adenocarcinoma cells. Am J Physiol Gastrointest Liver Physiol 287(4):G743–G748
60. Hormi-Carver K, Zhang X, Zhang HY, Whitehead RH, Terada LS, Spechler SJ et al (2009) Unlike esophageal squamous cells, Barrett's epithelial cells resist apoptosis by activating the nuclear factor-kappaB pathway. Cancer Res 69(2):672–677
61. Konturek PC, Nikiforuk A, Kania J, Raithel M, Hahn EG, Muhldorfer S (2004) Activation of NFkappaB represents the central event in the neoplastic progression associated with Barrett's esophagus: a possible link to the inflammation and overexpression of COX-2, PPARgamma and growth factors. Dig Dis Sci 49(7–8):1075–1083
62. Fitzgerald RC, Onwuegbusi BA, Bajaj-Elliott M, Saeed IT, Burnham WR, Farthing MJ (2002) Diversity in the oesophageal phenotypic response to gastro-oesophageal reflux: immunological determinants. Gut 50(4):451–459
63. Abdalla SI, Lao-Sirieix P, Novelli MR, Lovat LB, Sanderson IR, Fitzgerald RC (2004) Gastrin-induced cyclooxygenase-2 expression in Barrett's carcinogenesis. Clin Cancer Res 10(14):4784–4792
64. Shirvani V, Ouatu-Luscar R, Kaur B, Omary M, Traidafilopoulos G (2000) Cyclo-oxygenase 2 expression in Barrett's esophagus and adenocarcinoma. ex vivo induction by bile salts and acid exposure. Gastroenterology 118(3):487–496
65. Capello A, Moons LM, Van de Winkel A, Siersema PD, van Dekken H, Kuipers EJ et al (2008) Bile acid-stimulated expression of the farnesoid X receptor enhances the immune response in Barrett esophagus. Am J Gastroenterol 103(6):1510–1516
66. Yen CJ, Izzo JG, Lee DF, Guha S, Wei Y, Wu TT et al (2008) Bile acid exposure up-regulates tuberous sclerosis complex 1/mammalian target of rapamycin pathway in Barrett's-associated esophageal adenocarcinoma. Cancer Res 68(8):2632–2640
67. Grivennikov S, Karin M (2008) Autocrine IL-6 signaling: a key event in tumorigenesis? Cancer Cell 13(1):7–9
68. Watanabe S, Hojo M, Nagahara A (2007) Metabolic syndrome and gastrointestinal diseases. J Gastroenterol 42(4):267–274
69. Ryan AM, Healy LA, Power DG, Byrne M, Murphy S, Byrne PJ et al (2008) Barrett esophagus: prevalence of central adiposity, metabolic syndrome, and a proinflammatory state. Ann Surg 247(6):909–915
70. Han ES, Muller FL, Perez VI, Qi W, Liang H, Xi L et al (2008) The in vivo gene expression signature of oxidative stress. Physiol Genomics 34(1):112–126
71. Peng DF, Razvi M, Chen H, Washington K, Roessner A, Schneider-Stock R et al (2009) DNA hypermethylation regulates the expression of members of the Mu-class glutathione S-transferases and glutathione peroxidases in Barrett's adenocarcinoma. Gut 58(1):5–15
72. Boult J, Roberts K, Brookes MJ, Hughes S, Bury JP, Cross SS et al (2008) Overexpression of cellular iron import proteins is associated with malignant progression of esophageal adenocarcinoma. Clin Cancer Res 14(2):379–387
73. Corley DA, Kubo A, Levin TR, Block G, Habel L, Rumore GJ et al (2008) Hemochromatosis gene status as a risk factor for Barrett's esophagus. Dig Dis Sci 53(12):3095–3102
74. Fitzgerald RC (2006) Molecular basis of Barrett's oesophagus and oesophageal adenocarcinoma. Gut 55(12):1810–1820
75. Wild CP, Hardie LJ (2003) Reflux, Barrett's oesophagus and adenocarcinoma: burning questions. Nat Rev Cancer 3(9):676–684
76. Maley CC, Galipeau PC, Li X, Sanchez CA, Paulson TG, Reid BJ (2004) Selectively advantageous mutations and hitchhikers in neoplasms: p16 lesions are selected in Barrett's esophagus. Cancer Res 64(10):3414–3427
77. Barrett MT, Sanchez CA, Neshat K, Galipeau PC, Reid BJ (1996) Allelic loss of 9p21 and mutations of the CDKN2/p16 gene develop as early events in neoplastic progression in Barrett's esophagus. Gastroenterology 110:A489
78. Barrett MT, Sanchez CA, Prevo LJ, Wong DJ, Galipeau PC, Paulson TG et al (1999) Evolution of neoplastic cell lineages in Barrett oesophagus. Nat Genet 22(1):106–109

79. Hardie LJ, Darnton SJ, Wallis YL, Chauhan A, Hainaut P, Wild CP et al (2005) p16 Expression in Barrett's esophagus and esophageal adenocarcinoma: association with genetic and epigenetic alterations. Cancer Lett 217(2):221–230
80. Chao DL, Sanchez CA, Galipeau PC, Blount PL, Paulson TG, Cowan DS et al (2008) Cell proliferation, cell cycle abnormalities, and cancer outcome in patients with Barrett's esophagus: a long-term prospective study. Clin Cancer Res 14(21):6988–6995
81. Wong DJ, Paulson TG, Prevo LJ, Galipeau PC, Longton G, Blount PL et al (2001) p16(INK4a) lesions are common, early abnormalities that undergo clonal expansion in Barrett's metaplastic epithelium. Cancer Res 61(22):8284–8289
82. Lai LA, Paulson TG, Li X, Sanchez CA, Maley C, Odze RD et al (2007) Increasing genomic instability during premalignant neoplastic progression revealed through high resolution array-CGH. Genes Chromosomes Cancer 46(6):532–542
83. Huang Y, Peters CJ, Fitzgerald RC, Gjerset RA (2009) Progressive silencing of p14ARF in oesophageal adenocarcinoma. J Cell Mol Med 13(2):398–409
84. Baker SJ, Preisinger AC, Jessup JM, Paraskeva C, Markowitz S, Willson JK et al (1990) p53 Gene mutations occur in combination with 17p allelic deletions as late events in colorectal tumorigenesis. Cancer Res 50(23):7717–7722
85. Reid BJ, Prevo LJ, Galipeau PC, Sanchez CA, Longton G, Levine DS et al (2001) Predictors of progression in Barrett's esophagus II: baseline 17p (p53) loss of heterozygosity identifies a patient subset at increased risk for neoplastic progression. Am J Gastroenterol 96(10):2839–2848
86. Murray L, Sedo A, Scott M, McManus D, Sloan JM, Hardie LJ, Forman D, Wild CP (2006) TP53 and progression from Barrett's metaplasia to oesophageal adenocarcinoma in a UK population cohort. Gut 55(10):1390–1397
87. Hong MK, Laskin WB, Herman BE, Johnston MH, Vargo JJ, Steinberg SM et al (1995) Expansion of the Ki-67 proliferative compartment correlates with degree of dysplasia in Barrett's esophagus. Cancer 72(2):423–429
88. Sirieix P, O'Donovan M, Brown J, Save V, Coleman N, RC F (2003) Surface expression of mini-chromosome maintenance proteins provides a novel method for detecting patients at risk for developing adeocarcinoma in Barrett's oesophagus. Clin Cancer Res 9(7):2560–2566
89. Williams GH, Swinn R, Prevost AT, De Clive-Lowe P, Halsall I, Going JJ et al (2004) Diagnosis of oesophageal cancer by detection of minichromosome maintenance 5 protein in gastric aspirates. Br J Cancer 91(4):714–719
90. Galipeau P, Cowan D, Sanchez C, Barrett M, Emond M, Levine D et al (1996) 17p (p53) Allelic losses, 4N (G_2/tetraploid) populations, and progression to aneuploidy in Barrett's esophagus. Proc Natl Acad Sci U S A 93:7081–7084
91. Bani-Hani K, Martin IG, Hardie LJ, Mapstone N, Briggs JA, Forman D et al (2000) Prospective study of cyclin D1 overexpression in Barrett's esophagus: association with increased risk of adenocarcinoma. J Natl Cancer Inst 92(16):1316–1321
92. Lao-Sirieix P, Brais R, Lovat L, Coleman N, Fitzgerald RC (2004) Cell cycle phase abnormalities do not account for disordered proliferation in Barrett's carcinogenesis. Neoplasia 6:751–760
93. Maley CC, Galipeau PC, Li X, Sanchez CA, Paulson TG, Blount PL et al (2004) The combination of genetic instability and clonal expansion predicts progression to esophageal adenocarcinoma. Cancer Res 64(20):7629–7633
94. Vaughan TL, Dong LM, Blount PL, Ayub K, Odze RD, Sanchez CA, Rabinovitch PS, Reid BJ (2005) Non-steroidal anti-inflammatory drugs and risk of neoplastic progression in Barrett's oesophagus: a prospective study. Lancet Oncol 6:945–952
95. Galipeau PC, Prevo LJ, Sanchez CA, Longton GM, Reid BJ (1999) Clonal expansion and loss of heterozygosity at chromosomes 9p and 17p in premalignant esophageal (Barrett's) tissue. J Natl Cancer Inst 91(24):2087–2095
96. Maley CC, Galipeau PC, Finley JC, Wongsurawat VJ, Li X, Sanchez CA et al (2006) Genetic clonal diversity predicts progression to esophageal adenocarcinoma. Nat Genet 38(4):468–473
97. Muzeau F, Flejou JF, Belghiti J, Thomas G, Hamelin R (1997) Infrequent microsatellite instability in oesophageal cancers. Br J Cancer 75(9):1336–1339

98. Williams BR, Prabhu VR, Hunter KE, Glazier CM, Whittaker CA, Housman DE et al (2008) Aneuploidy affects proliferation and spontaneous immortalization in mammalian cells. Science 322(5902):703–709
99. Cestari R, Villanacci V, Rossi E, Della Casa D, Missale G, Conio M et al (2007) Fluorescence in situ hybridization to evaluate dysplasia in Barrett's esophagus: a pilot study. Cancer Lett 251(2):278–287
100. Chaves P, Crespo M, Ribeiro C, Laranjeira C, Pereira AD, Suspiro A et al (2007) Chromosomal analysis of Barrett's cells: demonstration of instability and detection of the metaplastic lineage involved. Mod Pathol 20(7):788–796
101. Rabinovitch PS, Longton G, Blount PL, Levine DS, Reid BJ (2001) Predictors of progression in Barrett's esophagus III: baseline flow cytometric variables. Am J Gastroenterol 96(11):3071–3083
102. Paulson TG, Maley CC, Li X, Li H, Sanchez CA, Chao DL et al (2009) Chromosomal instability and copy number alterations in Barrett's esophagus and esophageal adenocarcinoma. Clin Cancer Res 15(10):3305–3314
103. Li X, Galipeau PC, Sanchez CA, Blount PL, Maley CC, Arnaudo J et al (2008) Single nucleotide polymorphism-based genome-wide chromosome copy change, loss of heterozygosity, and aneuploidy in Barrett's esophagus neoplastic progression. Cancer Prev Res (Phila Pa) 1(6):413–423
104. Wang J, Qin R, Ma Y, Wu H, Peters H, Tyska M et al (2009) Differential gene expression in normal esophagus and Barrett's esophagus. J Gastroenterol 44(9):897–911
105. Selaru FM, Zou T, Xu Y, Shustova V, Yin J, Mori Y et al (2002) Global gene expression profiling in Barrett's esophagus and esophageal cancer: a comparative analysis using cDNA microarrays. Oncogene 21(3):475–478
106. Hourihan RN, O'Sullivan GC, Morgan JG (2003) Transcriptional gene expression profiles of oesophageal adenocarcinoma and normal oesophageal tissues. Anticancer Res 23(1A):161–165
107. Greenawalt DM, Duong C, Smyth GK, Ciavarella ML, Thompson NJ, Tiang T et al (2007) Gene expression profiling of esophageal cancer: comparative analysis of Barrett's esophagus, adenocarcinoma, and squamous cell carcinoma. Int J Cancer 120(9):1914–1921
108. Xu Y, Selaru FM, Yin J, Zou TT, Shustova V, Mori Y et al (2002) Artificial neural networks and gene filtering distinguish between global gene expression profiles of Barrett's esophagus and esophageal cancer. Cancer Res 62(12):3493–3497
109. Smith E, De Young NJ, Pavey SJ, Hayward NK, Nancarrow DJ, Whiteman DC et al (2008) Similarity of aberrant DNA methylation in Barrett's esophagus and esophageal adenocarcinoma. Mol Cancer 7:75
110. Schulmann K, Sterian A, Berki A, Yin J, Sato F, Xu Y et al (2005) Inactivation of p16, RUNX3, and HPP1 occurs early in Barrett's-associated neoplastic progression and predicts progression risk. Oncogene 24(25):4138–4148
111. Jin Z, Mori Y, Yang J, Sato F, Ito T, Cheng Y et al (2007) Hypermethylation of the nel-like 1 gene is a common and early event and is associated with poor prognosis in early-stage esophageal adenocarcinoma. Oncogene 26(43):6332–6340
112. Jin Z, Mori Y, Hamilton JP, Olaru A, Sato F, Yang J et al (2008) Hypermethylation of the somatostatin promoter is a common, early event in human esophageal carcinogenesis. Cancer 112(1):43–49
113. Maru DM, Singh RR, Hannah C, Albarracin CT, Li YX, Abraham R et al (2009) MicroRNA-196a is a potential marker of progression during Barrett's metaplasia–dysplasia–invasive adenocarcinoma sequence in esophagus. Am J Pathol 174(5):1940–1948
114. Esquela-Kerscher A, Slack FJ (2006) Oncomirs – microRNAs with a role in cancer. Nat Rev Cancer 6(4):259–269
115. El-Serag HB, Nurgalieva ZZ, Mistretta TA, Finegold MJ, Souza R, Hilsenbeck S et al (2009) Gene expression in Barrett's esophagus: laser capture versus whole tissue. Scand J Gastroenterol 44(7):787–795

116. Sabo E, Meitner PA, Tavares R, Corless CL, Lauwers GY, Moss SF et al (2008) Expression analysis of Barrett's esophagus-associated high-grade dysplasia in laser capture microdissected archival tissue. Clin Cancer Res 14(20):6440–6448
117. Marx J (2008) Cancer biology. All in the stroma: cancer's Cosa Nostra. Science 320(5872): 38–41
118. Bhowmick NA, Neilson EG, Moses HL (2004) Stromal fibroblasts in cancer initiation and progression. Nature 432(7015):332–337
119. Mueller MM, Fusenig NE (2004) Friends or foes – bipolar effects of the tumour stroma in cancer. Nat Rev Cancer 4(11):839–849
120. Bhowmick NA, Chytil A, Plieth D, Gorska AE, Dumont N, Shappell S et al (2004) TGF-beta signaling in fibroblasts modulates the oncogenic potential of adjacent epithelia. Science 303(5659):848–851
121. Hao Y, Triadafilopoulos G, Sahbaie P, Young HS, Omary MB, Lowe AW (2006) Gene expression profiling reveals stromal genes expressed in common between Barrett's esophagus and adenocarcinoma. Gastroenterology 131(3):925–933
122. Saadi A, Shannon N, Lao-Sirieix P, O'Dononvan M, Walker E, Clemons N et al (2010) Stromal genes discriminate preinvasive from invasive disease, predict outcome, and highlight inflammatory pathways in digestive cancers. Proc Natl Acad Sci U S A 107(5): 2177–2182
123 Onwuegbusi BA, Aitchison A, Chin SF, Kranjac T, Mills I, Huang Y et al (2006) Impaired transforming growth factor beta signalling in Barrett's carcinogenesis due to frequent SMAD4 inactivation. Gut 55(6):764–774
124. Onwuegbusi BA, Rees JR, Lao-Sirieix P, Fitzgerald RC (2007) Selective loss of TGFbeta Smad-dependent signalling prevents cell cycle arrest and promotes invasion in oesophageal adenocarcinoma cell lines. PLoS One 2(1):e177
125. Mantovani A (2009) Cancer: inflaming metastasis. Nature 457(7225):36–37
126. Peng D, Sheta EA, Powell SM, Moskaluk CA, Washington K, Goldknopf IL et al (2008) Alterations in Barrett's-related adenocarcinomas: a proteomic approach. Int J Cancer 122(6):1303–1310
127. Langer R, Ott K, Specht K, Becker K, Lordick F, Burian M et al (2008) Protein expression profiling in esophageal adenocarcinoma patients indicates association of heat-shock protein 27 expression and chemotherapy response. Clin Cancer Res 14(24):8279–8287
128. Cameron A, Zinsmeister A, Ballard D, Carney J (1990) Prevalence of columnar-lined (Barrett's) esophagus. Comparison of population-based clinical and autopsy findings. Gatsroenterology 99:1918–1922
129. Shaheen NJ, Sharma P, Overholt BF, Wolfsen HC, Sampliner RE, Wang KK et al (2009) Radiofrequency ablation in Barrett's esophagus with dysplasia. N Engl J Med 360(22): 2277–2288
130. Pouw RE, Wirths K, Eisendrath P, Sondermeijer CM, Kate FJ, Fockens P et al (2010) Efficacy of radiofrequency ablation combined with endoscopic resection for Barrett's esophagus with early neoplasia. Clin Gastroenterol Hepatol 8(1):23–29
131. Das D, Chilton AP, Jankowski JA (2009) Chemoprevention of oesophageal cancer and the AspECT trial. Recent Results Cancer Res 181:161–169
132. Medical Research Council Oesophageal Cancer Working Group (2002) Surgical resection with or without preoperative chemotherapy in oesophageal cancer: a randomised controlled trial. Lancet 359(9319):1727–1733
133. Jobe BA, Hunter JG, Chang EY, Kim CY, Eisen GM, Robinson JD et al (2006) Office-based unsedated small-caliber endoscopy is equivalent to conventional sedated endoscopy in screening and surveillance for Barrett's esophagus: a randomized and blinded comparison. Am J Gastroenterol 101(12):2693–2703
134. Bhardwaj A, Hollenbeak CS, Pooran N, Mathew A (2009) A meta-analysis of the diagnostic accuracy of esophageal capsule endoscopy for Barrett's esophagus in patients with gastroesophageal reflux disease. Am J Gastroenterol 104(6):1533–1539

135. Ramirez FC, Akins R, Shaukat M (2008) Screening of Barrett's esophagus with string-capsule endoscopy: a prospective blinded study of 100 consecutive patients using histology as the criterion standard. Gastrointest Endosc 68(1):25–31
136. Lao-Sirieix P, Boussioutas A, Kadri SR, O'Donovan M, Debiram I, Das M, Harihar L, Fitzgerald RC (2009) Non-endoscopic screening biomarkers for Barrett's oesophagus: from microarray analysis to the clinic. Gut 58:1451–1459
137. Lao-Sirieix P, Rous B, O'Donovan M, Hardwick RH, Debiram I, Fitzgerald RC (2007) Non-endoscopic immunocytological screening test for Barrett's oesophagus. Gut 56(7): 1033–1034
138. Sharma P, Dent J, Armstrong D, Bergman JJ, Gossner L, Hoshihara Y et al (2006) The development and validation of an endoscopic grading system for Barrett's esophagus: the Prague C & M criteria. Gastroenterology 131(5):1392–1399
139. Pepe MS, Etzioni R, Feng Z, Potter JD, Thompson ML, Thornquist M et al (2001) Phases of biomarker development for early detection of cancer. J Natl Cancer Inst 93(14):1054–1061
140. Galipeau PC, Li X, Blount PL, Maley CC, Sanchez CA, Odze RD et al (2007) NSAIDs modulate CDKN2A, TP53, and DNA content risk for progression to esophageal adenocarcinoma. PLoS Med 4(2):e67
141. Rygiel AM, Milano F, Ten Kate FJ, de Groot JG, Peppelenbosch MP, Bergman JJ et al (2008) Assessment of chromosomal gains as compared to DNA content changes is more useful to detect dysplasia in Barrett's esophagus brush cytology specimens. Genes Chromosomes Cancer 47(5):396–404
142. Borovicka J, Schonegg R, Hell M, Kradolfer D, Bauerfeind P, Dorta G et al (2009) Is there an advantage to be gained from adding digital image cytometry of brush cytology to a standard biopsy protocol in patients with Barrett's esophagus? Endoscopy 41(5):409–414
143. Lin X, Finkelstein SD, Zhu B, Ujevich BJ, Silverman JF (2009) Loss of heterozygosities in Barrett esophagus, dysplasia, and adenocarcinoma detected by esophageal brushing cytology and gastroesophageal biopsy. Cancer Cytopathol 117(1):57–66
144. Wongsurawat VJ, Finley JC, Galipeau PC, Sanchez CA, Maley CC, Li X et al (2006) Genetic mechanisms of TP53 loss of heterozygosity in Barrett's esophagus: implications for biomarker validation. Cancer Epidemiol Biomarkers Prev 15(3):509–516
145. Sato F, Jin Z, Schulmann K, Wang J, Greenwald BD, Ito T et al (2008) Three-tiered risk stratification model to predict progression in Barrett's esophagus using epigenetic and clinical features. PLoS One 3(4):e1890
146. Hsiung PL, Hardy J, Friedland S, Soetikno R, Du CB, Wu AP et al (2008) Detection of colonic dysplasia in vivo using a targeted heptapeptide and confocal microendoscopy. Nat Med 14(4):454–458
147. Prasad GA, Wang KK, Halling KC, Buttar NS, Wongkeesong LM, Zinsmeister AR et al (2008) Correlation of histology with biomarker status after photodynamic therapy in Barrett esophagus. Cancer 113(3):470–476
148. Prasad GA, Wang KK, Halling KC, Buttar NS, Wongkeesong LM, Zinsmeister AR et al (2008) Utility of biomarkers in prediction of response to ablative therapy in Barrett's esophagus. Gastroenterology 135(2):370–379
149. Babar M, Ennis D, Abdel-Latif M, Byrne PJ, Ravi N, Reynolds JV (2010) Differential molecular changes in patients with asymptomatic long-segment Barrett's esophagus treated by antireflux surgery or medical therapy. Am J Surg 199(2):137–143
150. Ouatu-Luscar R, Fitzgerald R, Triadafilopoulos G (1999) Differentiation and proliferation in Barrett's esophagus and the effects of acid suppression. Gatsroenterology 117:327–335
151. El-Serag HB, Aguirre TV, Davis S, Kuebeler M, Bhattacharyya A, Sampliner RE (2004) Proton pump inhibitors are associated with reduced incidence of dysplasia in Barrett's esophagus. Am J Gastroenterol 99(10):1877–1883
152. Hillman LC, Chiragakis L, Shadbolt B, Kaye GL, Clarke AC (2004) Proton-pump inhibitor therapy and the development of dysplasia in patients with Barrett's oesophagus. Med J Aust 180:387–391

153. Gatenby PA, Ramus JR, Caygill CP, Charlett A, Winslet MC, Watson A (2009) Treatment modality and risk of development of dysplasia and adenocarcinoma in columnar-lined esophagus. Dis Esophagus 22(2):133–142
154. De Jonge PJ, Siersema PD, Van Breda SG, Van Zoest KP, Bac DJ, Leeuwenburgh I et al (2008) Proton pump inhibitor therapy in gastro-oesophageal reflux disease decreases the oesophageal immune response but does not reduce the formation of DNA adducts. Aliment Pharmacol Ther 28(1):127–136
155. Lagergren J, Viklund P (2007) Is esophageal adenocarcinoma occurring late after antireflux surgery due to persistent postoperative reflux? World J Surg 31(3):465–469
156. Corley DA, Kerlikowske K, Verma R, Buffler P (2003) Protective association of aspirin/NSAIDs and esophageal cancer: a systematic review and meta-analysis. Gastroenterology 124(1):47–56
157. Heath EI, Canto MI, Piantadosi S, Montgomery E, Weinstein WM, Herman JG et al (2007) Secondary chemoprevention of Barrett's esophagus with celecoxib: results of a randomized trial. J Natl Cancer Inst 99(7):545–557
158. Dong LM, Kristal AR, Peters U, Schenk JM, Sanchez CA, Rabinovitch PS et al (2008) Dietary supplement use and risk of neoplastic progression in esophageal adenocarcinoma: a prospective study. Nutr Cancer 60(1):39–48
159. Torrance CJ, Jackson PE, Montgomery E, Kinzler KW, Vogelstein B, Wissner A et al (2000) Combinatorial chemoprevention of intestinal neoplasia. Nat Med 6(9):1024–1028
160. Rossi E, Grisanti S, Villanacci V, Casa DD, Cengia P, Missale G et al (2009) Her-2 overexpression/amplification in Barrett's esophagus predicts early transition from dysplasia to adenocarcinoma: a clinico-pathologic study. J Cell Mol Med 13(9B):3826–3833
161. Harris JC, Clarke PA, Awan A, Jankowski J, Watson SA (2004) An antiapoptotic role for gastrin and the gastrin/CCK-2 receptor in Barrett's esophagus. Cancer Res. 15;64(6):1915
162. Kadri AR, Lao-Sirieix P, O'Dononvan M, Debiram I, Blazeby JM et al. Acceptability and accuracy of a non-endoscopic screening test for Barrett's oesophagus in primary care: cohort study BMJ 2010;341:4372

Chapter 17
Helicobacter Infection: Infection, Immunity and the Progression of Lesions to Invasive Gastric Cancer

Evelyn Kurt-Jones and JeanMarie Houghton

Abstract Many malignancies that arise in areas of inflammation progress through a series of architectural changes prior to becoming frankly malignant. These changes are often times linked to the acquisition of distinct genetic defects, and predictably the appearance of distinctive lesions depends upon these changes. Gastric cancer arising from Helicobacter infection is associated with architectural changes similar to those seen in other inflammatory driven malignancies. Tissue progresses from chronic active inflammation to atrophy. Within atrophic mucosa, metaplastic cell types begin to appear, and with long standing disease, adenocarcinoma can result. While temporally associated, it is not clear if the progression of changes from "premalignant" to malignant are causally related. Here we describe the sequence of events leading to the mucosal changes seen, and explore the data which relates these changes to the eventual appearance of gastric adenocarcinoma.

Gastric Cancer: Background and History

Gastric cancer remains the second leading cause of cancer related deaths worldwide, accounting for 650,000 deaths per year. Until about 25 years ago, the cause of gastric cancer was largely an enigma. However with the discovery of *Helicobacter pylori*, our understanding of the etiology of gastric cancer, and particularly distal gastric cancer, has improved dramatically. Here we will review how Helicobacter colonization alters the gastric environment and impacts the mucosal architecture leading to preinvasive and invasive disease.

J.M. Houghton (✉)
Department of Cancer Biology, University of Massachusetts Medical School,
LRB 2nd floor 209, 364 Plantation Street, Worcester 01635, MA, USA
e-mail: jeanmarie.houghton@umassmed.edu

R.C. Fitzgerald (ed.), *Pre-Invasive Disease: Pathogenesis and Clinical Management*,
DOI 10.1007/978-1-4419-6694-0_17,

Helicobacter Infection: An Overview

Helicobacter pylori is a gram-negative microaerophilic bacterium which is perhaps the most common chronic infection in the world, competing with *Streptococcus mutans*, a leading cause of dental caries, for first place distinction. Warren and Marshall first identified and cultured *Helicobacter pylori* (then named *Campylobacter pylori*) in 1982 and developed their hypothesis that Helicobacter infection was the cause of peptic ulcer disease 1984. After attempts to infect piglets with the bacterium failed, Marshall ingested bacterial culture obtained from a patient's gastric biopsy and became the first documented acute *Helicobacter pylori* infection. He quickly developed symptomatic gastritis [1], thus opening a new direction of research in the field of gastroenterology. By the early to mid 1990s, *Helicobacter pylori* was accepted as the cause of antral gastritis, gastric and duodenal ulcers, gastric adenocarcinoma and gastric MALT lymphoma.

Since the discovery of a bacterial origin of gastric cancer, research has focused on several areas of interest including bacterial factors [2], immune response [3–7], environmental factors [8, 9] and host genetics [10–13]. This chapter will focus on the impact of mucosal changes and the relationship, and progression of premalignant to invasive disease.

General Bacterial Features

H. pylori is a microaerophilic gram-negative spiral bacterium, approximately 3 μm long and 0.5 μm wide. It contains a hydrogenase which is used to oxidizing molecular hydrogen produced by intestinal bacteria, for its own energy source. The bacterium also produces urease, oxidase and catalase. It is capable of forming biofilms, a complex protective matrix created by the bacteria which affords sessile bacteria protection from the local environment, allows growth in hostile environments, and alters host physiology [14]. The bacterium can exist as an active spiral form, or as a viable but metabolically inactive (and therefore poorly cultured and detectable) coccoid form. *H. pylori* possesses five major outer membrane protein (OMP) families. The largest family is the adhesins. Other families include porins, iron transporters, flagellum-associated proteins, and other proteins of unclear function [15]. *H. pylori* has a weak LPS, and elicits a weak immune response (relative to strong LPS producers such as *E. coli*) [16]. The O antigen of LPS may be fucosylated and mimic Lewis blood group antigens found on the gastric epithelium, further contributing to immune response to the bacteria [16]. *H. pylori* has 4–6 flagella making this organism highly motile, which is a necessary attribute for successful colonization [17].

Bacterial Colonization of the Stomach

The first step in the process of Hp induced mucosal alterations, begins with bacterial colonization. To successfully colonize the stomach, *H. pylori* must first survive the acidic pH of the stomach long enough to penetrate through the protective mucus layer and either adhere to or at least remain near the gastric epithelial cell surface. This task is accomplished effectively by several necessary attributes of the bacterium. Perhaps most important is the organisms highly motile nature. Bacterial flagella allow the rapid and directed movement of ingested bacteria through the mucus layer. By sensing pH gradients, the bacteria are able to migrate away from the acidic lumen, toward the more neutral pH at the cell surface. A combination of collagenases [18] and proteases secreted by the bacteria alter the viscosity of the mucus overlying the gastric mucosa making penetration easier. After successful penetration and colonization, direct contact of the bacteria with the gastric epithelium affects mucosal gene expression such that the type of mucus produced by epithelial cells [19] is altered. This change leads to further increased mobility of bacteria along the mucosal surface, allowing the bacterium to spread. The bacterium adheres to the epithelial layer using a large family of 32 related outer-membrane proteins (Hop proteins) that include the adhesions which bind to membrane-associated carbohydrates and lipids. One of the best characterized adhesin is BabA, encoded by the strain-specific gene *babA2*, a member of a highly conserved family of outer membrane proteins. BabA binds to the fucosylated Lewis B blood group antigen present on gastric epithelial cells and acts as a scaffold for bacterial growth. Bacterial strains which posses the *babA2* gene adhere more tightly to epithelial cells and promote a more aggressive clinical infection, higher incidence of preinvasive architectural changes in the mucosa and a higher incidence of gastric adenocarcinoma. Animal studies using transgenic mice carrying the Lewis B blood group antigen are more likely to develop severe gastritis, atrophy and anti-parietal cell antibodies when challenged with babA+ *H. pylori* strains then when challenged with babA- strains of bacteria [20]. It is presumed that this increase in clinical disease is due to increased bacterial adherence to mucosal cells causing an augmented host immune response. From these and other studies, a direct role for babA+ in cancer has been implied; however, it has not been conclusively proven.

Urease Production

In addition, *H. pylori* produces large amounts of the enzyme urease, which breaks down urea within the stomach. The breakdown of urea produces carbon dioxide and ammonia with the ultimate outcome of bicarbonate production which neutralizes gastric acid. The survival of *H. pylori* in the stomach is dependent on urease because the bacteria requires a neutral pH for continued growth and survival. In addition to changes in pH affecting the gastric mucosal environment, ammonia and other secreted products are toxic to epithelial cells and may lead directly to mucosal damage.

Clinical Disease Overview

Colonization of the stomach by *H. pylori* results in a chronic active gastritis, composed of both neutrophils and lymphocytes infiltrating the submucosa and intraepithelial space between gastric glands. Colonization elicits both an innate and adaptive response, with ineffective antibody production. Though there are reports of early spontaneous clearing of infection in some patients, the majority of patients have lifelong persistent infection.

Infected patients all develop a chronic active gastritis, however, the majority of patients remain asymptomatic. Though the risk varies with age, geographical location and ethnicity, overall fifteen to twenty percent of infected patients will develop gastric or duodenal ulcer disease and from less than 1% to 3% of patients will develop gastric adenocarcinoma [21, 22] or MALT lymphoma. Unfortunately, symptoms and disease are poorly correlated, and many cases of gastric cancer are detected late in disease progression, when they are incurable. Like many cancers which arise in chronically inflamed tissue, the progression to gastric cancer is associated with distinct histological changes within the mucosa. It is still debated if these alterations mark "at risk tissue," are direct precursors to cancer, or are merely associated with the same environment but not linked causally.

In order to understand the association of mucosal changes with the development of cancer, we must first understand the myriad of changes that occur during the course of Helicobacter infection. Infection induces a gastritis which can be broadly classified into one of two patterns – antral predominant gastritis and pan gastritis. The pattern of gastritis has been shown to correlate strongly with the risk of developing gastric adenocarcinoma and with the appearance of cellular changes thought to be premalignant. Patients who develop antral-predominant gastritis (the most common manifestation) are at a higher risk of developing duodenal ulcers, while those that develop corpus-predominant gastritis and multifocal atrophic gastritis are at a higher risk of developing gastric ulcers, and of progressing to intestinal metaplasia, dysplasia and adenocarcinoma [23].

Gastric cancers arising distal to the gastric cardia (which are considered more part of the spectrum of gastro-oesophageal adenocarcinomas) are divided into two histologically distinct types termed intestinal type adenocarcinoma and diffuse type adenocarcinoma [24]. Intestinal-type gastric adenocarcinoma forms gland-like structures [25] and arises after the mucosa has progressed through a stepwise series of changes from normal mucosa through atrophic gastritis, atrophy, and intestinal metaplasia. These have been termed the so called "premalignant lesions" though it must be stressed that this is an area of controversy. It is in the setting of atrophy and metaplasia that dysplasia arises, and overtime a stomach that contains these lesions my progress to adenocarcinoma [26], however the point of transition from a "premalignant" to "malignant" lesion has not been identified, nor is it clear if one lesion is actually a precursor of the next in the sequence of events. In contrast to intestinal type gastric cancer, diffuse-type gastric cancer is composed of individual neoplastic cells which infiltrate the gastric mucosa without forming glandular structures. There is no associated atrophy or intestinal metaplasia, and there is no stepwise progression as suggested in intestinal type cancer [27]. There is a stronger genetic component to the diffuse type of gastric cancer. For this chapter, we will focus our discussion on intestinal-type gastric adenocarcinoma, and the architectural changes that are associated with it.

Host Immunity Determines Disease Outcome

An important determinant of Helicobacter-related disease is the host immune response. And indeed- it is clear that chronic inflammation is necessary for both the mucosal alterations of atrophy/metaplasia/dysplasia and adenocarcioma. We will begin by defining what we know about the initial events in immune recognition of the bacterium, and outline how the polarity and strength of the adaptive response impacts disease outcomes by the effect it has on the mucosal architecture.

The Innate Immune Response to H. pylori

TLR 2 and TLR 4

Helicobacter activates several different classes of innate immune receptors including the Toll-like receptors (TLRs) on the cell surface (TLR2 and TLR4) and within endosomes (TLR9), as well as cytosolic NOD1 and helicase (RIG-I) receptors [28–30]. Whole Helicobacter bacteria (*H. pylori, H. hepaticus* and *H. felis*) activate immune response in macrophages by TLR2, but not TLR4, the classic Gram negative LPS receptor [28]. Indeed, expression of human TLR2 has been shown to be sufficient to confer responsiveness to intact Helicobacter bacteria, whereas TLR4 was not. Cag pathogenicity island genes may modulate the TLR2-agonist activity of *H. pylori* as CagA+ bacteria are more active on a per cell basis compared to cagA- bacteria when response is measured by IL-8 cytokine secretion [28]. In contrast, macrophages from both wild type and TLR-4 deficient mice produce a robust cytokine secretion response (IL-6 and MCP1) when stimulated with intact Helicobacter bacteria, while macrophages from TLR2-deficient mice were profoundly unresponsive to intact bacteria, failing to secrete cytokines even at high (100:1) bacteria-to-macrophage ratios. Because the quantity and strength of bacterial LPS is so weak, the involvement of TLR4 in clinical disease is unclear and in vitro and in vivo studies suggest that TLR2 may be the dominant innate immune receptor for recognition of gastrointestinal Helicobacter species [28].

Helicobacter produces a tetracylated LPS that is up to 10,000-folds less active then LPS of other gram-negative bacteria, such as *E. coli* [32–34]. While we know that LPS from gram-negative bacteria, such as *E. coli*, predominantly stimulate innate immunity through TLR4, the LPS of some gram negative organisms such as *Poryphorymonas gingivalis* activate TLR2 [35]. Data regarding *H. pylori* LPS are contradictory, with reports of activation of both TLR4 [36, 37] and TLR2 [29] in gastric epithelial cells. These contradictions may be explained by differences in bacterial strain, different bacterial concentrations used or trace contaminants in the LPS preparations such as peptidoglycan or lipopeptides, both which signal via TLR2 receptor.

TRL-5

Flagellin proteins are recognized by TLR-5, however a physiologic role for TLR-5 in Helicobacter recognition has not been established. In culture, gastric mucosal cells express low but detectable amounts of TLR-5 [38], but neither FlaA nor FlaB appear to have immunostimulatory potential on gastric cells. However the HEK293 (human embryonic kidney cells 293) cell line when transfected with TLR5 is able to respond to partially purified flagellin from *H. pylori* [29].

TLR9

Dendritic cells phagocytose Helicobacter bacteria and activate additional intracellular receptors including TLR9 in the endosomes, and NOD1 and RIG-I in the cytosol [30, 31]. NOD1 is a receptor for peptidoglycan while TLR9 is activated by CpG rich DNA. TLR9 is also triggered by the sugar backbone of dsDNA [39]. It is thought that the endosomal location of TLR9 prevent its activation by self-DNA while directing TLR9 to phagocytosed DNA [40].

Interaction between TLR9 and CpGs molecules in the endosome recruits the MyD88 adapter protein and triggers a strong Th1 immune response [40]. While there is no direct data linking the immune response to Helicobacter with Helicobacter-specific CpG sequences, a role for TLR9 in pathogenesis of Helicobacter related disease has been suggested. TLR2, like TLR9, is also linked to Th1 immune responses. A Th1 immune response, while associated with more severe damage, is also associated with decreased bacterial loads [41]. Oral administration of CpGs ODN concomitant with Helicobacter in a mouse model of infection limits the extent of *Helicobacter pylori* colonization [41]. Intragastric administration of a single dose of CpG ODN significantly increased the production of local chemokines and cytokines (MIP1alpha, MIP1beta, RANTES and IFN gamma inducible protein 10) in the stomach and small intestine, with reduced bacterial load in pre-established infection models. Consistent with a role for Th1 cytokines in initiating and perpetuating the mucosal damage of Helicobacter, mice infected with *H. pylori* and treated with CpGs ODN had higher levels of mucosal inflammation compared to controls which were infected but did not receive CpG ODN, or that received non-CpG ODN [41], suggesting that CpG from Helicobacter influences the immune response to acute and established Helicobacter infections.

Which Cells Act As the First Line of Recognition?

While the cell type responsible for initiation of the immune response has not been identified, it is possible that the gastric immune cells themselves act as the first line of recognition. Gastric epithelial cells reportedly fail to express TLR2 on their surface [42], but they do express TLR4 [37]. However, in vitro work suggests TLR2, -4, and -5 may all be expressed [29]. In addition to LPS acting locally, it may gain access to the blood stream to be detected by peripheral blood monocytes [43].

The innate immune response to Helicobacter, particularly the dendritic cell response, drives the adaptive immune response to the bacteria [31, 44, 45]. Differences in the response of different inbred mouse strains to Helicobacter infection have been suggested to reflect differences in expression and function of Toll-like receptors in dendritic cells from Balb/C (resistant host) and C57BL/6 (susceptible host) mice to the corresponding ligands [45]. Freshly isolated splenic dendritic cells from C57BL/6 express higher levels of TLR9 mRNA and lower levels of TLR2, -4, -5 and -6 mRNAs than Balb/C dendritic cells. LPS, lipoprotein, and CpG produced higher levels of IL-12 and lower levels of monocyte chemoattractant protein 1 (MCP-1) in C57BL/6 dendritic cells compared to those from the Balb/C. DC maturation markers such as CD40, CD86 and Stat4 are expressed in higher levels in DC from C57BL/6 mice then Balb/C mice [46]. These differences in innate immune response may help explain the subsequent differences in adaptive immunity to Helicobacter infection between the C57BL/6 and Balb/C mouse stains. TLRs signaling are required only for Th1 type of adaptive immunity, not for the development of Th2 type lymphocyte subsets. Th2 cells are most likely activated by another distinctive (but presently unknown) pathway. In the absence of induced IL-12 production by dendritic cells, a Th2 response appears to the "default" pathway [47]. Additional differences between the Balb/C and C57BL/6 mice include an exuberant PGE2 response by Balb/C macrophages, which may further inhibit a Th1 response upon LPS stimulation [48].

Adaptive Immunity to Helicobacter Infection

Most of our information regarding the effects of the immune system on gastric mucosal damage comes from mouse models of infection (Table 17.1). For example the role of the inflammatory response in the pathogenesis of gastric cancer began by determining that T-cells were vital for mucosal damage. Infection in recombinase activating gene (RAG) deficient mice, severe combined immunodeficiency (SCID) mice, and T-cell deficient mice failed to produce tissue damage or recreate the metaplasia-dysplasia-carcinoma sequence [3, 49] despite active bacterial colonization. B-cell responses are not necessary for mucosal disease as shown by infection in B cell-deficient mice (which retain a normal T-cell response) which develop infection and disease indistinguishable from that found in the wild type mice of the same strain. These findings stress a crucial role for CD4 T-lymphocytes in defining disease [49]. To further define the mechanism of disease progression, Th1/Th2 cytokine patterns were evaluated between different strains of mice and compared to their susceptibility to disease. Strains of mice

Table 17.1 Mouse models which have shaped our understanding of Helicobacter induced gastric cancer

Mouse model	Susceptible/resistant	Immune response/histology in response to Helicobacter infection
C57BL/6	Susceptible	Th1 response. "Classic" model for progression of mucosal changes to adenocarcinoma
Balb/C	Resistant	Th2 response. Immune infiltrates, with mucosal sparing. Develops MALT lymphoma
C3H	Mixed	Mixed Th1/Th2 cytokine pattern with mixed mucosal changes
SCID	Resistant	B cell and T cell deficient. Resistant to mucosal damage
Rag deficient	Resistant	B cell and T cell deficient. Resistant to mucosal damage
B-cell deficient	Susceptible	Lack mature B cell function. In the C57BL/6 background, maintain progression of mucosal changes to adenocarcinoma
IFN KO	Resistant	Immune infiltrates without parietal and chief cell loss (no atrophy). Resistant to adenocarcinoma
IL-10 KO	Susceptible	Severe unrelenting inflammation with mucosal damage and adenocarcinoma formation
T-bet KO	Resistant	Mixed mucosal cytokine pattern with elevated IL10 and low TNF-alpha and IL-1beta. Intermediate IFN gamma levels. Mucosal sparing
Fas Ag KO	Susceptible	Preservation of parietal and chief cells. Progression of metaplasia and dysplasia to adenocarcinoma
Fas L KO	Susceptible	Preservation of parietal and chief cells. Progression of metaplasia and dysplasia to adenocarcinoma

which are susceptible to helicobacter induced gastric atrophy and adenocarcinoma (such as the C57BL/6) mounts a strong Th1 response [5, 7] and strains such as the BALB/c which are resistant to developing atrophy and adenocarcinoma develop a polarized Th2 cytokine response [5]. Interestingly, strains such as the C3H, which have a mixed Th1/Th2 cytokine profile develop an intermediate pattern of disease and more closely represent the diverse disease presentation seen in humans. These findings suggest that cytokines within an immune response interact to form a continuum of disease rather than discrete disease states. Several studies have examined the role of individual cytokines in disease progression, however, these studies must be interpreted cautiously as over expression or knockout of an individual cytokine impacts the expression and function of other signaling cascades. Therefore, effects seen may be direct, or may be due to the effects of secondary pathways. For example, the IFN-γ knockout mouse does not develop Helicobacter induced atrophy [5, 7], while IFN-γ infusion into the infected C57BL/6 mouse accelerates disease progression [50]. The IL-10 knockout develops severe atrophic gastritis [5, 7], possibly due to the inability to contain the immune response. To further address this issue, we and others have physiologically manipulated the immune response within wild type strains. Infection of the susceptible strain, C57BL/6 with *Heligmosomoides polygyrus,* an intestinal helminth, skews the immune response to subsequent Helicobacter infection towards a Th2 polarized response and protects against atrophy and metaplasia [51]. Looking at the flip side of this immunological coin, co-infection with *Toxoplasma gondii* in the Balb/C mouse forces a Th1 skewed response to Helicobacter infection. These mice develop atrophy, metaplasia and dysplasia [52] essentially converting a resistant mouse strain to a susceptible strain. Additional work taking advantage of the T-bet knock out (T-bet KO) mouse has been done to sort out the impact of cytokines. T-bet is a member of the T-box family of transcription factors, and appears to regulate the commitment of Th cells to the Th1 lineage at least in part through transactivation of IFN-γ [53]. T-bet KO mice have several immune defects including the inability to mount a Th1 immune response and markedly impaired IFN-γ production in natural killer cells. IFN-γ production in cytotoxic CD8+ T cell remains intact. We used the T-bet KO mouse to directly assess Th1 responses in the C57BL/6 mouse model with minimal alterations of other immune functions, without the effects of global cytokine deficiency seen in other transgenic models and without the confounding effects of other coexisting infectious diseases. T-bet knockout mice in the C57BL/6 background or their wild type (WT) liter mates were infected with *Helicobacter felis* (*H. felis*) and followed for up to 15 months for disease progression. Analysis of mucosal cytokine patterns and *H. felis* specific IgG subclass analysis confirmed a blunted Th1 response in the T-bet KO mice. WT mice showed the expected progression of tissue alterations beginning with metaplasia and atrophy and continuing to dysplasia and carcinoma. In sharp contrast, the T-bet KO mice did not develop atrophy, and instead maintained parietal and chief cell populations, mucosal integrity and failed to develop adenocarcioma. Interestingly, when the composite cytokine profiles within the gastric mucosa were examined, there was a clear association between IL1-β and TNF-α in the pathogenesis of Helicobacter induced gastric adenocarcinoma [54]. Surprisingly, a direct role for IFN-γ was not shown. The cytokine pattern in these mouse models parallel cytokine patterns seen in susceptible human populations suggesting differences in T-bet regulation may underlie the mucosal alterations and susceptibility to gastric cancer in human populations.

Indeed, when one looks at the data emerging from human population based studies, interleukin-1 β, TNF-α and IL-10 emerge as key players. Patients with genetic polymorphisms that create a gastric inflammatory environment significant for high levels of IL-1β, TNF-α and low IL-10 have a 50-fold increased risk of gastric cancer as a result of Helicobacter infection [12, 13, 55].

Alterations in Gastric Mucosal Signaling; Regulation of Apoptotic and Proliferative Pathways Underlying the Development of Atrophy

How exactly do cytokines within the gastric mucosal environment effect the mucosal changes we characterize as "premalignant"? The host response to infection induces multiple changes within the gastric mucosa leading up to the formation of adenocarcinoma. Early on in infection, the balance between apoptosis and proliferation is distorted resulting in changes in the number and type of cells within the mucosa. Metaplastic lineages emerge, likely as a result of altered cell–cell signaling.

Helicobacter pylori in humans has been associated with both an increase and decrease in apoptosis, depending upon the cell population studied and the timing of the investigation [56, 57]. Increase in proliferation appears to be a universal finding. Apoptosis and proliferation are intimately linked physiologic processes and the regulation of these pathways is best discussed together. Apoptosis is a physiological process of cell death which is a defense against propagating damaged cells. High levels of apoptosis relative to proliferation, likely result in ulcer formation and the drop out of chief and parietal cells which are the hallmark of atrophy. On the other hand dysregulated proliferation may lead to transformation of cells leading to gastric adenocarcinoma. There are many pathways that regulate proliferation and apoptosis.

One pathway which has received the most attention with regard to Helicobacter induced disease is the Fas Ag (CD95) pathway which is responsible for the majority of apoptosis seen secondary to infection. *Helicobacter* bacteria directly and indirectly (through cytokine production) induces Fas Ag and Fas ligand expression on gastric epithelial cells. [56–61]. In non-transformed cell cultures, direct bacterial contact does not appear sufficient for induction and activation of the Fas Ag pathway, but instead requires cytokines generated by the host immune response to infection. On the other hand, *Helicobacter pylori* can directly induce and activate the Fas pathway in transformed cell lines [57] without the requirement of a conducive immune response, suggesting significant differences in the response by epithelial cells before and after malignant transformation. Importantly, Fas signaling can be utilized by metaplastic, dysplastic and malignant cells for proliferative signaling as well, essentially converting a tumor suppressor to a tumor promoter as disease progresses.

Our laboratory has shown that IL1-β, TNF-α and to a lesser degree IFN-γ within the gastric mucosa [54, 61] regulates surface Fas Ag expression on gastric mucosal cells. At low receptor abundance, activation of the Fas pathway leads to proliferation while at high receptor abundance, cells undergo apoptosis [62]. Parietal and chief cells appear to carry the highest levels of surface receptor and therefore are preferentially lost to apoptosis. This leads to several substantial alterations within the mucosa which have profound effects long term. Several mouse models have been used to investigate the role of Fas mediated apoptosis in gastric cancer. The B.6MRL-FAS^{lpr} (*lpr*) Fas Ag knockout mouse lacks Fas Ag protein and subsequently is deficient in all downstream signaling. This mouse is resistant to *Helicobacter* induced apoptosis and atrophy [60]. Long term infection in the mouse lacking Fas Ag presents the curious combination of intact parietal and chief cell lineages and an earlier onset of gastric cancer [63] suggesting that Fas mediated apoptosis not only eliminates parietal and chief cell populations, but may also function to remove cells at risk for neoplastic transformation. Fas L (gld) deficient mice show a similar phenotype, in that they develop more severe premalignant mucosal changes in response to infection with *H. pylori* [64] further supporting anti-apoptotic mechanisms in the development of gastric adenocarcinoma.

We hypothesize that in addition to apoptotic signaling, non-apoptotic Fas signaling is important in gastric mucosal disease. As the *lpr* mouse lacks all Fas signaling, it cannot be used as a model to address the contribution of alternate Fas signaling pathways in gastric disease, and this question will require additional models for study.

With ongoing tissue destruction, proliferation is increased and homeostasis is maintained at the cost of increased cell turnover. Persistent infection leads to metaplastic and dysplastic populations of cells which become resistant to Fas mediated apoptosis [65, 66] and may use the Fas pathway instead for proliferative signaling [62].

Once cells transform, factors that alter the immune-mediated removal of tumor cells may be important for continued tumor survival. Fas ligand is not normally expressed by gastric mucosal cells, but is highly expressed on the surface of intestinal type tumors, and at much lower abundance on diffuse type gastric carcinoma. The tumor cells themselves are apoptosis resistant through a variety of mechanisms [65–68]. Expression of Fas L on gastric mucosal cell which have acquired apoptosis resistance, may allow self-signaling, and stimulation of adjacent cells for proliferation. Also, lymphocytes infiltrating Fas L-bearing tumors undergo apoptosis at a high rate, implying that Fas L may be involved in a tumor initiated immune-counter attack [69–71]. This differential expression of Fas L suggests that intestinal and diffuse types of gastric carcinoma may arise through distinct mechanisms.

In addition to the Fas pathway, there are several other mechanisms for apoptotic cell death within the infected/inflamed gastric mucosa. TNF-α and IFN-γ can directly induce apoptosis [72–75] and nitric-oxide- can directly influence mitochondrial pathways of apoptosis [76], and contributes to signal transduction alterations at multiple levels during infections.

Expression of MHCII may play a role in gastric carcinogenesis. Cells expressing MHCII bind Helicobacter, process antigens and present them to lymphocytes to initiate and perpetuate the immune response. Under usual conditions, MHCII molecules are not expressed on gastric epithelial cells but they can be upregulated during Helicobacter infection by IFN-γ [68, 77–80]. MHCII expressing gastric mucosal cells are able to weakly present antigens [68, 80, 81]. Binding of *H. pylori* to MHCII induces apoptosis in cultured cells [79], suggesting alternate functions for this complex. Indeed, gastric mucosal cells co-expressing Fas Ag and MHCII molecules are resistant to Fas mediated apoptosis via impaired receptor aggregation and DISC (death inducing signal complex) formation [68]. Different MHCII alleles may interact with the bacterium and/or the Fas pathway differently, potentially explaining differences in gastric cancer susceptibility. For example, patients who have the MHC DQA1*0102 allele have an increased risk of intestinal type gastric adenocarcinoma [82], compared to patients without this allele.

Bacterial factors such as VacA, which has been reported to insert directly into the membrane of mitochondria, leading to cytochrome c release and apoptosis [83] may directly induce apoptosis of gastric mucosal cells. Apoptosis leads to cell loss, which is replaced through ramped up proliferation. Unlike normal proliferation, proliferation within areas of chronic injury and repair is an ongoing event, and not self limited. As such, many growth control mechanisms are bypassed, predisposing cells to acquiring and perpetuating mutations. Apoptosis also leads to an altered mucosal architecture. Parietal and chief cells are lost, and over time may be inadequately replaced. This loss of specialized cells, the hallmark of atrophy, likely results from a combination of events including reversible environmental influences on progenitor cell differentiation [84] and later on from permanent alterations to progenitor populations [85]. This atrophy has dire consequences for the gastric epithelium.

In addition to the immune response of the host regulating proliferation and apoptosis, bacterial products may also play a role in growth decisions. CagA protein interacts with the Ras/MEK/ERK pathway [86] and the Src family of protein-tyrosine kinases [87] which may explain differences in apoptosis/proliferation between individuals infected with different strains of *Helicobacter pylori* [57, 58, 88, 89]. Higher proliferation and lower apoptosis rates have been reported in patients infected with cagA+ isolates compared to those infected with cagA- strains, or uninfected controls [90, 91]. Also, activation of the Erk pathway in gastric epithelial cells may direct Fas signaling to proliferative signaling [92].

Endocrine Regulation of Proliferation

Gastrin is a peptide hormone produced primarily by G-cells located in the gastric antrum. G-cells are activated by neural and hormonal factors, intraluminal contents and by mechanical stimulation through protein kinase A activation, cAMP signaling and mitogen-activated protein kinase phosphorylation [93]. Alterations in gastrin levels seen during Helicobacter infection may be directly related to alterations in luminal acidity, direct effects of the bacteria and alterations in parietal cell number [94]. In addition to regulation of gastric acid secretion, gastrin has been shown to regulate oxyntic gland proliferation, and may directly synergize with *Helicobacter* to induce cell growth alterations and gastric tissue damage.

The gastrin expression pattern of the insulin-gastrin (INS-GAS) transgenic mouse mimics the serum G-17/G-gly profile seen in patients who develop gastric atrophy and cancer. Helicobacter infection in these mice produce an early increase in acid secretion followed over time by atrophy, achlorhydria, hyperplasia, metaplasia, dysplasia and invasive gastric cancer by 8 months of age [95].

Direct Effects of Inflammation on the Gastric Mucosa May Lead to Mutations Within Progenitor Cells

Ongoing inflammation generates mutagenic substances such as reactive nitrogen species (nitric oxide, peroxynitrite, nitrogen dioxide, nitrosoperoxy carbonate) [96] and reactive oxygen species (superoxide anions, hydrogen peroxide, hydroxyl and hydroperoxyl radicals) [97] which can directly damage DNA. These reactive nitrogen and oxygen species can also directly alter cell growth and cell death pathways [98–100]. *H. pylori* itself may also decrease the antioxidant properties of the gastric mucosa, thus leading to damage by these reactive species [101].

Cell–Cell Cross Talk and Signal Disruption Leading to Premalignant Disease

Parietal Cells as the Regulator of Cell Differentiation

Parietal cell loss is temporally associated with atrophy, mucous cell metaplasia and initiation of dysplastic changes [4], suggesting a cause and effect relationship. In addition to production of acid, the parietal cell regulates key differentiation decisions in the fundic oxyntic glands. Ablation of parietal cells is associated with the appearance and expansion of undifferentiated cell types. Is this coincidental parietal cell loss and abnormal differentiation of cells, only temporally related because of some environmental changes driving both phenotypes simultaneously? Or does parietal cell loss lead to these changes? The experimental data to date strongly supports the latter. Parietal cells secrete a number of factors which are important for the differentiation and growth of gastric progenitor cells. For example, parietal cells are a rich source of sonic hedge hog (Shh), one of a family of Hedgehog proteins which have a central role in embryonic development of the gut. Within the stomach, hedgehog signaling is responsible for gastric epithelial cell differentiation and maturation at least in part through Shh effect on bone morphogenic protein and hepatocyte nuclear factor 3β [102]. Parietal cells can also be induced to secrete a variety of growth factors. Cytokines such as IL-1β and hormones such as gastrin stimulate secretion of heparin binding epidermal growth factor and amphiregulin [103] from parietal cells, which in turn induces proliferation of surrounding epithelial cells. Early in helicobacter infection, parietal cell signaling is intact, and normal parietal signaling results in gastric mucosal cell proliferation, ordered differentiation and maturation of cells aimed at maintaining the injured or damaged epithelium. As infection progresses and parietal cells are lost to apoptosis, a severe distortion of differentiation signals leads to atrophy, metaplasia and disordered growth of gastric progenitor cells [104]. Indeed, dysregulated proliferation of poorly differentiated precursor cells is often associated with the appearance of a mucus neck cell lineage expressing trefoil factor 2 (TFF2) or spasmolytic polypeptide (SP). TFF2 is felt to have a physiological a role in cytoprotection and maintenance of mucosal integrity and repair [105, 106] because it is usually expressed at the edges of healing ulcers, with down regulation of expression once restitution and healing are complete. Continued expression of TFF2 is seen in mucous cell metaplasia and is associated with dysplasia and progression to cancer. However it is not clear if TFF2 marks a population of cells which have not down-regulated their "repair" phenotype, or if TFF2 expression is causally related to progression to premalignant histology. Parietal cell loss also leads to hypocholorhydria, hypergastrinemia, and bacterial overgrowth which may contribute independently to tissue damage and abnormal cell signaling.

Are "Premalignant Lesions" Really Premalignant?

Long-standing helicobacter infection is the leading cause of gastric cancer. Atrophy and intestinal metaplasia have been linked to progression to adenocarcinoma because both lesions can be found in the stomach with long-standing Helicobacter infection. But- does this mean these lesions are the direct precursor to the adenocarcinoma? While the association between these lesions and adenocarcinoma is present, direct cell progression through these stages has not been conclusively demonstrated. In order to directly prove this progression, researchers have sought to determine the mutations responsible for gastric cancer initiation and progression, and follow the acquisition of these mutations through various cell changes. To date, they have not been successful. We have been unable to identify a logical progression of acquired damage akin to what is seen in colorectal cancer [107]. What we do see is that p53 is most commonly mutated in gastric adenocarcinoma (60–70% of cancers) [108], while mutations in Ras and Myc are rare [109]. Other genetic abnormalities found at high frequency include deletions or suppression of the fragile histadine triad gene (*FHIT*) (60%), adenomatous polyposis coli gene (*APC*) (50%) and deleted in colorectal cancer gene (*DCC*) (50%), while overexpression/amplification of cyclooxygenase 2 (COX-2) (70%), HGF/SF (60%), VEGF (50%), c-met (45%), AIB-1 (40%), β-catenin (25%), microsatellite instability (25–40%) and DNA aneuploidy (60–75%) have also been demonstrated [110]. Unfortunately, most mutations studied to date appear to accumulate once the cell has undergone malignant transformation [111], and we do not see a pattern of mutations as the epithelium progresses through the various "premalignant" stages. The precise role, if any, these mutations play in initiating malignant transformation is therefore, not clear. In addition to the usually studied tumor suppressors and tumor promoters, there are proposed gastric specific tumor suppressor genes, specifically Trefoil factor family-1 TFF1 [112] and RUNX3 [113] have been identified. TFF1 has been shown to be a key gastric tumor-suppressor gene. Human gastric cancers typically lack TFF1 expression suggesting loss of this protein may be instrumental in cancer progression. Indeed, TFF1 knockout mice develop multiple gastric adenomas and carcinomas, solidifying this hypothesis [114]. RUNX3 is frequently inactivated in gastric cancer by hypermethylation leading to loss of expression or through aberrant protein localization [115]. These may represent "gatekeepers" of the gastric cancer pathway, and as such represent logical targets for further study. Investigations into these genes and their contributions to the gastric cancer phenotype will prove valuable to our understanding of disease progression.

Recent attention has been given to activation and silencing of developmental pathways in cancer initiation and progression [116]. Inappropriate activation of specific developmental pathways may be involved in the development of intestinal metaplasia – a predicted candidate precursor of intestinal-type gastric carcinomas. Caudal type homeobox transcription factor 2 (Cdx2) directs several events during early embryogenesis in mice including intestinal development. Cdx2 plays an important role in small bowel development and differentiation, and it is normally expressed in the proximal intestine, not the distal, and is not expressed in the stomach. Because intestinal metaplasia is characterized by the trans-differentiation of gastric epithelial cells to an intestinal phenotype, the role of small bowel specific developmental programs has been investigated. Ectopic expression of Cdx2 in the gastric mucosa in transgenic mice induces intestinal metaplasia [117], and is accompanied by the expression of intestine-specific genes; including MUC2, sucrase/isomaltase and carbonic anhydrase I. Ectopic expression of Cdx2 successfully produces ectopic intestinal tissue akin to "metaplasia," however, progression to dysplasia and cancer has not been noted. These findings suggesting that additional factors in the infected gastric milieu which favor intestinal cell development are responsible for transformation. Of interest, ectopic expression of Cdx2 has been shown in malignancies other than gastric adenocarcinoma; the most notable being acute myeloid leukemia (AML), where more than 85% of AML patient samples express ectopic Cdx2. Indeed ectopic expression of Cdx2 in murine bone marrow induces AML in mice and upregulate Hox genes in bone marrow progenitors [118, 119] further supporting a causative role. Perhaps the cell type (epithelial cell vs BM) in which it is expressed dictates whether Cdx2 expression will lead to terminal differentiation of on intestinal phenotype, or to malignancy.

What Is the Progression of Gastric Lesions Leading up to Gastric Cancer?

Most infected individuals never develop clinical symptoms though all have chronic gastritis. Approximately 10–20% develop gastric and duodenal ulcers [120], 1–2% will progress to gastric adenocarcinoma and less than 1% will develop gastric MALT lymphoma [120]. How can we predict which patients will progress to cancer? Is there a specific gastric lesion which accurately predicts who will progress, allowing us to reliably identify patients at highest risk? In order to address this, researchers began with the end product – namely chronically infected stomachs, and chronically infected stomachs which had developed gastric cancer, and began to work their way backwards. The presumption was that cancer arose in a "field" of abnormal tissue, therefore, if the cancer was the center of a chosen field – as one moved away for the center, you would encounter lesions which were premalignant, with the most highly associated lesions in closest proximity to the cancer, and lesions perhaps further back on the evolutionary time line – further away. The presence of gastric lesions adjacent to gastric adenocarcinoma was described first in surgical gastrectomy specimens which provided the largest and most complete map of the gastric mucosal changes, and later in endoscopic biopsy specimens, which only provide a limited "snap-shop" of the changes which are occurring. When these studies are looked at together, several important points emerge regarding the evolution of the stomach during infection to cancer (Fig. 17.1). Chronic active non-atrophic gastritis is the most common finding, followed over time by the presence of multifocal atrophy, then intestinal metaplasia (first complete, then incomplete). Long standing infection is associated with a small number of patients developing dysplasia and invasive carcinoma. These lesions are well-characterized histopathologically, though the distinction between dysplasia and cancer has not always been clear, and the diagnosis differs between pathologists. Though there is clearly an accumulation of these lesions as the time of infection progresses, it is still not clear if one lesion is a precursor to the next, and which lesion, if any, is a direct precursor of gastric adenocarcinoma.

Chronic Active Nonatrophic Gastritis

This lesion is characterized by infiltration of the gastric mucosa diffusely with neutrophils, lymphocytes, plasma cells, and macrophages with scattered eosinophils and mast cells. Inflammatory infiltrates as seen as small aggregates within both the submucosa and the epithelial layer, intercalating between glands and at times forming small intraglandular microabscesses. There is no loss of glands (atrophy) at this early stage of Helicobacter induced mucosal disease, and this lesion is termed "nonatrophic gastritis" [121]. For the most part, non-atrophic gastritis is found predominantly in the antrum, where it remains confined, and is not associated with "progression" to more advanced lesions. If patients are receiving acid suppression therapy however, this inflammation can become prominent in the corpus (oxyntic) mucosa as well. Interpretation of studies looking at the effects of bacterial eradication on progression of lesions or restoration of mucosal architecture in humans has been difficult to interpret for a variety of reasons including the inability to fully characterize the mucosal changes from small biopsy specimens, difficulty in determining the length of infection, genetic variability between patient populations and the relatively low number of patients who progress to dysplasia and carcinoma. For these reasons, we turned to animal models of Helicobacter infection to address the notion of progression and reversal of lesions. Studies done in the C57BL/6 mouse model of infection demonstrate that bacterial eradication at the stage of chronic active non-atrophic gastritis leads to complete regression of inflammation, restoration of normal mucosal architecture and the prevention of gastric adenocarcinoma [122].

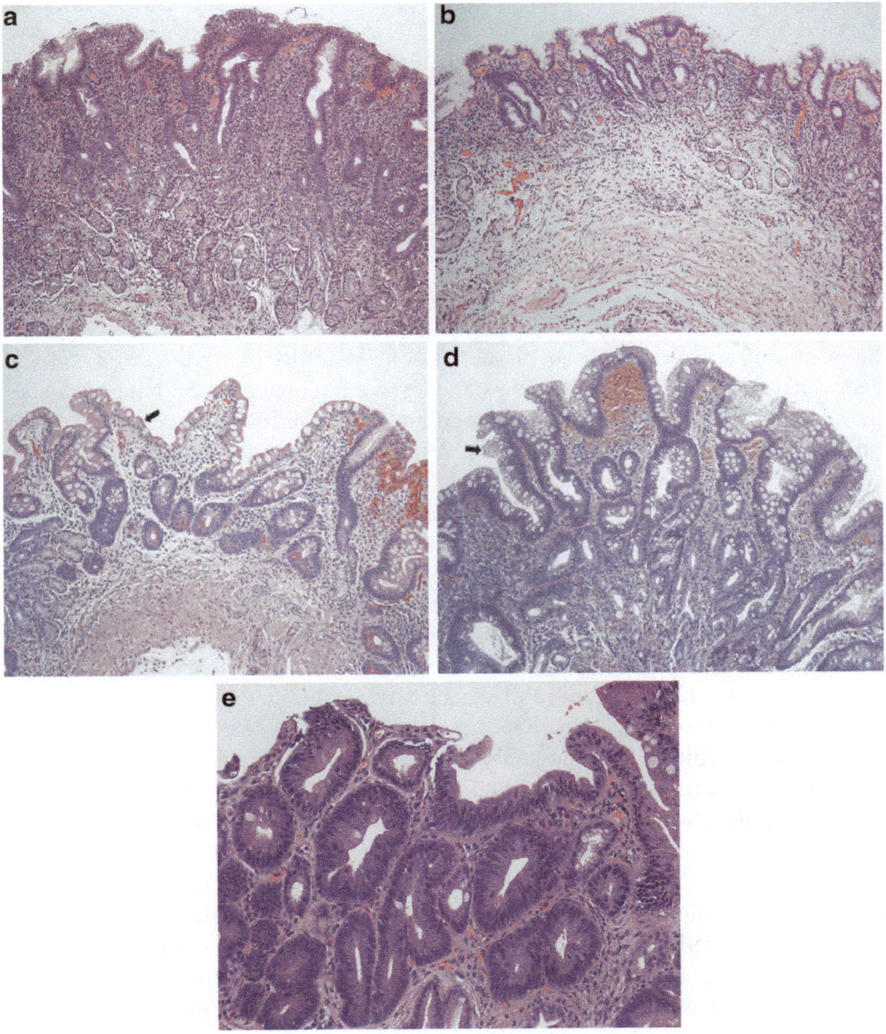

Fig. 17.1 Progression of mucosal changes in Helicobacter infection in the human stomach. (**a**) Nonatrophic gastritis. Antral gastric mucosa with diffuse mononuclear leukocytic infiltration and well-preserved glands. (**b**) Multifocal atrophic gastritis. The antral glands have disappeared from the center of the field and are replaced by fibrous tissue. Diffuse mononuclear leukocytic infiltrate is also observed in the lamina propria. (**c**) Multifocal atrophic gastritis with complete intestinal metaplasia. The *arrow* points to absorptive enterocytes with a brush border, markers of complete metaplasia. The original glands have disappeared from the center of the field and are replaced with metaplastic cells, extending to the surface. The metaplastic epithelium consists of eosinophilic absorptive enterocytes with a well-defined brush border. Well developed goblet cells are seen at regular intervals, and Paneth cells in the deep glands. (**d**) Multifocal atrophic gastritis with incomplete intestinal metaplasia. The epithelium consists of multiple, irregular goblet cells and there is an absence of brush border. The *arrow* points to goblet cells with several irregular vacuoles and without a brush border, markers of incomplete metaplasia. (**e**) Low-grade gastric dysplasia. Abnormal presence of irregular glands lined by epithelial cells with crowded, enlarged, hyperchromatic, pseudostratified nuclei, and frequent mitosis. The dysplastic changes extend to the surface epithelium but do not dip below the basement membrane

Multifocal Atrophic Gastritis

Some patients with longstanding infection will develop atrophic gastritis consisting of focal loss of glands (atrophy), first seen at the antrum–corpus junction and most prominently at the incisura angularis. This lesion is associated with more virulent bacterial strains and what has been termed a "permissive" host immune response (high levels of IL-1β, TNF-α and low levels of IL-10). It is also more frequently seen in populations at higher risk for gastric cancer. At this stage of mucosal alteration, it is believed the alterations in cell–cell signaling due to parietal and chief cell loss, and the expansion of stromal fibrous tissue leads to an influx of bone marrow derived stem cells which (at least in the mouse model) are the precursor cells for adenocarcinoma [85]. Indeed, this concept of recruited bone marrow derived stem cells to areas of inflammation was tested in the C57BL/6 mouse model of gastric cancer. We hypothesized that bone marrow derived stem cells represent the ultimate uncommitted adult stem cell and are the ideal candidate for transformation if placed in a favorable environment. For these studies, C57BL/6J mice were irradiated and transplanted with gender-mismatched bone marrow from mice that express a non-mammalian beta-galactosidase enzyme [C57BL/*6JGtrosa26* (ROSA 26)], mice that expressed green fluorescent protein [C57BL/6J-*beta-actin-EGFP* (GFP)], or control C57BL/6J liter mates. A variety of detection methods were used to verify engrafted cells were of donor origin, including specific B-galactosidase immunohistochemistry (IHC) detection of LacZNeo fusion gene sequence by PCR, GFP detected by fluorescence activated cell sorting, GFP immunohistochemistry and X/Y chromosome fluorescent in situ hybridization and the epithelial lineage confirmed by specific cytokeratin staining, and the absence of the leukocyte marker CD45 [85]. As would be predicted, infection is associated with an influx of marrow derived inflammatory cells. At early time points, we did not detect any engraftment or differentiation of BMDCs to an epithelial cell phenotype. At 30 weeks of infection, when antralized glands (SPEM) and metaplastic cells were prominent, the metaplastic cells at the squamocolumnar junction were replaced by marrow derived cell. By 1 year of infection, invasive neoplastic glands were seen in nearly all the mice. These intraepithelial neoplastic lesions arose from donor marrow cells, supporting an inherent vulnerability of the marrow derived stem cell is population to malignant progression. In addition to epithelial cells within the tumor, BMDCs also contributed to activated fibroblasts, endothelial cells and adipose tissue within the tumor stroma and within seemingly uninvolved epithelium and subepithelial spaces adjacent to the tumors (Fig. 17.2).

Intestinal Metaplasia

In the context of mucosal atrophy, original gastric glands and specialized epithelial cells are replaced by cells with an intestinal phenotype. Initially, metaplastic cells resemble small intestinal mucosa with absorptive cells containing well developed

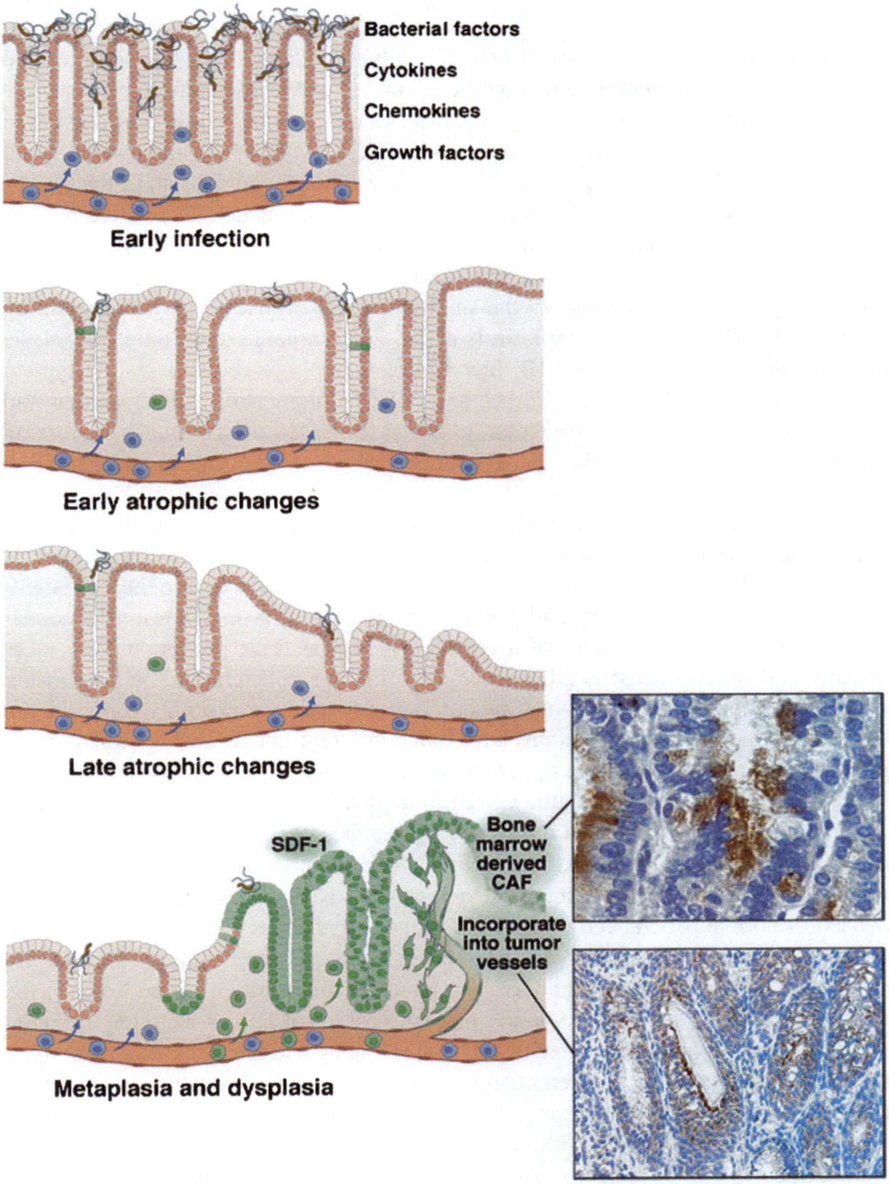

Fig. 17.2 The role of BMDC in mucosal disease and repair. Bacterial factors and host factors recruit inflammatory cells to the gastric mucosa. Lone BMDC rarely engraft as differentiated cells (shown here marked in *green*) in early infection when cell loss is minimal. With ongoing inflammation and damage, the mucosa becomes atrophic and peripheral stem cell loss is evident. With time, chemokines such as SDF-1 recruit BMDC into the stem cell niche (shown here for an antral gland). These stem cells divide and repopulate entire gastric units. With time, BMDC acquire mutations and transform. BMDC also contribute to cancer-associated fibroblasts and incorporate into tumor vasculature. The illustration on the left depicts these events. The photomicrographs on the right demonstrate beta-galactosidase-labeled BMDC (brown cytoplasmic staining), which are dysplastic, and comprise entire glandular units

microvilli and mucin-filled goblet cells. This type of metaplasia has been termed small intestinal type, type I, and "complete," metaplasia because these cells secrete the normal set of digestive enzymes. [123] Complete metaplasia has decreased levels of expression of "gastric" mucins (MUC1, MUC5AC, and MUC6) and expresses MUC2, an intestinal mucin. Complete metaplastic cells stain for intestinal type of acid mucins (Alcian blue at pH 2.5) and sulfated HID-positive mucins and not for colonic mucins (sulfomucins with high iron diamine (HID)).

As injury and repair continue, the metaplastic phenotype changes to a more colonic type of tissue with loss of the small bowel absorptive cells, while retaining goblet cells. This type of metaplasia is called "incomplete" or colonic metaplasia and includes both types II and III. Incomplete metaplasia coexpresses the typical "gastric mucins" (MUC1, MUC5AC, and MUC6) along with MUC2 mucin and also expresses the large intestine marker Das-112. Based on the mucin expression pattern, it does not appear that there is sequential pathway of intestinal metaplasia from type I to types II and III [124].

Examination of small presumably early carcinoma may reveal areas of incomplete metaplasia surrounding the tumor. Larger more extensive carcinomas do not show this association. The evolution of mucosal alterations of the infected gastric mucosa begins with inflammation and atrophy and gradually progresses from small intestinal metaplasia to a metaplasia with more of a colonic phenotype. This process usually takes decades and once initiated is progressive. It is difficult to determine the progression from one lesion to the next in human studies, or to determine reversibility with bacterial eradication. Indeed, different groups have found different findings using biopsy specimens from patients undergoing upper endoscopy [125–131]. Mouse models of infection demonstrate that at least in the C57BL/6 model, eradication of Helicobacter after metaplasia has been established results in reappearance of parietal and chief cells, and diminution of metaplasia, though not a complete restoration of normal architecture. In the setting of bacterial eradication, metaplasia and dysplasia/carcinoma exist in the context of normal parietal cell populations suggesting the loss of specialized cells and the appearance of metaplastic cells may occur temporally, but may not be causally related [122]. Alternately, though there is not a clear cut evolution of one lesion to the next, these findings support the notion that environmental factors including bacterial products, dietary components, loss of cell–cell signaling and the cytokine environment may initially act to disturb differentiation decisions of progenitor cells via epigenetic changes. These changes may be reversible with bacterial eradication and restoration of a normal immune response. With time however, permanent changes in the stem cell compartment are likely to have occurred and are irreversible and progressive.

SPEM in Humans

The presence of glands with gastric antrum phenotype in the oxyntic mucosa has been described as "antralization" or "pseudopyloric metaplasia."[132] and has been given the name spasmolytic polypeptide expressing metaplasia (SPEM). This lesion was first recognized in the mouse model of disease, and was uncommonly reported in human specimens. For a while, it was felt to be a unique pre-cancerous lesion in the rodent model with questionable relevance to human disease. Recently however, this metaplasia has received renewed attention. Studies have been carried out predominantly in Asian populations who have developed gastric reminant carcinoma years after gastric resection for benign ulcer disease or gastric carcinoma. Spasmolytic polypeptide expressing metaplasia (SPEM) was found to be ubiquitously expressed in the mucosa surrounding the remnant carcinomas and in dysplastic and neoplastic cells whereas intestinal metaplasia was found in only about half of the cancer specimens [125], making the association of SPEM and gastric adenocarcinoma stronger than the association between intestinal metaplasia and carcinoma.

Dysplasia

In dysplasia nuclei become enlarged, hyperchromatic, irregular in shape, and lose their basal polarity. The architecture becomes highly irregular, but the atypical changes are confined to the mucosal layer and are not found below the basement membrane. Dysplasia is classified as low grade or high-grade, based on the degree of nuclear atypia and architectural distortion. Once abnormal cells are found below the basement membrane, they are classified as invasive carcinomas. It is generally agreed that dysplastic epithelium is in fact neoplastic, and as such, dysplasia is termed intraepithelial neoplasia [133]. High grade dysplasia has been reported to progress to invasive cancer from 60 to 85% if left untreated. Interestingly, when one looks at the mouse model of infection, dysplasia progresses uniformly to invasive cancer. Eradication therapy slows the progression to invasive lesions and symptomatic cancer, however the risk of histological progression is not completely eliminated suggesting there may be a "point of no return" in the progression of lesions [122].

Summary

The leading cause of gastric cancer is infection with *Helicobacter pylori*. The chronic inflammatory environment of the infected stomach combined with host genetics and environmental factors leads to a series of mucosal alterations with adenocarcinoma the most dreaded end point of changes. Similar to the changes which occur in the colonic mucosa prior to colon cancer, examination of the gastric mucosa reveals a series of changes ranging from inflammation and hyperplasia to atrophy, metaplasia, dysplasia and cancer. Unlike colon cancer however, there is no clear evidence that one lesion leads to the next in an orderly progression, nor has a progressive accumulation of genetic mutations been mapped out which is necessary for the progression from benign to malignant disease. The strongest association between mucosal alterations and progression to adenocarcinoma appears to be with SPEM. Examination of resected gastric carcinoma specimens showed a 100% correlation between adenocarcinoma and the presence of surrounding SPEM lesions clearly establishing association. Direct progression from suspected premalignant lesions to malignancy however, has still has not been conclusively shown. Delineating the point in the progression where elimination of infection/inflammation leads to regression of disease, and identifying points in the progression where the genetic changes dictate progressive disease will allow a more effective approach to gastric cancer prevention and treatment.

References

1. Marshall BJ, Armstrong JA, McGechie DB et al (1985) Attempt to fulfill Koch's postulates for pyloric Campylobacter. Med J Aust 142(8):436–439
2. Peek RM Jr, Miller GG, Tham KT et al (1995) Heightened inflammatory response and cytokine expression in vivo to cagA+ *Helicobacter pylori* strains. Lab Invest 73:760–770
3. Eaton KA, Mefford M, Thevenot T (2001) The role of T cell subsets and cytokines in the pathogenesis of *Helicobacter pylori* gastritis in mice. J Immunol 66:7456–7461
4. Wang TC, Goldenring JR, Dangler C et al (1998) Mice lacking secretory phospholipase A2 show altered apoptosis and differentiation with *Helicobacter felis* infection. Gastroenterology 14:675–689
5. Sutton P, Kolesnikov T, Danon S et al (2000) Dominant nonresponsiveness to *Helicobacter pylori* infection is associated with production of interleukin 10 but not gamma interferon. Infect Immun 68:4802–4804
6. Roth KA, Kapadia SB, Martin SM et al (1999) Cellular immune responses are essential for the development of Helicobacterelis-associated gastric pathology. J Immunol 63:1490–1497
7. Smythies LE, Waites KB, Lindsey JR et al (2000) *Helicobacter pylori*-induced mucosal inflammation is Th1 mediated and exacerbated in IL-4 but not IFN-gamma, gene-deficient mice. J Immunol 165:1022–1029
8. Chen SY, Liu TY, Shun CT et al (2004) Modification effects of GSTM1, GSTT1 and CYP2E1 polymorphisms on associations between raw salted food and incomplete intestinal metaplasia in a high-risk area of stomach cancer. Int J Cancer 108:606–612
9. Fox JG, Dangler CA, Taylor NS et al (1999) High-salt diet induces gastric epithelial hyperplasia and parietal cell loss, and enhances *Helicobacter pylori* colonization in C57BL/6 mice. Cancer Res 59:4823–4828
10. El-Omar EM, Oien K, Murray LS et al (2000) Increased prevalence of precancerous changes in relatives of gastric cancer patients: critical role of *H. pylori*. Gastroenterology 118:22–30
11. Enders KW, Chan WY, Auyeung A et al (2002) Increased frequency of pre-malignant gastric lesions in first degree relatives of stomach cancer patients [abstract]. Gastroenterology 122(Suppl 1):136
12. El-Omar EM, Carrington M, Chow WH et al (2000) Interleukin 1 polymorphisms associated with increased risk of gastric cancer. Nature 404:398–402
13. El-Omar EM, Rabkin CS, Gammon MD et al (2003) Increased risk of noncardia gastric cancer associated with proinflammatory cytokine gene polymorphisms. Gastroenterology 124:1193–1201
14. Coticchia J, Sugawa C, Tran V et al (2006) J Gastrointest Surg. http://www.sciencedirect.com/science?_ob=ArticleURL&_udi=B6W8T-4K51GKS-G&_user=115184&_

coverDate=06%2F30%2F2006&_rdoc=1&_fmt=high&_orig=article&_cdi=6663&_sort=v&_docanchor=&view=c&_ct=33108&_acct=C000009258&_version=1&_urlVersion=0&_userid=115184&md5=95d6cf2b35d080646ce13a90254b519f. Accessed 29 July 2009
15. Yamaoka Y, Alm R (2008) *Helicobacter pylori*: molecular genetics and cellular biology – *Helicobacter pylori* outer membrane proteins. Caister Academic Press, Linton, England
16. Moran A, Trent S (2008) *Helicobacter pylori*: molecular genetics and cellular biology – *Helicobacter pylori* lipopolysaccharides and Lewis antigens. Caister Academic Press, Linton, England
17. Rust M, Schweinitzer T, Josenhans C (2008) *Helicobacter pylori:* molecular genetics and cellular biology – *Helicobacter* flagella, motility and chemotaxis. Caister Academic Press, Linton, England
18. Covacci A, Rappuoli R (2003) *Helicobacter pylori*: after the genomes, back to biology. J Exp Med 197:807–811
19. Schmitz JM, Durham CG, Ho SB et al (2009) Gastric mucus alterations associated with murine Helicobacter infection. J Hisotochem Cytochem 57:457–467
20. Guruge JL, Falk PG, Lorenz RG et al (1998) Epithelial attachment alters the outcome of *Helicobacter pylori* infection. Proc Natl Acad Sci U S A 95:3925–3930
21. Peek RM Jr, Blaser MJ (2002) *Helicobacter pylori* and gastrointestinal tract adenocarcinomas. Nat Rev Cancer 2:28–37
22. Suerbaum S, Michetti P (2002) *Helicobacter pylori* infection. N Engl J Med 347:1175–1186
23. Dixon MF (2001) Prospects for intervention in gastric carcinogenesis: reversibility of gastric atrophy and intestinal metaplasia. Gut 49:2–4
24. Lauren P (1965) The two histological main types of gastric carcinoma: diffuse and so-called intestinal-type carcinoma. Acta Pathol Microbiol Scand 64:31–49
25. Fuchs CS, Mayer RJ (1995) Gastric carcinoma. N Engl J Med 333:32–41
26. Correa P (1992) Human gastric carcinogenesis: a multistep and multifactorial process – first American Cancer Society Award Lecture on Cancer Epidemiology and Prevention. Cancer Res 52:6735–6740
27. Sipponen P, Marshall BJ (2000) Gastritis and gastric cancer. Western countries. Gastroenterol Clin North Am 29:579–592
28. Mandell L, Moran AP, Cocchiarella A et al (2004) Intact Gram-negative *Helicobacter hepaticus*, *Helicobacter pylori* and *Helicobacter felis* bacteria activate innate immunity via Toll-like receptor-2 not Toll-like receptor 4. Infect Immun 72(11):6446–6454
29. Smith MF Jr, Mitchell A, Li G et al (2003) Toll-like receptor (TLR) 2 and TLR5, but not TLR4, are required for *Helicobacter pylori*-induced NF-kappa B activation and chemokine expression by epithelial cells. J Biol Chem 278:32552–32560
30. Chaouche-Drider N, Kaparakis M, Karrar A et al (2009) A commensal Helicobacter sp. Of the rodent intestinal flora activates TLR2 and NOD1 responses in epithelial cells. PLos One 4(4):e5396
31. Rad R, Ballhorn W, Voland P et al (2009) Extracellular and intracellular pattern recognition receptors cooperate in the recognition of *Helicobacter pylori.* Gastroenterology 136: 2247–2257
32. Moran AP, Lindner B, Walsh EJ (1997) Structural characterization of the lipid A component of *Helicobacter pylori* rough- and smooth-form lipopolysaccharides. J Bacteriol 179: 6453–6463
33. Muotiala A, Helander IM, Pyhala L et al (1992) Low biological activity of *Helicobacter pylori* lipopolysaccharide. Infect Immun 60:1714–1716
34. Bliss CM Jr, Golenbock DT, Keates S et al (1998) *Helicobacter pylori* lipopolysaccharide binds to CD14 and stimulates release of interleukin-8, epithelial neutrophil-activating peptide 78, and monocyte chemotactic protein 1 by human monocytes. Infect Immun 66:5357–5363
35. Martin M, Katz J, Vogel SN et al (2001) Differential induction of endotoxin tolerance by lipopolysaccharides derived from *Porphyromonas gingivalis* and *Escherichia coli.* J Immunol 167:5278–5285

36. Kawahara T, Kuwano Y, Teshima-Kondo S et al (2001) *Helicobacter pylori* lipopolysaccharide from type I, but not type II strains, stimulates apoptosis of cultured gastric mucosal cells. J Med Invest 48:167–174
37. Kawahara T, Teshima S, Oka A et al (2001) Type I *Helicobacter pylori* lipopolysaccharide stimulates toll-like receptor 4 and activates mitogen oxidase 1 in gastric pit cells. Infect Immun 69:4382–4389
38. Lee SK, Stack A, Katzowitsch E et al (2003) *Helicobacter pylori* flagellins have very low intrinsic activity to stimulate human gastric epithelial cells via TLR5. Microbes Infect 5:45–56
39. Haas T, Metzger J, Schmitz F et al (2008) The DNA sugar backbone 2' deoxyribose determines toll-like receptor 9 activation. Immunity 28:315–323
40. Latz E, Verma A, Visintin A (2007) Ligand-induced conformational changes allosterically activate Toll-like receptor 9. Nat Immunol 8:772–779
41. Raghavan S, Nystrom J, Fredriksson M et al (2003) Orally administered CpG oligodeoxynucleotide induces production of CXC and CC chemokines in the gastric mucosa and suppresses bacterial colonization in a mouse model of *Helicobacter pylori* infection. Infect Immun 71:7014–7022
42. Ortega-Cava CF, Ishihara S, Rumi MA et al (2003) Strategic compartmentalization of Toll-like receptor 4 in the mouse gut. J Immunol 170:3977–3985
43. Chen ZT, Li SL, Cai EQ et al (2003) LPS induces pulmonary intravascular macrophages producing inflammatory mediators via activating NF-kappaB. J Cell Biochem 89: 1206–1214
44. Rad R et al (2007) Toll-like receptor-dependent activation of antigen-presenting cells affects adaptive immunity to *Helicobacter pylori*. Gastroenterology 133:150–163
45. Liu T, Matsuguchi T, Tsuboi N et al (2002) Differences in expression of toll-like receptors and their reactivities in dendritic cells in BALB/c and C57BL/6 mice. Infect Immun 70:6638–6645
46. Visintin A, Mazzoni A, Spitzer JH et al (2001) Regulation of Toll-like receptors in human monocytes and dendritic cells. J Immunol 166:249–255
47. Schnare M, Barton GM, Holt AC et al (2001) Toll-like receptors control activation of adaptive immune responses. Nat Immunol 2:947–950
48. Kuroda E, Yamashita U (2003) Mechanisms of enhanced macrophage-mediated prostaglandin E2 production and its suppressive role in Th1 activation in Th2-dominant BALB/c mice. J Immunol 170:757–764
49. Roth KA, Kapadia SB, Martin SM et al (1999) Cellular immune responses are essential for the development of *Helicobacter felis*-associated gastric pathology. J Immunol 163: 1490–1497
50. Cui G, Houghton J, Finkel N et al (2003) IFN-gamma infusion induces gastric atrophy, metaplasia and dysplasia in the absence of Helicobacter infection – a role for immune response in Helicobacter disease [abstract]. Gastroenterology 24:A19
51. Fox JG, Beck P, Dangler CA et al (2000) Concurrent enteric helminth infection modulates inflammation and gastric immune responses and reduces helicobacter-induced gastric atrophy. Nat Med 6:536–542
52. Stoicov C, Whary M, Rogers AB et al (2004) Co-infection modulates inflammatory response and clinical outcomes of *Helicobacter felis* and *Toxoplasma gondii* infection. J Immunol 173(5):3329–3336
53. Szabo SJ, Kim ST, Costa GL (2000) A novel transcription factor, T-bet, directs Th1 lineage commitment. Cell 100:655–669
54. Stoicov C, Fan X, Liu JH et al (2009) T-bet knockout prevents *Helicobacter felis* induced gastric cancer. J Immunol 183:642–649
55. Macarthur M, Hold LG, El-Omar EM (2004) Inflammation and Cancer II. Role of chronic inflammation and cytokine gene polymorphisms in the pathogenesis of gastrointestinal malignancy. Am J Physiol Gastrointest Liver Physiol 286:515–520
56. Wagner S, Beil W, Westermann J et al (1997) Regulation of gastric epithelial cell growth by *Helicobacter pylori*: evidence for a major role of apoptosis. Gastroenterology 113:1836–1847

57. Jones NL, Shannon PT, Cutz E et al (1997) Increase in proliferation and apoptosis of gastric epithelial cells early in the natural history of *Helicobacter pylori* infection. Am J Pathol 151:1695–1703
58. Rudi J, Kuck D, Strand S et al (1998) Involvement of the CD95 (APO-1/Fas) receptor and ligand system in *Helicobacter pylori*-induced gastric epithelial apoptosis. J Clin Invest 102:1506–1514
59. Houghton J, Korah RM, Kim CMR et al (1999) Apoptosis in *Helicobacter pylori*-associated gastric and duodenal ulcer disease is mediated via the Fas antigen pathway. Dig Dis Sci 44:465–478
60. Houghton JM, Bloch LM, Goldstein M et al (2000) In vivo disruption of the Fas pathway abrogates gastric growth alterations secondary to Helicobacter infection. J Infect Dis 182:856–864
61. Houghton J, Macera-Bloch LS, Harrison L et al (2000) Tumor necrosis factor alpha and interleukin 1beta up-regulate gastric mucosal Fas antigen expression in *Helicobacter pylori* infection. Infect Immun 68:1189–1195
62. Li H, Stoicov C, Houghton J (2003) Fas antigen ligation signal for apoptosis or proliferation in gastric mucosal cells – the importance of receptor abundance [abstract]. Gastroenterology 124:A595
63. Cai X, Stoicov C, Li H et al (2005) Overcoming Fas mediated apoptosis accelerates Helicobacter induced gastric cancer in the mouse. Cancer Res 65(23):10912–10919
64. Jones NL, Day AS, Jennings H et al (2002) Enhanced disease severity in *Helicobacter pylori*-infected mice deficient in Fas signaling. Infect Immun 70:2591–2597
65. Lee SH, Shin MS, Park WS et al (1999) Immunohistochemical localization of FAP-1, an inhibitor of Fas mediated apoptosis, in normal and neoplastic human tissues. APMIS 107:1101–1108
66. Lee SH, Kim HS, Kim SY et al (2003) Increased expression of FLIP, an inhibitor of Fas mediated apoptosis, in stomach cancer. APMIS 111:309–314
67. Li H, Stoicov C, Houghton J et al (2003) Hyperosmolarity shifts signaling pathway from apoptosis to proliferation by activation of p38 in gastric mucosal cell [abstract]. Gastroenterology 124:A460
68. Stoicov C, Cai X, Li H et al (2005) Major histocompatibility complex class II inhibits Fas antigen-mediated gastric mucosal cell apoptosis through actin-dependent inhibition of receptor aggregation. Infect Immun 73(10):6311–6321
69. Kim R, Emi M, Tanabe K et al (2004) The role of Fas ligand and transforming growth factor beta in tumor progression. Cancer 100:2281–2291
70. Zheng HC, Sun JM, Wei ZL et al (2003) Expression of Fas ligand and caspase-3 contributes to formation of immune escape in gastric cancer. World J Gastroenterol 9:1415–1420
71. Bennett MW, O'connell J, O'sullivan GC, Roche D et al (1999) Expression of Fas ligand by human gastric adenocarcinomas: a potential mechanism of immune escape in stomach cancer. Gut 44:156–162
72. Furuta S, Goto H, Niwa Y et al (2002) Interferon-gamma regulates apoptosis by releasing soluble tumor necrosis factor receptors in a gastric epithelial cell line. J Gastroenterol Hepatol 17:1283–1290
73. Lehmann FS, Terracciano L, Carena I et al (2002) In situ correlation of cytokine secretion and apoptosis in *Helicobacter pylori*-associated gastritis. Am J Physiol Gastrointest Liver Physiol 283:481–488
74. Huber C, Zanner R, Pohlinger A et al (2002) Tumor necrosis factor-alpha effects on rat gastric enterochromaffin-like cells. Digestion 65:87–102
75. Shimada M, Ina K, Kyokane K et al (2002) Upregulation of mucosal soluble Fas ligand and interferon-gamma may be involved in ulcerogenesis in patients with *Helicobacter pylori*-positive gastric ulcer. Scand J Gastroenterol 37:501–511
76. Mannick JB, Hausladen A, Liu L et al (1999) Fas-induced caspase denitrosylation. Science 284:651–654

77. Archimandritis A, Sougioultzis S, Foukas PG et al (2000) Expression of HLA-DR, costimulatory molecules B7-1, B7-2, intercellular adhesion molecule-1 (ICAM-1) and Fas ligand (FasL) on gastric epithelial cells in *Helicobacter pylori* gastritis; influence of *H. pylori* eradication. Clin Exp Immunol 119:464–471
78. Fan X, Crowe SE, Behar S et al (1998) The effect of class II major histocompatibility complex expression on adherence of *Helicobacter pylori* and induction of apoptosis in gastric epithelial cells: a mechanism for T helper cell type 1-mediated damage. J Exp Med 187: 1659–1669
79. Fan X, Gunasena H, Cheng Z et al (2000) *Helicobacter pylori* urease binds to class II MHC on gastric epithelial cells and induces their apoptosis. J Immunol 165:1918–1924
80. Ye G, Barrera C, Fan X et al (1997) Expression of B7-1 and B7-2 costimulatory molecules by human gastric epithelial cells: potential role in CD4+ T cell activation during *Helicobacter pylori* infection. J Clin Invest 99:1628–1636
81. Barrera C, Ye G, Espejo R et al (2001) Expression of cathepsins B, L, S, and D by gastric epithelial cells implicates them as antigen presenting cells in local immune responses. Hum Immunol 62:1081–1091
82. Azuma T, Ito S, Sato F et al (1998) The role of the HLA-DQA1 gene in resistance to atrophic gastritis and gastric adenocarcinoma induced by *Helicobacter pylori* infection. Cancer 82:1013–1018
83. Galmiche A, Rassow J, Doye A et al (2000) The N-terminal 34 kDa fragment of *Helicobacter pylori* vacuolating cytotoxin targets mitochondria and induces cytochrome c release. EMBO J 19:6361–6370
84. Goldenring J, Nomura S (2006) Differentiation of the gastric mucosa III animal models of oxyntic atrophy and metaplasia. Am J Physiol Gastrointest Liver Physiol 291:G999–G1004
85. Houghton J, Stoicov C, Nomura S et al (2004) Gastric cancer originating from bone marrow-derived cells. Science 306(5701):1568–1571
86. Mimuro H, Suzuki T, Tanaka J et al (2002) Grb2 is a key mediator of *Helicobacter pylori* CagA protein activities. Mol Cell 10:745–755
87. Tsutsumi R, Higashi H, Higuchi M et al (2003) Attenuation of *Helicobacter pylori* CagA × SHP-2 signaling by interaction between CagA and C-terminal Src kinase. J Biol Chem 278:3664–3670
88. Moss SF, Calam J, Agarwal B et al (1996) Induction of gastric epithelial apoptosis by *Helicobacter pylori*. Gut 38:498–501
89. Kohda K, Tanaka K, Aiba Y et al (1999) Role of apoptosis induced by *Helicobacter pylori* infection in the development of duodenal ulcer. Gut 44:456–462
90. Peek RM Jr, Moss SF, Tham KT et al (1997) *Helicobacter pylori* cagA+ strains and dissociation of gastric epithelial cell proliferation from apoptosis. J Natl Cancer Inst 89:863–868
91. Rokkas T, Ladas S, Liatsos C et al (1999) Relationship of *Helicobacter pylori* CagA status to gastric cell proliferation and apoptosis. Dig Dis Sci 44:487–493
92. Li H, Cai X, Fan X et al (2008) Fas Ag-FasL coupling leads to ERK1/2-mediated proliferation of gastric mucosal cells. Am J Physiol Gastrointestintest Liver Physiol 294(1): G263–G275
93. Kidd M, Hauso Ø, Drozdov I et al (2009) Delineation of the chemomechanosensory regulation of gastrin secretion using pure rodent G cells. Gastroenterology 137:231–241
94. Schubert ML, Peura DA (2008) Control of gastric acid secretion in health and disease. Gastroenterology 134:1842–1860
95. Wang TC, Dangler CA, Chen D et al (2000) Synergistic interaction between hypergastrinemia and Helicobacter infection in a mouse model of gastric cancer. Gastroenterology 118:36–47
96. Fu S, Ramanujam KS, Wong A et al (1999) Increased expression and cellular localization of inducible nitric oxide synthase and cyclooxygenase 2 in *Helicobacter pylori* gastritis. Gastroenterology 116:1319–1329
97. Baik SC, Youn HS, Chung MH et al (1996) Increased oxidative DNA damage in *Helicobacter pylori*-infected human gastric mucosa. Cancer Res 56:1279–1282
98. Williams GM, Weisburger JH (1983) Carcinogen risk assessment. Science 221:4605–4606

99. Pitot HC, Goldsworthy T, Moran S (1981) The natural history of carcinogenesis: implications of experimental carcinogenesis in the genesis of human cancer. J Supramol Struct Cell Biochem 17:133–146
100. Kolaja KL, Stevenson DE, Walborg EF Jr et al (1996) Selective dieldrin promotion of hepatic focal lesions in mice. Carcinogenesis 17:1243–1250
101. Rokkas T, Liatsos C, Petridou E et al (1999) Relationship of *Helicobacter pylori* CagA(+) status to gastric juice vitamin C levels. Eur J Clin Invest 29:56–62
102. van den Brink GR, Hardwick JC, Tytgat GN et al (2001) Sonic hedgehog regulates gastric gland morphogenesis in man and mouse. Gastroenterology 121:317–328
103. Beales ILP (2004) Gastrin and interleukin-1β stimulate growth factor secretion from cultured rabbit gastric parietal cells. Life Sci 75:2983–2995
104. Stepan V, Ramamoorthy S, Nitsche H et al (2005) Regulation and function the sonic hedgehog signal transduction pathway in isolated gastric parietal cells. J Biol Chem 280:15700–15708
105. Mashimo H, Wu DC, Podolsky DK et al (1996) Impaired defense of intestinal mucosa in mice lacking intestinal trefoil factor. Science 274:262–265
106. Farrell JJ, Taupin D, Koh TJ et al (2002) TFF2/SP-deficient mice show decreased gastric proliferation, increased acid secretion, and increased susceptibility to NSAID injury. J Clin Invest 109:193–204
107. Maesawa C, Tamura G, Suzuki Y et al (1995) The sequential accumulation of genetic alterations characteristic of the colorectal adenoma-carcinoma sequence does not occur between gastric adenoma and adenocarcinoma. J Pathol 176:249–258
108. Kim JH, Takahashi T, Chiba I et al (1991) Occurrence of p53 gene abnormalities in gastric carcinoma tumors and cell lines. J Natl Cancer Inst 83:938–943
109. Victor T, Du Toit R, Jordaan AM et al (1990) No evidence for point mutations in codons 12, 13, and 61 of the ras gene in a high-incidence area for esophageal and gastric cancers. Cancer Res 50:4911–4914
110. Stemmermann G, Heffelfinger SC, Noffsinger A et al (1994) The molecular biology of esophageal and gastric cancer and their precursors: oncogenes, tumor suppressor genes, and growth factors. Hum Pathol 25:968–981
111. Farinati F, Cardin F, Di Mario F et al (1987) Early and advanced gastric cancer during follow-up of apparently benign gastric ulcer: significance of the presence of epithelial dysplasia. J Surg Oncol 36:263–267
112. Park WS, Oh RR, Park JY et al (2000) Somatic mutations of the trefoil factor family 1 gene in gastric cancer. Gastroenterology 119:691–698
113. Li QL, Ito K, Sakakura C et al (2002) Causal relationship between the loss of RUNX3 expression and gastric cancer. Cell 109:113–124
114. Karam SM, Tomasetto C, Rio MC (2008) Amplification and invasiveness of epithelial progenitors during gastric carcinogenesis in trefoil factor 1 knockout mice. Cell Proliferation 41(6):923–935
115. Ito K, Liu Q, Salto-Tellez M et al (2005) RUNX3 a novel tumor suppressor is frequently inactivated in gastric cancer by protein mislocalization. Cancer Res 65:7743–7750
116. Yuasa Y (2003) Control of gut differentiation and intestinal-type gastric carcinogenesis. Nat Rev Cancer 3:592–600
117. Silberg DG, Sullivan J, Kang E et al (2002) Cdx2 ectopic expression induces gastric intestinal metaplasia in transgenic mice. Gastroenterology 122:689–696
118. Rawat VP, Cusan M, Deshpande A et al (2004) Ectopic expression of the homeobox gene Cdx2 is the transforming event in a mouse model of t(12;13)(p13;q12) acute myeloid leukemia. Proc Natl Acad Sci U S A. doi:10.1073/pnas.0305555101
119. Scholl C, Bansal D, Döhner K et al (2007) The homeobox gene CDX2 is aberrantly expressed in most cases of acute myeloid leukemia and promotes leukemogenesis. J Clin Invest. doi:10.1172/JCI30182
120. Hansson LE, Nyren O, Hsing AW et al (1996) The risk of stomach cancer in patients with gastric or duodenal ulcer disease. N Engl J Med 335:242

121. Dixon MF, Genta RM, Yardley JH et al (1994) Classification and grading of gastritis. The updated Sydney System. International Workshop on the Histopathology of Gastritis. Am J Surg Pathol 20:1161–1181
122. Cai X, Carlson J, Stoicov C et al (2005) *Helicobacter felis* eradication restores normal architecture and inhibits gastric cancer progression in C57BL/6 mice. Gastroenterology 128:1937–1952
123. Matsukura N, Suzuki K, Kawachi T et al (1980) Distribution of marker enzymes and mucin in intestinal metaplasia in human stomach and relation to complete and incomplete types of intestinal metaplasia to minute gastric carcinomas. J Natl Cancer Inst 65:231–240
124. Reis CA, David L, Correa P et al (1999) Intestinal metaplasia of human stomach displays distinct patterns of mucin (MUC1, MUC2, MUC5AC, and MUC6) expression. Cancer Res 59:1003–1007
125. de Vries AC, Haringsma J, Kuipers EJ (2007) The detection, surveillance and treatment of premalignant gastric lesions related to *Helicobacter pylori* infection. Helicobacter 12:1–15
126. Uemura N, Okamoto S, Yamamoto S et al (2001) *Helicobacter pylori* infection and the development of gastric cancer. N Engl J Med 345:784–789
127. Kato M, Asaka M, Nakamura T et al (2006) *Helicobacter pylori* eradication prevents the development of gastric cancer - results of a long-term retrospective study in Japan. Aliment Pharmacol Ther 24:203–206
128. Ley C, Mohar A, Guarner J et al (2004) *Helicobacter pylori* eradication and gastric preneoplastic conditions: a randomized, double-blind, placebo-controlled trial. Cancer Epidemiol Biomarkers Prev 13:4–10
129. Wong BC, Lam SK, Wong WM, China Gastric Cancer Study Group et al (2004) *Helicobacter pylori* eradication to prevent gastric cancer in a high-risk region of China: a randomized controlled trial. JAMA 291:187–194
130. Leung WK, Lin SR, Ching JY et al (2004) Factors predicting progression of gastric intestinal metaplasia: results of a randomised trial on *Helicobacter pylori* eradication. Gut 53:1244–1249
131. You WC, Brown LM, Zhang L et al (2006) Randomized double-blind factorial trial of three treatments to reduce the prevalence of precancerous gastric lesions. J Natl Cancer Inst 98:974–983
132. Yamaguchi H, Goldenring JR, Kaminishi M et al (2002) Association of spasmolytic polypeptide – expressing metaplasia with carcinogen administration and oxyntic atrophy in rats. Lab Invest 82:1045–1052
133. Hamilton SR, Aaltonen LA (2000) World Health Organization Classification of Tumours. Pathology and genetics. Tumours of the digestive system. IARC, Lyon, France

Chapter 18
Pathways and Crossroads to Colorectal Cancer

Elisa Cattaneo, Michael Baudis, Federico Buffoli, Maria Antonia Bianco, Fausto Zorzi, and Giancarlo Marra

Abbreviations

ACFs	aberrant crypt foci
APC	adenomatous polyposis coli
CIN	chromosomal instability
CIMP	CpG island methylator phenotype
MMR	DNA mismatch repair
FAP	familial adenomatous polyposis
GCSPs	goblet-cell serrated polyps
HP	hyperplastic polyposis
IBD	inflammatory bowel disease
MSI	microsatellite instability
MVSPs	microvesicular serrated polyps
SAs	serrated adenomas
SSAs	sessile serrated adenomas

Introduction

Colorectal tumorigenesis is one of the best known processes of cellular transformation in humans. Its characterization has moved ahead by leaps and bounds during the last three decades thanks to major advances in the fields of endoscopy, histology and molecular pathology. And as often happens when a human disease is subjected to in-depth investigation, what originally appeared to be a single entity turns out to include several distinct clinical, histologic, and molecular phenotypes. Among other things, tumor phenotypes can tell us a great deal about the route taken by the tumor cells on their journey toward malignancy. Not surprisingly, some tumors develop

G. Marra (✉)
Institute of Molecular Cancer Research, University of Zurich, Zurich, Switzerland
e-mail: marra@imcr.uzh.ch

R.C. Fitzgerald (ed.), *Pre-Invasive Disease: Pathogenesis and Clinical Management*, DOI 10.1007/978-1-4419-6694-0_18,

along pathways that are "heavily trafficked" (and for this reason, relatively well known); others follow the "roads less traveled." But if obstacles arise along the way, tumor cells are adept at exploiting alternative routes that permit them to continue their journey toward cancer, and these deviations can give rise to mixed phenotypes. These phenotypes are nonetheless consistent with the concept of carcinogenesis as a nonrandom – and therefore, predictable – process. Each pathway, each crossroads is the result of a specific set of genetic or epigenetic alterations. Many are already well defined, others are only partially characterized, and some are still in the realm of hypothesis. Thus far, we have fairly reliable maps of at least two of the major pathways to colorectal cancer, but with increasingly sophisticated molecular analysis of preinvasive lesions, there is little doubt that we will eventually identify variants of these pathways and uncover others whose existence was not even suspected.

In this chapter, we have attempted to provide an overview of the enormous amount of work and progress that has characterized this field over the past 30 years or so – a challenging task that has involved a number of difficult choices. Some aspects undeniably deserved much more attention than they have received, and important references have regrettably been omitted. We have kept our focus on the basic pathogenesis of preinvasive lesions of the colorectum; as for their clinical management, there are several excellent articles that can and should be consulted [1–10].

On the Way to Cancer

Preinvasive lesions of the human colorectum are small areas of tissue that alter the surface contour of the gut mucosa. They are conventionally referred to as "polyps," which indicates growth protruding into the intestinal lumen, and this is indeed a fair description of most premalignant colorectal lesions. But we now know that there are also others, which are only slightly raised above the mucosal surface, or flat, or even depressed. Standard colonoscopy is performed to identify and resect these benign lesions in the belief that some of them will progress to cancer. Figure 18.1 illustrates the conventional pathway by which this progression is thought to occur. The first step is the development of early morphologic changes in discrete clusters of epithelial crypts. The benign polypoid lesion in panel C is believed to represent an intermediate stage between these aberrant crypt foci (ACFs) and invasive adenocarcinoma. The transformation process summarized in the figure has never been directly documented – when a preinvasive neoplasm is found at

Fig. 18.1 (continued) and longer with initial signs of branching and infolding of the epithelium. The epithelial lining presents low-grade dysplasia (mild mucin depletion, hyperchromatic nuclei, initial signs of nuclear enlargement, occasional areas of stratification). In the lower left corner, the crypt lumens are enlarged – a frequent finding at the borders of ACFs. (**c**) The adenomatous polypoid lesion shows a prevalent tubular growth pattern with some villous projections. The degree of dysplasia varies from low-grade (left half of the lesion) to high-grade (*right half*, *superficial*). In the lower left corner is present a portion of normal mucosa of the stalk. (**d**) (adenocarcinoma): irregular branching of glands showing atypical epithelium. They are surrounded by stroma composed of dense fibrous tissue comprising spindle cells in a collagenuos and inflammatory background (desmoplastic reaction). (Magnification: Normal mucosa, 10×; ACF, 10×; Adenoma, 2×; Adenocarcinoma, 10×)

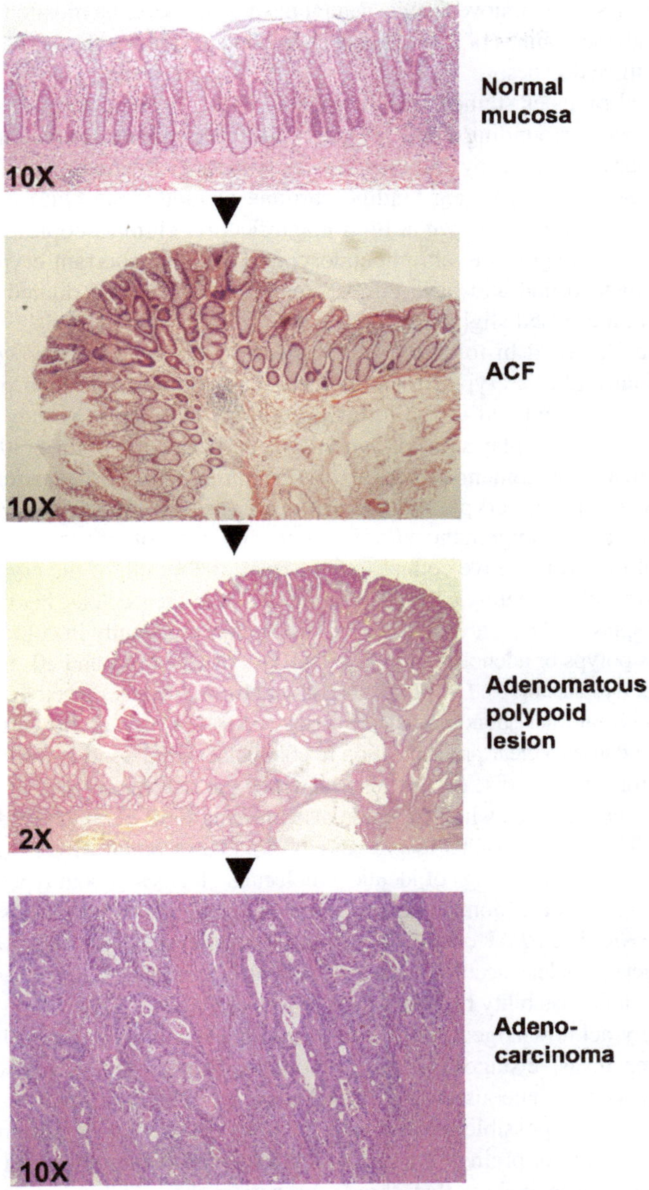

Fig. 18.1 A simplified 4-stage model of the transformation of normal colorectal mucosa into adenocarcinoma. The figure shows the histologic features of the four stages of the adenoma-carcinoma pathway to colorectal cancer: (**a**) normal mucosa; (**b**) aberrant crypt focus (ACF); (**c**) tubulo-villous adenoma with epithelial dysplasia; and (**d**) invasive adenocarcinoma. The dysplastic ACF shown in panel B came from the colon of a patient with colon cancer (H&E staining, 25× magnification). The photomicrogram shows approximately 12 of the 50 or so aberrant crypts included in the ACF, which is slightly raised above (≈500 μm) the surface of the gut mucosa. Compared with the surrounding normal crypts (*right*, *upper corner*), the aberrant crypts are larger

endoscopy, it has to be removed, so its natural history can never be monitored – but it is consistent with the findings of innumerable endoscopic and histologic studies performed over the last three decades.

In mucosal biopsies stained with methylene blue, ACFs appear darker than the normal mucosa surrounding them [11]. In situ, these minute lesions are invisible during standard colonoscopy, but they are easily identified when magnifying endoscopes are used with dyes (e.g., indigo carmine or methylene blue) that enhance mucosal detail, a process known as high-magnification-chromoscopic-colonoscopy or, more simply, magnifying chromoendoscopy [12]. The aberrant crypts are usually larger than normal and have thicker epithelial linings and dilated or slit-like openings that are raised slightly above the adjacent mucosa.

ACFs are classified histologically as dysplastic and nondysplastic. Apart from their size, nondysplastic crypts are not remarkably abnormal, and their proliferative compartments are confined to the lower portion of the glands, as they should be. However, they often display signs of hyperplasia and infolding of the epithelium into the crypt lumen, a phenomenon referred to as *serration,* which is discussed in greater detail below. Dysplastic crypts, in contrast, present signs of cellular atypia (mucin depletion, nuclear enlargement, stratification, and loss of polarity) and upward expansion of the proliferative compartment toward the mouth of the crypts.

Around 60% of all healthy adults have a few ACFs in their colons, but these lesions are rarely dysplastic. ACFs are encountered much more frequently in colons harboring adenomatous polyps or adenocarcinomas (80–100% of all cases), and 20–50% of these show signs of dysplasia [13]. Dysplastic ACFs are also frequently detected in the colons of patients with familial adenomatous polyposis (FAP) [14], a high-penetrance genetic condition that causes a clear predisposition to colorectal cancer. And in ulcerative colitis (a chronic inflammatory disease that also increases the risk for colorectal cancer), the number of ACFs increases when the colon also presents signs of epithelial dysplasia or cancer [15]. The view of ACFs as probable precursors of preinvasive colorectal neoplasms is supported by findings of identical molecular changes in both types of lesions. Indeed, although they are more common features of premalignant neoplasms, mutations involving the *KRAS* or *BRAF* oncogene or the adenomatous polyposis coli (*APC*) tumor-suppressor gene, nuclear accumulation of β-catenin, aberrant DNA methylation, and low-level genomic instability have also been reported in some ACFs.

It is widely acknowledged that, while a few ACFs will progress to the preinvasive and, later, invasive stages (adenocarcinomas), others will not, and some might actually regress spontaneously [16]. These lesions are so small and so numerous that it is virtually impossible to eliminate them by endoscopic resection (which is no problem with larger preinvasive lesions), but they do seem to respond to chemoprevention [13]. The weight that should be assigned to ACFs – their presence, number, and type – in planning surveillance colonoscopy is currently unclear, but the increasing use of magnifying chromoendoscopy is expected to provide important information on this question.

Preinvasive neoplasms – the next stage – are also a frequent finding. They are identified in roughly one third of all asymptomatic adults undergoing standard colonoscopy, but, like ACFs, some may regress on their own, and only a fraction will be transformed into cancers. The progression process generally involves increases in size and in the degree of cellular atypia. Lesions over 1 cm in diameter with high-grade dysplasia (referred to as *advanced adenomas*) are the ones farthest along on the road toward malignancy. (The term *adenoma* is used hereafter to refer to neoplasms – regardless of their macroscopic appearance – that display epithelial dysplasia.)

Several lines of evidence indicate that some of these preinvasive lesions will indeed give rise to colorectal cancers. For one thing, the frequency of these benign neoplasms and that of colorectal cancers both increase with age, but the age/prevalence curve for the former is shifted to the left by ~10 years. The regional distribution of cancers within the colon also parallels that of large adenomas. In addition, the expected incidence of colorectal cancer is substantially reduced by colonoscopy with polypectomy (even though 10–20% of all premalignant lesions, mainly those with diameters <5 mm, are likely to be missed on standard endoscopy) [17]. And finally, there is the impressive frequency at which invasive adenocarcinomas are detected within an advanced adenoma, especially those displaying villous growth patterns and particularly severe dysplasia. About half of all adenocarcinomas are elevated above the surrounding mucosa, and in the other half growth occurs at or below the surface of the normal tissue, so it seems that both polypoid and nonpolypoid benign lesions give rise to cancer.

Breaking Convention: The Contributions of Modern Endoscopy and Histology

For decades, all preinvasive colorectal lesions were referred to as polyps. Pre-neoplastic growth that did not protrude into the gut lumen was first detected in the eighties by Japanese endoscopists [18]. Once these nonprojecting lesions were recognized, they were reported with increasing frequency in other countries as well, where they represented 10–40% of all the preinvasive neoplasms encountered during screening colonoscopy [19].

Since then, attempts have been made to reclassify preinvasive lesions of the digestive tract. These efforts have been more or less successful, but older terms are still encountered, and they can be a source of considerable confusion. When possible, we will give preference in this chapter to the newer, more precise terminology, which refers to all protruding lesions as *polypoid* and sub-classifies them as *pedunculated* (attached with a pedicle or stalk) or *sessile* (attached by a broad base). At the other end of the spectrum are the *nonpolypoid* lesions. They are still widely referred to as "flat" although most are actually slightly elevated (<2.5 mm above the surface of the gut mucosa); those that are completely flat or slightly depressed are rare, but even when they are small, they are generally farther along on the road to cancer (Fig. 18.2) [20]. O'Brien et al. highlighted the impact of the new terminology in their recent reassessment of 1,505 superficial neoplasms classified as polyps in the United States' National Polyp Study. Around 30% – specifi-

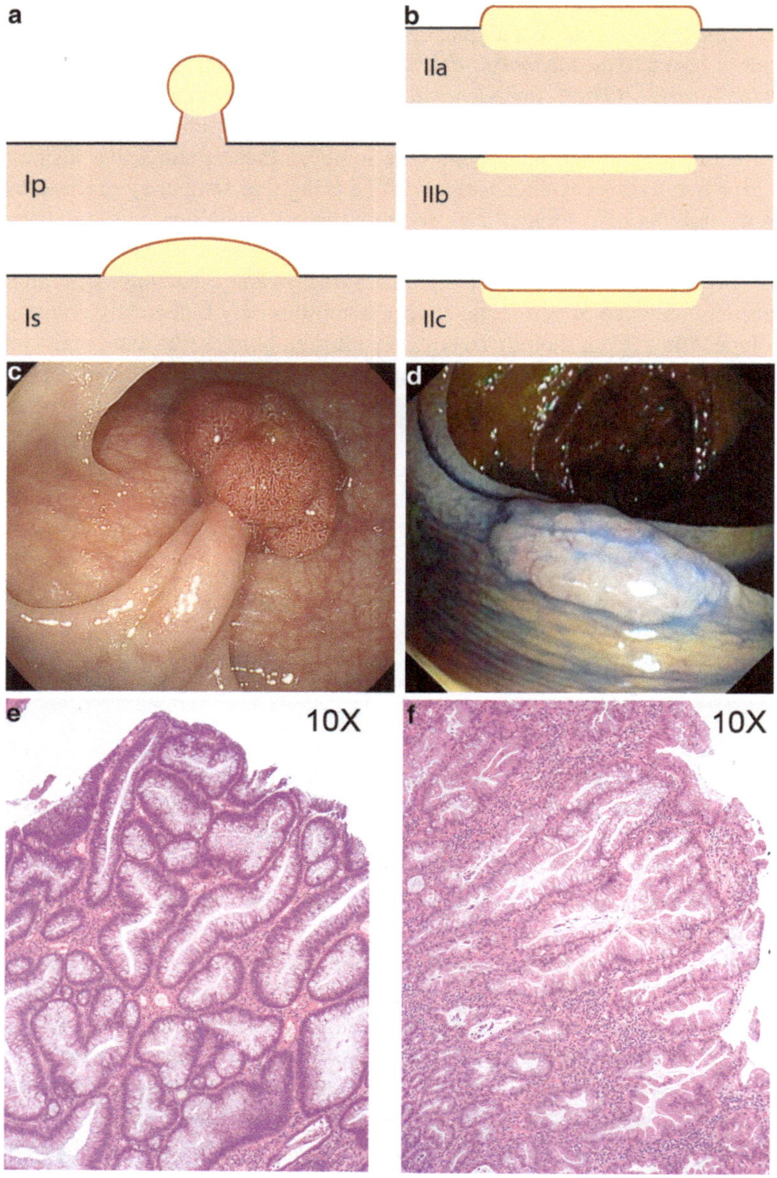

Fig. 18.2 Polypoid and nonpolypoid preinvasive lesions of the colorectum. (**a**, **b**), Types of tumor growth associated with the development of colorectal neoplasia (Paris classification, ref. [20]). Polypoid (**a**) lesions can be pedunculated *(Type Ip)* or sessile (*Type Is*); most nonpolypoid (**b**) lesions are slightly elevated (*Type IIa*), but some are completely flat (*Type IIb*) or depressed (*Type IIc*). Mixed growth patterns can also be found. The endoscopic appearances of polypoid (pedunculated) and nonpolypoid (slightly elevated) lesions are shown in panel (**c**) and (**d**), respectively. Histological examination shows conventional adenomatous features

cally, two-thirds of those originally considered *sessile polyps* – met the new criteria for *nonpolypoid* neoplasms [21].

These lesions had all been detected in the 1980s with standard colonoscopy. In a more recent study based on high-magnification chromoendoscopy, 38% of the adenomatous lesions were nonpolypoid [22]. This approach also allows accurate in vivo classification of lesions based on surface morphology. The shape of the colon crypt lumen in particular (the so-called pit pattern) has proved to be a very reliable predictor of a lesion's histologic features [23]. These newer techniques are becoming increasingly popular, and their use will undoubtedly improve the accuracy of endoscopic diagnoses. Nevertheless, high-quality standard colonoscopy – that is, *complete* examination of a clean colon, all the way to the cecum, with slow, careful withdrawal and re-examination of potential blind spots – is still widely regarded as a reliable tool for detecting preinvasive lesions and preventing colorectal cancer.

The more accurate endoscopic classification of preinvasive colorectal lesions led to some important observations. While true polypoid lesions were more frequently detected in the left colon (from the splenic flexure to rectum), nonpolypoid neoplasms were more common in the right colon (from the cecum to the splenic flexure). Even more important was the discovery that, while most of the latter lesions had classic adenomatous features, others presented a peculiar histologic pattern characterized by infolding of the glandular epithelium. As noted earlier, this phenomenon is referred to as *serration*, because it produces a saw-toothed (or serrated) pattern in longitudinally sectioned crypts [24] (Fig. 18.2e, f). On cross-section, the serrated crypt has a star-shaped appearance, and this feature can also be discerned in vivo by careful examination of crypt mouths with magnification chromoendoscopy.

Serrated crypt architecture proved to be typical of lesions that were then (and sometimes still are) being referred to as *hyperplastic polyps*. They had long been considered innocuous with a negligible risk for progression to cancer, mainly because, in spite of their architectural abnormality, they showed no clear signs of epithelial dysplasia. The term *hyperplastic polyp* is gradually being abandoned in favor of *nondysplastic serrated polyp* (although in both cases, the term "polyp" is a misnomer since many of these lesions are nonpolypoid). It is also becoming increasingly clear that this category includes morphologically and molecularly distinct subsets with different propensities for malignant transformation.

Three major histologic subtypes have been identified thus far (see [25] for details). *Goblet-cell serrated polyps* (GCSPs) have the fewest architectural anomalies, and it is generally agreed that they are unlikely to progress to cancer. These lesions are found primarily in the left colon, and most are small rectal lesions. They contain enlarged, nonbranching crypts displaying little or no epithelial infolding. Their main abnormality consists in an increased goblet cell/columnar cell ratio that

Fig. 18.2 (continued) (tubular proliferation withlow-grade epithelial dysplasia) in a pedunculated polyp (**e**; magnification, 10×) and the serrated pattern (irregular shape of the crypts with serration of glandular lumens) in a nonpolypoid lesion (**f**; magnification, 10×). (See text for description of the histotypes.) Either of these histological patterns can be found in polypoid and nonpolypoid lesions

affects the entire length of the gland. *Microvesicular serrated polyps* (MVSPs) are more common than GCSPs. They are found throughout the colon, although their frequency is also highest in the left colon and rectum. The crypts are elongated and funnel-shaped, but the proliferative compartment is normally confined to the bottom of the gland. The upper crypts contain numerous microvacuolated columnar cells. The upper two-third of the crypt (and less commonly the crypt base as well) typically presents epithelial serration. The third subset comprises lesions that are still widely referred to as *sessile serrated adenomas* (SSAs). The term is imprecise: first, because the group includes both sessile polyps and nonpolypoid lesions, and second, because the dysplasia that is the hallmark of an adenoma is absent in these lesions. SSAs are generally found in the right colon. They are characterized by L-shaped or inverted-T shaped crypts lined with infolded epithelium from base to mouth. The proliferative compartment is sometimes expanded, but as noted, there is no real cytologic dysplasia.

Histologic and molecular findings (detailed in the next section) suggest that SSAs evolve from MVSPs and that some do eventually become dysplastic. But at this point, they are usually referred to as *serrated adenomas* (SAs). The histologic definition of this term is still a matter of debate among pathologists so their diagnosis displays substantial interobserver variation. Because cellular dysplasia is an essential feature of SAs, some are likely to be classified as conventional adenomas. Mixed lesions containing serrated areas interspersed with areas displaying conventional adenomatous changes can also be found [26].

In a recent study [27], 65% of the premalignant lesions resected during standard colonoscopy were conventional adenomas. The other 35% displayed serrated architecture and were generally classified as "hyperplastic polyps." Most of the latter were MVSPs or GCSPs (30%), a few were SSAs (~4%), and less than 2% were dysplastic. Similar figures (~60% conventional adenomas, ~40% serrated lesions) emerged from another study based on magnifying chromoendoscopy [28]. Nine percent of all lesions removed in this study were SSAs, and 2.4% were dysplastic (SAs). The coexistence of adenomatous and serrated lesions in the same patient is a common finding.

Therefore, alongside the conventional adenoma-carcinoma pathway illustrated in Fig. 18.1, there seems to be a second, less-frequented route, the serrated pathway, which also leads to the development of colorectal adenocarcinoma (Fig. 18.3). There is evidence of its existence at both ends of the transformation process. Serrated/stellate crypt morphology has, in fact, been described in some nondysplastic (or hyperplastic) ACFs [29], and ~10% of all colorectal cancers have predominantly serrated histologic patterns (the serrated adenocarcinomas) [30] or contain peripheral remnants of serrated adenoma [31]. The mixed (serrated and conventionally adenomatous) histology observed in some preinvasive lesions suggests that the two pathways have somehow intersected or merged during tumorigenesis.

In summary, two out of three preinvasive colorectal lesions discovered at endoscopy are classic adenomas with tubular and/or villous architecture and some degree of dysplasia (Figs. 18.1 and 18.2e). The third will present a serrated histological pattern, in rare cases combined with dysplastic changes (Fig. 18.2f). The classic adenomas are usually pedunculated (or less frequently, sessile) polyps, but around

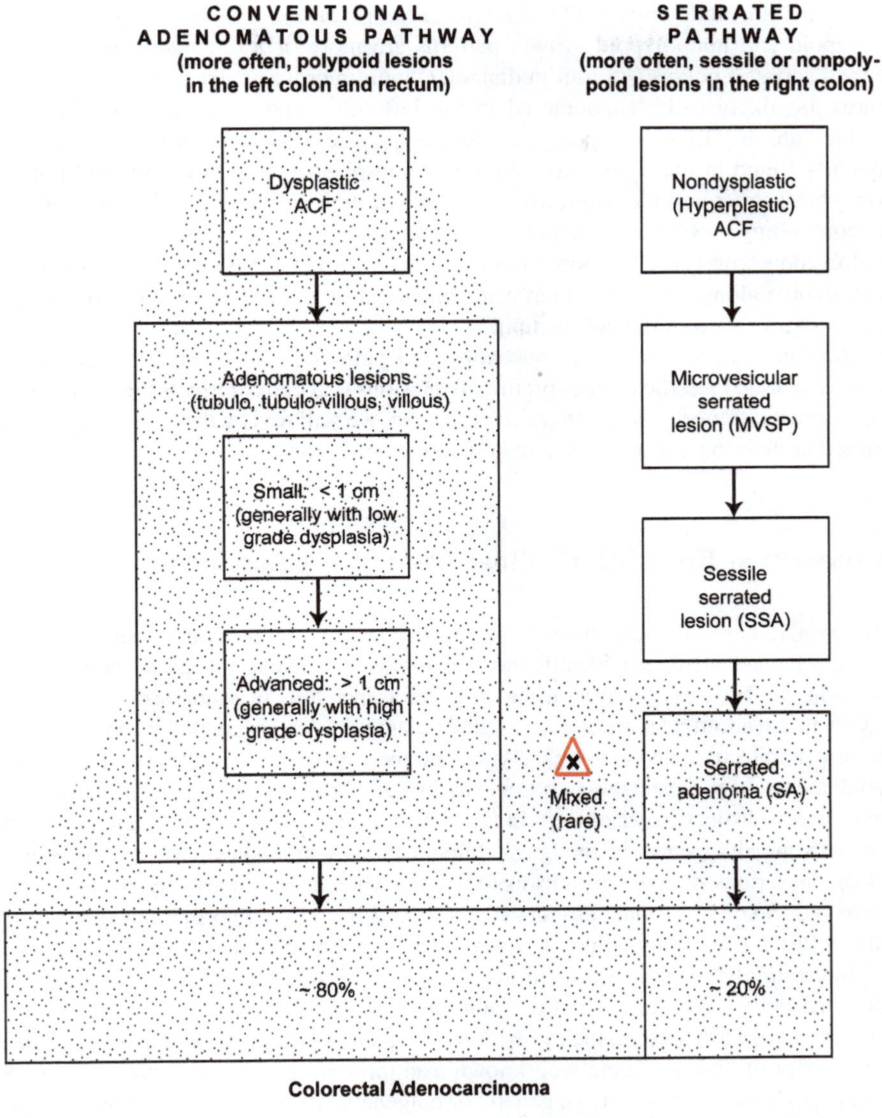

Fig. 18.3 The best characterized pathways to colorectal adenocarcinoma. The conventional adenomatous pathway is the most common route to adenocarcinoma. The cancers that arise through this pathway can be located anywhere in the colorectum, but they are more frequent in the left colon and rectum. Progressively severe cellular and architectural dysplasia (shaded region) is the hallmark of this pathway. It can already be found in the earliest-stage lesions, such as ACFs. The putative stations in the "less traveled" serrated pathway are shown on the right. Architectural abnormalities are an early feature of this pathway, whereas cellular dysplasia appears late (details in the text). Among the lesions that develop through this pathway, those most likely to develop into cancer are located in the right colon

one-third are nonpolypoid [22, 27, 28] (Fig. 18.2a–d). Among serrated lesions, polypoid and nonpolypoid growth patterns are more or less equally represented. Small serrated polyps (<5 mm in diameter) with microvesicular or goblet-cell features are likely to be encountered in the left colon and rectum. Larger MVSPs (which are usually sessile polyps or nonpolypoid lesions) and SSAs are more frequently found in the right colon. As for the dysplastic serrated lesions (SA), over two-thirds are polypoid, and most are located in the left colon [32]. However, there is compelling molecular evidence (see next section) that their less common, right-colon counterparts are far more important: these proximal SAs seem to be the ones that evolve along the serrated pathway, presumably giving rise to ~20% of adenocarcinomas found in the colorectum.

Advances in the fields of endoscopy and pathology have provided us with a more accurate classification of preinvasive lesions that better reflects their relevance in colorectal tumorigenesis. In the next section, we will review the results of studies aimed at defining the molecular features of these lesions.

Convention-Breaking Findings from Molecular Biology

The availability of tissue samples of preinvasive lesions removed during endoscopy or surgery fuelled attempts to identify the crucial molecular events that allow these lesions to form and progress toward cancer. In general, increases in lesion size – from tiny ACFs to advanced adenomas over 1 cm in diameter – are paralleled by increasingly bizarre architectural and cytologic atypia, and the larger lesions (polypoid or nonpolypoid) are the ones most likely to become malignant. Analyzing lesions of different sizes thus reveals distinct stages or steps in the transformation process. And when molecular changes are discovered in malignant tumors (adenocarcinomas), we can backtrack along the various steps of the pathway to find out when (and perhaps why) the alteration appeared. Some abnormalities can even be traced back to the normal mucosa, where they reflect a genetically- and/or environmentally-determined field defect.

Interestingly, molecular alterations considered highly relevant to the transformation process in the colon are often found in some but not all premalignant lesions, and when they are present, their prevalence frequently correlates poorly with the size or severity of lesions. Some well known examples are oncogene mutations (*KRAS* and *BRAF*) and more extensive genetic or epigenetic alterations, such as microsatellite instability or the methylator phenotype (see below). The fact that some of these changes appear to be mutually exclusive suggests that pre-cancerous cells can be transformed into invasive cancer cells by different sequences of mutations.

Nevertheless, there does seem to be a common denominator in the onset and progression of most, if not all, pre-cancerous lesions of the colorectum: aberrant activation of the Wnt signaling cascade. Canonical Wnt signaling is a crucial driver of epithelial-cell division within the lower third of the intestinal crypt, which represents one of the simplest self-renewing biological entities in mammals [33]. In this proliferative compartment of the gland, secreted Wnt proteins interact with serpentine receptors of the frizzled family and low-density lipid receptors 5 or 6 expressed by the dividing epithelial cells. Signal transduction activated by this binding inhibits the formation of a cytoplasmic complex whose core components include APC (a multidomain protein encoded by the adenomatous polyposis coli gene), glycogen synthase kinase-3β, the scaffolding protein axin, and casein kinase 1. This so-called destruction complex catalyzes the phosphorylation of β-catenin, thereby targeting it for ubiquitin-mediated degradation. In its absence, β-catenin accumulates in the cytoplasm and eventually translocates into nucleus, where it encounters DNA-binding proteins of the T-cell factor (TCF)/lymphoid enhancer factor (LEF) family. β-catenin binding converts the TCF and LEF1 proteins from transcription repressors to transcription activators. Among their targets are genes whose products play fundamental roles in maintaining stem- and cycling-cell populations at the bases of colon crypts (other transcription factors like CMYC, the cell cycle kinase activator cyclin D, and matrix metalloproteinase 7, to name a few). Cells in the upper two-thirds of the crypt are not stimulated by Wnt signaling proteins, so the β-catenin in these cells is recruited to the destruction complex and promptly degraded. This leaves the upper-crypt cells free to differentiate as they migrate upward toward the intestinal lumen.

Constitutive Wnt signaling leads to an expansion of the proliferative compartment of the crypt, destroying the equilibrium between proliferation and differentiation, and this loss generally coincides with the development of precancerous lesions. In virtually all colorectal tumors (preinvasive and invasive), this inappropriate signaling reflects abnormal stabilization of β-catenin, and in 60–80%, the cause is homozygous mutation of the well-known tumor suppressor gene *APC* [34–37] (Fig. 18.4), which presumably occurs in the progenitor stem cells at the crypt base [38, 39]. *APC* mutation is therefore a frequent event in the initial stages of colon tumorigenesis, but it is not the only cause of the altered stability and distribution of β-catenin that characterize colorectal tumors. Wnt signaling can also be constitutively activated by somatic changes affecting other crucial pathway components. They can be genetic (e.g., mutations involving the gene that encodes β-catenin, which generally result in substitution of serine or threonine residues whose phosphorylation allows the protein to be degraded by the destruction complex [40–42]) or epigenetic (transcriptional silencing of the *SFRP1* gene [43], which encodes a receptor that normally inhibits Wnt signaling).

APC and β-catenin mutations are mutually exclusive in colorectal neoplasms, but other genetic and epigenetic changes in Wnt-pathway components are often found together in the same tumor. Many human tumors develop and evolve as a result of the deregulation of multiple signaling pathways, and this is undoubtedly true of colorectal tumors as well, but colorectal tumorigenesis also seems to be characterized by the selection of repeated alterations (or "hits") involving the Wnt pathway. These observations suggest that Wnt signalling dysregulation itself may be modulated during transformation to meet the specific needs of the tumor at various points in its journey.

Changes of this type can naturally have an impact on the tumor phenotype. For example, biallelic mutation of tumor suppressor genes is generally envisioned as

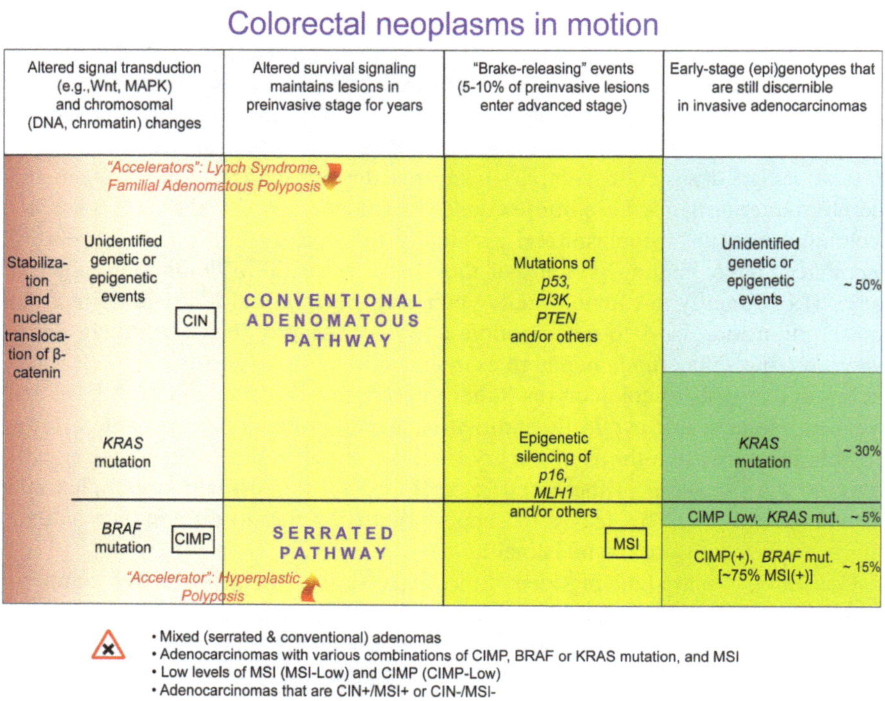

Fig. 18.4 Molecular pathways and crossroads in colorectal transformation. The conventional adenomatous pathway and the serrated pathway are currently the best characterized stepwise models of colorectal carcinogenesis. In both, dysregulation of Wnt signaling (β-catenin stabilization and nuclear translocation) is an early event. It can be caused by different (epi)mutations. (In the conventional adenomatous pathway, the most frequent cause is *APC* mutation). Other early events have also been documented, including mutations affecting components of the MAPK/ERK cascades (i.e., *KRAS* or *BRAF* mutations, which are mutually exclusive) and chromosomal changes, like CIN (lower-level compared to that seen in advanced adenocarcinomas) or CIMP. And there are undoubtedly others that have yet to be discovered. They account for roughly half of all adenocarcinomas, i.e., those with no evidence of the early alterations listed above (far right column – light blue segment). Mutations involving "survival signaling" cascades (e.g., MAPK/ERK) alter the normal homeostatic equilibrium between proliferation, checkpoint repair of DNA damage, and apoptosis, allowing preinvasive lesions to survive for years. Additional mutations are necessary to allow the tumor to move on into the advanced stage, where malignancy is imminent. The nature of these "brake-releasing" events differs, depending on which pathway the tumor is moving along. Crossroad warning sign: Examples from the literature [26, 55–58, 64] of "molecular deviation" from the original pathway, a phenomenon that can occur at almost any stage of carcinogenesis. Accelerators: Colon cancer predisposition syndromes – each represents high-speed transformation along one of the pathways shown in this figure: the adenomatous pathway in Lynch syndrome and familial adenomatous polyposis; the serrated pathway in hyperplastic polyposis. The information reported in this figure is based on rates of detection of a dozen or so genetic and epigenetic alterations in preinvasive colorectal lesions and their persistence in advanced adenocarcinomas. The relative frequency of a given alteration or combination of alterations can vary considerably from study to study owing to differences in inclusion criteria (i.e., types of lesion studied), in the number and type of molecular changes investigated, and in the method(s)

causing loss of protein function, but in the case of *APC*, the mutant gene products are usually stable, truncated proteins that may well retain some ability to interact with β-catenin, for example [44]. The mutant alleles (i.e., the first and second hits) seem to be co-selected to achieve a level of aberrant Wnt signaling that is "optimal" for tumor cell proliferation and DNA replication. During tumor progression, however, one of the two *APC* alleles may develop a second mutation – a "third hit" that readjusts the level or characteristics of the dysregulated signaling to meet the tumor's current needs [45].

The quality of the dysregulated signaling also changes when one pathway component instead of another is altered. For instance, compared with tumors bearing β-catenin mutations, those with abnormal APC function are thought to be more prone to DNA ploidy changes, because APC is also involved in mitotic spindle formation and chromosome segregation, processes that are essential for the maintenance of chromosomal stability [46]. Low-level chromosomal instability has in fact been detected in adenomatous polyps (mainly gains of chromosome 7 and 20, as well as deletions in multiple regions) and in dysplastic ACFs of patients with APC mutations [47, 48], although no genomic imbalances were found when a small series of adenomas with biallelic *APC* mutations were recently subjected to comparative genomic hybridization analysis [49].

The RAS/RAF/MEK/ERK (or MAPK/ERK) cascade is another signaling pathway that is frequently dysregulated in colorectal carcinogenesis, and it, too, transforms extracellular signals into transcriptional regulation. The MAPK/ERK cascade is a classical "survival" pathway, in that it promotes cell proliferation and prevents apoptosis. Two of its gene components, *KRAS* and *BRAF*, are known oncogenes that often present gain-of-function mutations in preinvasive colorectal lesions. The hyperactive mutant kinases they encode ($KRAS^{G12D}$ and $BRAF^{V600E}$, for example) maintain a state of chronically activated "survival signaling" in premalignant cells.

The level of this aberrant MAPK/ERK activity has yet to be well defined, but the balance between cellular proliferation and apoptosis undoubtedly differs from that observed in the normal mucosa. Loss of this normal homeostatic equilibrium seems to be associated with a substantial increase in DNA replication stress. Unlike the proliferating cells of normal colorectal crypts, premalignant epithelial cells with oncogene-activated survival signaling display classic examples of cellular responses to DNA damage, including phosphorylation of checkpoint kinase CHK2 and the histone protein H2AX, or signs of telomere attrition [50, 51]. These events halt the cells at a specific stage of the cell cycle so that the DNA damage can be repaired. This checkpoint repair system is probably one of several mechanisms that put a brake on the progression of tumorigenesis and allow lesions to remain in the preinvasive stage for years (Fig. 18.4).

BRAF and *KRAS* oncogene mutations are early mutually exclusive events that can already be detected in ACFs [29]. The former is more frequent in serrated ACFs, and the latter is more common in ACFs that lack serration. Interestingly

Fig. 18.4 (continued) employed to detect these changes. Abbreviations: CIN (chromosomal instability); CIMP (CpG island methylator phenotype); MIN: microsatellite instability

enough, this difference is maintained as transformation progresses. In fact, *BRAF* mutations are found in over two-thirds of all MVSPs, SSAs, and dysplastic SAs, and they are also present in ~15% of all adenocarcinomas, mainly those right-colon cancers that develop along the serrated pathway. *KRAS* mutations are detected in 30–40% of conventional adenomas and in approximately one-third of all adenocarcinomas [31, 52] (Fig. 18.4).

Therefore, although KRAS is located immediately upstream to BRAF in the MAPK/ERK signaling pathway and each intermediate is frequently mutated in preinvasive colorectal lesions, the phenotypic consequences of these mutations are quite different. (We saw the same thing above, when we looked at mutations of APC and β-catenin in the Wnt pathway.) The distinctive effects of mutations involving two components of a given pathway, even those that are adjacent to one another in the signaling cascade, are not surprising, because each component is transduced differently downstream and each interacts in its own way with factors of other signaling pathways (e.g., cross-talk between components of the MAPK/ERK and PTEN/PI3K/AKT/mTOR pathways [53]).

While activating mutation of *KRAS* or *BRAF* seems to be an early event in the process of colorectal transformation, 50–60% of all colorectal adenocarcinomas show no sign of either mutation (Fig. 18.4). If, as it seems, oncogene activation of survival signaling allows preinvasive lesions to avoid cell death for many years, it seems reasonable to expect that benign lesions without *KRAS* or *BRAF* mutation would have mutations/alterations involving other oncogenes. To date, however, none have been identified.

The end of this more or less lengthy preinvasive stage and the onset of true malignancy is believed to be caused by the addition of one or more new genetic or epigenetic alterations. The "brake-releasing" events are nonrandom, but they may differ, depending on the nature of the preinvasive neoplasm. Some lesions are set in motion by mutation of the tumor-suppressor gene *TP53*, which is often altered in advanced colorectal tumors; in others, the crucial event affects another survival signaling pathway (e.g., mutation of *PIK3CA* or *PTEN* in the PTEN/PI3K/AKT/mTOR pathway [54]) or another Wnt signaling protein; and in others, the brake-releasing hit targets a gene needed for genomic stability (the DNA mismatch repair gene, *MLH1*, for example). The type of event(s) necessary to provoke the transition to invasiveness seems to be dictated at least in part by the original genetic features of the premalignant lesion. (Somatic *MLH1* silencing, for instance, seems to be the most common trigger for progression of *BRAF*-mutated serrated lesions.)

Analysis of a dozen or more different genetic and epigenetic alterations in a substantial number of colorectal neoplasms has revealed at least two clearly discernable paths toward the invasive stage (Fig. 18.4). Each includes a number of molecular crossroads, however, and the tumor-in-motion can thus be deviated toward a different pathway by biological obstacles encountered during progression (most of which have yet to be characterized). Route changes of this type can result in mixed phenotypes [55–58].

The serrated pathway shown in Fig. 18.4 generates colorectal neoplasms that are phenotypically distinct from those that develop through the conventional, APC-driven, adenoma-carcinoma sequence. *BRAF*-mutated, serrated lesions give rise to sporadic *MLH1*-deficient cancers of the right colon, which are more frequent in women and occur later than other sporadic colorectal cancers (peak prevalence between the ages of 70 and 80 years). A frequent feature of these neoplasms is the CpG island methylator phenotype (CIMP), which is characterized by nonrandom transcriptional silencing of several cancer-relevant gene promoters, like those of *p16* and *MLH1* [31, 59–66]. Relatively rare in conventional adenomas, the CIMP is found in 70–80% of all dysplastic serrated lesions of the right colon, and it is closely associated with *BRAF* mutations. The basis of this association is unknown, and it is also unclear why CIMP-positive tumors prefer the right colon of women. The latter aspect presumably highlights roles played by hormonal and environmental factors (including cigarette smoking [67] and hypoxia [68, 69]).

High-throughput sequencing technology and system biology studies (based on genomics, transcriptomics, and proteomics, and other more specific – omics) will certainly improve mutation detection, providing us with a more precise picture of the colorectal oncogenetic tree [70, 71] than the one represented in Fig. 18.4. These advances will bring us several steps closer to the goal of type-specific treatment for colorectal cancers. The different phenotypes might also have specific mechanisms for developing resistance to treatment regimens, so detailed knowledge of a given phenotype might also facilitate the early detection and prompt treatment of tumors that are no longer responding to treatment.

Fast-Track Transformation Models: Inherited Syndromes and Inflammatory Bowel Disease

The adenomatous and serrated pathways of colorectal transformation can be discerned within three inherited syndromes that are major risk factors for the development of colon cancer. Because the susceptibility to cancer is inherited, tumorigenesis generally begins earlier and proceeds more rapidly than it does in sporadic disease, and mutation carriers frequently develop adenocarcinomas between the third and fifth decades of life.

Familial adenomatous polyposis – Less than 1% of all colorectal cancers are related to familial adenomatous polyposis (FAP), but this syndrome provides us with an invaluable "fast-forward" view of mutant APC-driven transformation through the adenomatous pathway. Individuals with FAP are born with a heterozygous germ-line mutation in *APC*, and by adolescence or early adulthood, their colons are filled with hundreds or thousands of classical adenomatous polyps. They also develop extracolonic disease, such as congenital hypertrophy of the retinal pigment epithelium, desmoid tumors of the abdomen, upper gastrointestinal adenomas and carcinomas, and, less frequently, osteomas, dental abnormalities, lipomas, and epidermoid cysts. Malignant tumors of the brain, thyroid, and hepatobiliary tract have also been associated with FAP.

FAP is transmitted in an autosomal dominant fashion, although ~30% of all patients represent new cases in the family (i.e., de novo mutations). There is also a milder variant, attenuated FAP, characterized by later disease onset and a smaller number of colorectal polyps (conventionally, fewer than 100) [72]. But since approximately 5% of all adenomas eventually become cancers, the probability of colorectal cancer by the age of 40–50 years is 100% even in these patients. FAP adenomas do not seem to be more prone to transformation than their sporadic counterparts. The accelerated tumorigenesis associated with this syndrome appears to be related primarily to the prodigious numbers of polyps that form and the early age at which they appear.

APC encodes a 2843-amino-acid protein with several functional domains, including several that bind with β-catenin and others that interacts with axin. As mentioned in the previous section, nonsense germ-line *APC* mutations usually generate partially functional N-terminal APC fragments lacking one or more of these domains. Variability in the domain make-up of these truncated proteins is reflected by different degrees of Wnt signaling dysregulation, which produce different effects on cell–cell adhesion, cell migration, cell division, and chromosomal stability [73]. This is the basis for the genotype–phenotype association model of FAP (reviewed in [74]), which holds that the severity of the disease – in terms of number and onset of colorectal adenomas and extracolonic manifestations – depends on the location of the germ-line mutation within the *APC* gene.

The model has some obvious shortcomings. For one thing, past analyses have been largely restricted to the mutation cluster region of *APC*, and this may have provided a skewed picture of the mutational spectrum in this gene. Furthermore, the transformation process within single lesions can also be influenced by the characteristics of second and (in some cases) third hits involving *APC* at the somatic level (as discussed in the previous section). Numerous studies have revealed inconsistencies and contradictions in the genotype-phenotype association model, the most striking of which is the fact that, in 30–50% of patients with FAP or attenuated FAP phenotypes, current testing methods reveal no *APC* mutations at all! In some of these cases, bi-allelic germ-line mutations involving the base excision repair gene *MYH* have been detected. They represent a recessively inherited variant of FAP (or attenuated FAP), in which the development of adenomatous polyposis is believed to be triggered by *somatic APC* mutations resulting from defective processing of oxidative DNA damage by the base excision repair system [75–77].

Lynch syndrome – This is the most common colorectal cancer predisposition syndrome of known etiology and the cause of ~3% of all adenocarcinomas of the colon. Like FAP, Lynch syndrome is a model of accelerated transformation along the conventional adenomatous pathway, but the driving force here is completely different. Lynch syndrome patients generally harbor a heterozygous germ-line mutation involving one of four genes that are essential for DNA mismatch repair (MMR): *MSH2*, *MSH6*, *MLH1*, and *PMS2*. As a result, base/base mismatches and strand misalignments generated during DNA replication by polymerase δ or ε go unrepaired, and the rate of mutations rises markedly (reviewed in [78]). This defect results in what is known as a *mutator phenotype* characterized by the accumulation of large numbers of mutations in the genome.

MMR is normally initiated when a mispair or misalignment is bound by the mismatch recognition complex, MSH2/MSH6. The heterodimer then undergoes an ATP-driven conformational change, which allows it to interact with another MMR protein heterodimer, MLH1/PMS2. This interaction activates the endonucleolytic function of PMS2, which nicks the newly synthesized DNA strand on the 3′ and 5′ sides of the mismatch. Exonuclease 1 then degrades the mispair-containing segment, beginning at the 5′ nick, and the resulting gap is then filled in with the correct sequence by replicating DNA polymerase δ or ε.

Genes whose germ-line mutations cause inherited forms of cancer are often found to be somatically altered in certain sporadic tumors, and the MMR genes are no exception [79]. This is especially true of *MLH1*. Loss of MLH1 expression is found in approximately 10% of all colorectal carcinomas, and the vast majority are unrelated to Lynch syndrome. Sporadic, MLH1-defective tumors are in fact the most common MMR-defective colorectal cancers. These are the cancers discussed in the previous section, the ones that are almost always found in the right colon. They arise through the serrated pathway and are often characterized by *BRAF* mutations and CIMP-positivity, which leads to somatic silencing of *MLH1* via bi-allelic methylation of its promoter.

In contrast, the inherited MMR-defective colorectal cancers associated with Lynch syndrome develop along the conventional adenomatous pathway. The first hit – heterozygous germ-line mutation of one of the MMR genes – predisposes the carrier to MMR deficiency, but the system remains proficient until some somatic event leads to the mutation or loss of the wild-type allele of this gene. So, the disease is inherited as an autosomal dominant predisposition, but it is recessive at the somatic level. Consequently, the affected MMR protein is fully expressed in normal tissue, where heterozygosity has been maintained, but absent in tumor cells, where the wild-type allele has been lost.

When does this second hit occur in the epithelial cells of the colon? Heterozygosity is generally believed to be lost fairly early in the pre-cancerous adenomatous polyp stage [80]. Failure of the MMR system gives rise to a mutator phenotype and microsatellite instability, which should markedly accelerate the adenoma's transformation, and Lynch syndrome adenomas do indeed progress to adenocarcinoma more rapidly (within 2–5 years) and at a higher frequency than their sporadic counterparts. As noted above, adenoma formation itself seems to be triggered by dysregulation of Wnt signaling, which is a very early event in colorectal tumorigenesis (Fig. 18.4). In fact, although the temporal relationships between the various events are still fairly obscure, aberrant Wnt signaling almost certainly precedes the loss of the wild type *MMR* allele. The adenomatous polyps associated with Lynch syndrome are by no means as numerous as those seen in FAP. In most cases, the patient presents with a single adenoma, and there are rarely more than five or six. It seems then that these early dysplastic lesions somehow favor the loss of MMR in heterozygous cells.

In summary, the MMR-defective colorectal cancers associated with the Lynch syndrome arise from isolated adenomatous lesions, which undergo "fast-track" transformation driven by high-rate mutation that often targets tumor suppressor genes [81, 82]. This mechanism probably predominates over chromosomal instability (another frequent driver of carcinogenesis), since MMR-deficient tumors have few chromosomal gains and losses and are often near-diploid (Fig. 18.4). Later on, their aggressiveness and invasiveness are fortunately curbed by a strong antitumor immune response. The molecular components of this response are now under investigation [70], but the trigger seems to consist in the presentation of novel antigens produced by highly mutable, MMR-defective tumor cells.

Hyperplastic polyposis – The paradigm of "fast-track transformation" along the serrated pathway is the syndrome known as *hyperplastic polyposis* (HP), a rare (and underdiagnosed) condition that is often associated with $BRAF^{V600E}$ and the CIMP. HP is diagnosed when there are [83]:(a) at least five histologically diagnosed hyperplastic polyps proximal to the sigmoid colon, including two with diameters exceeding 10 mm; (b) any number of hyperplastic polyps proximal to the sigmoid colon plus first-degree kinship with a patient known to have HP; or (c) over 30 hyperplastic polyps distributed throughout the colon. HP presents with a variety of preinvasive lesions, which include not only hyperplastic polyps but also larger SSAs and even classical adenomas. The syndrome is now known to confer an increased risk for malignant transformation, although the reported magnitude of this risk varies to some extent from study to study [84–86]. HP-related colorectal cancers show a predilection for the proximal colon, and their onset occurs roughly 10 years earlier than that of sporadic colorectal cancers and about two decades later than those related to the Lynch syndrome.

Fewer than 150 cases of HP have been reported to date, and the picture that is emerging is that of a heterogeneous entity. Some authors have suggested [87] that there are actually two different phenotypes. They advocate reserving the term "hyperplastic polyposis" for cases characterized by multiple, small, pancolonic hyperplastic polyps and using "serrated adenomatous polyposis" when there are smaller numbers of relatively large, proximal, hyperplastic polyps with features of SSA. Familial aggregation has been documented in relatively few cases. When present, it seems to reflect dominant transmission of an unidentified genetic predisposition to CIMP, which frequently leads to somatic methylation of the *MLH1* promoter [88, 89]. Compared with patients harboring sporadic serrated lesions, those with HP have a significantly higher frequency of methylated alleles in the normal colon mucosa [90, 91], and this finding is also consistent with the possibility of genetically determined CIMP.

Inflammatory bowel disease – Third on the list of conditions conferring high risk for colorectal cancer – after the Lynch syndrome and FAP – is inflammatory bowel disease (IBD). Ulcerative colitis and Crohn's disease are chronic disorders with an onset peak between the second and fourth decades of life. They are caused by the combined effects of genetic, immune, and environmental factors – most of which are still poorly characterized. Strong evidence supports the view that both involve a dysregulated immune response to commensal bacteria in genetically susceptible individuals [92, 93]. The risk for IBD has been linked to variations in numerous genes [94].

Both ulcerative colitis and Crohn's disease confer an increased risk for colorectal cancer, but this risk varies with disease duration, the extent of colonic involvement, age at diagnosis, the severity of inflammation, family history of colon cancer, and the presence or absence of primary sclerosing cholangitis. The cumulative risk in patients with ulcerative colitis was recently estimated to be 8% at 20 years and 18% at 30 years; similar figures have been reported for Crohn's disease [95, 96]. Most of what we know about colitis-associated carcinogenesis comes from studies of ulcerative colitis, so the rest of this section will focus mainly on this IBD.

The mechanism that links chronic inflammation to carcinogenesis has never been precisely defined. However, persistent inflammation is believed to trigger and sustain oxidative stress that increases proliferation and eventually leads to dysplasia [97]. Two important features of colitis-associated dysplasia are macroscopic heterogeneity and multifocality [98]. Elevated lesions (sometimes referred to as DALM [dysplasia-associated lesion or mass]) range from circumscribed, pedunculated or sessile polyps that resemble noncolitic adenomas to nonadenoma-like lesions that are irregular, broad-based, or poorly circumscribed. These latter lesions often contain ulcerated or hemorrhagic foci, and the flat mucosa surrounding them is also frequently dysplastic. They have often been referred to as "invisible dysplasia," because they are usually undetectable with standard colonoscopy. The only way to demonstrate their existence was to collect large numbers of biopsies from randomly selected sites throughout the colon, and this approach is still used today. However, thanks to the introduction of magnifying chromoendoscopy, these flat lesions can be identified and biopsied, and this advance has greatly facilitated the demonstration of IBD-related dysplasia [99].

The finding of flat or elevated areas of high-grade dysplasia in a patient with ulcerative colitis is an indication for proctocolectomy because these lesions are likely to be multifocal, and their presence is associated with a high risk (~50%) for concurrent or imminent colorectal cancer [100]. Prophylactic surgery for low-grade dysplasia is more controversial [101], in part because there is no real consensus on the criteria for a pathologic diagnosis of this type. Endoscopic detection of preinvasive lesions and histologic assessment of dysplasia are problematic in settings of chronic inflammation, but thus far colorectal carcinogenesis in ulcerative colitis also seems to involve the development of dysplastic ACFs followed by low-grade and then high-grade dysplastic lesions that are eventually transformed into cancers. The identification of molecular markers of these stages will undoubtedly improve the quality of the clinical choices during the follow up of these patients.

Numerous studies have analyzed the molecular profiles of colitis-associated preinvasive lesions and the nonlesional inflamed mucosa. The typical approach involves the search for molecular abnormalities found in noncolitic carcinogenesis – the chromosomal and microsatellite instability, epigenetic alterations, and oncogene and tumor-suppressor-gene mutations mentioned in the previous sections. As expected, most have also been detectable in colitis-associated mucosal lesions, but in many cases it is still unclear how their frequency and timing differ from those observed in the absence of chronic inflammation.

The discrepancies that have arisen were to be expected for several reasons. The availability of tissue samples of colitis-associated lesions is limited, and the linear correlation between lesion size and disease severity observed in noncolitic tumori-

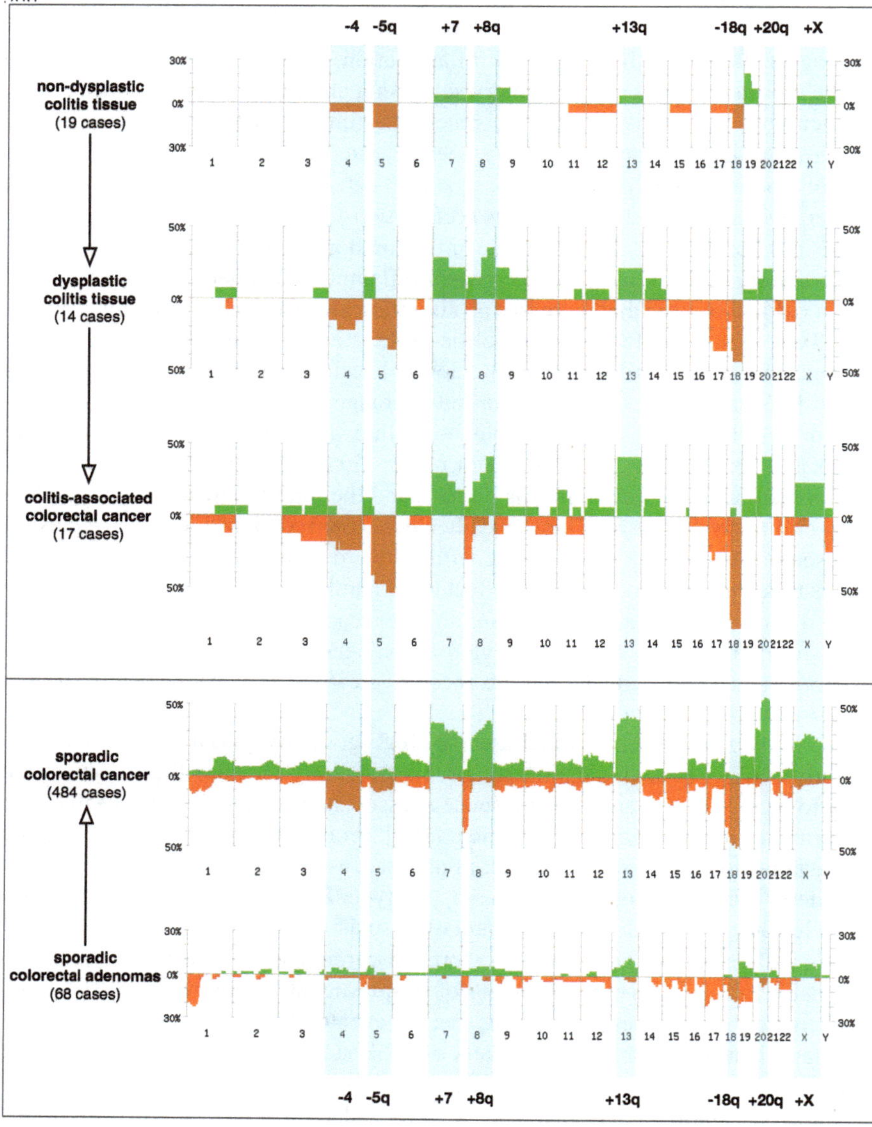

Fig. 18.5 Chromosomal instability in preinvasive and invasive colorectal lesions from patients with and without ulcerative colitis. Histograms show the frequency of genomic imbalances in selected colorectal tissue samples (gains appear in green above the baseline; losses appear below in red). In ulcerative colitis (upper panel), chromosomal aberrations leading to clonal imbalances can already be observed in nondysplastic tissues. Examples are the recurring deletions involving the long arms of chromosomes 5 and 18, which increase in frequency as malignancy progresses. Interestingly, both aberrations are earlier and more frequent events in tumorigenesis associated with ulcerative colitis than in sporadic adenomatous tumorigenesis (two lower panels) or FAP-related tumorigenesis, where 5q deletions are rarely detected (data not shown). During progression, colitis-associated lesions accumulate most of the other genomic imbalances observed in sporadic tumors, namely gains of chromosomes 7, 8q, 13q, 20 and X, as well as deletions of chromosomes 4 and 8p. The data was extracted from the Progenetix database (www.progenetix.net; [109])

genesis tends to break down in IBD, where small lesions are often advanced and molecular changes can also be found in the inflamed, nonneoplastic mucosa. The molecular analyses were also marred by selection biases related to the difficulties mentioned above in the endoscopic detection and histologic classification of colitis-associated lesions, as well as other methodologic flaws that had hampered the molecular investigation of noncolitic lesions (analysis restricted to the most frequently mutated regions of genes, the use of different – sometimes incomplete – marker panels for the detection of specific phenotypes, suboptimal diagnostic reliability of most of the methods used).

Nevertheless, certain differences with respect to noncolitic carcinogenesis have emerged from these studies. *KRAS* and *APC* mutations, for example, are rare in IBD-related carcinogenesis, whereas *TP53* mutations are frequently encountered in the early stages and are sometimes found even in nondysplastic mucosa [15, 102–104]. DNA methylation [105] and microsatellite instability [106] seem to play less important roles, but chromosomal instability is very common and appears to be an early event that probably stems from *TP53* mutations and inflammation-triggered DNA damage [107]. Genome-wide screening with comparative genomic hybridization has revealed several recurrent genomic imbalances. Losses of chromosome 5q and 18q, for example, were found in nondysplastic colitis tissue [108] (Fig. 18.5), but their frequency was higher in dysplastic colitis tissue and higher still in colitis-associated colorectal cancer. Progression was also associated with the accumulation of other genomic imbalances typical of colorectal cancer such as –4, +7, +8q, +13q, +20q and +X. Changes detected in premalignant colitis tissue were encountered more often in colitis-associated colorectal cancers than in their sporadic counterparts (for example: –5q: 53% vs. 10%; −18q: 76% vs. 49%; Fig. 18.5) (data through www.progenetix.net; [109]). The presence of specific genomic changes in colon tissues from patients with ulcerative colitis is evidence of preinvasive clonal expansion, and it might someday serve as an additional marker for disease monitoring in these patients.

In conclusion, magnifying chromoendoscopy and the analysis of *TP53* mutations and chromosomal abnormalities in endoscopic biopsies are important tools that can substantially improve early diagnosis of colorectal cancer in patients with ulcerative colitis. The challenge is to implement these adjunctive diagnostic modalities in the surveillance of all patients with long-standing ulcerative in a way that optimizes the cost-benefit ratio.

Acknowledgements E.C. is supported by grants received by G.M. from the Swiss National Science Foundation. G.M. also gratefully acknowledges the generous financial support of the Zurich Cancer League. The authors wish to thank Luca Roncucci for photos illustrating the histologic features of ACFs, Jana Rojickova for editing the figures, and Marian Kent for editing the text.

References

1. Winawer SJ, Zauber AG, Fletcher RH et al (2006) Guidelines for colonoscopy surveillance after polypectomy: a consensus update by the US Multi-Society Task Force on Colorectal Cancer and the American Cancer Society. Gastroenterology 130:1872–1885
2. Levine JS, Ahnen DJ (2006) Clinical practice. Adenomatous polyps of the colon. N Engl J Med 355:2551–2557
3. Gupta S (2008) Colorectal polyps: the scope and management of the problem. Am J Med Sci 336:407–417
4. Young GP, Cole SR (2009) Which fecal occult blood test is best to screen for colorectal cancer? Nat Clin Pract Gastroenterol Hepatol 6(3):140–141
5. Psaty BM, Potter JD (2006) Risks and benefits of celecoxib to prevent recurrent adenomas. N Engl J Med 355:950–952
6. Schoenfeld P, Cash B, Flood A et al (2005) Colonoscopic screening of average-risk women for colorectal neoplasia. N Engl J Med 352:2061–2068
7. Neklason DW, Thorpe BL, Ferrandez A et al (2008) Colonic adenoma risk in familial colorectal cancer – a study of six extended kindreds. Am J Gastroenterol 103:2577–2584
8. Hendriks YM, de Jong AE, Morreau H et al (2006) Diagnostic approach and management of Lynch syndrome (hereditary nonpolyposis colorectal carcinoma): a guide for clinicians. CA Cancer J Clin 56:213–225
9. Vasen HF, Moslein G, Alonso A et al (2008) Guidelines for the clinical management of familial adenomatous polyposis (FAP). Gut 57:704–713
10. Ahmadi A, Polyak S, Draganov PV (2009) Colorectal cancer surveillance in inflammatory bowel disease: the search continues. World J Gastroenterol 15:61–66
11. Roncucci L, Stamp D, Medline A, Cullen JB, Bruce WR (1991) Identification and quantification of aberrant crypt foci and microadenomas in the human colon. Hum Pathol 22:287–294
12. Hurlstone DP, Karajeh M, Sanders DS, Drew SK, Cross SS (2005) Rectal aberrant crypt foci identified using high-magnification-chromoscopic colonoscopy: biomarkers for flat and depressed neoplasia. Am J Gastroenterol 100:1283–1289
13. Takayama T, Katsuki S, Takahashi Y et al (1998) Aberrant crypt foci of the colon as precursors of adenoma and cancer. N Engl J Med 339:1277–1284
14. Takayama T, Ohi M, Hayashi T et al (2001) Analysis of K-ras, APC, and beta-catenin in aberrant crypt foci in sporadic adenoma, cancer, and familial adenomatous polyposis. Gastroenterology 121:599–611
15. Kukitsu T, Takayama T, Miyanishi K et al (2008) Aberrant crypt foci as precursors of the dysplasia-carcinoma sequence in patients with ulcerative colitis. Clin Cancer Res 14:48–54
16. Schoen RE, Mutch M, Rall C et al (2008) The natural history of aberrant crypt foci. Gastrointest Endosc 67:1097–1102
17. Winawer SJ (2007) The multidisciplinary management of gastrointestinal cancer. Colorectal cancer screening. Best Pract Res Clin Gastroenterol 21:1031–1048
18. Muto T, Kamiya J, Sawada T et al (1985) Small "flat adenoma" of the large bowel with special reference to its clinicopathologic features. Dis Colon Rectum 28:847–851
19. Kudo S, Lambert R, Allen JI et al (2008) Nonpolypoid neoplastic lesions of the colorectal mucosa. Gastrointest Endosc 68:S3–47
20. Endoscopic Classification Review Group (2005) Update on the Paris classification of superficial neoplastic lesions in the digestive tract. Endoscopy 37:570–578
21. O'Brien MJ, Winawer SJ, Zauber AG et al (2004) Flat adenomas in the National Polyp Study: is there increased risk for high-grade dysplasia initially or during surveillance? Clin Gastroenterol Hepatol 2:905–911
22. Hurlstone DP, Cross SS, Adam I et al (2003) A prospective clinicopathological and endoscopic evaluation of flat and depressed colorectal lesions in the United Kingdom. Am J Gastroenterol 98:2543–2549
23. Kudo S, Rubio CA, Teixeira CR, Kashida H, Kogure E (2001) Pit pattern in colorectal neoplasia: endoscopic magnifying view. Endoscopy 33:367–373

24. Snover DC, Jass JR, Fenoglio-Preiser C, Batts KP (2005) Serrated polyps of the large intestine: a morphologic and molecular review of an evolving concept. Am J Clin Pathol 124:380–391
25. O'Brien MJ (2007) Hyperplastic and serrated polyps of the colorectum. Gastroenterol Clin North Am 36:947–968, viii
26. Jass JR, Baker K, Zlobec I et al (2006) Advanced colorectal polyps with the molecular and morphological features of serrated polyps and adenomas: concept of a 'fusion' pathway to colorectal cancer. Histopathology 49:121–131
27. Carr NJ, Mahajan H, Tan KL, Hawkins NJ, Ward RL (2009) Serrated and non-serrated polyps of the colorectum: their prevalence in an unselected case series and correlation of BRAF mutation analysis with the diagnosis of sessile serrated adenoma. J Clin Pathol 62(6):516–518
28. Spring KJ, Zhao ZZ, Karamatic R et al (2006) High prevalence of sessile serrated adenomas with BRAF mutations: a prospective study of patients undergoing colonoscopy. Gastroenterology 131:1400–1407
29. Rosenberg DW, Yang S, Pleau DC et al (2007) Mutations in BRAF and KRAS differentially distinguish serrated versus non-serrated hyperplastic aberrant crypt foci in humans. Cancer Res 67:3551–3554
30. Makinen MJ (2007) Colorectal serrated adenocarcinoma. Histopathology 50:131–150
31. O'Brien MJ, Yang S, Mack C et al (2006) Comparison of microsatellite instability, CpG island methylation phenotype, BRAF and KRAS status in serrated polyps and traditional adenomas indicates separate pathways to distinct colorectal carcinoma end points. Am J Surg Pathol 30:1491–1501
32. Oka S, Tanaka S, Hiyama T et al (2004) Clinicopathologic and endoscopic features of colorectal serrated adenoma: differences between polypoid and superficial types. Gastrointest Endosc 59:213–219
33. Clevers H (2006) Wnt/beta-catenin signaling in development and disease. Cell 127:469–480
34. Powell SM, Zilz N, Beazer-Barclay Y et al (1992) APC mutations occur early during colorectal tumorigenesis. Nature 359:235–237
35. Groden J, Thliveris A, Samowitz W et al (1991) Identification and characterization of the familial adenomatous polyposis coli gene. Cell 66:589–600
36. Su LK, Kinzler KW, Vogelstein B et al (1992) Multiple intestinal neoplasia caused by a mutation in the murine homolog of the APC gene. Science 256:668–670
37. Iwamoto M, Ahnen DJ, Franklin WA, Maltzman TH (2000) Expression of beta-catenin and full-length APC protein in normal and neoplastic colonic tissues. Carcinogenesis 21:1935–1940
38. Barker N, Ridgway RA, van Es JH et al (2009) Crypt stem cells as the cells-of-origin of intestinal cancer. Nature 457:608–611
39. Zhu L, Gibson P, Currle DS et al (2009) Prominin 1 marks intestinal stem cells that are susceptible to neoplastic transformation. Nature 457:603–607
40. Ilyas M, Tomlinson IP, Rowan A, Pignatelli M, Bodmer WF (1997) Beta-catenin mutations in cell lines established from human colorectal cancers. Proc Natl Acad Sci U S A 94: 10330–10334
41. Morin PJ, Sparks AB, Korinek V et al (1997) Activation of beta-catenin-Tcf signaling in colon cancer by mutations in beta-catenin or APC. Science 275:1787–1790
42. Samowitz WS, Powers MD, Spirio LN et al (1999) Beta-catenin mutations are more frequent in small colorectal adenomas than in larger adenomas and invasive carcinomas. Cancer Res 59:1442–1444
43. Suzuki H, Watkins DN, Jair KW et al (2004) Epigenetic inactivation of SFRP genes allows constitutive WNT signaling in colorectal cancer. Nat Genet 36:417–422
44. Schneikert J, Grohmann A, Behrens J (2007) Truncated APC regulates the transcriptional activity of beta-catenin in a cell cycle dependent manner. Hum Mol Genet 16:199–209
45. Segditsas S, Rowan AJ, Howarth K et al (2009) APC and the three-hit hypothesis. Oncogene 28:146–155
46. Alberici P, Fodde R (2006) The role of the APC tumor suppressor in chromosomal instability. Genome Dyn 1:149–170
47. Cardoso J, Molenaar L, de Menezes RX et al (2006) Chromosomal instability in MYH- and APC-mutant adenomatous polyps. Cancer Res 66:2514–2519

48. Luo L, Li B, Pretlow TP (2003) DNA alterations in human aberrant crypt foci and colon cancers by random primed polymerase chain reaction. Cancer Res 63:6166–6169
49. Sieber OM, Heinimann K, Gorman P et al (2002) Analysis of chromosomal instability in human colorectal adenomas with two mutational hits at APC. Proc Natl Acad Sci U S A 99:16910–16915
50. Bartkova J, Rezaei N, Liontos M et al (2006) Oncogene-induced senescence is part of the tumorigenesis barrier imposed by DNA damage checkpoints. Nature 444:633–637
51. Raynaud CM, Jang SJ, Nuciforo P et al (2008) Telomere shortening is correlated with the DNA damage response and telomeric protein down-regulation in colorectal preneoplastic lesions. Ann Oncol 19:1875–1881
52. Vogelstein B, Fearon ER, Hamilton SR et al (1988) Genetic alterations during colorectal-tumor development. N Engl J Med 319:525–532
53. Grant S (2008) Cotargeting survival signaling pathways in cancer. J Clin Invest 118:3003–3006
54. Wood LD, Parsons DW, Jones S et al (2007) The genomic landscapes of human breast and colorectal cancers. Science 318:1108–1113
55. Sweeney C, Boucher KM, Samowitz WS et al (2009) Oncogenetic tree model of somatic mutations and DNA methylation in colon tumors. Genes Chromosomes Cancer 48:1–9
56. Shen L, Toyota M, Kondo Y et al (2007) Integrated genetic and epigenetic analysis identifies three different subclasses of colon cancer. Proc Natl Acad Sci U S A 104:18654–18659
57. Samowitz WS, Slattery ML, Sweeney C et al (2007) APC mutations and other genetic and epigenetic changes in colon cancer. Mol Cancer Res 5:165–170
58. Goel A, Arnold CN, Niedzwiecki D et al (2003) Characterization of sporadic colon cancer by patterns of genomic instability. Cancer Res 63:1608–1614
59. Toyota M, Ahuja N, Ohe-Toyota M et al (1999) CpG island methylator phenotype in colorectal cancer. Proc Natl Acad Sci U S A 96:8681–8686
60. O'Brien MJ, Yang S, Clebanoff JL et al (2004) Hyperplastic (serrated) polyps of the colorectum: relationship of CpG island methylator phenotype and K-ras mutation to location and histologic subtype. Am J Surg Pathol 28:423–434
61. Chan TL, Zhao W, Leung SY, Yuen ST (2003) BRAF and KRAS mutations in colorectal hyperplastic polyps and serrated adenomas. Cancer Res 63:4878–4881
62. Nosho K, Irahara N, Shima K et al (2008) Comprehensive biostatistical analysis of CpG island methylator phenotype in colorectal cancer using a large population-based sample. PLoS ONE 3:e3698
63. Kambara T, Simms LA, Whitehall VL et al (2004) BRAF mutation is associated with DNA methylation in serrated polyps and cancers of the colorectum. Gut 53:1137–1144
64. Weisenberger DJ, Siegmund KD, Campan M et al (2006) CpG island methylator phenotype underlies sporadic microsatellite instability and is tightly associated with BRAF mutation in colorectal cancer. Nat Genet 38:787–793
65. Goel A, Nagasaka T, Arnold CN et al (2007) The CpG island methylator phenotype and chromosomal instability are inversely correlated in sporadic colorectal cancer. Gastroenterology 132:127–138
66. Menigatti M, Truninger K, Gebbers JO et al (2009) Normal colorectal mucosa exhibits sex- and segment-specific susceptibility to DNA methylation at the hMLH1 and MGMT promoters. Oncogene 28:899–909
67. Samowitz WS, Albertsen H, Sweeney C et al (2006) Association of smoking, CpG island methylator phenotype, and V600E BRAF mutations in colon cancer. J Natl Cancer Inst 98:1731–1738
68. Laiho P, Kokko A, Vanharanta S et al (2007) Serrated carcinomas form a subclass of colorectal cancer with distinct molecular basis. Oncogene 26:312–320
69. Lee SH, Kim J, Kim WH, Lee YM (2009) Hypoxic silencing of tumor suppressor RUNX3 by histone modification in gastric cancer cells. Oncogene 28:184–194
70. di Pietro M, Sabates Bellver J, Menigatti M et al (2005) Defective DNA mismatch repair determines a characteristic transcriptional profile in proximal colon cancers. Gastroenterology 129:1047–1059

71. Sabates-Bellver J, Van der Flier LG, de Palo M et al (2007) Transcriptome profile of human colorectal adenomas. Mol Cancer Res 5:1263–1275
72. Knudsen AL, Bisgaard ML, Bulow S (2003) Attenuated familial adenomatous polyposis (AFAP). A review of the literature. Fam Cancer 2:43–55
73. Schneikert J, Behrens J (2007) The canonical Wnt signalling pathway and its APC partner in colon cancer development. Gut 56:417–425
74. Sabates Bellver J, Cattaneo E, Heinimann K, Jiricny J, Marra G (2007) Getting familiar with familial colon cancer. In: Gasche C (ed) Intestinal inflammation and colorectal cancer (FALK Symposium 158). Springer, New York, pp 27–60
75. Al-Tassan N, Chmiel NH, Maynard J et al (2002) Inherited variants of MYH associated with somatic G:C→T:A mutations in colorectal tumors. Nat Genet 30:227–232
76. Sieber OM, Lipton L, Crabtree M et al (2003) Multiple colorectal adenomas, classic adenomatous polyposis, and germ-line mutations in MYH. N Engl J Med 348:791–799
77. Marra G, Jiricny J (2003) Multiple colorectal adenomas – is their number up? N Engl J Med 348:845–847
78. Marra G, Jiricny J (2005) DNA mismatch repair and colon cancer. In: Nigg E (ed) Genome instability in cancer development (advances in experimental medicine and biology). Springer, New York, pp 85–123
79. Truninger K, Menigatti M, Luz J et al (2005) Immunohistochemical analysis reveals high frequency of PMS2 defects in colorectal cancer. Gastroenterology 128:1160–1171
80. de Jong AE, Morreau H, Van Puijenbroek M et al (2004) The role of mismatch repair gene defects in the development of adenomas in patients with HNPCC. Gastroenterology 126:42–48
81. Markowitz S, Wang J, Myeroff L et al (1995) Inactivation of the type II TGF-beta receptor in colon cancer cells with microsatellite instability. Science 268:1336–1338
82. Rampino N, Yamamoto H, Ionov Y et al (1997) Somatic frameshift mutations in the BAX gene in colon cancers of the microsatellite mutator phenotype. Science 275:967–969
83. Burt RW, Jass JR (2000) Hyperplastic polyposis. In: Hamilton SR, Aaltonen LA (eds) World Health Organization classification of tumors. Pathology and genetics. Tumors of the digestive system. Springer, Berlin, pp 135–136
84. Jass JR (2000) Familial colorectal cancer: pathology and molecular characteristics. Lancet Oncol 1:220–226
85. Ferrandez A, Samowitz W, DiSario JA, Burt RW (2004) Phenotypic characteristics and risk of cancer development in hyperplastic polyposis: case series and literature review. Am J Gastroenterol 99:2012–2018
86. Lage P, Cravo M, Sousa R et al (2004) Management of Portuguese patients with hyperplastic polyposis and screening of at-risk first-degree relatives: a contribution for future guidelines based on a clinical study. Am J Gastroenterol 99:1779–1784
87. Torlakovic E, Snover DC (2006) Sessile serrated adenoma: a brief history and current status. Crit Rev Oncog 12:27–39
88. Jass JR (2008) Colorectal polyposes: from phenotype to diagnosis. Pathol Res Pract 204:431–447
89. Beach R, Chan AO, Wu TT et al (2005) BRAF mutations in aberrant crypt foci and hyperplastic polyposis. Am J Pathol 166:1069–1075
90. Minoo P, Baker K, Goswami R et al (2006) Extensive DNA methylation in normal colorectal mucosa in hyperplastic polyposis. Gut 55:1467–1474
91. Young J, Jass JR (2006) The case for a genetic predisposition to serrated neoplasia in the colorectum: hypothesis and review of the literature. Cancer Epidemiol Biomarkers Prev 15:1778–1784
92. Cho JH (2008) The genetics and immunopathogenesis of inflammatory bowel disease. Nat Rev Immunol 8:458–466
93. Xavier RJ, Podolsky DK (2007) Unravelling the pathogenesis of inflammatory bowel disease. Nature 448:427–434
94. Budarf ML, Labbe C, David G, Rioux JD (2009) GWA studies: rewriting the story of IBD. Trends Genet 25(3):137–146
95. Eaden JA, Abrams KR, Mayberry JF (2001) The risk of colorectal cancer in ulcerative colitis: a meta-analysis. Gut 48:526–535

96. Canavan C, Abrams KR, Mayberry J (2006) Meta-analysis: colorectal and small bowel cancer risk in patients with Crohn's disease. Aliment Pharmacol Ther 23:1097–1104
97. Itzkowitz SH, Yio X (2004) Inflammation and cancer IV. Colorectal cancer in inflammatory bowel disease: the role of inflammation. Am J Physiol Gastrointest Liver Physiol 287:G7–17
98. Itzkowitz SH, Harpaz N (2004) Diagnosis and management of dysplasia in patients with inflammatory bowel diseases. Gastroenterology 126:1634–1648
99. Kiesslich R, Goetz M, Lammersdorf K et al (2007) Chromoscopy-guided endomicroscopy increases the diagnostic yield of intraepithelial neoplasia in ulcerative colitis. Gastroenterology 132:874–882
100. Kornbluth A, Sachar DB (1997) Ulcerative colitis practice guidelines in adults. American College of Gastroenterology, Practice Parameters Committee. Am J Gastroenterol 92:204–211
101. Lewis JD (2003) The many faces of low-grade dysplasia. Gastroenterology 125:1531–1533
102. Yin J, Harpaz N, Tong Y et al (1993) p53 point mutations in dysplastic and cancerous ulcerative colitis lesions. Gastroenterology 104:1633–1639
103. Brentnall TA, Crispin DA, Rabinovitch PS et al (1994) Mutations in the p53 gene: an early marker of neoplastic progression in ulcerative colitis. Gastroenterology 107:369–378
104. Fujii S, Fujimori T, Chiba T (2003) Usefulness of analysis of p53 alteration and observation of surface microstructure for diagnosis of ulcerative colitis-associated colorectal neoplasia. J Exp Clin Cancer Res 22:107–115
105. Konishi K, Shen L, Wang S et al (2007) Rare CpG island methylator phenotype in ulcerative colitis-associated neoplasias. Gastroenterology 132:1254–1260
106. Risques RA, Rabinovitch PS, Brentnall TA (2006) Cancer surveillance in inflammatory bowel disease: new molecular approaches. Curr Opin Gastroenterol 22:382–390
107. Risques RA, Lai LA, Brentnall TA et al (2008) Ulcerative colitis is a disease of accelerated colon aging: evidence from telomere attrition and DNA damage. Gastroenterology 135:410–418
108. Willenbucher RF, Aust DE, Chang CG et al (1999) Genomic instability is an early event during the progression pathway of ulcerative-colitis-related neoplasia. Am J Pathol 154:1825–1830
109. Baudis M, Cleary ML (2001) Progenetix.net: an online repository for molecular cytogenetic aberration data. Bioinformatics 17:1228–1229

Chapter 19
Precursor Lesions of Pancreatic Cancer

Hanno Matthaei and Anirban Maitra

Abstract Pancreatic ductal adenocarcinoma (a.k.a. PDAC) is a disease of near-uniform lethality. Multiple lines of evidence suggest that PDAC does not arise de novo. Several distinct subtypes of non-invasive precursors of PDAC have been identified in the past two decades, including the microscopic Pancreatic intraepithelial neoplasia (PanIN), which is by far the most common precursor lesion, followed by the macroscopic (cystic) precursor lesions, comprised of Intraductal Papillary Mucinous Neoplasm (IPMN) and Mucinous Cystic Neoplasm (MCN). In this review, we discuss the diagnostic features for each of these PDAC precursor subtypes, and present the salient molecular alterations underlying their pathogenesis and progression to invasive neoplasia. Finally, the translational implications of identifying PDAC precursor lesions are discussed, particularly in the context of early detection of PDAC in at-risk populations.

Introduction

Pancreatic ductal adenocarcinoma (a.k.a. PDAC) is a cancer of near uniform lethality. The American Cancer Society estimates that in 2009, the incidence of PDAC will be 42,470 in the United States, whereas the cancer-related mortality will be 35,240, reinforcing the dire prognosis of this disease [1]. The high mortality of PDAC stems primarily from the fact that nearly 80% of patients present with either distant metastatic or locally advanced disease that is not amenable to surgical resection [2]. Current chemo-radiation therapeutic strategies are largely ineffective in ameliorating the natural history observed in most patients following diagnosis. Therefore, it is paramount that PDAC is identified at an early, and hence potentially curable, stage of the disease.

A. Maitra (✉)
The Sol Goldman Pancreatic Cancer Research Center, Johns Hopkins University School of Medicine, 1550 Orleans Street, CRB-2, Suite 345, 21231, Baltimore, MD, USA
e-mail: amaitra1@jhmi.edu

R.C. Fitzgerald (ed.), *Pre-Invasive Disease: Pathogenesis and Clinical Management*, DOI 10.1007/978-1-4419-6694-0_19,

Table 19.1 Clinical features of PDAC precursor lesions

	PanIN	IPMN	MCN
Predominant age	Prevalence increases with age	60–70 yeears	40–50 years
Gender ratio (female: male)	1:1	2:3	20:1
Predominant intrapancreatic localization	Head > body/tail	Head	Body/tail
Multifocal growth	Often	In 20–30%	Rare
Communication of the cysts with larger pancreatic ducts	N/A	Arises in major or branch ducts	Rare
Stroma	Collagen-rich	Collagen-rich	Ovarian-type
Cyst fluid quality	N/A	Mucoid	Mucoid
Muzin oozing from papilla	No	Yes	No
Characteristic ERCP finding	Normal	Dilated pancreatic duct and filling defects	Displaced or compressed pancreatic duct

As elegantly outlined throughout this textbook, most epithelial cancers arise through a multistep progression, initiating as non-invasive precursor lesions that undergo increasing degrees of epithelial atypia within the confines of the basement membrane, eventually culminating in invasive neoplasia. Several lines of evidence, including meticulous morphological studies and molecular analyses, have established that PDAC follows this general trend of multistep progression. Understanding the biology and natural history of precursor lesions of epithelial cancer is not simply a matter of academic interest, but rather forms the underlying basis for designing rational early detection and chemoprevention strategies. This has been exemplified time and again in the context of numerous epithelial malignancies like colorectal, cervical and breast cancers [3–6]. In this chapter, we will discuss the three common subtypes of PDAC precursor lesions, beginning with Pancreatic Intraepithelial Neoplasia or PanINs followed by the two macroscopic (cystic) precursor lesions, Intraductal Papillary Mucinous Neoplasm (IPMN) and Mucinous Cystic Neoplasm (MCN). A comparison of their most characteristic features is shown in Table 19.1.

Pancreatic Intraepithelial Neoplasia

Clinical Features and Morphology of PanINs

Ductal epithelial changes consistent with PanIN lesions were first described over a century ago in the European literature [7]. However, their recognition as bona fide precursors to invasive PDAC, including their detailed molecular characterization and a consensus nomenclature, has only become established over the past two decades. PanINs represent the most frequently observed epithelial precursor lesion in the pancreas, with an increasing prevalence with age, such that autopsy studies have documented that more than 50% of the population older than 65 years harbor these lesions [8, 9]. Of note, these "incidental" PanIN lesions are almost always low-grade, and it is unusual to find higher-grade lesions in the absence of a neoplasm in the pancreas. For example, Cubilla and Fitzgerald analyzed 227 pancreata of patients with PDAC, as well as 100 pancreata of patients without cancer [8]. Lesions corresponding to intermediate grade PanINs were observed three times more often in association with, than in the absence of, a carcinoma, while the highest grade "carcinoma-in situ" lesions (corresponding to PanIN-3, *see below*) were found exclusively in pancreata with concomitant PDAC. PanINs are more frequently located in the pancreatic head than the tail, which mirrors the distribution of PDAC. PanINs are also found with a higher propensity in the setting of chronic pancreatitis, which might explain the epidemiological association between long standing pancreatitis and an increased risk of subsequent malignancy. Thus, Andea et al. examined 234 pancreata, and found PanIN lesions in 60% of the pancreata with chronic pancreatitis (4% of which were PanIN-3), and in 82% of the pancreata with invasive cancers (40% corresponding to PanIN-3). In contrast, only 16% of normal pancreata harbored PanIN lesions [10].

Morphologically, PanINs are microscopic lesions found in the smaller pancreatic ducts with a diameter less than 0.5 cm [11, 12]. They are divided into three grades with respect to their grade of cytologic atypia and architecture (Fig. 19.1). PanIN-1A lesions have a flat epithelium consisting of columnar mucin producing cells with basally located uniform nuclei; PanIN-1B lesions are similar to PanIN-1A lesions, except for a more papillary growth pattern. PanIN-2 lesions demonstrate somewhat greater architectural complexity than PanIN-1 lesions, as well as nuclear abnormalities, including loss of nuclear polarity, hyperchromasia (i.e., darker nuclei), pleomorphism (i.e., differences in nuclear sizes), and "pseudostratification" (i.e. piling up of nuclei, as opposed to an organized basal orientation). PanIN-3 lesions ("carcinoma-in situ") show marked architectural and cytological atypia, such as "cribriforming" (the formation of so-called "Roman bridges" between tufts), severe loss of nuclear polarity, hyperchromasia, and presence of mitotic figures, including occasional abnormal mitotic figures. PanINs need to be distinguished from IPMNs, which are typically larger lesions visible on radiology and by gross examination as cystic structures in the pancreas [12]. As described subsequently, IPMNs harbor more prominent papillary structures and a distinct immunohistochemical and molecular profile compared to PanIN lesions. Nevertheless, occasional lesions fall into an "intermediate" category, leading to an emerging concept that some PanIN lesions might undergo transition over time into IPMNs.

One newly described feature associated with PanINs has emerged as an example of how meticulous morphological observations can be translated into clinical care. Thus, Brune et al. and Detlefsen et al. have described a characteristic "lobulo-centric atrophy" in the pancreatic parenchyma surrounding PanINs, including low-grade lesions (Fig. 19.2) [13, 14]. Lobulocentric atrophy represents an area of localized pancreatitis,

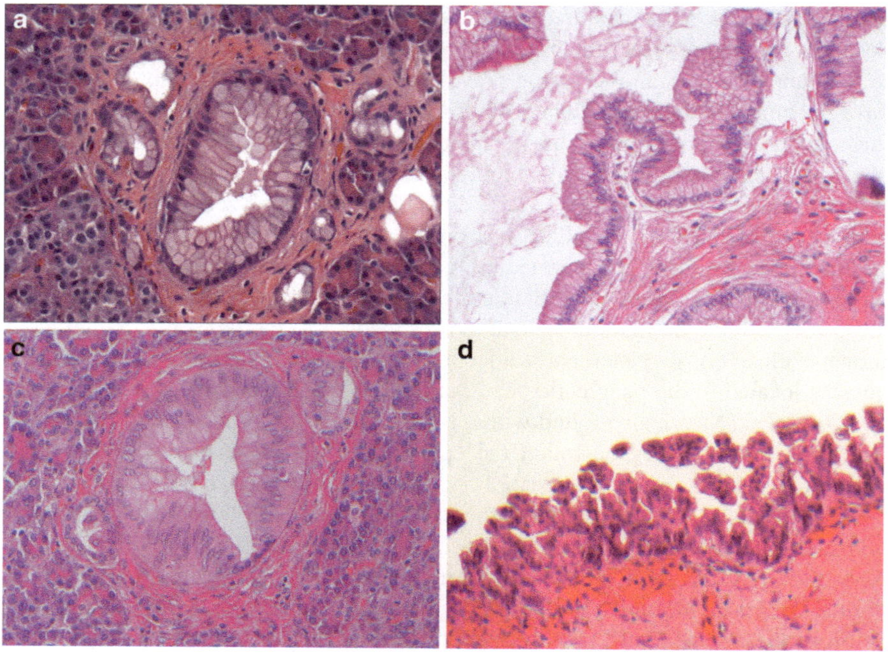

Fig. 19.1 Histological grades of PanIN lesions, including PanIN-1A (panel **a**), PanIN-1B (panel **b**), PanIN-2 (panel **c**), and PanIN-3 (panel **d**)

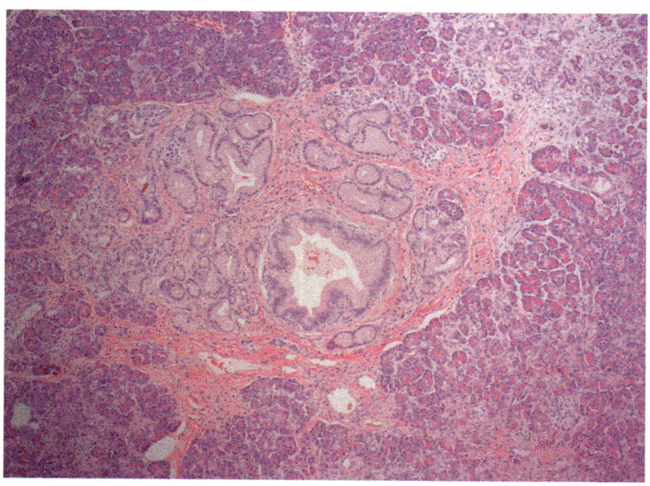

Fig. 19.2 An example of lobulo-centric atrophy in the pancreatic parenchyma adjacent to a PanIN lesion. Multifocal PanINs and associated lobulo-centric atrophy can be present in pancreata of individuals belonging to high-risk familial PDAC kindred, and is visualized on endoscopic ultrasound (EUS) as a diffuse chronic pancreatitis-like pattern. Photomicrograph courtesy of Professor Ralph Hruban, Sol Goldman Pancreatic Cancer Research Center, Johns Hopkins University School of Medicine, Baltimore, Maryland

likely because the intraductal PanIN lesion hampers the flow of secretions, resulting in the secondary release of acinar enzymes into the surrounding parenchyma. In patients with multifocal PanIN lesions (for example, as is observed in patients with a family history of PDAC, *see below*), the associated multifocal lobulocentric atrophy can be visualized by imaging as a distinctive pattern, providing a relatively non-invasive basis for monitoring early pancreatic neoplasia [15].

Molecular Alterations in PanINs

A large compendium of studies in the past decade has cataloged the molecular alterations in PanIN lesions and demonstrated that histological progression is mirrored by progressive accumulation of genetic changes [16–23]. A "PanINgram" model of genetic progression delineates changes that are observed more frequently in early, intermediate and later grades of PanIN lesions (Fig. 19.3); nevertheless, it is important to stress that the alterations may not necessarily occur in a linear sequence in all instances during the progression to cancer.

Multiple oncogenes have been identified that contribute to pancreatic carcinogenesis, but none are probably as near-ubiquitous in PDAC as activating point mutations in the *KRAS2* gene [24, 25]. The *RAS* family of proto-oncogenes encodes for small GTP-binding proteins. Mutations of *KRAS2* causes activation of downstream effector cascades, including mitogen-activated protein kinase (MAPK), PI-3-Kinase/AKT,

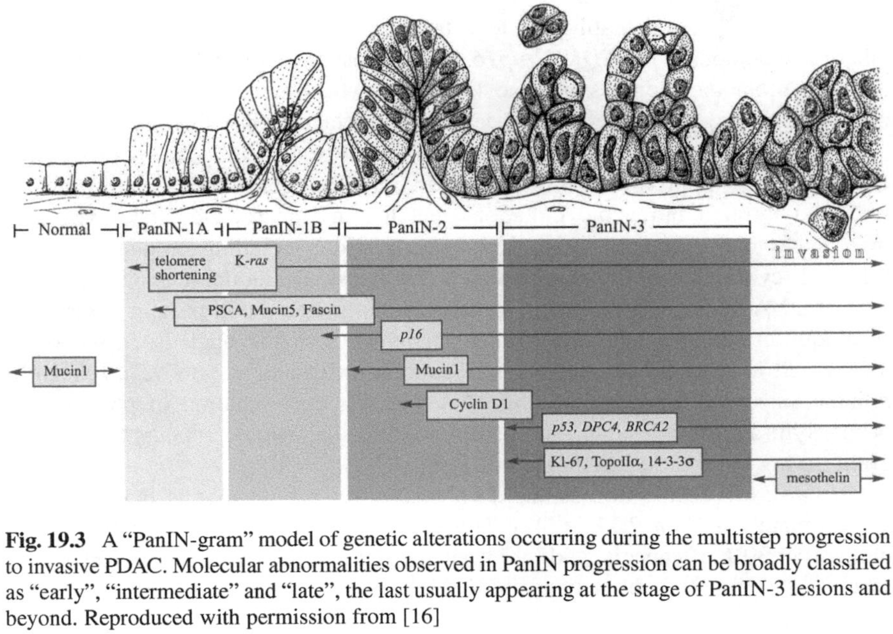

Fig. 19.3 A "PanIN-gram" model of genetic alterations occurring during the multistep progression to invasive PDAC. Molecular abnormalities observed in PanIN progression can be broadly classified as "early", "intermediate" and "late", the last usually appearing at the stage of PanIN-3 lesions and beyond. Reproduced with permission from [16]

and the RalGDS pathways, which promote cancer development [26, 27]. Mutations of *KRAS2* in PDAC and PanINs are almost always restricted to codons 12 or 13. The frequency of *KRAS2* mutations increases from low to high grade PanIN lesions (for example, 36, 44 and 87% in PanIN-1A, PanIN-1B and PanIN 2/3 lesions, respectively, in one study) [28]. The importance of *KRAS2* to PanIN formation is underscored by recently developed mouse models of PDAC, where expression of a mutant $Kras^{G12D}$ allele from its endogenous promoter leads to formation of murine PanIN (mPanIN) lesions with near uniform penetrance in mice (*see below*) [29, 30].

Tumor suppressor genes (TSGs) encode for proteins that inhibit cell growth and proliferation [31]. As the recent sequencing of the PDAC genome has demonstrated, loss of function of three TSGs – *CDKN2A/p16* (on chromosome 9p21), *TP53* (on chromosome 17p13), and *DPC4/SMAD4* (on chromosome 18q21) are observed in the majority of invasive adenocarcinomas [24]. Not surprisingly, alterations at these TSG loci are also observed in PanIN lesions. For example, an immunohistochemical analysis for p16 protein expression during PanIN progression by Wilentz and colleagues revealed that 30% of PanIN-1A lesions, 55% of PanIN-1B and PanIN-2 lesions, and 71% of PanIN-3 lesions display loss of p16 expression [32]. At the genetic level, inactivation of *CDKN2A/p16* in PDAC occurs through multiple mechanisms, including homozygous deletion (40%), intragenic mutations with loss of the second allele (40%) and epigenetic silencing (15%) [33, 34]. Accordingly, aberrant methylation of the *CDKN2A/p16* promoter has been reported in 12% of PanIN-1A lesions, 4.5% of PanIN-2 lesions, and in 21.4% of PanIN-3 lesions [21]. Similarly, loss of heterozygosity (LOH) at the chromosome 9p21 *CDKN2A/p16* locus has been reported in PanIN lesions [17]. The p16 protein causes cell-cycle arrest through binding to the cyclin dependent kinases, CDK4 and CDK6. As a result, loss of protein function leads to reduced phosphorylation of the retinoblastoma protein Rb-1, facilitating G1 to S transition of the cell cycle [35]. Notably, inherited mutations in the *CDKN2A/p16* gene are responsible for the familial atypical multiple mole melanoma syndrome (FAMM), wherein individuals carrying the mutation harbor an increased risk of developing melanoma and PDACs [36, 37].

Comparable to other solid cancers, inactivation of *TP53* is also relatively frequent in PDAC (approximately 50–75%) [38, 39]. This genetic alteration is mostly mediated through intragenic mutations and loss of the second allele. The p53 protein has multifaceted roles in tumor suppression, including regulation of the G1/S cell-cycle checkpoint, maintaining G2/M arrest, and inducing apoptosis in the face of DNA damage [40]. Owing to the fact that mutated p53 protein is resistant to ubiquitin-mediated degradation and accumulates in the nucleus, immunohistochemical assessment for nuclear p53 expression has proven to be a relatively reliable surrogate for genetic status [41]. Nuclear accumulation of p53 is seen primarily in PanIN-3 lesions, and therefore, *TP53* inactivation appears to be a late event during pancreatic carcinogenesis [16].

DPC4/SMAD4 on chromosome 18q21 is another TSG that is inactivated in approximately 55% of PDACs [42]. This inactivation is mediated by homozygous deletion in 30% of cancers, and by intragenic mutation combined with loss of the second allele in 25% of patients [43]. The protein encoded by *DPC4/SMAD4* transduces growth inhibitory signals that are caused by the binding of transforming growth factor β (TGF-β) ligand to its surface receptors [44]. Thus, inactivation of Smad4 function results in escape from TGF-β mediated growth inhibition. Similar to TP53, inactivation of DPC4/SMAD4 occurs relatively late in the multistep progression of PanINs to PDAC [16, 45].

In addition to oncogenes and TSGs, a third category of genes implicated in tumorigenesis are the so-called "caretaker" genes, which are responsible for maintenance of genomic stability [31]. Of particular interest in the context of PDAC is the breast and ovarian cancer susceptibility gene (*BRCA2*) on chromosome 13q, a member of the Fanconi anemia gene family. The product of *BRCA2* contributes to DNA repair by a mechanism known as homologous recombination repair, where it partners with other member proteins of the Fanconi anemia family in a multi-protein complex at sites of DNA damage [46]. Germline mutations of *BRCA2* are detected in 5–10% of familial PDAC and are particularly common in PDAC patients of Ashkenazi Jewish heritage [47]; recent studies have identified germline mutations of the *BRCA2* binding and localizing partner *PALB2* in a minor fraction of familial PDAC cases [48]. Loss of *BRCA2* (assessed by LOH on chromosome 13q) is observed mainly in PanIN-3 lesions, suggesting that this is a relatively late alteration in progression [49].

Chromosomal instability (CIN), characterized by structural and numerical chromosomal aberrations, is a hallmark of PDAC [50, 51]. It is postulated that structural integrity of chromosomes is maintained by protective caps of hexameric DNA repeats, known as telomeres, which prevent chromosomal ends from sticking together during mitosis [52]. Telomere length is maintained by the enzyme telomerase, for the discovery of which Elizabeth Blackburn and Carol Greider received the 2009 Nobel prize in Medicine [53]; telomerase is typically silent in most somatic cells but is reactivated in cancers. Loss of telomere function (as assessed by decreased telomere length using a fluorescence in situ hybridization technique, TEL-FISH) is observed in greater of 90% of PanIN lesions, including PanIN-1, rendering it as one of the earliest demonstrable somatic molecular alterations in PDAC pathogenesis [54]. While loss of telomere integrity is, in and of itself, unlikely to be a tumor promoter, it likely facilitates onset of CIN within the incipient PanIN epithelium, and accelerates tumorigenesis through secondary loss of TSG function. This possibly explains why LOH events are observed even in the earliest PanIN lesions, and can precede the acquisition of somatic point mutations [22].

Epigenetic regulation of gene expression through differential promoter methylation has emerged as an important mechanism of transcriptional regulation in mammalian cells [55]. In fact, aberrant hypermethylation of gene promoters appears to be the most common mechanism through which cancer cells abrogate TSG function. Not surprisingly, hypermethylation of TSG promoters is frequently observed in PDAC [34, 56, 57] and epigenetic silencing of a subset of these genes is also found in the non-invasive precursor lesions [21, 58–60]. For example, Goggins and colleagues determined the methylation status of 8 genes frequently altered in invasive adenocarcinomas (*ST14*, *CDH3*, *CLDN5*, *LHX1*, *NPTX2*, *SARP2*, *SPARC*, and *Reprimo*) in a series of 65 PanIN lesions, and found at least one of these genes to be aberrantly methylated in 71% of

PanIN-1 lesions. Furthermore, PanIN-3 lesions demonstrated a significant increase in methylated loci compared to PanIN-1 and 2 lesions, underscoring the paradigm that epigenetic abnormalities, like their genetic counterparts, also mirror the histological progression of PanINs to adenocarcinoma [60]. The clinical implications of studying epigenetic alterations in PanINs stems from the potential for utilizing aberrantly methylated DNA as biomarkers for early pancreatic neoplasia in clinical specimens, like pancreatic juice or cyst fluid samples [61–63].

In addition to genetic and epigenetic abnormalities, solid cancers and their precursors also harbor a compendium of aberrantly expressed transcripts discernible through global expression profiling [64]. In some instances, transcript overexpression has an underlying genomic component (for example, a copy number gain or promoter *hypo*methylation) [65–68], and in other instances, it is secondary to abnormal activation of transcription factors that drive expression [69]. In the past decade, a number of global expression profiling studies have been conducted in PDACs, and have identified a consistent repertoire of genes that are aberrantly expressed in this neoplasm [24, 70–74]. Subsequent analyses of PanIN lesions have confirmed aberrant upregulation of the corresponding protein products during multistep progression [16]. It is not only critical that we catalog these transcriptomic abnormalities in PanIN lesions, but clearly elucidate at which point in the "PanINgram" model these alterations are observed, as this has direct relevance for the design of biomarker and chemoprevention strategies. For example, prostate stem cell antigen (PSCA) and mesothelin transcripts are both upregulated in the majority of PDACs, as confirmed by more than profiling technology [70, 75, 76]. PSCA protein is detected in 30% of PanIN-1 lesions, 40% of PanIN-2, and 60% of PanIN-3 lesions. In contrast to PSCA, mesothelin is expressed essentially in high-grade PanIN-3 lesions and in invasive adenocarcinomas [16]. Thus, overexpression of mesothelin in either biopsy samples or in juice specimens possibly represents a more ominous lesion than PSCA alone.

A class of cell surface proteins that have both biological and diagnostic significance for PanIN lesions are the cellular apomucins (MUC proteins) [77]. PanINs typically express a profile comprised of MUC1, MUC4, and MUC5AC, whereas MUC2 is usually not expressed [78]. The expression of apomucins also demonstrates a stepwise progression, suggesting an association with increased potential for invasive neoplasia. Thus, MUC4 expression was detected in 17% of PanIN-1 lesions, 36% of PanIN-2 lesions, 85% of PanIN-3 lesions, and 89% of PDACs, respectively [79]. From a diagnostic standpoint, the apomucin pattern of PanINs differs from that IPMNs (specifically the intestinal subtypes, *see below*), in that PanINs are MUC1+, MUC2-, while IPMNs are typically MUC1-, MUC2+ [80, 81]. This can be a useful ancillary parameter for the differential diagnosis of IPMNs vs. PanINs in tissue or cytology specimens. From a biological context, PDAC arising in the background of MUC1-expressing precursors tend to be inherently more aggressive than the PDAC that arise in the backdrop of MUC2-expressing IPMNs, suggesting a dichotomy in terms of pathway to invasive neoplasia of the exocrine pancreas [82].

Finally, we will conclude the discussion on molecular pathology of PanINs with reference to so-called developmental or embryonic signaling pathways, principally the Hedgehog (Hh) and Notch pathways. These two pathways are required for developmental patterning, as well as for mature tissue homeostasis [83, 84]. Reactivation of Hh and Notch signaling has been reported at the earliest stages of PDAC initiation in animal models (i.e., in murine PanINs) [29, 85–87], and aberrant expression of pathway components is also observed in corresponding human precursor lesions [88, 89]. A global profiling study of low-grade human PanINs found an RNA expression profile that recapitulated what is observed with ectopic activation of Hh signaling in pancreatic ductal cells, validating the notion that this pathway has a role at the earliest stages of human PDAC [90]. Recently, Bardeesy and colleagues have demonstrated the potential chemopreventive utility of targeting Notch signaling in a genetically engineered PDAC model [91]; both the frequency of high-grade mPanINs and of invasive carcinomas were significantly reduced in mice receiving an orally bioavailable Notch inhibitor. The Hh and Notch pathways appear to not only play a role in tumor initiation, but also in tumor maintenance. Thus, small molecule inhibitors of these pathways have been shown to inhibit primary tumor growth and metastases in animal models of PDAC [91–95], and this new class of drugs has very recently entered the clinic for evaluation in patients with solid cancers [96].

Intraductal Papillary Mucinous Neoplasms

Clinical Appearance and Morphology of IPMNs

IPMNs are mucin-producing epithelial lesions arising from the main pancreatic duct (Fig. 19.4a) or from one of its side branches [97, 98]. They are generally located in the pancreatic head rather than in the pancreatic body or tail. In contrast to MCNs (see below), IPMNs occur somewhat more commonly in men than in women. The observation that invasive IPMNs are more frequent in older patients, and that patients often suffer from abdominal symptoms for a long period of time prior to their final diagnosis suggests a critical diagnostic window for detecting and treating IPMNs before they can progress to invasive cancer [99]. This is underscored by studies that show that the ~90% 5-year survival of patients with non-invasive IPMNs drops to ~50% survival with concomitant invasion [100, 101]. Symptoms reported by patients presenting with IPMN are generally non-specific (e.g. abdominal discomfort, nausea and vomiting, and back pain), highlighting the difficulty for early detection in the absence of an antecedent risk factor like family history.

Since IPMNs are frequently larger than 1 cm in maximum diameter they account for grossly visible and, most importantly, radiologically detectable precursor lesions. Partly owing to the improvements in imaging techniques and the greater inclusion of the pancreas in imaging studies for symptoms outside of the epigastric region, a dramatic increase in the number of asymptomatic or incidental pancreatic cysts has been noted [102, 103]. In case the underlying pancreatic cyst is an IPMN, computerized tomography typically shows a cystic lesion with dilatation of the

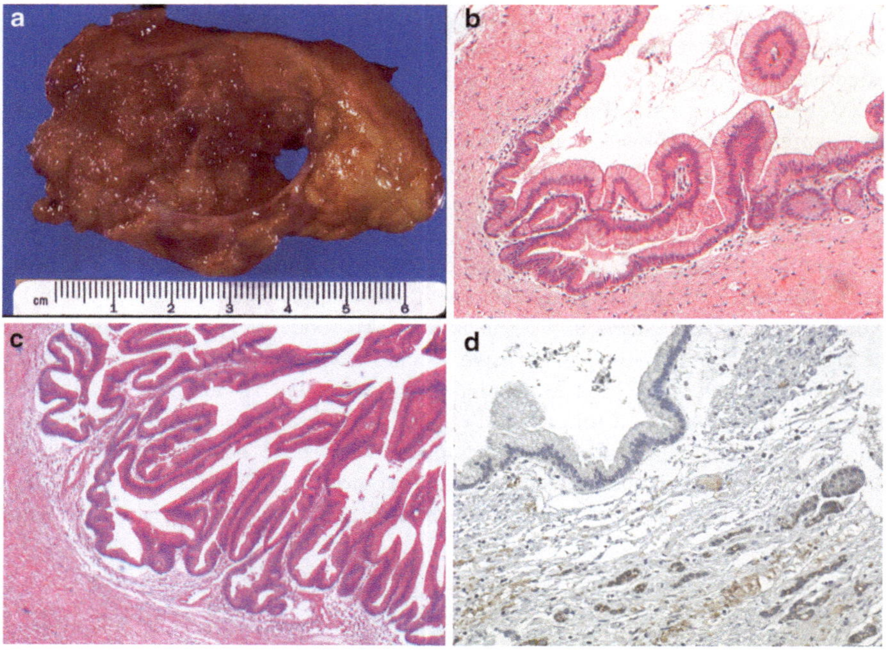

Fig. 19.4 Gross appearance of a surgically resected Intraductal papillary mucinous neoplasm (IPMN) of the pancreas (panel **a**). Note the dilated main pancreatic duct within which the IPMN has arisen, and the glistening surface of the neoplasm consistent with extruded mucin. Photomicrographs of IPMNs demonstrating examples of low-grade dysplasia (panel **b**) and high-grade dysplasia (panel **c**), respectively. An IPMN lesion with loss of Lkb1 expression in the neoplastic epithelium (panel **d**)

main pancreatic duct or several cystic lesions as a consequence of dilated branch ducts. A virtually diagnostic sign during upper gastrointestinal endoscopy is mucin oozing from a patulous ampulla of Vater. Apart from dilated pancreatic ducts, endoscopic retrograde cholangiopancreaticography (ERCP) occasionally shows mural nodules. Serum levels of tumor markers such as carcinoembryonic antigen (CEA) or CA19-9 are usually not elevated in non-invasive IPMN lesions [104], but CEA levels in cyst fluid aspirate can be elevated in up to two thirds of patients, and can provide ancillary diagnostic information [105, 106].

Two major clinical subtypes of non-invasive IPMN lesions are the main duct type and the branch duct type IPMNs, based on the epicenter of the lesion [107]. A combined main and branch duct involvement may be seen in some patients [108]. The location of the IPMN has histopathological and clinical implications, as discussed below. Based on the degree of architectural and cytological atypia, IPMNs are graded into mild dysplasia (adenoma; Fig. 19.4b), moderate dysplasia and severe dysplasia (carcinoma in situ, Fig. 19.4c). IPMN lesions of the main duct type tend to exhibit a higher degree of dysplasia and are more frequently observed in association with an invasive carcinoma compared to IPMNs of branch duct type.

Based on these data, a recent international consensus conference has outlined criteria for management of pancreatic cysts determined to be IPMNs based on radiology and/or preoperative biopsy diagnosis [109]. Specifically, the recommendations include surgical resection of all main duct IPMNs, and those branch duct lesions that are greater than 3 cm in diameter, or contain mural nodules, or are symptomatic. Most of the other branch duct lesions that do not meet these so-called "Tanaka criteria" for resection can be conservatively followed [110, 111]. An important caveat vis-à-vis IPMNs pertains to their multifocality in the pancreas; therefore even if the primary cyst is removed by partial pancreatectomy, the remnant pancreas remains at risk for progression of existing synchronous lesions, or the development of new metachronous lesions, including invasive cancer [112–114]. As a result, patients who retain a portion of their pancreas following an IPMN diagnosis need lifelong imaging and follow up.

Based on the morphology of their papillary epithelium in the resection specimen, IPMNs are recognized as gastric type, intestinal type, or pancreatobiliary type [115]. Main duct IPMNs are typically intestinal or pancreatobiliary types, while the branch duct IPMNs are almost always gastric type. Every IPMN epithelial type expresses a characteristic pattern of apomucin: thus, the intestinal type expresses MUC2, the pancreatobiliary type expresses MUC1, and the gastric type expresses MUC5AC but typically lacks MUC1 and MUC2 expression [81, 116]. Approximately one third of IPMNs are associated with an invasive carcinoma, which can either be so-called "colloid" carcinomas or garden-variety ductal adenocarcinoma. The "colloid" cancers are characterized by abundant extracellular pools of mucin, in which floating neoplastic epithelium can be observed [117]. Colloid cancers generally arise in the backdrop of MUC2-expressing intestinal type IPMNs, while the ductal adenocarcinomas are associated with MUC1-expressing pancreatobiliary type lesions. The gastric type IPMNs are only infrequently associated with malignant progression, further justifying a conservative treatment approach to most branch-duct IPMNs where this epithelium is usually present [118]. Nonetheless, given the rather dramatic differences in 5-year survival rates between non-invasive IPMNs and those with invasion (90% vs. 50%, respectively) [119], it is essential that the presence of an invasive component be excluded by meticulous histopathological assessment of the sample, including submission of the entire specimen, if warranted.

Molecular Alterations in IPMNs

It is becoming increasingly apparent that the spectrum of genetic alterations in IPMNs differs from that observed in PanINs. We have already alluded to the distinct apomucin patterns in IPMNs vs. PanINs. The incidence of *KRAS2* mutations is lower in IPMNs than in PanINs, and is typically present in cysts with higher grades of epithelial dysplasia [120]. Loss of *DPC4/SMAD4* is rarely observed in non-invasive IPMNs, and is essentially seen in the invasive component [121]. IPMNs also tend to harbor alterations that are rarely observed in PanINs, or ductal adenocarcinomas.

For example, the serine threonine kinase encoding gene *STK11/LKB1*, which is mutated in the germline in patients with the Peutz-Jeghers polyposis syndrome, is inactivated in up to a quarter of IPMNs (Fig. 19.4d) [122, 123]. Similarly, the *PIK3CA* gene, whose product is an essential component of Akt oncogenic signaling pathway, is mutated in 10% of IPMNs [124]. Recent transcriptomic studies of IPMNs using oligonucleotide microarrays have identified a number of differentially expressed genes (*claudin 4, CXCR4, S100A4*, and *mesothelin*) that are selectively overexpressed in the invasive compared to non-invasive IPMN lesions [125]. Thus, the products of these transcripts might be involved in facilitating progression of the non-invasive epithelium towards stromal invasion.

MicroRNAs (miRNAs) are 21-23 nucleotide long non-coding RNAs that are involved in translational regulation of coding transcripts [126]. Aberrant miRNA expression has emerged as a hallmark of human neoplasia, including PDAC [127–129]. Habbe et al. assessed relative expression levels of a panel of twelve miRNAs known to be upregulated in PDAC in 15 non-invasive IPMNs, with miR-21 (mean 12.1-fold) and miR-155 (mean 11.6-fold) identified as the most promising candidates [130]. Furthermore, upregulation of miR-155 transcripts were observed in 6 of 10 (60%) IPMN-associated cyst fluid specimens compared to 0 of 5 (0%) disease controls. Therefore, aberrant miRNA expression in clinical material like cyst fluid samples might serve as an ancillary diagnostic tool for IPMNs.

Mucinous Cystic Neoplasms

Clinical Appearance and Morphology of MCNs

MCNs are the least common of the three known precursor lesions of PDAC. MCNs are epithelial cystic neoplasms with mucinous and sometimes hemorrhagic cyst content. These neoplasms are significantly more common in women than in men (9:1 ratio) and patients are usually between 40 and 50 years at primary diagnosis [131]. Symptoms of an underlying MCN can be vague and comprise of abdominal discomfort or sensations of an epigastric mass. Comparable to IPMNs, non-invasive MCNs are on average detected in younger patients, whereas MCNs with an associated invasive carcinoma occurs approximately a decade later in life [119]. On imaging, MCN presents as a well circumscribed cystic lesion, which is usually multiloculated. In contrast to IPMNs, there is no dilatation of the main pancreatic duct, and the lesion does not demonstrate any obvious communication with the ductal system. The lesions are mostly located in the pancreatic body or tail rather than in the head. Circulating tumor markers such as carcinoembryonic antigen (CEA) or cancer antigen 19-9 (CA 19-9) are not elevated in the absence of an invasive carcinoma, although these may be elevated in the cyst fluid aspirate [132, 133].

Histologically, the epithelial lining of MCN consists of mucin-producing columnar cells with a varying degree of dysplasia [134]. Thus, MCN adenomas (mild dysplasia) demonstrate minimal architectural and cytological atypia. The lining cells contain abundant mucin overlying basally oriented nuclei, and are strongly positive for MUC5AC labeling. In MCNs with moderate dysplasia, the nuclei begin to lose polarity and vary in morphology and size. MCN lesions with severe dysplasia (carcinoma in situ) demonstrate marked architectural and cytological abnormalities; one curious feature that may be observed in the cyst lining is an abrupt transition between areas of severe and mild dysplasia. A diagnostic sine qua non of MCNs is the presence of an ovarian-like stroma underlying the neoplastic epithelium [135]. The stroma expresses progesterone and estrogen receptors, and can even undergo luteinization akin to the actual ovarian stroma. Comparable to IPMNs, one third of MCNs are associated with an invasive adenocarcinoma, which are of the usual ductal type [119]. Patients who undergo resection for an MCN with an associated invasive cancer have a 5-year survival of 50–60%. In comparison, patients with a non-invasive MCN usually have an excellent outcome, with a disease-specific 5-year survival rate of almost 100% [136, 137]. In contrast to IPMNs (*see above*), MCNs are typically unifocal lesions. Therefore, documenting the presence of an invasive component is critical in the resection specimen, since non-invasive MCNs, including those harboring severe dysplasia, are essentially cured following surgical resection [134, 136, 137].

Molecular Alterations in MCNs

The molecular pathology of MCNs is a work in progress due to the infrequency of these lesions. Activating *KRAS2* mutations are observed even in lower grades of dysplasia, while *TP53* and *DPC4/SMAD4* mutations usually occur at a later stage, including in the invasive component [138, 139]. The expression of cellular apomucins MUC5AC and MUC2 are observed in non-invasive MCNs, while appearance of MUC1 expression is associated with acquisition of invasive properties [140]. Global expression profiling has detected a range of differentially expressed transcripts in either the epithelium or the ovarian-like stroma of MCNs [141]. Thus, potential oncogenic transcripts like *S100P*, *PSCA*, *MYC*, *MET*, and *cathepsin E* are upregulated in the neoplastic epithelial cells, while the steroidogenic acute regulatory protein (STAR) and estrogen receptor-1 (ESR-1) are expressed in the stroma. Furthermore, transcripts corresponding to Jagged-1 and Hes1, key components of Notch signaling, are overexpressed, suggesting a reactivation of this "druggable" pathway in MCN.

Genetically Engineered Models of PDAC and Precursor Lesions

The pancreas was one of the first organs in which transgenesis was attempted in mouse models [142, 143]. Unfortunately, most of these early models developed carcinomas of acinar cell origin, which are rare neoplasms in humans, and did not

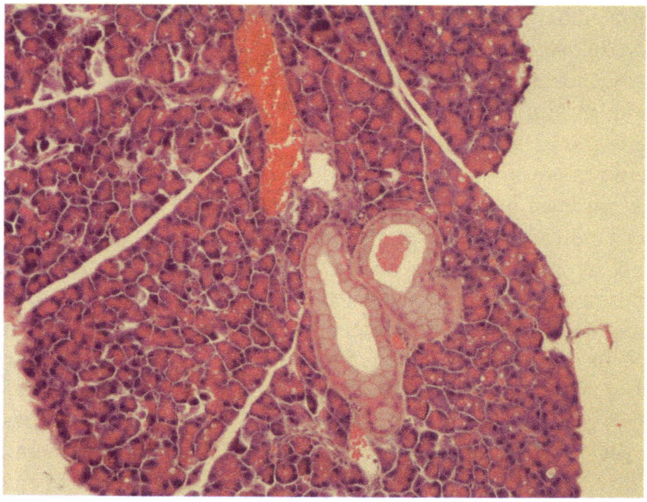

Fig. 19.5 A murine PanIN (mPanIN) lesion occurring in a genetically engineered mouse model of PDAC

manifest the multistep progression observed in the cognate disease. The first series of models that recapitulated human PDAC progression were generated in 2003 by conditional expression of a mutant *Kras*^{G12D} (or *Kras*^{G12V}) "knock-in" allele from its endogenous promoter [29]. Expression of the mutant allele was activated by Cre-mediated recombination during pancreas development, by driving recombinase within the *Pdx1* expression domain. Pdx1 is a developmental transcription factor expressed within the entire pancreatic anlage [144]. Mice with pancreas specific mutant *Kras* expression develop the entire histological compendium of ductal precursor lesions, designated as murine PanINs or "mPanINs" (Fig. 19.5) [145]. A minor fraction of these mice (<10%) develops invasive neoplasia and metastatic disease. However, when additional genetic hits (such as expression of a dominant negative *Trp53*^{R72H} allele, or conditional bi-allelic knockout of *Inka4a/Arf*) are superimposed, the mice rapidly progress to invasive adenocarcinomas with near uniform penetrance [30, 146, 147]. These studies have reinforced a critical requirement for mutant Kras expressed at endogenous (physiologic) levels in order for mPanIN development ("tumor initiation"), with the cooperating genetic hits serving to accelerate progression to invasive adenocarcinoma and metastases.

The choice of the cooperating genetic hit does appear to influence the morphology of additional precursor-like lesions that develops in these mice. For example, Schmid and colleagues generated mice that combined pancreas-specific mutant *Kras* expression with overexpression of the transforming growth factor α (TGFα), which resulted in accelerated development of metastatic adenocarcinomas in the backdrop of mPanINs [148]. At the same time, cystic papillary lesions resembling human IPMNs were identified in the pancreata of compound heterozygous mice. Similarly, Hingorani and colleagues generated mice that express mutant *Kras* with hemi-allelic deletion of *Smad4* in the pancreas, resulting in the development of grossly visible cystic neoplasms in the body and tail [149]. On histopathological assessment, the murine pancreata harbored "classic" mPanINs as well as cystic lesions with histological characteristics comparable to that of human MCNs; loss of the second Smad4 allele is associated with progression invasive PDAC and metastases in these mice.

The genetically engineered models of PDAC and associated murine precursor lesions have proven to be a rich seedbed for preclinical translational studies with direct relevance to the human disease. For example, these models have been utilized to generate a proteomic signature of early pancreatic neoplasia using circulating biomarkers identified by a mass spectrometry-based approach [29, 150, 151]. The validation of these markers in human serum samples confirms the utility of this comparative proteomics approach. More recently, the genetically engineered models have been utilized to test the efficacy of chemoprevention strategies aimed at ameliorating the progression of mPanIN lesions to invasive cancers [91, 152, 153]; pharmacological agents such as the cyclooxygenase inhibitor aspirin and the angiotensin receptor antagonist enalapril have been shown to be efficacious in stemming the progression to PDAC in this model, a finding that can be translated with relative ease to high-risk cohorts such as familial PDAC kindred or those harboring germline mutations in PDAC-predisposing genes [154].

In addition to studies with clinical relevance, the genetically engineered models have provided unique biological insights into the cellular origins of mPanIN, and by extension, human PanINs. In the "classic" models of mPanIN and PDAC, recombination and expression was enabled in the Pdx1-expression domain during development [29, 30, 146, 147]. Since Pdx1 is expressed in the entire pancreatic anlage, the precise cell of origin transforming into mPanIN lesions was undetermined. A series of subsequent studies have confirmed the striking plasticity of terminally differentiated cells in the mature pancreas, which have the ability to generate mPanIN lesions in the appropriate genetic context. For example, Guerra et al. and Habbe et al. demonstrated the ability of elastase-expressing mature acinar cells to generate mPanINs upon expression of mutant *Kras* allele in these cells [155, 156]; of note, the former study required the concomitant induction of chronic pancreatits in order to initiate mPanINs, while this phenomenon was spontaneously observed in the latter study. More recently Jacks and colleagues have extended this phenomenon even further, by expressing mutant *Kras* in several discrete compartments of the mature pancreas using tamoxifen-inducible Cre "driver" mice [157]; in their study, a mature *Pdx1* expressing population, likely residing within the exocrine compartment, demonstrated the highest efficiency of spontaneous mPanIN generation. Even insulin-positive endocrine cells retained the ability to generate mPanINs with a low efficiency (accelerated upon chronic pancreatitis induction), underscoring the rather remarkable ability of mature pancreatic cells of all lineages to potentially transdifferentiate into the mPanIN phenotype.

Clinical Implications of Pancreatic Cancer Precursor Lesions

The identification of tangible precursor lesions for a highly aggressive, often fatal, neoplasm like PDAC has engendered the promise of early detection and secondary prevention of invasive neoplasia. At the same time, the dictum of "primum non nocere" mandates that physicians avoid the pitfall of over-treatment and surgical resection for those precursor lesions that have minimal, if any risk for progression. The standards for conservative vs. interventional therapies for PDAC precursor lesions remain a work in progress; however, it is becoming increasingly apparent that a multi-disciplinary team approach, including surgeons, gastroenterologists, radiologists, pathologists, and molecular diagnosticians, will be required for the appropriate risk stratification and management of these lesions [158]. Population screening for PDAC is confounded by the relative infrequency of the neoplasm, and the inaccessibility of the source organ compared to superficial sites such as the breast and cervix. Nonetheless, at least two "at-risk" subgroups have been identified where intensive screening efforts clearly have a role. The first are individuals that belong to high-risk familial pancreatic cancer kindred [47, 159]. In some instances the underlying germline mutation predisposing to inherited disease risk is known [48], while other kindred are simply identified on the basis of multiple affected family members and the disease-predisposing mutation remains undetermined [159]. The significantly increased risk of prospective, often metastatic, pancreatic cancers in these high-risk kindred is unequivocal [160]. Many tertiary centers in the United States and other countries now screen asymptomatic family members for early pancreatic neoplasia using sophisticated imaging techniques like endoscopic ultrasound (EUS). For example, Canto et al. screened 78 asymptomatic individuals with a family history of pancreatic cancer using computerized tomography and EUS. PDAC precursor lesions, including high-grade IPMN and PanIN lesions and at least one micro-invasive carcinoma, were found in 10% of individuals [161]. These pancreata typically harbor multifocal PanIN lesions (simulating "polyposis" of the pancreas), secondarily resulting in multifocal "lobulo-centric atrophy" of the adjacent parenchyma, as described above; such a pattern of diffuse echogenicity can be discerned by EUS and provides a radiographic readout of inherited risk for PDAC in affected individuals [15, 162].

A second "at-risk" category pertains to individuals identified as harboring an asymptomatic pancreatic cyst ("pancreatic incidentaloma"). With improvements in imaging techniques and the widespread use of CT scans, approximately 1% of the general population undergoing abdominal scans are diagnosed with an incidental pancreatic cyst [163–165]; the proportion of individuals harboring such cysts rises even further with advancing age [103, 166]. Histological examination of surgically resected cysts has established that a little over half of those lesions harbor one of the two mucinous precursors of PDAC (IPMN or MCN, respectively) [165, 166]. The last decade has seen considerable inter-institutional variations in the management of incidental pancreatic cysts, with some centers aggressively resecting any lesion deemed on radiology as a potential precursor, and others implementing a more conservative approach. The confusion has abated to some extent in recent years with the publication of the so-called "Tanaka criteria" for determining cyst resectability (*see above*) [109], and the subsequent validation of these criteria in independent studies [110, 111, 167, 168]. Nonetheless, these criteria are not perfect, and in spite of guidelines, the management of patients with small cystic lesions remains problematic. This was exemplified in a study by Tada et al., wherein 7 of 197 patients harboring a pancreatic cystic lesion eventually developed invasive pancreatic cancer [169]. Notably, three of the invasive cysts were ≤1 cm in maximum diameter. This prevailing uncertainty provides an opportunity for developing ancillary molecular markers, including methylation and miRNA profiles of cyst fluid [130, 170], in order to enable better stratification of malignancy risk in pancreatic cysts. By far, this is one of the most intensive areas of research in the field of PDAC precursor lesions [119].

Finally, we will mention two clinical caveats that are particular to the entity of IPMNs. The first, which was discussed above, pertains to the multifocal nature of these precursor lesions, such that patients undergoing partial pancreas resections are at lifetime risk for recurrence in the remnant organ [112–114]. In a series by Chari et al. 5 of 60 patients relapsed after partial pancreatectomy for non-invasive IPMN [112]. In contrast, thirteen patients who underwent total pancreatectomy did not develop a recurrent lesion. The second unique characteristic for IPMNs is that patients may also develop extrapancreatic malignancies [171–175]. To quote selected examples, Kamisawa et al. described that 12 out of 79 patients with IPMN suffered from synchronous or metachronous gastric cancer and 7 patients had colorectal cancer [176]. In another study Eguchi et al. of 69 IPMN patients 3 (4%) had a history of gastric and another ten patients (12%) had a history of colorectal cancer [177]. Follow-up examination must therefore include a systemic check-up in patients who received surgery for IPMNs, even in those with tumor-free resection margins.

Conclusions

With significant advances in understanding carcinogenesis of pancreatic cancer, translation of our current knowledge into early detection and treatment before the onset of malignancy remains a major clinical challenge of the next years. Ongoing studies addressing early detection aim for screening methods on molecular basis whereas no cost effective screening method has been established so far. The dramatic increase of pancreatic "incidentalomas" diagnosed through improved imaging represents a double-edged sword. On the one hand, even tiny morphologic irregularities may be detected enabling early detection. On the other hand, in many individuals clinically irrelevant lesions attract undeserved attention. Selection of patients eligible for surgery should be performed carefully because in spite of significant advances in operative and perioperative treatment pancreatic surgery still harbors a risk for severe morbidity. Conclusively, there is a need for appropriate prospective studies and subsequent evidence based guidelines for the management of pancreatic incidentaloma. Last not least, the authors emphasize that the management of patients with pancreatic lesions should be performed by an experienced multidisciplinary team in centers of high patient volume.

Acknowledgement This work was supported by R01CA113669, P50CA62924, P01CA134292, the Sol Goldman Pancreatic Cancer Research Center and the Michael Rolfe Foundation for Pancreatic Cancer Research. Hanno Matthaei is supported by a grant from the Mildred-Scheel-Stiftung, Deutsche Krebshilfe, Bonn, Germany.

References

1. Jemal A, Siegel R, Ward E, Hao Y, Xu J, Thun MJ (2009) Cancer statistics, 2009. CA Cancer J Clin 59:225–249
2. Maitra A, Hruban RH (2008) Pancreatic cancer. Annu Rev Pathol 3:157–188
3. Lieberman DA (2009) Clinical practice. Screening for colorectal cancer. N Engl J Med 361:1179–1187
4. Schiffman M, Castle PE, Jeronimo J, Rodriguez AC, Wacholder S (2007) Human papillomavirus and cervical cancer. Lancet 370:890–907
5. 16-year mortality from breast cancer in the UK Trial of Early Detection of Breast Cancer (1999) Lancet 353:1909–1914.
6. Berry DA, Cronin KA, Plevritis SK et al (2005) Effect of screening and adjuvant therapy on mortality from breast cancer. N Engl J Med 353:1784–1792
7. Hulst SPL (1905) Zur kenntnis der genese des adenokarzinoms und karzinoms des pankreas. Virchows Arch 180:288–316
8. Cubilla AL, Fitzgerald PJ (1976) Morphological lesions associated with human primary invasive nonendocrine pancreas cancer. Cancer Res 36:2690–2698
9. Kozuka S, Sassa R, Taki T et al (1979) Relation of pancreatic duct hyperplasia to carcinoma. Cancer 43:1418–1428
10. Andea A, Sarkar F, Adsay VN (2003) Clinicopathological correlates of pancreatic intraepithelial neoplasia: a comparative analysis of 82 cases with and 152 cases without pancreatic ductal adenocarcinoma. Mod Pathol 16:996–1006
11. Hruban RH, Adsay NV, Albores-Saavedra J et al (2001) Pancreatic intraepithelial neoplasia: a new nomenclature and classification system for pancreatic duct lesions. Am J Surg Pathol 25:579–586
12. Hruban RH, Takaori K, Klimstra DS et al (2004) An illustrated consensus on the classification of pancreatic intraepithelial neoplasia and intraductal papillary mucinous neoplasms. Am J Surg Pathol 28:977–987
13. Brune K, Abe T, Canto M et al (2006) Multifocal neoplastic precursor lesions associated with lobular atrophy of the pancreas in patients having a strong family history of pancreatic cancer. Am J Surg Pathol 30:1067–1076
14. Detlefsen S, Sipos B, Feyerabend B, Kloppel G (2005) Pancreatic fibrosis associated with age and ductal papillary hyperplasia. Virchows Arch 447:800–805
15. Hruban RH, Takaori K, Canto M et al (2007) Clinical importance of precursor lesions in the pancreas. J Hepatobiliary Pancreat Surg 14:255–263
16. Maitra A, Adsay NV, Argani P et al (2003) Multicomponent analysis of the pancreatic adenocarcinoma progression model using a pancreatic intraepithelial neoplasia tissue microarray. Mod Pathol 16:902–912
17. Yamano M, Fujii H, Takagaki T, Kadowaki N, Watanabe H, Shirai T (2000) Genetic progression and divergence in pancreatic carcinoma. Am J Pathol 156:2123–2133

18. Biankin AV, Kench JG, Morey AL et al (2001) Overexpression of p21(WAF1/CIP1) is an early event in the development of pancreatic intraepithelial neoplasia. Cancer Res 61:8830–8837
19. Lohr M, Kloppel G, Maisonneuve P, Lowenfels AB, Luttges J (2005) Frequency of K-ras mutations in pancreatic intraductal neoplasias associated with pancreatic ductal adenocarcinoma and chronic pancreatitis: a meta-analysis. Neoplasia 7:17–23
20. Maitra A, Ashfaq R, Gunn CR et al (2002) Cyclooxygenase 2 expression in pancreatic adenocarcinoma and pancreatic intraepithelial neoplasia: an immunohistochemical analysis with automated cellular imaging. Am J Clin Pathol 118:194–201
21. Fukushima N, Sato N, Ueki T et al (2002) Aberrant methylation of preproenkephalin and p16 genes in pancreatic intraepithelial neoplasia and pancreatic ductal adenocarcinoma. Am J Pathol 160:1573–1581
22. Luttges J, Galehdari H, Brocker V et al (2001) Allelic loss is often the first hit in the biallelic inactivation of the p53 and DPC4 genes during pancreatic carcinogenesis. Am J Pathol 158:1677–1683
23. Koorstra JB, Hong SM, Shi C et al (2009) Widespread activation of the DNA damage response in human pancreatic intraepithelial neoplasia. Mod Pathol 22:1439–1445
24. Jones S, Zhang X, Parsons DW et al (2008) Core signaling pathways in human pancreatic cancers revealed by global genomic analyses. Science 321:1801–1806
25. Almoguera C, Shibata D, Forrester K, Martin J, Arnheim N, Perucho M (1988) Most human carcinomas of the exocrine pancreas contain mutant c-K-ras genes. Cell 53:549–554
26. Deramaudt T, Rustgi AK (2005) Mutant KRAS in the initiation of pancreatic cancer. Biochim Biophys Acta 1756:97–101
27. Hingorani SR, Tuveson DA (2003) Ras redux: rethinking how and where Ras acts. Curr Opin Genet Dev 13:6–13
28. Moskaluk CA, Hruban RH, Kern SE (1997) p16 and K-ras gene mutations in the intraductal precursors of human pancreatic adenocarcinoma. Cancer Res 57:2140–2143
29. Hingorani SR, Petricoin EF, Maitra A et al (2003) Preinvasive and invasive ductal pancreatic cancer and its early detection in the mouse. Cancer Cell 4:437–450
30. Hingorani SR, Wang L, Multani AS et al (2005) Trp53R172H and KrasG12D cooperate to promote chromosomal instability and widely metastatic pancreatic ductal adenocarcinoma in mice. Cancer Cell 7:469–483
31. Vogelstein B, Kinzler KW (2004) Cancer genes and the pathways they control. Nat Med 10:789–799
32. Wilentz RE, Geradts J, Maynard R et al (1998) Inactivation of the p16 (INK4A) tumor-suppressor gene in pancreatic duct lesions: loss of intranuclear expression. Cancer Res 58:4740–4744
33. Caldas C, Hahn SA, da Costa LT et al (1994) Frequent somatic mutations and homozygous deletions of the p16 (MTS1) gene in pancreatic adenocarcinoma. Nat Genet 8:27–32
34. Ueki T, Toyota M, Sohn T et al (2000) Hypermethylation of multiple genes in pancreatic adenocarcinoma. Cancer Res 60:1835–1839
35. Sherr CJ (2004) Principles of tumor suppression. Cell 116:235–246
36. Lal G, Liu L, Hogg D, Lassam NJ, Redston MS, Gallinger S (2000) Patients with both pancreatic adenocarcinoma and melanoma may harbor germline CDKN2A mutations. Genes Chromosom Cancer 27:358–361
37. Rulyak SJ, Brentnall TA, Lynch HT, Austin MA (2003) Characterization of the neoplastic phenotype in the familial atypical multiple-mole melanoma-pancreatic carcinoma syndrome. Cancer 98:798–804
38. Berrozpe G, Schaeffer J, Peinado MA, Real FX, Perucho M (1994) Comparative analysis of mutations in the p53 and K-ras genes in pancreatic cancer. Int J Cancer 58:185–191
39. Redston MS, Caldas C, Seymour AB et al (1994) p53 mutations in pancreatic carcinoma and evidence of common involvement of homocopolymer tracts in DNA microdeletions. Cancer Res 54:3025–3033
40. Sherr CJ, McCormick F (2002) The RB and p53 pathways in cancer. Cancer Cell 2:103–112

41. Baas IO, Mulder JW, Offerhaus GJ, Vogelstein B, Hamilton SR (1994) An evaluation of six antibodies for immunohistochemistry of mutant p53 gene product in archival colorectal neoplasms. J Pathol 172:5–12
42. Hahn SA, Schutte M, Hoque AT et al (1996) DPC4, a candidate tumor suppressor gene at human chromosome 18q21.1. Science 271:350–353
43. Wilentz RE, Su GH, Dai JL et al (2000) Immunohistochemical labeling for dpc4 mirrors genetic status in pancreatic adenocarcinomas: a new marker of DPC4 inactivation. Am J Pathol 156:37–43
44. Siegel PM, Massague J (2003) Cytostatic and apoptotic actions of TGF-beta in homeostasis and cancer. Nat Rev 3:807–821
45. Wilentz RE, Iacobuzio-Donahue CA, Argani P et al (2000) Loss of expression of Dpc4 in pancreatic intraepithelial neoplasia: evidence that DPC4 inactivation occurs late in neoplastic progression. Cancer Res 60:2002–2006
46. D'Andrea AD, Grompe M (2003) The Fanconi anaemia/BRCA pathway. Nat Rev 3:23–34
47. Shi C, Hruban RH, Klein AP (2009) Familial pancreatic cancer. Arch Pathol Lab Med 133:365–374
48. Jones S, Hruban RH, Kamiyama M et al (2009) Exomic sequencing identifies PALB2 as a pancreatic cancer susceptibility gene. Science 324:217
49. Goggins M, Hruban RH, Kern SE (2000) BRCA2 is inactivated late in the development of pancreatic intraepithelial neoplasia: evidence and implications. Am J Pathol 156:1767–1771
50. Griffin CA, Hruban RH, Long PP, Morsberger LA, Douna-Issa F, Yeo CJ (1994) Chromosome abnormalities in pancreatic adenocarcinoma. Genes Chromosom Cancer 9:93–100
51. Moskovitz AH, Linford NJ, Brentnall TA et al (2003) Chromosomal instability in pancreatic ductal cells from patients with chronic pancreatitis and pancreatic adenocarcinoma. Genes Chromosom Cancer 37:201–206
52. Sharpless NE, DePinho RA (2004) Telomeres, stem cells, senescence, and cancer. J Clin Invest 113:160–168
53. Greider CW, Blackburn EH (1996) Telomeres, telomerase and cancer. Sci Am 274:92–97
54. van Heek NT, Meeker AK, Kern SE et al (2002) Telomere shortening is nearly universal in pancreatic intraepithelial neoplasia. Am J Pathol 161:1541–1547
55. Jones PA, Baylin SB (2007) The epigenomics of cancer. Cell 128:683–692
56. Omura N, Li CP, Li A et al (2008) Genome-wide profiling of methylated promoters in pancreatic adenocarcinoma. Cancer Biol Ther 7:1146–1156
57. Tan AC, Jimeno A, Lin SH, et al. (2009) Characterizing DNA methylation patterns in pancreatic cancer genome. Mol Oncol 3(5–6):425–438
58. Jansen M, Fukushima N, Rosty C et al (2002) Aberrant methylation of the 5' CpG island of TSLC1 is common in pancreatic ductal adenocarcinoma and is first manifest in high-grade PanlNs. Cancer Biol Ther 1:293–296
59. Sato N, Fukushima N, Matsubayashi H, Iacobuzio-Donahue CA, Yeo CJ, Goggins M (2006) Aberrant methylation of Reprimo correlates with genetic instability and predicts poor prognosis in pancreatic ductal adenocarcinoma. Cancer 107:251–257
60. Sato N, Fukushima N, Hruban RH, Goggins M (2008) CpG island methylation profile of pancreatic intraepithelial neoplasia. Mod Pathol 21:238–244
61. Sato N, Fukushima N, Maitra A et al (2003) Discovery of novel targets for aberrant methylation in pancreatic carcinoma using high-throughput microarrays. Cancer Res 63:3735–3742
62. Fukushima N, Walter KM, Uek T et al (2003) Diagnosing pancreatic cancer using methylation specific PCR analysis of pancreatic juice. Cancer Biol Ther 2:78–83
63. Matsubayashi H, Canto M, Sato N et al (2006) DNA methylation alterations in the pancreatic juice of patients with suspected pancreatic disease. Cancer Res 66:1208–1217
64. Porter D, Polyak K (2003) Cancer target discovery using SAGE. Expert Opin Ther Targets 7:759–769
65. Myllykangas S, Junnila S, Kokkola A et al (2008) Integrated gene copy number and expression microarray analysis of gastric cancer highlights potential target genes. Int J Cancer 123:817–825

66. Lin J, Gan CM, Zhang X et al (2007) A multidimensional analysis of genes mutated in breast and colorectal cancers. Genome Res 17:1304–1318
67. Irizarry RA, Ladd-Acosta C, Wen B et al (2009) The human colon cancer methylome shows similar hypo- and hypermethylation at conserved tissue-specific CpG island shores. Nat Genet 41:178–186
68. Feinberg AP (2004) The epigenetics of cancer etiology. Semin Cancer Biol 14:427–432
69. Dang CV, O'Donnell KA, Zeller KI, Nguyen T, Osthus RC, Li F (2006) The c-Myc target gene network. Semin Cancer Biol 16:253–264
70. Iacobuzio-Donahue CA, Ashfaq R, Maitra A et al (2003) Highly expressed genes in pancreatic ductal adenocarcinomas: a comprehensive characterization and comparison of the transcription profiles obtained from three major technologies. Cancer Res 63: 8614–8622
71. Iacobuzio-Donahue CA, Maitra A, Olsen M et al (2003) Exploration of global gene expression patterns in pancreatic adenocarcinoma using cDNA microarrays. Am J Pathol 162: 1151–1162
72. Logsdon CD, Simeone DM, Binkley C et al (2003) Molecular profiling of pancreatic adenocarcinoma and chronic pancreatitis identifies multiple genes differentially regulated in pancreatic cancer. Cancer Res 63:2649–2657
73. Crnogorac-Jurcevic T, Efthimiou E, Capelli P et al (2001) Gene expression profiles of pancreatic cancer and stromal desmoplasia. Oncogene 20:7437–7446
74. Crnogorac-Jurcevic T, Missiaglia E, Blaveri E et al (2003) Molecular alterations in pancreatic carcinoma: expression profiling shows that dysregulated expression of S100 genes is highly prevalent. J Pathol 201:63–74
75. Argani P, Rosty C, Reiter RE et al (2001) Discovery of new markers of cancer through serial analysis of gene expression: prostate stem cell antigen is overexpressed in pancreatic adenocarcinoma. Cancer Res 61:4320–4324
76. Argani P, Iacobuzio-Donahue C, Ryu B et al (2001) Mesothelin is overexpressed in the vast majority of ductal adenocarcinomas of the pancreas: identification of a new pancreatic cancer marker by serial analysis of gene expression (SAGE). Clin Cancer Res 7:3862–3868
77. Ringel J, Lohr M (2003) The MUC gene family: Their role in diagnosis and early detection of pancreatic cancer. Mol Cancer 2:9
78. Levi E, Klimstra DS, Andea A, Basturk O, Adsay NV (2004) MUC1 and MUC2 in pancreatic neoplasia. J Clin Pathol 57:456–462
79. Swartz MJ, Batra SK, Varshney GC et al (2002) MUC4 expression increases progressively in pancreatic intraepithelial neoplasia. Am J Clin Pathol 117:791–796
80. Nagata K, Horinouchi M, Saitou M et al (2007) Mucin expression profile in pancreatic cancer and the precursor lesions. J Hepatobiliary Pancreat Surg 14:243–254
81. Moriya T, Kimura W, Semba S et al (2005) Biological similarities and differences between pancreatic intraepithelial neoplasias and intraductal papillary mucinous neoplasms. Int J Gastrointest Cancer 35:111–119
82. Adsay NV, Merati K, Andea A et al (2002) The dichotomy in the preinvasive neoplasia to invasive carcinoma sequence in the pancreas: differential expression of MUC1 and MUC2 supports the existence of two separate pathways of carcinogenesis. Mod Pathol 15:1087–1095
83. Ruiz i Altaba A, Sanchez P, Dahmane N (2002) Gli and hedgehog in cancer: tumours, embryos and stem cells. Nat Rev 2:361–372
84. Artavanis-Tsakonas S, Rand MD, Lake RJ (1999) Notch signaling: cell fate control and signal integration in development. Science 284:770–776
85. Pasca di Magliano M, Sekine S, Ermilov A, Ferris J, Dlugosz AA, Hebrok M (2006) Hedgehog/Ras interactions regulate early stages of pancreatic cancer. Genes Dev 20:3161–3173
86. Morton JP, Mongeau ME, Klimstra DS et al (2007) Sonic hedgehog acts at multiple stages during pancreatic tumorigenesis. Proc Natl Acad Sci U S A 104:5103–5108
87. De La OJ, Emerson LL, Goodman JL et al (2008) Notch and Kras reprogram pancreatic acinar cells to ductal intraepithelial neoplasia. Proc Natl Acad Sci U S A 105:18907–18912

88. Thayer SP, di Magliano MP, Heiser PW, et al. Hedgehog is an early and late mediator of pancreatic cancer tumorigenesis. Nature 2003; doi:10.1038/nature02009
89. Miyamoto Y, Maitra A, Ghosh B et al (2003) Notch mediates TGF alpha-induced changes in epithelial differentiation during pancreatic tumorigenesis. Cancer Cell 3:565–576
90. Prasad NB, Biankin AV, Fukushima N et al (2005) Gene expression profiles in pancreatic intraepithelial neoplasia reflect the effects of Hedgehog signaling on pancreatic ductal epithelial cells. Cancer Res 65:1619–1626
91. Plentz R, Park JS, Rhim AD, et al (2009) Inhibition of gamma-secretase activity inhibits tumor progression in a mouse model of pancreatic ductal adenocarcinoma. Gastroenterology 136(5):1741–1749
92. Rubin LL, de Sauvage FJ (2006) Targeting the Hedgehog pathway in cancer. Nat Rev Drug Discov 5:1026–1033
93. Yauch RL, Gould SE, Scales SJ et al (2008) A paracrine requirement for hedgehog signalling in cancer. Nature 455:406–410
94. Feldmann G, Dhara S, Fendrich V et al (2007) Blockade of hedgehog signaling inhibits pancreatic cancer invasion and metastases: a new paradigm for combination therapy in solid cancers. Cancer Res 67:2187–2196
95. Mullendore ME, Koorstra JB, Li YM, et al (2009) Ligand-dependent notch signaling is involved in tumor initiation and tumor maintenance in pancreatic cancer. Clin Cancer Res 15(7):2291–2301
96. Von Hoff DD, Lorusso PM, Rudin CM et al (2009) Inhibition of the hedgehog pathway in advanced Basal-cell carcinoma. N Engl J Med 361:1164–1172
97. Ohhashi K, Murakami F, Maruyama M (1982) Four cases of mucous secreting pancreatic cancer. Prog Dig Endosc 203:348–351
98. Belyaev O, Seelig MH, Muller CA, Tannapfel A, Schmidt WE, Uhl W (2008) Intraductal papillary mucinous neoplasms of the pancreas. J Clin Gastroenterol 42:284–294
99. Ferrone CR, Correa-Gallego C, Warshaw AL et al (2009) Current trends in pancreatic cystic neoplasms. Arch Surg 144:448–454
100. Sohn TA, Yeo CJ, Cameron JL et al (2004) Intraductal papillary mucinous neoplasms of the pancreas: an updated experience. Ann Surg 239:788–797, discussion 97–99
101. Salvia R, Fernandez-del Castillo C, Bassi C et al (2004) Main-duct intraductal papillary mucinous neoplasms of the pancreas: clinical predictors of malignancy and long-term survival following resection. Ann Surg 239:678–685, discussion 85–87
102. Fernandez-del Castillo C, Targarona J, Thayer SP, Rattner DW, Brugge WR, Warshaw AL (2003) Incidental pancreatic cysts: clinicopathologic characteristics and comparison with symptomatic patients. Arch Surg 138:427–423, discussion 33–34
103. Laffan TA, Horton KM, Klein AP et al (2008) Prevalence of unsuspected pancreatic cysts on MDCT. AJR Am J Roentgenol 191:802–807
104. Fernandez-del Castillo C, Alsfasser G, Targarona J, Brugge WR, Warshaw AL (2006) Serum CA 19-9 in the management of cystic lesions of the pancreas. Pancreas 32:220
105. Brugge WR, Lewandrowski K, Lee-Lewandrowski E et al (2004) Diagnosis of pancreatic cystic neoplasms: a report of the cooperative pancreatic cyst study. Gastroenterology 126: 1330–1336
106. Allen PJ, Qin LX, Tang L, Klimstra D, Brennan MF, Lokshin A (2009) Pancreatic cyst fluid protein expression profiling for discriminating between serous cystadenoma and intraductal papillary mucinous neoplasm. Ann Surg 250(5):754–760
107. Bassi C, Sarr MG, Lillemoe KD, Reber HA (2008) Natural history of intraductal papillary mucinous neoplasms (IPMN): current evidence and implications for management. J Gastrointest Surg 12:645–650
108. Tanaka M, Kobayashi K, Mizumoto K, Yamaguchi K (2005) Clinical aspects of intraductal papillary mucinous neoplasm of the pancreas. J Gastroenterol 40:669–675
109. Tanaka M, Chari S, Adsay V et al (2006) International consensus guidelines for management of intraductal papillary mucinous neoplasms and mucinous cystic neoplasms of the pancreas. Pancreatology 6:17–32

110. Rodriguez JR, Salvia R, Crippa S et al (2007) Branch-duct intraductal papillary mucinous neoplasms: observations in 145 patients who underwent resection. Gastroenterology 133:72–79, quiz 309–310
111. Salvia R, Crippa S, Falconi M et al (2007) Branch-duct intraductal papillary mucinous neoplasms of the pancreas: to operate or not to operate? Gut 56:1086–1090
112. Chari ST, Yadav D, Smyrk TC et al (2002) Study of recurrence after surgical resection of intraductal papillary mucinous neoplasm of the pancreas. Gastroenterology 123:1500–1507
113. Kobayashi G, Fujita N, Noda Y et al (2005) Mode of progression of intraductal papillary-mucinous tumor of the pancreas: analysis of patients with follow-up by EUS. J Gastroenterol 40:744–751
114. Salvia R, Partelli S, Crippa S et al (2009) Intraductal papillary mucinous neoplasms of the pancreas with multifocal involvement of branch ducts. Am J Surg 198:709–714
115. Furukawa T, Kloppel G, Volkan Adsay N et al (2005) Classification of types of intraductal papillary-mucinous neoplasm of the pancreas: a consensus study. Virchows Arch 447: 794–799
116. Yonezawa S, Nakamura A, Horinouchi M, Sato E (2002) The expression of several types of mucin is related to the biological behavior of pancreatic neoplasms. J Hepatobiliary Pancreat Surg 9:328–341
117. Adsay NV, Pierson C, Sarkar F et al (2001) Colloid (mucinous noncystic) carcinoma of the pancreas. Am J Surg Pathol 25:26–42
118. Adsay NV, Merati K, Basturk O et al (2004) Pathologically and biologically distinct types of epithelium in intraductal papillary mucinous neoplasms: delineation of an "intestinal" pathway of carcinogenesis in the pancreas. Am J Surg Pathol 28:839–848
119. Crippa S, Fernandez-Del Castillo C, Salvia R, et al (2009) Mucin-producing neoplasms of the pancreas: an analysis of distinguishing clinical and epidemiological characteristics. Clin Gastroenterol Hepatol 8(2):213–219
120. Schonleben F, Qiu W, Bruckman KC et al (2007) BRAF and KRAS gene mutations in intraductal papillary mucinous neoplasm/carcinoma (IPMN/IPMC) of the pancreas. Cancer Lett 249:242–248
121. Iacobuzio-Donahue CA, Klimstra DS, Adsay NV et al (2000) Dpc-4 protein is expressed in virtually all human intraductal papillary mucinous neoplasms of the pancreas: comparison with conventional ductal adenocarcinomas. Am J Pathol 157:755–761
122. Sahin F, Maitra A, Argani P et al (2003) Loss of Stk11/Lkb1 expression in pancreatic and biliary neoplasms. Mod Pathol 16:686–691
123. Sato N, Rosty C, Jansen M et al (2001) STK11/LKB1 Peutz-Jeghers gene inactivation in intraductal papillary-mucinous neoplasms of the pancreas. Am J Pathol 159:2017–2022
124. Schonleben F, Qiu W, Ciau NT et al (2006) PIK3CA mutations in intraductal papillary mucinous neoplasm/carcinoma of the pancreas. Clin Cancer Res 12:3851–3855
125. Sato N, Fukushima N, Maitra A et al (2004) Gene expression profiling identifies genes associated with invasive intraductal papillary mucinous neoplasms of the pancreas. Am J Pathol 164:903–914
126. Croce CM, Calin GA (2005) miRNAs, cancer, and stem cell division. Cell 122:6–7
127. Szafranska AE, Davison TS, John J et al (2007) MicroRNA expression alterations are linked to tumorigenesis and non-neoplastic processes in pancreatic ductal adenocarcinoma. Oncogene 26:4442–4452
128. Lee EJ, Gusev Y, Jiang J et al (2007) Expression profiling identifies microRNA signature in pancreatic cancer. Int J Cancer 120:1046–1054
129. Bloomston M, Frankel WL, Petrocca F et al (2007) MicroRNA expression patterns to differentiate pancreatic adenocarcinoma from normal pancreas and chronic pancreatitis. JAMA 297:1901–1908
130. Habbe N, Koorstra JB, Mendell JT, et al (2009) MicroRNA miR-155 is a biomarker of early pancreatic neoplasia. Cancer Biol Ther 8(4):340–346
131. Klimstra DS (2005) Cystic, mucin-producing neoplasms of the pancreas: the distinguishing features of mucinous cystic neoplasms and intraductal papillary mucinous neoplasms. Semin Diagn Pathol 22:318–329

132. Buscaglia JM, Giday SA, Kantsevoy SV et al (2009) Patient- and cyst-related factors for improved prediction of malignancy within cystic lesions of the pancreas. Pancreatology 9:631–638
133. Garcea G, Ong SL, Rajesh A et al (2008) Cystic lesions of the pancreas. A diagnostic and management dilemma. Pancreatology 8:236–251
134. Fernandez-del Castillo C (2008) Mucinous cystic neoplasms. J Gastrointest Surg 12:411–413
135. Wilentz RE, Albores-Saavedra J, Hruban RH (2000) Mucinous cystic neoplasms of the pancreas. Semin Diagn Pathol 17:31–42
136. Wilentz RE, Albores-Saavedra J, Zahurak M et al (1999) Pathologic examination accurately predicts prognosis in mucinous cystic neoplasms of the pancreas. Am J Surg Pathol 23:1320–1327
137. Crippa S, Salvia R, Warshaw AL et al (2008) Mucinous cystic neoplasm of the pancreas is not an aggressive entity: lessons from 163 resected patients. Ann Surg 247:571–579
138. Jimenez RE, Warshaw AL, Z'Graggen K et al (1999) Sequential accumulation of K-ras mutations and p53 overexpression in the progression of pancreatic mucinous cystic neoplasms to malignancy. Ann Surg 230:501–509, discussion 9–11
139. Iacobuzio-Donahue CA, Wilentz RE, Argani P et al (2000) Dpc4 protein in mucinous cystic neoplasms of the pancreas: frequent loss of expression in invasive carcinomas suggests a role in genetic progression. Am J Surg Pathol 24:1544–1548
140. Luttges J, Feyerabend B, Buchelt T, Pacena M, Kloppel G (2002) The mucin profile of noninvasive and invasive mucinous cystic neoplasms of the pancreas. Am J Surg Pathol 26:466–471
141. Fukushima N, Sato N, Prasad N, Leach SD, Hruban RH, Goggins M (2004) Characterization of gene expression in mucinous cystic neoplasms of the pancreas using oligonucleotide microarrays. Oncogene 23:9042–9051
142. Ornitz DM, Hammer RE, Messing A, Palmiter RD, Brinster RL (1987) Pancreatic neoplasia induced by SV40 T-antigen expression in acinar cells of transgenic mice. Science 238:188–193
143. Quaife CJ, Pinkert CA, Ornitz DM, Palmiter RD, Brinster RL (1987) Pancreatic neoplasia induced by ras expression in acinar cells of transgenic mice. Cell 48:1023–1034
144. Jonsson J, Carlsson L, Edlund T, Edlund H (1994) Insulin-promoter-factor 1 is required for pancreas development in mice. Nature 371:606–609
145. Hruban RH, Adsay NV, Albores-Saavedra J et al (2006) Pathology of genetically engineered mouse models of pancreatic exocrine cancer: consensus report and recommendations. Cancer Res 66:95–106
146. Aguirre AJ, Bardeesy N, Sinha M et al (2003) Activated Kras and Ink4a/Arf deficiency cooperate to produce metastatic pancreatic ductal adenocarcinoma. Genes Dev 17:3112–3126
147. Bardeesy N, Aguirre AJ, Chu GC et al (2006) Both p16(Ink4a) and the p19(Arf)-p53 pathway constrain progression of pancreatic adenocarcinoma in the mouse. Proc Natl Acad Sci U S A 103:5947–5952
148. Siveke JT, Einwachter H, Sipos B, Lubeseder-Martellato C, Kloppel G, Schmid RM (2007) Concomitant pancreatic activation of Kras(G12D) and Tgfa results in cystic papillary neoplasms reminiscent of human IPMN. Cancer Cell 12:266–279
149. Izeradjene K, Combs C, Best M et al (2007) Kras(G12D) and Smad4/Dpc4 haploinsufficiency cooperate to induce mucinous cystic neoplasms and invasive adenocarcinoma of the pancreas. Cancer Cell 11:229–243
150. Harsha HC, Kandasamy K, Ranganathan P et al (2009) A compendium of potential biomarkers of pancreatic cancer. PLoS Med 6:e1000046
151. Faca VM, Song KS, Wang H et al (2008) A mouse to human search for plasma proteome changes associated with pancreatic tumor development. PLoS Med 5:e123
152. Funahashi H, Satake M, Dawson D et al (2007) Delayed progression of pancreatic intraepithelial neoplasia in a conditional Kras(G12D) mouse model by a selective cyclooxygenase-2 inhibitor. Cancer Res 67:7068–7071

153. Fendrich V, Chen NM, Neef M, et al (2009) The Angiotensin-I-converting enzyme inhibitor enalapril and aspirin delay progression of pancreatic intraepithelial neoplasia and cancer formation in a genetically engineered mouse model of pancreatic cancer. Gut 59(5):630–637
154. Brand RE, Lerch MM, Rubinstein WS et al (2007) Advances in counselling and surveillance of patients at risk for pancreatic cancer. Gut 56:1460–1469
155. Guerra C, Schuhmacher AJ, Canamero M et al (2007) Chronic pancreatitis is essential for induction of pancreatic ductal adenocarcinoma by K-Ras oncogenes in adult mice. Cancer Cell 11:291–302
156. Habbe N, Shi G, Meguid RA et al (2008) Spontaneous induction of murine pancreatic intraepithelial neoplasia (mPanIN) by acinar cell targeting of oncogenic Kras in adult mice. Proc Natl Acad Sci U S A 105:18913–18918
157. Gidekel Friedlander SY, Chu GC, Snyder EL et al (2009) Context-dependent transformation of adult pancreatic cells by oncogenic K-Ras. Cancer Cell 16:379–389
158. Pawlik TM, Laheru D, Hruban RH et al (2008) Evaluating the impact of a single-day multidisciplinary clinic on the management of pancreatic cancer. Ann Surg Oncol 15: 2081–2088
159. Petersen GM, de Andrade M, Goggins M et al (2006) Pancreatic cancer genetic epidemiology consortium. Cancer Epidemiol Biomark Prev 15:704–710
160. Klein AP, Brune KA, Petersen GM et al (2004) Prospective risk of pancreatic cancer in familial pancreatic cancer kindreds. Cancer Res 64:2634–2638
161. Canto MI, Goggins M, Hruban RH et al (2006) Screening for early pancreatic neoplasia in high-risk individuals: a prospective controlled study. Clin Gastroenterol Hepatol 4:766–781, quiz 665
162. Brune K, Abe T, Canto M et al (2006) Multifocal neoplastic precursor lesions associated with lobular atrophy of the pancreas in patients having a strong family history of pancreatic cancer. Am J Surg Pathol 30:1067–1076
163. Allen PJ, Brennan MF (2007) The management of cystic lesions of the pancreas. Adv Surg 41:211–228
164. Fasanella KE, McGrath K (2009) Cystic lesions and intraductal neoplasms of the pancreas. Best practice & research 23:35–48
165. Kiely JM, Nakeeb A, Komorowski RA, Wilson SD, Pitt HA (2003) Cystic pancreatic neoplasms: enucleate or resect? J Gastrointest Surg 7:890–897
166. Winter JM, Cameron JL, Lillemoe KD et al (2006) Periampullary and pancreatic incidentaloma: a single institution's experience with an increasingly common diagnosis. Ann Surg 243:673–680, discussion 80–83
167. Fritz S, Warshaw AL, Thayer SP (2009) Management of mucin-producing cystic neoplasms of the pancreas. Oncologist 14:125–136
168. Guarise A, Faccioli N, Ferrari M et al (2008) Evaluation of serial changes of pancreatic branch duct intraductal papillary mucinous neoplasms by follow-up with magnetic resonance imaging. Cancer Imaging 8:220–228
169. Tada M, Kawabe T, Arizumi M et al (2006) Pancreatic cancer in patients with pancreatic cystic lesions: a prospective study in 197 patients. Clin Gastroenterol Hepatol 4:1265–1270
170. Hong SM, Kelly D, Griffith M et al (2008) Multiple genes are hypermethylated in intraductal papillary mucinous neoplasms of the pancreas. Mod Pathol 21:1499–1507
171. Riall TS, Stager VM, Nealon WH et al (2007) Incidence of additional primary cancers in patients with invasive intraductal papillary mucinous neoplasms and sporadic pancreatic adenocarcinomas. J Am Coll Surg 204:803–813, discussion 13–14
172. Reid-Lombardo KM, Mathis KL, Wood CM, Harmsen WS, Sarr MG (2009). Frequency of extrapancreatic neoplasms in intraductal papillary mucinous neoplasm of the pancreas: implications for management. Ann Surg 251(1):64–69
173. Baumgaertner I, Corcos O, Couvelard A et al (2008) Prevalence of extrapancreatic cancers in patients with histologically proven intraductal papillary mucinous neoplasms of the pancreas: a case-control study. Am J Gastroenterol 103:2878–2882

174. Yoon WJ, Ryu JK, Lee JK et al (2008) Extrapancreatic malignancies in patients with intraductal papillary mucinous neoplasm of the pancreas: prevalence, associated factors, and comparison with patients with other pancreatic cystic neoplasms. Ann Surg Oncol 15:3193–3198
175. Choi MG, Kim SW, Han SS, Jang JY, Park YH (2006) High incidence of extrapancreatic neoplasms in patients with intraductal papillary mucinous neoplasms. Arch Surg 141:51–56, discussion 6
176. Kamisawa T, Tu Y, Egawa N, Nakajima H, Tsuruta K, Okamoto A (2005) Malignancies associated with intraductal papillary mucinous neoplasm of the pancreas. World J Gastroenterol 11:5688–5690
177. Eguchi H, Ishikawa O, Ohigashi H et al (2006) Patients with pancreatic intraductal papillary mucinous neoplasms are at high risk of colorectal cancer development. Surgery 139:749–754

Chapter 20
Breast: Ductal Carcinoma In Situ (DCIS)

John P. Brown and Sarah E. Pinder

Introduction

Ductal carcinoma in situ (DCIS) of the breast is a proliferation of malignant epithelial cells within parenchymal structures of the breast, which is distinguished from invasive carcinoma by the absence of stromal invasion through the limiting basement membrane. Although the incidence of DCIS has apparently increased over the last 20 years, this is interpreted as a result of the enhanced detection through mammographic breast screening programmes rather than a true increase in frequency of the disease. However, despite the increased numbers of radiologically identified and surgically excised cases, less is understood about the biological and clinical aspects of DCIS than invasive breast cancer. Indeed, research into all aspects, including risk factors, genetics, biology, biomarkers, prognostic factors and the clinical management, of DCIS all lapse behind the significant translational knowledge gained into invasive breast cancer in the last decade.

Precursors of Invasive Breast Cancer

The presence of an epithelial proliferation within the breast parenchymal structures is associated with an increased risk of the subsequent development of invasive breast cancer. It is clear that for some intraductal epithelial proliferations, such as moderate or florid usual epithelial hyperplasia, this risk may only be marginally increased (less than 2×) over the general population level, whilst other, atypical, intraductal and intralobular lesions confer a more significant risk for the individual. For example, atypical ductal hyperplasia (ADH) confers a 4–5× increased risk [1]. This is greater if there is also a family history of breast carcinoma, when the relative risk can be approximately 10× that of the general population [1, 2].

S.E. Pinder (✉)
Professor of Breast Pathology, Research Oncology, Division of Cancer Studies,
King's College London, 3rd Floor, Bermondsey Wing, Guy's Hospital, Great Maze Pond,
SE1 9RT, London, UK
e-mail: sarah.pinder@kcl.ac.uk

R.C. Fitzgerald (ed.), *Pre-Invasive Disease: Pathogenesis and Clinical Management*,
DOI 10.1007/978-1-4419-6694-0_20,

ADH is an uncommon lesion, although it has long been recognised that it is seen with increased frequency as a result of microcalcification detected in mammographic breast screening programmes [3]. Its relevance in the context of a chapter on DCIS is that the condition was modeled on small cell DCIS of cribriform and micropapillary architecture. Thus histological features of low grade DCIS, including a uniform population of cells, smooth geometric spaces between cells or micropapillary formations with evenly placed cells and hyperchromatic nuclei were used to define the ADH lesion [1]. In essence, ADH is a small, microfocal lesion which shows some, but not all of the features of low grade DCIS, or all of the features in less than two complete duct spaces (or less than 2 mm in size [4]). Although immunohistochemical assays for oestrogen receptor [5] and basal type cytokeratins (e.g. Ck5 and Ck14 [6]) show homogeneous staining, inferring clonality, in an ADH or low grade DCIS lesion compared to heterogeneous expression in usual epithelial hyperplasia, there are no markers of value in distinguishing ADH from low grade DCIS. Similarly, studies showing loss of heterozygosity in low grade DCIS and ADH have, unsurprisingly, revealed similar genetic changes in the two processes, whilst the frequency of loss of heterozygosity in cases of usual hyperplasia is much lower [7]. More recently, DNA microarrays applied to microdissected tissue showed small numbers of genes ($n=61$) which were differentially expressed between ADH and DCIS and the expression differences were reproduced in an independent cohort of lesions by quantitative real-time PCR [8]. Whilst such findings are reassuring diagnostically they are not surprising, given that the diagnosis of ADH is based on its morphological (and immunohistochemical) equivalence to a small focus of low grade DCIS and to some extent are therefore a self-fulfilling prophecy. What is less explicable biologically, however, is the bilateral increased risk of developing invasive breast cancer seen following a diagnosis of ADH [9], compared to the unilateral risk of progression to invasive breast carcinoma of DCIS, see below.

DCIS, Precursor Risk

The outcome of DCIS treated by biopsy alone, and thus inference of the frequency and rate at which invasive carcinoma develops, remains debated; series of cases treated in this manner are generally small and are from the era when only large cell (high grade) comedo type of disease was recognised. The most widely quoted of the series (from the 1930s and 1940s) demonstrated a 50% rate of progression to invasive carcinoma after three years when DCIS was treated by biopsy alone [10]. Reviews of the natural history of lesions originally classified as benign and treated by biopsy alone [11, 12] often show lower frequencies of recurrence and progression to invasive carcinoma with approximately 20–30% of patients developing invasive cancer and doing so over a longer time, of

15–20 years. However, the invasive lesion occurs in the same area as the original lesion, indicating a true precursor process [11, 13]. Of note, these latter series were predominantly of morphologically different lesions to those of the early studies of high grade DCIS and comprised mostly small cell (low grade) DCIS that was missed on initial histological examination. As described below, there is convincing evidence that low grade and high grade DCIS have different genetic and biological profiles and it is not surprising if they have somewhat dissimilar clinical behaviour.

Apart from the limited availability of clinical evidence of the precursor risk of DCIS, there is support from the routine morphological assessment of the disease that DCIS progresses to invasive breast cancer. Cytonuclear grade of DCIS is most commonly the same as that of invasive disease when present synchronously; thus, in tumours composed of both invasive carcinoma and DCIS, there is a significant correlation between the grade of the DCIS and that of the invasive portion [14, 15]. Indeed, no progression in grade is seen between the in situ, invasive, locally recurrent and metastatic phases of a breast carcinoma [16], in keeping with the concept that there is, non-obligate, progression. Perhaps more robust evidence regarding the precursor nature of DCIS comes from comparative genomic hybridization series which confirm that, when DCIS and invasive carcinoma are synchronously present, there is a high degree of genetic homology between the in situ and invasive components [17, 18].

Presentation

The mode of clinical presentation of DCIS has changed considerably in the last 20 years or so. Prior to mammography, DCIS usually presented as a palpable mass or with nipple discharge, often bloodstained. However, all forms of DCIS have a propensity to undergo microcalcification, either within inspissated secretion or within comedo-type necrosis in the remaining luminal space of the duct. This allows detection of the disease as fine or coarse microcalcification, respectively, which can be seen radiologically. Prior to the widespread use of mammographic breast screening programmes, DCIS constituted 5% or less of cases of breast cancer but in the era of mammography, its frequency is typically 15–20% [19–21]. DCIS may also still present as a mass in the breast, or as Paget's disease of the nipple. This latter disease is clinically similar to eczema or non-specific dermatitis but is a manifestation of, typically high grade, DCIS when it involves subareolar ducts and extends, still within the confines of the duct and epidermal basement membrane, into the epidermis. Indeed, high grade DCIS is almost always identified in at least one subareolar duct in such cases, with careful scrutiny. A proportion of patients will also have developed associated invasive carcinoma derived from the DCIS; thus between 35 and 50% of patients are reported to have associated invasive adenocarcinoma in older series [22].

Biology (see also Chap. 5)

DCIS is a unicentric process and typically involves one duct system [23]. Unlike some other in situ cancers this disease does not appear to arise in an extensive area of "field change" involving all of one, or both, breasts. Indeed, stereoscopic examination showing a multifocal distribution is very uncommon; a gap of 40 mm or more between foci was seen in only one of 60 mastectomy specimens in the most thorough examination published [24]. In particular, although 8% of DCIS has apparent "gaps" of more than 10 mm between histologically identifiable foci within a duct system, this is most common in low grade disease, whilst high grade DCIS tends to have a continuous growth pattern.

This understanding of the unicentricity and distribution of DCIS has significant implications for therapeutic management; the optimum treatment of DCIS is surgical excision with clear margins [25], although the optimal width of uninvolved surrounding tissue is a matter of significant controversy [26]. Local "recurrence" of DCIS typically occurs at the site of previous excision and it is therefore better interpreted as residual disease, as demonstrated by studies showing concordance of genetic pattern with comparative genomic hybridization (CGH) in primary and recurrent lesions [27]. Particularly as approximately half of the recurrences after wide local excision for DCIS are as invasive disease [28], it is essential to adequate excise and treat the primary DCIS/precursor lesion.

However, DCIS is typically impalpable and invisible to the naked eye and thus poses problems in surgical excision by therapeutic breast conserving surgery and also laboratory assessment. The site of the radiological microcalcifications are "marked" by the insertion of one or more wires by the radiologist, generally under stereotactic or ultrasound guidance, to enable the surgeon to identify the area requiring therapeutic excision. Subsequent specimen radiography is then used intraoperatively to determine whether the radiological calcification has been removed with a rim of surrounding normal tissue. However, not all of a DCIS lesion is generally visible on X-ray; 85% of comedo/solid DCIS is seen mammographically but only 50% of the area of micropapillary/cribriform disease may be evident [29]. Radiology tends therefore to underestimate the size of DCIS, particularly low grade disease, with the associated risk that the apparently "normal" tissue surrounding the mammographic calcifications may still bear DCIS. This discrepancy is less than 20 mm in 80–85% of the cases if modern mammography, including magnification views, is used [23]. However, thorough pathological sampling of the lesion, including both the non-calcified areas close to the radiological abnormality and the margins of the surgical specimen, may result in the discovery of a greater extent of disease than suspected by X-ray. As a result further surgery to obtain complete excision of the process is more often required than for invasive breast cancer. Guidelines on pathology specimen handling and reporting, including methods for the estimation of DCIS size and margin width have been outlined in an excellent recent College of American Pathologists protocol document and will not be described in detail in this chapter [30].

Histological Features

DCIS is a markedly heterogeneous disease in almost all aspects, including histological appearance. As a result, a number of systems for categorisation have been described; historically DCIS was classified based on the architectural growth pattern into comedo, cribriform, micropapillary, solid or mixed types. This system provides some information regarding likely extent of disease; micropapillary DCIS is more often multiquadrant (71%) than comedo-type disease (8%) [31]. However, lesions are frequently (62%) of mixed architecture [32], and the reproducibility of this classification is poor. Other systems utilising nuclear grade alone, which is less often variable within a case (15.7%), or nuclear grade in combination with the presence of comedo-type necrosis, have therefore proven popular.

High nuclear grade DCIS (Fig. 20.1) is composed of large atypical pleomorphic epithelial cells that usually show a lack of polarisation. The nuclei of the disease are typically more than two and a half erythrocytes in size [30]. The nuclear chromatin is typically coarse. Large, often multiple, nucleoli are common. Frequent mitoses are seen and atypical forms may be identified. Architecturally the disease typically forms a solid growth pattern, although cribriform and micropapillary architecture may occur. Central comedo-type necrosis (often, at least focally, calcifying, due to the release of high levels of calcium from damaged cell membranes) is seen within a duct distended by the malignant cells. Periductal chronic inflammation and fibrosis may be present (Fig. 20.2).

At the other end of the spectrum, low nuclear grade DCIS is composed of evenly spaced cells with small, regular nuclei that are typically between one and a half to

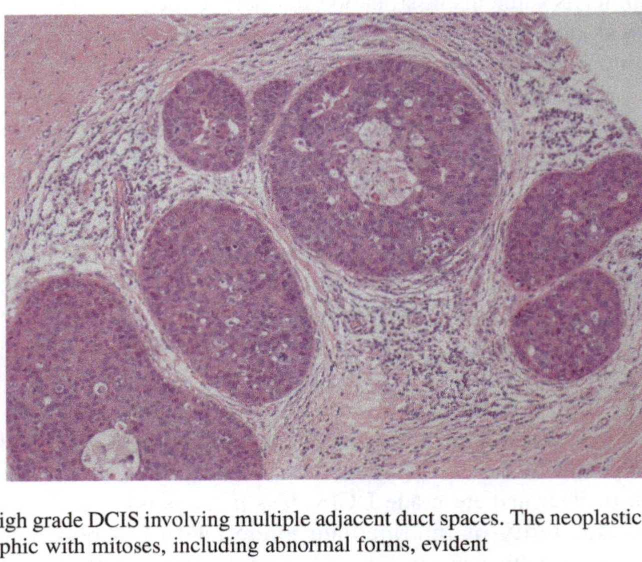

Fig. 20.1 High grade DCIS involving multiple adjacent duct spaces. The neoplastic cells are large and pleomorphic with mitoses, including abnormal forms, evident

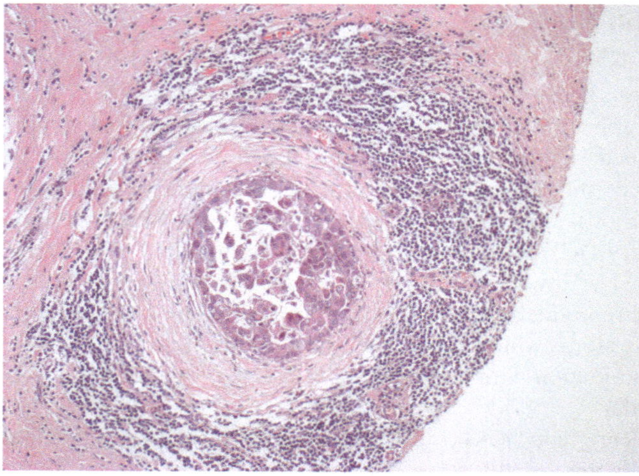

Fig. 20.2 High grade DCIS in a single duct space, with surrounding periductal fibrosis and chronic inflammatory infiltrate

two times the size of an erythrocyte [30]. Nucleoli, if present, are indistinct and the chromatin pattern is fine and evenly distributed in the nucleus. The malignant cells are typically polarized around the classical "punched-out" cribriform spaces or the intraluminal bulbous projections of the micropapillary architecture. These two growth patterns are commonly seen admixed in a single lesion. Indeed the architecture of a DCIS lesion is frequently of mixed type growth pattern, as noted above [32] which limits its value in classification for therapeutic purposes. A solid growth pattern of low grade DCIS is less frequently seen. Mitoses are infrequent and necrosis is uncommon. Unlike high grade DCIS, the small islands of laminated microcalcification present is seen in luminal secretions corresponding to the clusters of fine granular microcalcification present mammographically. Of interest, there is some suggestion that pure DCIS in males (i.e. in the absence of invasive breast cancer) is especially rare and is usually of low nuclear grade [33].

The nuclei in intermediate nuclear grade DCIS (Fig. 20.3) show less pleomorphism than in high-grade disease and lack the uniformity of the low-grade type. The nuclei are between 2 and 2.5 red blood cells in size [30]. Nucleoli may be present but usually are not large. Necrosis may be present, but is not extensive. There may be some cell polarization. The architectural pattern may be solid, cribriform, or micropapillary. Thus the diagnosis of intermediate grade DCIS is largely one of exclusion; the features are not those of high grade, or low grade, disease. Indeed this is highlighted by the document from the College of American Pathologists [30] which lists "intermediate" for all relevant features for the classification of intermediate grade DCIS. It is perhaps not surprising, therefore, that the reproducibility of intermediate grade DCIS has poor agreement in the UK National Health Service Breast Screening Programme External Quality

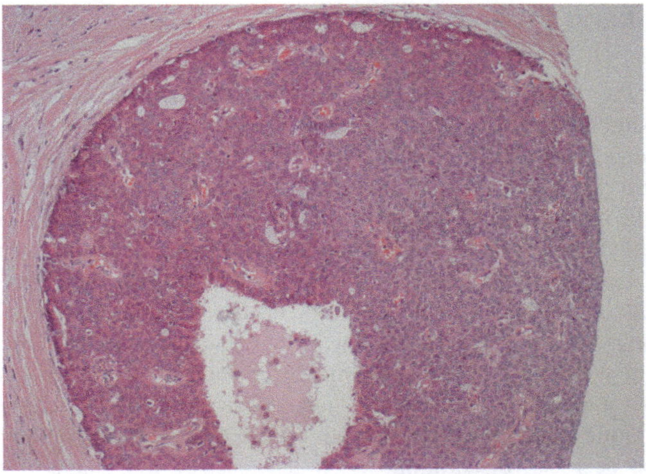

Fig. 20.3 Intermediate grade DCIS of solid papillary architecture (seen as fibrovascular cores bearing erythrocytes)

Assurance Scheme (kappa value = 0.23), although the agreement for classification as high grade DCIS is moderate (kappa = 0.51) [34]. Overall this system of classification by assessment of cytonuclear grade has clinical relevance and shows reasonable reproducibility [35]. Nevertheless, the reproducibility of grade of DCIS does not typically reach that of invasive breast cancer, which has more strictly defined criteria and cut-offs for each component; further research and application to developing and defining the grading system of DCIS is warranted.

Other systems for typing of DCIS have been proposed and are in use. In particular forms of categorisation based on a combination of nuclear grade and the presence of comedo-type necrosis have some support because of the good reproducibility of classification [36, 37]. Such categorisation, into high-grade, non-high-grade with necrosis, and non-high-grade without necrosis has, as with nuclear grade, been shown to be associated with local recurrence and disease-free survival [38].

In addition to classification according to the preferred system for grading of DCIS, rare morphological types can be seen either in pure form, or admixed with more typical variants, including apocrine, signet ring, neuroendocrine and cystic hypersecretory DCIS. The genetic alterations associated with these forms, and any clinical relevance of the different histology, are poorly understood; these forms are at present of greatest relevance in relation to the potential for difficulties or errors in histological diagnosis. Thus, whilst overtly malignant apocrine epithelial proliferations showing marked nuclear pleomorphism and comedo-type necrosis are easy to diagnose as high grade DCIS, lesions with lesser degrees of apocrine atypia can be difficult to categorise [39] and the clinical behaviour is even more difficult to predict than "classical" forms of the disease.

Treatment and Prognostic Factors

Historically the treatment for DCIS was mastectomy, which conferred a 98–99% cure rate. Although, breast-conserving surgery is associated with a higher rate of local recurrence than mastectomy it is now recognized to be appropriate for many DCIS lesions, dependent on the lesion extent, the patient's wishes and breast size. In essence the choice of surgical options is related to the likelihood of obtaining a good cosmetic result balanced with completely excising the lesion with surrounding normal tissue margin. It is now established that radiotherapy after wide local excision reduces the risk of local recurrence of disease by approximately half [40, 41]. However, in addition to radiotherapy, a number of prognostic markers of DCIS have been identified in randomized clinical trials and in other series [40, 42–46]. These factors include the width of the surrounding, uninvolved, margin of tissue, the nuclear grade and architectural growth pattern of the DCIS and the presence of comedo-type necrosis. In addition, larger lesion size, young age of patient and symptomatic detection have been recognised to be poor prognostic factors and to correlate with increased likelihood of local recurrence of disease. However, although there is clearly importance in developing these, and more sophisticated, markers to predict which patients with DCIS are at high risk of recurrence after conservative surgery and potentially a group who could avoid adjuvant radiotherapy, relatively little research has been undertaken into combinations of markers, or describing molecular or genetic signatures.

In addition to being a prognostic marker, the nuclear grade of DCIS in core biopsy specimens is also clinically relevant with regard to the likelihood of there being radiologically undetected invasion; if more than 40 flecks of calcification are seen on the mammogram and core biopsy demonstrates high grade DCIS, the risk of an invasive focus that has not been identified radiologically (as, for example, an associated mass lesion), approaches 50% [47]. For this reason assessing the nuclear grade of DCIS in pre-operative specimens may be valuable as such patients may benefit from a sentinel lymph nodes procedure at the time of primary breast surgery, rather than awaiting the discovery of invasive disease and requiring a second surgical procedure. However, in the vast majority of patients with localized DCIS, no axillary node surgery is required, or indeed recommended. Axillary nodal involvement is described in older symptomatic series of DCIS at frequencies of only around 1–2%, usually in association with extensive disease in which small foci of invasive carcinoma may be missed histologically, presumably due to the difficulties of extensively examining very large lesions.

Biomarkers in DCIS

As described above, it is clear that different histological forms of DCIS exist and that these have varying clinical and radiological presentation and morphological appearance which is reflected in differing likely clinical outcomes. That these different

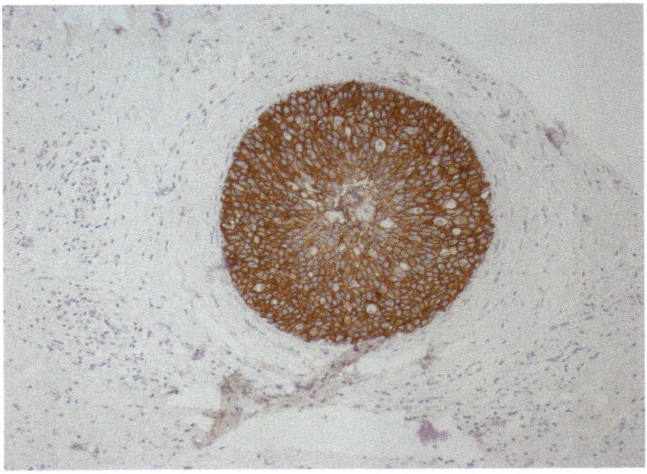

Fig. 20.4 HER2 positive high grade DCIS

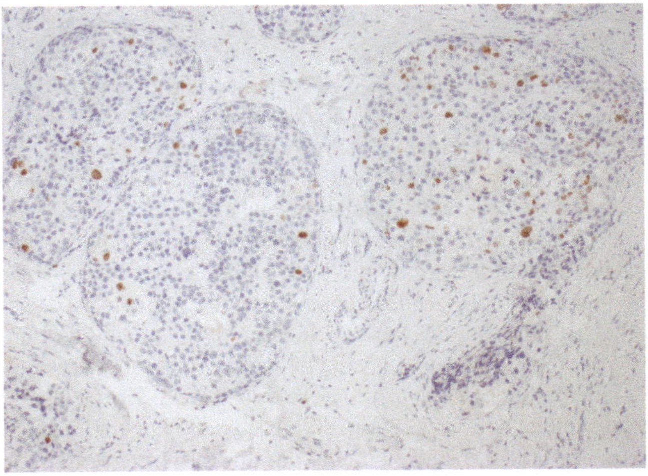

Fig. 20.5 Ki67 expression in high grade DCIS

morphological forms of DCIS reflect true biological variation, rather than histological mirage, is supported by the findings of a range of biomarkers. Thus, it has long been recognized that high grade DCIS is often positive for HER2 (Fig. 20.4) and p53 and to have an intermediate or high proliferation index (Fig. 20.5), whilst conversely it may be negative for oestrogen receptor, progesterone receptor and bcl-2 [48–50]. This is not invariably the case and high grade DCIS is often ER positive (see Fig. 20.6). Conversely, however, examples of low-grade DCIS are typically negative for HER2 and p53 and have a low proliferation rate, whilst being typically strongly positive for oestrogen receptor, as well as progesterone receptor and bcl-2. This is essentially similar to the patterns of these markers and histological grade in invasive breast carcinoma.

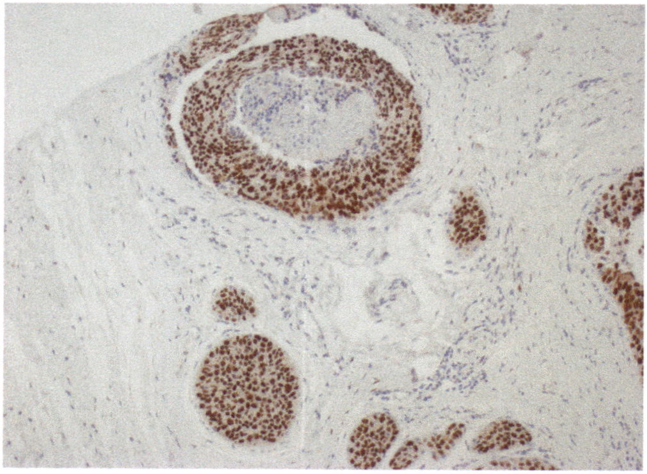

Fig. 20.6 High grade DCIS showing extensive (approaching 100%) nuclear positivity with oestrogen receptor

Numerous series have reported on the frequency and pattern of expression of a range of markers in, albeit often small numbers of, cases of DCIS. However, assessment of the literature regarding the clinical significance of such differences in marker expression is hampered by the use of different antibodies, methodologies and cut-offs, as is often the case with immunohistochemical series of invasive cancers from any organ. The nature of the cases included also makes interpretation difficult; some authors have examined series of pure DCIS whilst others have compared expression of matched DCIS with associated synchronous invasive carcinoma. In particular, although some studies have included only patients with pure DCIS, the size of the disease, the margins of excision of surrounding uninvolved tissue and the cytonuclear grade frequencies (i.e. other known prognostic factors) have varied enormously, subsequent adjuvant treatment (e.g. radiotherapy or hormone therapy or none) has varied within the study population, and differing lengths of follow-up information have been available, significantly confounding the results.

Nevertheless, such histological and cytogenetic studies as there are, largely support the concept that morphological forms of DCIS express different markers and suggest that there are different routes by which low grade and high grade invasive carcinomas evolve from this precursor lesion. Indeed, genetic studies suggest that low and high grade DCIS have different alterations, in keeping with the concept that this is a group of pre-invasive processes, rather than a single disease [51]. Thus most authorities support the view that it is not the case that low grade DCIS progresses to high grade DCIS and that lesion subsequently develops into invasive breast carcinoma. Rather, low grade DCIS generally progresses to grade 1 invasive cancer [52] and high grade DCIS to grade 2 and grade 3 invasive lesions. Whilst it has been reported that a mixture of grades and of biomarker expression may frequently be seen within an individual case of DCIS [53], this is not widely recorded. Indeed reconciliation of this suggestion with more established data indicating genetic homology between DCIS and invasive carcinoma [54, 55] is problematic.

DCIS appears to bear most of the molecular and genetic changes that characterize invasive breast cancer [56–62]. Partly for this reason, the search has turned to examination of potential genomic differences between DCIS and invasive carcinoma which may provide a clue to genes involved in the invasive transition (rather than genes associated with the malignant phenotype). More recent studies have examined the gene expression patterns of cells from pure DCIS, DCIS matched with co-existing invasive carcinoma and invasive carcinoma. As might be predicted, the cells from the pure DCIS have been reported to exhibit the most divergent molecular profile whilst those from the in situ component of lesions with co-existing invasive carcinoma were very similar to cells from invasive lesions [63]. However, some groups have identified potential genes of interest; Castro et al [63], for example, found 147 genes differentially expressed between pure DCIS and the in situ component of lesions with co-existing invasion, and which, they suggested, could discriminate samples representative of the in situ component of lesions present in association with invasive carcinoma from 60% of pure DCIS samples. Among these genes, LOX and SULF-1 were potential participants. As is frequently the case with series of DCIS, such data is intriguing, but is based on small numbers of a heterogeneous and complex entity; in the series of Castro et el [63] only five cases of pure DCIS were assessed, three were of high grade and one of mixed intermediate and high grade whilst the cytonuclear grade of one was not determined.

Advances in invasive breast cancer genomics have shown that at least four major categories of invasive breast cancer can be identified by gene expression profiling, and that these are associated with different clinical outcome [64, 65]. The categorisation of invasive breast cancer into groups according to histological tumour type and grade is straightforward and routinely performed, but additional information can be obtained by assessment of the gene profile with carcinomas typically grouped into: luminal A, luminal B, HER2 and basal-like invasive breast carcinomas. Such molecular sub-typing is now widely accepted. The prevalence of these gene expression groups in DCIS is clearly more difficult to assess, in particular because access to frozen tissue is more difficult to obtain and fewer cells are present when such material is available. Researchers have therefore resorted to comparing immunohistochemical profiles, which are recognized to be roughly equivalent to the genomic types in invasive carcinoma [66] but now also in assessing DCIS. For example, Tamini et al found that the prevalence of the "molecular phenotypes" differed significantly between DCIS ($n=272$) and invasive breast cancers ($n=2,249$) when immunohistochemical profiles from tissue microarray sections were examined [67]. These authors found that the luminal A immunophenotype was significantly more frequent among invasive cancers (73.4%) than among DCIS (62.5%), whilst the luminal B and HER2 immunophenotypes were both more frequently seen in DCIS (13.2 and 13.6%) compared to invasive lesions (5.2 and 5.7%). Interestingly, the basal-like phenotype was (non-significantly) more frequent among the invasive cancers (10.9%) than in DCIS (7.7%). As described above, these authors confirmed that high grade DCIS was more likely to be HER2 positive, but also to be basal-like, than low or intermediate grade lesions. The question of why the frequency of the phenotype groups differs between DCIS and invasive carcinoma requires further investigation, but it is likely that the low grade invasive pathway is contributed to by other precursors, such as lobular in situ neoplasia and flat epithelial atypia.

Such immunohistochemical profiling is far simpler and less expensive to undertake that gene profiling, particularly in cases of DCIS, and confirms that the molecular immunophenotypes described in invasive breast cancer are also seen among cases of DCIS. As with immunohistochemical assessment of series of invasive breast carcinoma, the reported frequency of the types varies, according to the criteria and definitions of the "profile" required (as well almost certainly as the nature of the cases recruited). For example, although Livasy et al [68] found that 8% of cases were "basal-like", defined as ER negative, HER2 negative, EGFR positive (Fig. 20.7) and/or cytokeratin 5/6 positive and Bryan et al [69] similarly reported that 8% of cases were "triple negative" (ER negative, PR negative and HER2 negative), the latter authors also noted that 32% showed expression of any basal marker (CK5/6, Ck14 or Ck17). Thus, although examination of panels of immunohistochemical markers has a significant attraction for categorisation of groups of DCIS, the absence of any consensus regarding the antibodies to be examined, the methodology and assessment has proven disappointing to date in the classification of both DCIS and of invasive breast cancer.

In conclusion, DCIS is a complex and heterogeneous lesion. Translational research into pre-invasive breast disease is hampered by limited funding [70], but especially by availability of sufficient numbers and quantity of high quality tissue samples, particularly fresh material, from patients with adequate length of follow-up

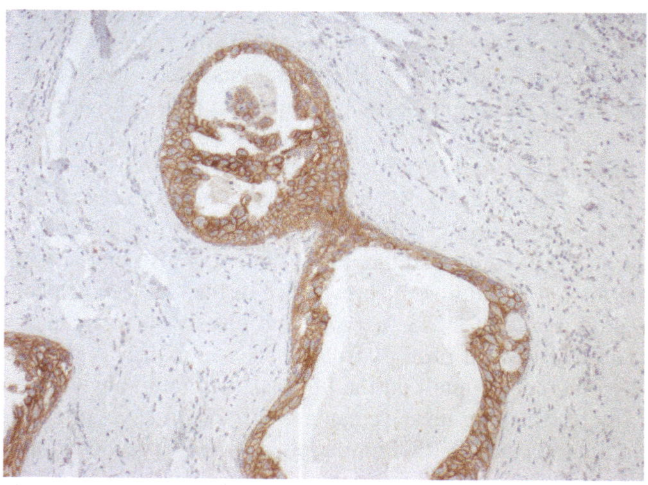

Fig. 20.7 EGFR expression in high grade DCIS; both membrane and cytoplasmic reactivity is seen in all neoplastic cells

for meaningful comparison of outcome. As described in the Breast Cancer Campaign analysis of gaps in current knowledge in breast cancer research [70], there remains a substantial challenge to understand the causative factors underlying progression of DCIS to invasive breast cancer and factors related to recurrence, a lack of biomarkers for selection of therapies (e.g. endocrine treatment and/or radiotherapy) and for recognition of targets to potentially subvert progression into invasive breast cancer.

References

1. Page DL, Dupont WD, Rogers LW, Rados MS (1985) Atypical hyperplastic lesions of the female breast. A long-term follow-up study. Cancer 55:2698–2708, which is greater in pre-menopausal women (approaching a sixfold risk)
2. London SJ, Connolly JL, Schnitt SJ, Colditz GA (1992) A prospective study of benign breast disease and the risk of breast cancer. JAMA 267:941–944
3. Stomper PC, Cholewinski SP, Penetrante RB, Harlos JP, Tsangaris TN (1993) Atypical hyperplasia: frequency and mammographic and pathologic relationships in excisional biopsies guided with mammography and clinical examination. Radiology 189:667–671
4. Tavassoli FA, Norris HJ (1990) A comparison of the results of long-term follow-up for atypical intraductal hyperplasia and intra-ductal hyperplasia of the breast. Cancer 65:518–529
5. Gillett CE, Lee AHS, Millis RR, Barnes DM (1998) Cyclin D1 and associated proteins in mammary ductal carcinoma in situ and atypical ductal hyperplasia. J Pathol 184: 396–400
6. Otterbach F, Bànkfalvi A, Bergner S, Decker T, Krech R, Boecker W (2000) Cytokeratin 5/6 immunohistochemistry assists the differential diagnosis of atypical proliferations of the breast. Histopathology 37:232–240
7. Lakhani SR, Collins N, Stratton MR, Sloane JP (1995) Atypical ductal hyperplasia of the breast: clonal proliferation with loss of heterozygosity on chromosomes 16q and 17p. J Clin Pathol 48:611–615
8. Emery LA, Tripathi A, King C (2009) Early dysregulation of cell adhesion and extracellular matrix pathways in breast cancer progression. Am J Pathol 175:1292–1302
9. Dupont WD, Page DL (1985) Risk factors for breast cancer in women with proliferative breast disease. N Engl J Med 312:146–151
10. Geschickter CF, Lewis D (1938) Comedo carcinomas of the breast. Arch Surg 33:225–244
11. Page DL, Dupont WD, Rogers LW, Landenberger M (1982) Intraductal carcinoma of the breast: Follow up after biopsy alone. Cancer 49:751–758
12. Rosen PP, Braun DW Jr, Kinne DW (1980) The clinical significance of preinvasive breast carcinoma. Cancer 46:919–925
13. Betsill WLJ, Rosen PP, Lieberman PH, Robbins GF (1978) Intraductal carcinoma. Long-term follow-up after treatment by biopsy alone. JAMA 239:1863–1867
14. Lampejo OT, Barnes DM, Smith P, Millis RR (1994) Evaluation of infiltrating ductal carcinomas with a DCIS component: correlation of the histologic type of the in situ component with grade of the infiltrating component. Semin Diagn Pathol 11:215–222
15. Gupta SK, Douglas-Jones AG, Fenn N, Morgan JM, Mansel RE (1997) The clinical behavior of breast carcinoma is probably determined at the preinvasive stage (ductal carcinoma in situ). Cancer 80:1740–1745
16. Millis RR, Barnes DM, Lampejo OT, Egan MK, Smith P (1998) Tumour grade does not change between primary and recurrent mammary carcinoma. Eur J Cancer 34:548–553

17. Buerger H, Otterbach F, Simon R et al (1999) Different genetic pathways in the evolution of invasive breast cancer are associated with distinct morphological subtypes. J Pathol 189: 521–526
18. Boecker W, Buerger H, Schmitz K et al (2001) Ductal epithelial proliferations of the breast: a biological continuum? Comparative genomic hybridization and high-molecular-weight cytokeratin expression patterns. J Pathol 195:415–421
19. Andersson I, Aspegren K, Janzon L et al (1988) Mammographic screening and mortality from breast cancer: the Malmo mammographic screening trial. Br Med J 297:943–948
20. Anderson TJ, Lamb J, Donnan P et al (1991) Comparative pathology of breast cancer in a randomised trial of screening. Br J Cancer 64:108–113
21. Gibbs NM (1985) Comparative study of the histopathology of breast cancer in a screened and unscreened population investigated by mammography. Histopathology 9:1307–1318
22. Haagensen CD (1986) Diseases of the breast. WB Saunders, Philadelphia
23. Holland R, Hendriks JH, Vebeek AL, Mravunac M, Schuurmans Stekhoven JH (1990) Extent, distribution, and mammographic/histological correlations of breast ductal carcinoma in situ. Lancet 335:519–522
24. Faverly DR, Burgers L, Bult P, Holland R (1994) Three dimensional imaging of mammary ductal carcinoma in situ: clinical implications. Semin Diagn Pathol 11:193–198
25. Meijnen P, Gilhuijs KG, Rutgers EJ (2008) The effect of margins on the clinical management of ductal carcinoma in situ of the breast. J Surg Oncol 98:579–584
26. MacDonald HR, Silverstein MJ, Mabry H et al (2005) Local control in ductal carcinoma in situ treated by excision alone: incremental benefit of larger margins. Am J Surg 190: 521–525
27. Waldman FM, DeVries S, Chew KL, Moore DH 2nd, Kerlikowske K, Ljung BM (2000) Chromosomal alterations in ductal carcinomas in situ and their in situ recurrences. J Natl Cancer Inst 92:313–320
28. Sakorafas GH, Farley DR (2003) Optimal management of ductal carcinoma in situ of the breast. Surg Oncol 12:221–240
29. Holland R, Hendriks JH (1994) Microcalcifications associated with ductal carcinoma in situ: mammographic-pathologic correlation. Semin Diagn Pathol 11:181–192
30. Lester SC, Bose S, Chen Y-Y et al (2009) Protocol for the examination of specimens from patients with ductal carcinoma in situ of the breast. Arch Pathol Lab Med 133:15–25
31. Bellamy CO, McDonald C, Salter DM, Chetty U, Anderson TJ (1993) Noninvasive ductal carcinoma of the breast: the relevance of histologic categorization. Hum Pathol 24:16–23
32. Quinn CM, Ostrowski JL (1997) Cytological and architectural heterogeneity in ductal carcinoma in situ of the breast. J Clin Pathol 50:596–599
33. Hittmair A, Lininger RA, Tavassoli FA (1998) Ductal carcinoma in situ (DCIS) in the male breast. Cancer 83:2139–2149
34. Ellis IO, Coleman D, Wells C et al (2006) Impact of a National External Quality Assurance Scheme for breast pathology in the United Kingdom. J Clin Pathol 59:138–145
35. Badve S, A'Hern RP, Ward AM et al (1998) Prediction of local recurrence of ductal carcinoma in situ of the breast using five histological classifications: A comparative study with long follow-up. Hum Pathol 29:915–923
36. Silverstein MJ, Poller DN, Waisman JR et al (1995) Prognostic classification of breast ductal carcinoma-in-situ. Lancet 345:1154–1157
37. Poller DN, Silverstein MJ, Galea M et al (1994) Ductal carcinoma in situ of the breast. A proposal for a new simplified histological classification. Association between cellular proliferation and c-erbB-2 protein expression. Mod Pathol 7:257–262
38. Silverstein MJ, Lagios MD, Craig PH et al (1996) A prognostic index for ductal carcinoma in situ of the breast. Cancer 77:2267–2274
39. O'Malley FP, Bane A (2008) An update on apocrine lesions of the breast. Histopathology 52:3–10
40. EORTC Breast Cancer Cooperative Group; EORTC Radiotherapy Group, Bijker N, Meijnen P, Peterse JL et al. (2006) Breast-conserving treatment with or without radiotherapy in ductal carcinoma-in-situ: ten-year results of European Organisation for Research and Treatment of

Cancer randomized phase III trial 10853 – a study by the EORTC Breast Cancer Cooperative Group and EORTC Radiotherapy Group. J Clin Oncol 24:3381–3387.

41. UK Coordinating Committee on Cancer Research Ductal Carcinoma In Situ Working Party (2003) Radiotherapy and tamoxifen in women with completely excised ductal carcinoma in situ of the breast in the UK, Australia, and New Zealand: randomised controlled trial. Lancet 362:95–102
42. Di Saverio S, Catena F, Santini D et al (2008) 259 Patients with DCIS of the breast applying USC/Van Nuys prognostic index: a retrospective review with long term follow up. Breast Cancer Res Treat 109:405–416
43. Vargas C, Kestin L, Go N et al (2005) Factors associated with local recurrence and cause-specific survival in patients with ductal carcinoma in situ of the breast treated with breast-conserving therapy or mastectomy. Int J Radiat Oncol Biol Phys 63:1514–1521
44. Ringberg A, Nordgren H, Thorstensson S et al (2007) Histopathological risk factors for ipsilateral breast events after breast conserving treatment for ductal carcinoma in situ of the breast – results from the Swedish randomised trial. Eur J Cancer 43:291–298
45. Fisher ER, Dignam J, Tan-Chiu E et al (1999) Pathologic findings from the National Surgical Adjuvant Breast Project (NSABP) eight-year update of Protocol B-17: intraductal carcinoma. Cancer 86:429–438
46. Sahoo S, Recant WM, Jaskowiak N, Tong L, Heimann R (2005) Defining negative margins in DCIS patients treated with breast conservation therapy: The University of Chicago experience. Breast J 11:242–247
47. Bagnall MJ, Evans AJ, Wilson AR et al (2001) Predicting invasion in mammographically detected microcalcification. Clin Radiol 56:828–832
48. Bobrow LG, Happerfield LC, Gregory WM et al (1994) The classification of ductal carcinoma in situ and its association with biological markers. Semin Diagn Pathol 11:199–207
49. Poller DN, Roberts EC, Bell JA et al (1993) p53 protein expression in mammary ductal carcinoma in situ: relationship to immunohistochemical expression of estrogen receptor and c-erbB-2 protein. Hum Pathol 24:463–468
50. Poller DN, Snead DR, Roberts EC et al (1993) Oestrogen receptor expression in ductal carcinoma in situ of the breast: relationship to flow cytometric analysis of DNA and expression of the c-erbB-2 oncoprotein. Br J Cancer 68:156–161
51. Roylance R, Gorman P, Hanby A, Tomlinson I (2002) Allelic imbalance analysis of chromosome 16q shows that grade I and grade III invasive ductal breast cancers follow different genetic pathways. J Pathol 196:32–36
52. Abdel-Fatah TM, Powe DG, Hodi Z, Reis-Filho JS, Lee AH, Ellis IO (2008) Morphologic and molecular evolutionary pathways of low nuclear grade invasive breast cancers and their putative precursor lesions: further evidence to support the concept of low nuclear grade breast neoplasia family. Am J Surg Pathol 32:513–523
53. Allred DC, Wu Y, Mao S et al (2008) Ductal carcinoma in situ and the emergence of diversity during breast cancer evolution. Clin Cancer Res 14:370–378
54. Buerger H, Otterbach F, Simon R et al (1999) Different genetic pathways in the evolution of invasive breast cancer are associated with distinct morphological subtypes. J Pathol 189:521–526
55. Boecker W, Buerger H, Schmitz K et al (2001) Ductal epithelial proliferations of the breast: a biological continuum? Comparative genomic hybridization and high-molecular-weight cytokeratin expression patterns. J Pathol 195:415–421
56. Vincent-Salomon A, Lucchesi C, Gruel N et al (2008) Integrated genomic and transcriptomic analysis of ductal carcinoma in situ of the breast. Clin Cancer Res 14:1956–1965
57. Bijker N, Peterse JL, Duchateau L et al (2001) Histological type and marker expression of the primary tumour compared with its local recurrence after breast-conserving therapy for ductal carcinoma in situ. Br J Cancer 84:539–544
58. Meeker AK, Hicks JL, Gabrielson E et al (2004) Telomere shortening occurs in subsets of normal breast epithelium as well as in situ and invasive carcinoma. Am J Pathol 164: 925–935
59. Mommers EC, Leonhart AM, Falix F et al (2001) Similarity in expression of cell cycle proteins between in situ and invasive ductal breast lesions of same differentiation grade. J Pathol 194:327–333

60. Ottesen GL (2003) Carcinoma in situ of the female breast. A clinico-pathological, immunohistological, and DNA ploidy study. APMIS 108:1–67
61. Shackney SE, Silverman JF (2003) Molecular evolutionary patterns in breast cancer. Adv Anat Pathol 10:278–290
62. Cornfield DB, Palazzo JP, Schwartz GF et al (2004) The prognostic significance of multiple morphologic features and biologic markers in ductal carcinoma in situ of the breast: a study of a large cohort of patients treated with surgery alone. Cancer 100:2317–2327
63. Castro NP, Osório CABT, Torres C et al (2008) Evidence that molecular changes in cells occur before morphological alterations during the progression of breast ductal carcinoma. Breast Cancer Res 10:R87
64. Perou CM, Sorlie T, Eisen MB et al (2000) Molecular portraits of human breast tumours. Nature 406:747–752
65. Sorlie T, Perou CM, Tibshirani R et al (2001) Gene expression patterns of breast carcinomas distinguish tumor subclasses with clinical implications. Proc Natl Acad Sci U S A 98:10869–10874
66. Abd El-Rehim DM, Ball G, Pinder SE et al (2005) High-throughput protein expression analysis using tissue microarray technology of a large well-characterised series identifies biologically distinct classes of breast cancer confirming recent cDNA expression analyses. Int J Cancer 116:340–350
67. Tamimi RM, Baer HJ, Marotti J et al (2008) Comparison of molecular phenotypes of ductal carcinoma in situ and invasive breast cancer. Breast Cancer Res 10:R67
68. Livasy CA, Perou CM, Karaca G et al (2007) Identification of a basal-like subtype of breast ductal carcinoma in situ. Hum Pathol 38:197–204
69. Bryan BB, Schnitt SJ, Collins LC (2006) Ductal carcinoma in situ with basal-like phenotype: a possible precursor to invasive basal-like breast cancer. Mod Pathol 19:617–621
70. Thompson A, Brennan K, Cox A et al (2008) Evaluation of the current knowledge limitations in breast cancer research: a gap analysis. Breast Cancer Res 10:R26

Chapter 21
Molecular Pathogenesis, Detection and Clinical Management of Pre-invasive Cervical Lesions

Wen-Chung Chen, Barbara Ma, Chih-Ping Mao, and T-C Wu

Abstract The major public health burden of cervical cancer and its associated lesions warrants the development of effective preventive measures and successful therapies. Cervical cancer is the second most common female cancer worldwide, with approximately 493,000 diagnoses and 270,000 deaths annually. The disease can be detected early by cervical cytology in the pre-malignant phase, in the form of high-grade squamous intraepithelial lesions, and treated by a variety of methods including loop electrosurgical excision procedure. As human papillomavirus (HPV) has been identified as the major causative agent of cervical dysplasia and cervical cancer, HPV DNA testing and genotyping are also valuable in enhancing the sensitivity and specificity of cervical cancer screening. Advances in the understanding of HPV pathogenesis have led to the concept that persistent infection with high-risk HPV (hrHPV) genotypes is recognized as a necessary though not sufficient step in causing cervical cancer. This has led to the identification of tumor-promoting markers that may be required in cervical carcinogenesis. Further investigation of these markers may potentially be useful for risk stratification in screening. The knowledge of HPV virology and its role in cervical carcinogenesis leads to the potential prevention and treatment of cervical cancer. The current status of HPV vaccines is also discussed.

T.-C. Wu (✉)
Department of Pathology, The Johns Hopkins Medical Institutions, Cancer Research Building II, Rm 309, 1550 Orleans Street, Baltimore, MD, USA
and
Department of Obstetrics and Gynecology, The Johns Hopkins Medical Institutions, Baltimore, MD, USA
and
Department of Molecular Microbiology and Immunology, The Johns Hopkins Medical Institutions, Orleans Street, Baltimore, MD, USA
and
Department of oncology, The Johns Hopkins Medical Institutions, Baltimore, MD, USA
e-mail: wutc@jhmi.edu

R.C. Fitzgerald (ed.), *Pre-Invasive Disease: Pathogenesis and Clinical Management*, DOI 10.1007/978-1-4419-6694-0_21,

Introduction

Cervical cancer is the second most common cancer in women worldwide, with approximately 493,000 women diagnosed and 270,000 deaths annually [1]. The incidence of cervical cancer among countries is greatly influenced by the effectiveness of population-based screening programs. In developed countries such as the United States, the incidence and mortality rate of invasive cervical cancer has declined over the past decades as a result of the introduction of effective cytology screening programs [1]. The majority of cervical cancer cases (>80%) come from developing countries, where medical facilities are limited.

Premalignant Cervical Lesions

Cervical cancer arises from premalignant cervical lesions. The premalignant cervical lesions are classified according to their histopathologic features, clinical behavior and the current concepts regarding its pathogenesis. In 1932, carcinoma in situ was believed to be the precursor of invasive cervical cancer [2]. Carcinoma in situ is characterized by the replacement of the entire thickness of normal epithelium with markedly dysplastic cells, but an intact basement membrane and was considered to have progressed to cancer following the invasion of tumor cells into and beyond the basement membrane. Later on, other types of noninvasive cervical lesions were recognized. These lesions had epithelial abnormalities that were cytologically and histologically less severe than carcinoma in situ. They were classified as mild, moderate and severe dysplasia. In 1969, Dr. Ralph M. Richart hypothesized that cervical cancer developed in a linear, multi-step progression from non-invasive stages and that all types of precursor lesions represented a disease process [3]. On the basis of this concept, Dr. Richart introduced the terminology of cervical intraepithelial neoplasia (CIN) [4].

The CIN terminology divided cervical cancer precursors into three stages (Fig. 21.1). CIN 1 is the stage where undifferentiated, basaloid cells occupy the lower third of the epithelium, corresponding to mild dysplasia. CIN 2 is the stage where undifferentiated, basaloid cells occupy the lower third to two-thirds of the epithelium, corresponding to moderate dysplasia. CIN 3 describes the stage where undifferentiated, basaloid cells occupy two-thirds to the entire thickness of the epithelium, corresponding to severe dysplasia and carcinoma in situ; CIN 3 includes both severe dysplasia and carcinoma in situ because pathologists cannot usually distinguish these two consistently [5]. It was believed that CIN lesions of all grades were precursors and that all, even CIN 1 lesions in very unusual situations, had the potential to progress to invasive cancer if untreated.

However, advances in the understanding of cervical cancer pathogenesis has now found that the spectrum of histopathologic changes referred to as CIN does not represent a single disease process at different stages but instead two distinct entities: (1) productive HPV infection and (2) a true neoplastic process (cancerous precursors) [5]. In the majority of patients, productive HPV infections are self-limiting and

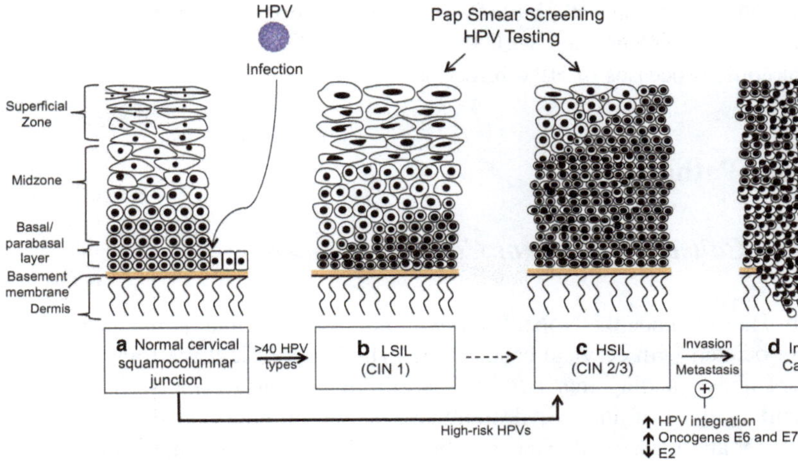

Fig. 21.1 Cervical squamous intraepithelial lesions (SILs) and HPV-associated pathogenesis. The two distinct pathways of HPV-associated pathogenesis: productive viral infection (**b**) and cancerous precursors (**c**, **d**) are shown above as bolded arrows, accompanied by corresponding histopathologic lesions. (**a**) The normal cervical squamocolumnar junction. The layer of basal cells rests on the basement membrane, which is the normal barrier of epithelium and its underlying stromal tissue. The parabasal cells form layers of one to two cells thick just above the basal cell layer. Normal squamous epithelium differentiates as shown, with decreasing nuclear/cytoplasmic ratio toward the surface. The squamocolumnar junction is the most common site for the development of cervical cancer. (**b**) Low-grade squamous intraepithelial lesions. Productive HPV infections produce low-grade squamous intraepithelial lesions (LSILs), which are also known as cervical intraepithelial neoplasia (CIN) 1, in which the basaloid cells occupy the lower third of the epithelium. (**c**) High-grade squamous intraepithelial lesions. Cancerous precursor pathway is usually initiated by a significant fraction of high-risk HPV infections (hrHPV) and produce high-grade squamous intraepithelial lesions (HSILs) also known as CIN 2/3. HSILs show less cellular differentiation and the basaloid cells occupy the lower one-third to full-thickness of the epithelium. Pap smear and HPV tests can be used to detect SILs. (**d**) Invasive cancer. If untreated, premalignant lesions can progress into microinvasive or invasive cancer, in which tumor cells break the basement membrane. The process is associated with integration of the HPV genome into the host chromosomes, loss of *E2* and upregulation of viral oncogene expression and genomic instability (modified from [16])

result in CIN 1 in the form of flat or exophytic lesions (condylomata acuminata). The flat lesions can be caused by any of the more than 40 different HPV types that infect the human anogenital tract [6–9]. In contrast, for true neoplastic processes, it is well recognized that invasive squamous cell carcinomas and adenocarcinomas of the cervix and their premalignant lesions are highly associated with high-risk HPV (hrHPV), including HPV-16, 18, 31, 45 and 56 [6–10].

To better reflect the biologic processes underlying these precancerous cervical lesions, the terminology was changed to the Bethesda System for reporting results of cervical cytology and histology [11]. This two-tiered classification system uses "low-grade squamous intraepithelial lesion" (LSIL) for lesions previously named as CIN 1 and "high-grade squamous intraepithelial lesion" (HSIL) for lesions previously classified as CIN 2 and CIN 3 [11, 12]. This terminology reflects our current knowledge of the pathobiology of HPV infection. Figure 21.1 shows the correlation of this terminology with the old terminology and the corresponding distinct biologic processes of HPV infection.

Molecular Pathogenesis

HPV As a Causative Agent of Cervical Cancer

Harald zur Hausen made the Nobel Prize-winning discovery that human papillomavirus is associated with cervical cancer [13, 14]. His work laid the foundation for our current understanding that HPV is the etiologic agent of almost all cervical cancers and a subset of anogenital malignancies and oropharyngeal cancers [15], accounting for about 5% of all cancer cases worldwide [1]. More than 100 different HPV genotypes have been identified and can be classified into low- or high-risk by their inclination to cause cervical cancer. Low-risk (lr) HPV types, typified by types 6 and 11, produce benign genital warts. High-risk (hr) types, most notably types 16 and 18, are associated with cervical cancers. Although HPV-16 accounts for about 50% of all cervical cancers, and HPV-18 an additional 15–20%, there are at least 15 known oncogenic HPV types [16]. Molecular studies have also revealed the deregulated expression of viral oncogenes, HPV E6 and E7, as necessary factors for the malignant phenotype of cervical cancer cells.

Molecular Biology of HPV

HPV are epithelial-tropic, non-enveloped DNA viruses with a double-stranded genome of around 8,000 base pairs. The HPV genome consists of at least six early genes (E1, E2, E4, E5, E6, E7), two late genes (L1, L2) and a non-coding long control region. The early genes encode protein that are expressed before the onset of viral DNA replication and then regulate viral DNA replication. The two late genes, L1 and L2, encode two structural proteins comprising the major and minor viral capsid proteins, respectively. The non-coding region contains regulatory elements. Three of the early genes (E5, E6 and E7) mediate the transformation process of HPV. E4 facilitates cytoskeletal reorganization. E1 and E2 are two regulatory proteins, which regulate replication and transcription. Importantly, E2 is the transcriptional repressor of E6 and E7 [17].

HPV-Associated Pathogenesis

While infection with hrHPV is necessary for the progression of cervical cancer, it is not sufficient. Most hrHPV infections are subclinical, with only a minority of hrHPV infections producing squamous intraepithelial lesions (SILs) [18], and a small fraction of SILs leading to cervical cancers. It has been shown that most HPV infections and HPV-related intraepithelial lesions are cleared, probably by immune mechanisms [19, 20]. While these immune mechanisms are not clearly understood, a more comprehensive picture of viral carcinogenesis has emerged from many studies. It may be possible to differentiate between benign lesions that do not progress to cervical cancer and precursor lesions that may progress to cervical cancer as the onset of cancer depends predominantly on the deregulation of viral gene expression of E6 and E7 oncoproteins. Therefore, as previously mentioned, the currently accepted model for HPV-associated pathogenesis can be classified into two distinct

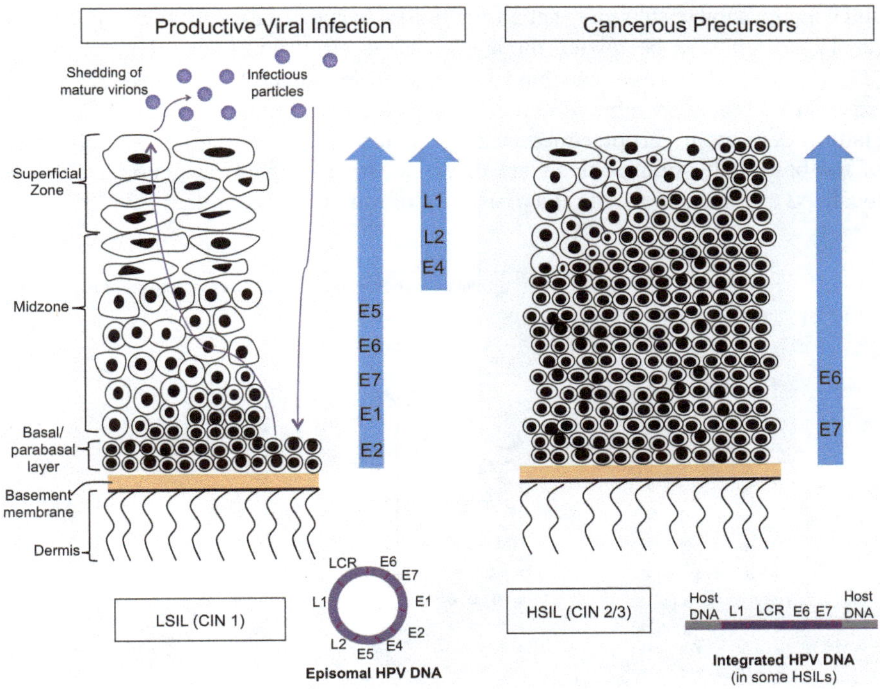

Fig. 21.2 Two pathways of HPV-associated pathogenesis. Basal cells in the cervical epithelium rest on the basement membrane, which is supported by the dermis. Human papillomavirus (HPV) is thought to access the basal cells through micro-abrasions in the cervical epithelium. In productive viral infection, the early HPV genes E1, E2, E4, E5, E6 and E7 are expressed and the viral DNA replicates from episomal DNA. In the upper layers of epithelium (the midzone and superficial zone) the viral genome is replicated further, and the late genes L1 and L2, and E4 are expressed. L1 and L2 encapsidate the viral genomes to form progeny virions in the nucleus. The shed virus can then initiate a new infection. Low-grade intraepithelial lesions support productive viral replication. There may be episomal DNA or integrated DNA in high-grade cervical intraepithelial neoplasia (cancerous precursors). Integration of the HPV genome into the host chromosomes is associated with loss or disruption of E2, and subsequent upregulation of E6 and E7 oncogene expression. LCR, long control region

pathways: (1) productive viral infection (associated with LSILs and rarely progress to neoplasia) or (2) cancerous precursors (associated with HSILs) (Fig. 21.2).

Productive Viral Infection

Papillomavirus infection requires infection of the basal cells, which are the only cells in the squamous epithelium able to undergo long-term cell division. It is believed that microtrauma to the cervical epithelium of the transformation zone is required to provide access of the virus to the basal cells. Virions bind first to the basement membrane at sites of trauma, undergo a conformational change in which L2 minor capsid protein is cleaved by a proprotein convertase (PC), furin, or PC5/6, and undergo another subsequent conformational change that exposes L2 neutralization (aa 17–36) epitope, bestowing the ability of the virion to bind to the cell surface [21] (Fig. 21.3). Virions can bind to heparan sulfate proteoglycans [22] of the exposed basement membrane and enter into the basal cells of the epithelium via clathrin-dependent, receptor-mediated endocytosis [23, 24]. Within the endosomes of the basal cell, viral particles are disassembled and the viral genomic DNA is localized to the nucleus with the assistance of minor capsid protein L2 [23].

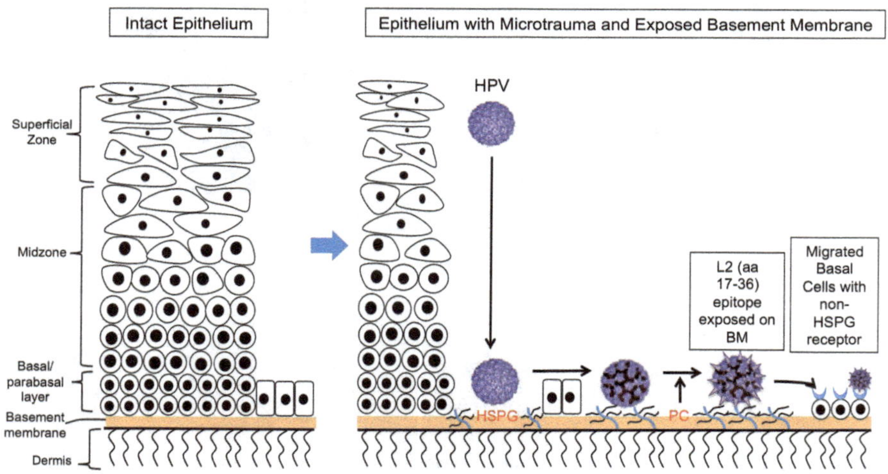

Fig. 21.3 Initial steps leading to HPV infection. HPV infection requires infection of the basal cells, which are the only cells in the squamous epithelium able to undergo long-term cell division. It is believed that microtrauma to the cervical epithelium of the transformation zone is required to provide access of the virus to the basal cells. Virions bind first to the basement membrane at sites of trauma, undergo a conformational change in which L2 minor capsid protein is cleaved by a proprotein convertase (PC), furin, or PC5/6, and undergo another subsequent conformational change that exposes L2 neutralization (aa 17–36) epitope, bestowing the ability of the virion to bind to the cell surface. Virions can bind to heparan sulfate proteoglycans (HSPG) of the exposed basement membrane and enter into the migrated basal cells of the epithelium via endocytosis (Virion not drawn to scale. Modified from [21])

The replicative phase of the HPV life cycle is closely associated with the differentiation of the infected squamous epithelium (Fig. 21.2). As mentioned above, initial infection occurs in the basal cells and the HPV genome is maintained as a low copy number episome in the nuclei of infected host cells. Hence, HPV infection is established with the expression of viral replication proteins E1 and E2, which are required for genomic amplification. The cells above the basal layer are forced into a state of increased proliferation to support the production of HPV virions. As the keratinocytes differentiate, the early HPV genes E1, E2, E4, E5, E6, and E7 are expressed while the viral DNA continues to replicate from the episomal DNA. The binding of E2 protein to the HPV genome recruits E1 helicase to the viral origin of replication and leads to the association of E1 protein with other host factors required for viral DNA replication, such as DNA polymerase α primase and protein A [25–28]. It is also believed that E2 behaves as a transcriptional activator when present at low levels in the cell [29]. As the amount of E2 increases during maturation of the infected keratinocytes, binding of E2 to HPV DNA causes displacement of transcription factors such as TATA-binding protein and Sp1, which are essential for promoter activation, and therefore inhibit expression of the E6 and E7 viral oncoproteins [30]. Consequently, the levels of HPV E6 and E7 are invariably downregulated as the infection progresses. In terminally differentiated cells, the virus replicates to a high copy number and the expression of E6/E7 is effectively repressed by E2. The L1 and L2 capsid proteins are also expressed in terminally differentiated cells and serve to package the viral genomes to form progeny virions in the nucleus. E4 associates with keratin intermediate filaments and mediates cytoskeletal changes for the release of virions [31]. The shed infectious viral particles can then initiate a new infection.

In HPV-infected cells, HPV E5, E6, E7 induce cell proliferation. Specifically, E5, located on the endoplasmic reticulum of the infected cell, stimulates cell growth by forming a complex with epidermal growth factor receptor, the platelet-derived growth factor β receptor and the colony-stimulating factor 1 receptor [32]. E5 can also increase phosphorylation of epidermal growth factor receptor and prolong signaling necessary for the maintenance of an environment favorable for cell proliferation [33], potentially through inhibiting the acidification of endosomes by associating with and disrupting the function of ATPase-driven proton pumps on the endosomal membrane [34, 35].

E6 and E7 normally inhibit p53 and retinoblastoma (Rb) tumor suppressor pathways, respectively. Therefore, the repression of E6 and E7 mediated by E2 in productive viral infection results in the reactivation of the tumor suppressor genes, inducing cell cycle arrest and cellular senescence. Unlike their role in the cancerous precursor pathway, E6 and E7 do not act as viral oncoproteins in the productive viral infection pathway. Rather, they are associated with facilitating viral replication and promoting cervical cell proliferation. It has been shown that E6 and E7 of low-risk HPV types are important for the maintenance of episomal viral DNA [36] and the maintenance of extrachromosomal forms of HPV in undifferentiated basal cells [37]. While the specific mechanisms of E6 and E7 in low-risk HPV types are not fully elucidated in the context of the viral life cycle, it is likely that HPV must block normal cellular checkpoints to allow for the persistence of viral episomes since the presence of extrachromosomal DNA in normal cells is likely sensed as DNA damage. More studies are required to understand the role of E6 and E7 in productive viral infection.

The production of progeny virions is usually limited to LSIL lesions, as the full viral replication cycle is tied to the differentiation process. LSIL lesions often contain low-risk HPVs that are unlikely to cause cervical cancer [9]. Even in the cases where LSIL lesions harbor high-risk HPV types, viral gene expression analysis frequently indicates productive viral infection rather than cancerous precursors [38, 39]. Hence, LSIL is associated with the maintenance of the viral genome as an episome and low-level expression of E6 and E7. The pathogenesis pathway of productive viral infection may be seen as one in which the virus productively amplifies itself within the host but does not induce malignant transformation of infected cells.

Cancerous Precursors

The cancerous precursor pathway refers to cases of HPV infection that result in HSIL lesions that will progress to malignant cancer. One of the key steps of HPV-induced cervical carcinogenesis is the integration of the HPV genome into host-cell genome, resulting in the deletion of several viral genes (E2, E4, E5, L1, L2). The role of E5 in cervical carcinogenesis has been explored in several studies as it has transformative properties [40–43]. However, since E5 is often deleted upon integration and is not obligatory in late events of HPV-mediated carcinogenesis, the main focus of cervical carcinogenesis has been on the primary oncoproteins expressed in cervical cancer cells – E6 and E7. As E2 is the transcriptional repressor protein of E6 and E7, the loss of E2 leaves E6 and E7 as the principal proteins expressed within the infected cell [44]. The interference of viral genes E6 and E7 with cellular pathways essential to cell cycle regulation may result in genomic instability, leading to the continuous and deregulated expression of viral oncogenes E6/E7 in infected basal cells. These cells therefore have a greater chance of acquiring secondary genomic abnormalities that may drive malignant progression to cancer (for a review, see [45]).

The transforming activity of the E6 viral oncoprotein is attributed to its interaction with p53. E6 targets p53 tumor suppressor protein, which governs G1 arrest and DNA repair, for proteasomal degradation by complexing with ubiquitin ligase E6-AP. E6 also interacts with and degrades the proapoptotic protein Bak. The downregulation of p53 and Bak by E6 leads to progression through the cell cycle, resistance to apoptosis, and chromosomal instability [46–48]. In addition, E6 activates telomerase and may inhibit proteolysis of the SRC-family kinases to further stimulate cell growth and proliferation [49]. While the downregulation of p53 by E6 is associated with high-risk HPV types, some evidence suggests that E6 of low-risk HPV types may also bind to p53 with lower affinity [50–52]. However, it has also been shown that low-risk HPV E6 have significantly lower transforming activity in that they do not interact efficiently with p53 [52], are incompetent for p53 degradation [53], and do not induce telomerase activity [54]. More recently, it has been found that E6 also promotes carcinogenesis by epigenetically silencing production of interferon-kappa, an immune protein produced in keratinocytes important in the stimulation of innate immunity [55].

The transforming activity of E7 is attributed to its interaction with the Rb protein. Specifically, E7 binds and degrades the hypophosphorylated form of Rb complex, which releases the transcription factor E2F and allows the infected cells to remain active in the S phase of the cell cycle as they leave the basal layer [56]. The release of transcription factor E2F upregulates cyclin-dependent kinase inhibitor INK4A (also known as p16) and accumulation of E2F may lead to apoptosis in E7-expressing cells. While low-risk forms of E7 have been shown to bind to Rb, they do so with a lower affinity compared to high-risk forms of E7 [57–59] and do not destabilize Rb [60, 61]. High-risk forms of E7 also stimulate S-phase genes cyclin A and cyclin E [62] and inactivate cyclin-dependent kinase inhibitors WAF1 (also known as p21) and KIP1 (also known as p27) [63–65], while low-risk E7 proteins have no such effect [66]. Interestingly, E7 may also exert an antiapoptotic effect by upregulating serine/threonine kinase AKT [67]. However, it is not clear whether anti-apoptotic or apoptosis-promoting effects are dominant in E7.

The functions of the HPV oncoproteins E6 and E7 complement one another to induce efficient malignant transformation of normal cells (for review, see [17]). While E6 and E7 are independently able to immortalize various human cell types in tissue culture, their efficiency is increased when they are expressed together [68]. The transforming activities of E6 are blocked by p16, a protein inhibitor of cyclin D1-CDK complexes, which blocks progression into S-phase of the cell cycle by inhibiting expression of cyclin E. However, E7 is able to bypass this obstacle by directly stimulating expression of cyclins E and A. The cell is therefore driven through the cell cycle without much resistance. Furthermore, although E7-mediated activation of E2F may contribute to the onset of apoptotic signals in the cell, E6 causes degradation of the apoptosis-promoting proteins p53 and Bak, thereby disrupting the transmission of these signals to downstream effector molecules [62, 69]. High-risk forms of E6 and E7 deregulate the key cell cycle checkpoints (G1/S, G2/M) and their persistent viral oncogenic E6/E7 activity in cervical cells represents an essential step in cervical carcinogenesis.

The cancerous precursors are best characterized by, and likely a result of, a dramatic, uncontrolled E6/E7 expression that can occur as a result of integration of viral DNA into host genome [38, 39]. The exact molecular mechanisms accounting for the deregulated increase in E6/E7 production are not completely understood, though experiments with epithelial raft cultures have indicated that aberrant histone deacetylation may be a potential underlying factor [70]. Other mechanisms, such as promoter methylation and direct mutation of E2 may also be responsible for upregulation of E6/E7 [71–73].

Tumor-Promoting Risk Factors

The onset of cervical dysplasia and cancer requires not only persistent infection with a high-risk type of HPV, but also the presence of a tumor-promoting risk factor. The transformative ability of high risk HPV types was discovered by findings that demonstrated that human primary keratinocytes could be immortalized by the expression of E6 and E7 [74–77] and that culturing these cells for extended periods of time resulted in the emergence of tumorigenic clones [78, 79]. Several in vitro models have identified principal characteristics of HPV-transformed epithelial cells: prolonged lifespan, immortalization, anchorage-independent proliferation, and tumorigenicity. These characteristics are recessive and arise from deregulation of tumor suppressor pathways [78, 79]. Also, for all of these properties, in vitro complementation assays have been performed, and the chromosomal changes likely responsible for each one have been proposed. Remarkably, these changes correlate closely with those observed in cervical cancer samples derived from human patients, suggesting that a conserved set of genetic alterations underlie both in vitro HPV-induced cellular transformation and in vivo cervical carcinogenesis [78, 79].

Immortalization

Although HPV-infected cells with deregulated E6/E7 expression are able to resist entry into cellular senescence [46, 80], these cells are often observed to undergo crisis, a condition in which the majority of cells die and immortal clones emerge at low frequency. Passage through crisis and the attainment of an immortal status is likely attributable to the activation of the telomerase reverse transcriptase enzyme [81, 82].

Telomerase activity is an important HPV-dependent effect strongly induced in cancer cells. Each round of DNA replication leads to erosion of the telomeric ends of chromosomes, serving as a mechanism for restricting the proliferative capacity of normal cells [83]. Since telomerase adds on hexamer repeats to the telomeric ends of chromosomes, increased telomerase activity can prolong the life of cells. Telomerase activity is upregulated in cancer cells and depends on the expression level of human telomerase reverse transcriptase (hTERT), the catalytic subunit of this enzyme [84]. The importance of hTERT in the immortalization of hrHPV-infected cells is demonstrated by experiments in which HPV-16 and HPV-18-containing epithelial cells ectopically expressing hTERT were resistant to telomere erosion and apoptotic effects of crisis [85]. While E6 is implicated in hTERT production [54], the susceptibility to crisis of hrHPV-infected cells (without ectopic introduction of hTERT) suggests that other cellular changes are necessary for telomerase activation [81, 85, 86]. Several groups have conducted experiments in which regions of human chromosomes 2, 3, 4, and 6 were transferred into HPV-immortalized cells, leading to growth arrest [85, 87–90]. These findings suggest that some host cell genes have the potential to suppress telomerase activation, and that the loss of these genes may facilitate, in conjunction with E6, the immortalization of high risk HPV-infected cells. Later reports identified portions of chromosomes 3, 4, and 6 to directly exert a suppressive effect on telomerase activity [85, 87]. For example, ectopic expression of hTERT counteracted growth arrest mediated by chromosome 6 in HPV16^{+} cells, showing that parts of this chromosome interfere with telomerase function.

These in vitro data correlate strongly with information derived from clinical specimens. Elevated hTERT expression and subsequent increased telomerase activity has been reported in nearly all cervical squamous cell carcinomas and in about 40% of CIN 3 lesions but not in CIN 1 [91]. Furthermore, in these HSIL+ lesions with increased telomerase activity, allelic imbalances were widely observed on chromosome 6 [92], implicating the presence of a telomerase suppressor on this chromosome. Furthermore, deletions at chromosomes 3, 4, and 10 are commonly found in cervical carcinomas and in HSILs [88, 89, 92]. Although additional studies are necessary to identify specific genes on these chromosomes responsible for their presumed antiproliferative function, it is clear that they play important roles in repressing cellular immortalization.

Tumorigenicity and Anchorage-Independent Proliferation

In vitro studies have suggested that the tumorigenicity of cervical cancer cells is dependent on loss or suppression of certain genes at chromosome 11, as treatment of the cells with this chromosome rendered them incapable of establishing tumors in nude mice [93]. These results are verified by clinical observations of chromosome 11 deletions in a variety of cervical carcinomas [94]. Further exploration into this phenomenon has recently revealed that the tumor suppressor in lung cancer 1 (TSLC1) gene in particular may be lost in cervical cancer cells [95], which confers the properties of tumorigenicity and anchorage-independent proliferation to these cells. The TSLC1 gene encodes an immunoglobulin-like cell surface protein called Necl-2, which helps mediate cell-cell adhesion by homotypic or heterotypic interactions [96]. The lack of TSLC1 in epithelial cells eliminates their adhesive potential and contributes to their anchorage-independent cell growth. In addition, Necl-2 interacts with class I-restricted T cell-associated molecule (CRTAM) – a receptor protein expressed on activated $CD8^+$ T cells and natural killer cells – and thereby can promote an anticancer immune response [97]. Thus, the loss of Necl-2 in cervical cancer cells is likely to increase their tumorigenicity by facilitating a state of immunological privilege.

The importance of TSLC1 in HPV-mediated cervical cancer progression is supported by several clinical studies. For example, it has been shown that this gene is repressed in approximately 90% of cervical cancer cell lines due to allelic loss or promoter hypermethylation [95]. Similar results were noted in about 60% of cervical carcinomas and 40% of HSILs, but not in LSILs. Additionally, ectopic TSLC1 protected against tumor formation in nude mice and abolished anchorage-independent proliferation of cervical cancer cell lines [95]. Altogether, these findings suggest that loss of TSLC1 occurs during cervical carcinogenesis, disrupting cell–cell contacts and potentially facilitating tumor immune escape. However, it is unlikely that changes in expression of this one gene alone are sufficient for inducing tumorigenicity in cervical cancer cells.

It has also been found that alterations in the composition of the AP-1 complex are also important for tumorigenicity [98–100]. The AP-1 transcription factor, which consists of the subunits c-Jun, c-Fos, or Fra-1 associated as homo or heterodimers, regulates multiple cellular pathways, including differentiation and proliferation. In normal cells, AP-1 exists predominately as Jun/Fra-1 complexes, but in cervical cancer cells, c-Fos is constitutively expressed (with concomitant reduction of Fra-1 levels), resulting in a significant shift towards Jun/c-Fos [98, 99]. It is probable that this change affects the ability of transformed cells to form tumors in vivo, since ectopic expression c-Fos in nontumorigenic cell lines drove the cells towards a tumorigenic phenotype [98]. Reports of upregulation of c-Fos in human cervical carcinomas [101] also support a role for abnormal AP-1 composition in HPV-mediated cervical carcinogenesis.

Furthermore, gain of chromosomal segment 3q is frequently observed in cases of cervical carcinoma and oftentimes marks the shift from dysplasia to invasive cancer [102]. Although the specific genes present on 3q that contribute to tumorigenesis are currently unknown, it is likely that this region of the chromosome contains one or more oncogenes.

Screening and Detection of Pre-malignant Cervical Lesions

Because of the long latency between the development of cervical dysplasia and the development of invasive cancer, it is possible to prevent the development of precursor lesions into malignant cancer through early detection and treatment methods.

Conventional Pap Smear

Premalignant cervical lesions are generally screened by cervical cytologic smears. Papanicolaou tests, also known as Pap smears, were created by Dr. George Papanicolaou and Dr. Herbert Traut in 1941, when they demonstrated that exfoliative cytology could be used to detect in situ and invasive cervical carcinomas [103]. The Pap smear involves the examination of cells collected from the cervix for the presence of any cellular abnormalities (multinucleation, koilocytosis, abnormal mitosis) that may be associated with cancerous precursor lesions or cancer. Pap smear screening performed yearly is estimated to reduce a woman's risk of invasive cervical cancer by 93% [104]. However, despite its effectiveness, a single cervical smear has low sensitivity for detecting cervical cancer precursors [105]. More recently, the guidelines for cervical screening have changed to lessen the frequency of screening. Current general guidelines recommend that women should have a Pap test every 2 years starting at the age of 21 years as opposed to the yearly screening that women have had in years past [106]. In women 30 years and older who have had three normal Pap results in a row, they may reduce frequency of Pap smear screening to every 3 years if they have no history of moderate or severe dysplasia, are not immune-deficient, were not exposed to diethylstilbestrol before birth and are not infected with HIV. The guidelines were revised based on studies that have shown that risk of cervical cancer is same in women who have screening every 2 years compared with women annually screened.

The results of a Pap smear are reported using the Bethesda System of terminology. Pap smear samples that have no cell abnormalities are negative for intraepithelial lesions. Atypical squamous cells (ASC) refer to samples where atypical squamous cell changes cannot be reliably distinguished as normal or clearly abnormal [107]. In 2001, ASC was subdivided into atypical squamous cells of undetermined significance (ASC-US) and atypical squamous cells – "cannot rule out high grade squamous intraepithelial lesion" (ASC-H) [108], with ASC-H indicating a higher probability of precancerous lesions than ASC-US. Atypical glandular cells (AGC) imply abnormal changes to the mucus-producing glandular cells located in the upper cervix or uterus. LSIL and HSIL are diagnostic terms, as described earlier in Premalignant Cervical Lesions section.

One of the most powerful advances in the recent decade for collection and preparation of cytologic specimens has been the introduction of liquid-based cytology (LBC). To date, there are currently three FDA-approved LBC methods – ThinPrep Pap Test (Hologic (merged with Cytyc Corp in 2007), Bedford, MA, USA), SurePath™ Pap Test (Becton, Dickinson and Company (acquired TriPath Imaging Inc in 2006), Franklin Lakes, NJ, USA), MonoPrep System (MPPT; MonoGen, Lincolnshire, IL, USA) [105, 109–112]. Whereas conventional Pap smear involves smearing the sample onto a microscope slide, LBC transfers all cervical tissue collected on the sampling device (cervical brush) into a preservative solution, producing a cell suspension. The cells are fixed immediately and can be well preserved at room temperature for several weeks. Many reports have showed significant improvement of diagnostic sensitivity compared to conventional cytology [113–116]. Moreover, less unsatisfactory slides are found using LBC [114, 115]. Since only a small aliquot of cell suspension is removed for preparing cytologic glass slides, LBC technique is also advantageous in providing a residual specimen for additional tests such as cervical cancer testing, HPV testing, chlamydia testing and gonorrhea testing. In particular, ThinPrep Pap Test is the only pap test that is FDA-approved for additional testing from a single pap sample [111]. These supplementary tests may further improve the specificity and sensitivity of the screening tests and offer more accurate risk stratification for women whose cytological interpretations are controversial, such as atypical squamous cells of undetermined significance (ASC-US).

HPV Testing

The concept that infection with hrHPV is a necessary though insufficient step in cervical carcinogenesis provides the rationale for the development of molecular techniques to identify oncogenic HPV in cervical sample and improve the quality of cervical screening. For example, cross sectional and large randomized studies had proven the use of hrHPV testing for triage in abnormal Pap smears [117–119]. Women with ASC-US are best managed by HPV testing, with women positive for HPV triaged to colposcopy and women negative for HPV safely placed in a 12-month cytology follow-up [120, 121]. However, the high rate of HPV-positive LSIL and low specificity of HPV testing in this group of cytologic interpretation preclude the HPV testing in the triage of LSIL [117, 122, 123]. Subsequently, other large studies expand the roles of hrHPV testing and verify its clinical use in post-colposcopy management of women referred for ASC-US, ASC-H, AGC, LSIL not found to have CIN2, 3 or cancer (CIN2+) or adenocarcinoma in situ (AIS) at initial colposcopy, in post-treatment of CIN 2+ surveillance, and in co-testing with the Pap smear of women age 30 and over (for review, see [119]).

The development of assays to accurately diagnose the HPV infection currently relies on the detection of HPV genome in cervical specimens. There are a wide variety of methods for HPV DNA testing in cytological specimens, which can be divided into two broad categories – with or without amplification. Two methods of HPV testing without amplification are Southern blot and in situ hybridization and use nucleic acid probes. However, these two methods are largely replaced in clinical use by amplification techniques due to the disadvantages of low sensitivity and labor intensiveness [109, 124]. Amplification techniques can be further divided into those using target amplification (such as PCR, which amplifies a target nucleic acid) and those using signal amplification (a signal generated from each probe is amplified by a compound-probe). The analytic sensitivity and reproducibility of results by PCR are different and depend on the methods used to detect the amplification product (such as nucleic acid hybridization, restriction fragment length polymorphism or sequencing). PCR assays can also be greatly affected by various unrelated substances that can inhibit the amplification reaction [109].

Two currently commercially available hrHPV DNA tests are Digene Hybrid Capture 2 HPV DNA Test (Qiagen, (formerly Digene), Gaithersburg, MD, USA) and Roche Amplicor® HPV test (Roche Molecular Systems, Branchburg, NJ, USA). Digene HC2 is the only non-type-specific HPV DNA testing kit currently approved by the US Food and Drug Administration (FDA). HC2 uses the principle of signal amplification by utilizing a RNA probe cocktail that detects 13 hrHPV types (16, 18, 31, 33, 35, 39, 45, 51, 52, 56, 58, 59, 68) and 5 lrHPV types (6, 11, 42, 43, 44). Digene HC2 is currently the most commonly used and clinically validated assay and is becoming a standard of care for cervical cancer prevention for use together with Pap test in women age 30 and older. It is also less vulnerable to error than the Pap smear and the combination of both identifies 95–100% of women who are later confirmed to have advanced cervical disease [125]. Digene HC2 has become the standard of care in the United States.

Roche Amplicor® HPV test has demonstrated comparable results in comparison to Digene HC2 in detecting HPV DNA in cervical samples [126]. In contrast to Digene HC2, Roche Amplicor® uses a target amplification method to detect the same 13 hrHPV types. However, Amplicor® is not yet FDA approved for use in the United States, though it is registered for use in the European Union, Canada and Japan [127]. As both Amplicor® and Digene HC2 are not type-specific, they can only differentiate the presence of hrHPV infection or no hrHPV infection. Neither one can recognize potential multiple types of hrHPV infection in one specimen nor allow for the identification of type-specific persistent HPV infection.

Recently, in March 2009, FDA approved two HPV tests, the Invader 14-type HPV DNA panel test, Cervista™ HPV HR Test [128] and the type-specific Cervista™ HPV 16/18 test (Hologic, Bedford, MA, USA) for clinical use [129]. Cervista™ HPV HR detects 14 hrHPV types using three probe sets. The probe set A5/A6 detects HPV types 51, 56 and 66. Whereas the probe set A7 detects HPV subtypes often found in glandular lesions (HPV types 18, 39, 45, 59 and 68), the probe set A9 detects HPV subtypes found more frequently in squamous lesions (HPV types 16, 31, 33, 35, 52 and 58). The results from the probe set gives an indication of which group of types the infection may be derived from and also helps facilitate subsequent clinical management [119]. The Cervista™ HPV 16/18 test is the first HPV test approved for genotyping for HPV types 16 and 18. The Cervista™ HPV HR and Cervista™ HPV 16/18 tests are both based on Invader chemistry, a patented technology owned by Hologic that uses the principle of signal amplification [130]. Both tests are approved for use utilizing the sample collected with the ThinPrep Pap Test, offering additional convenience for the healthcare provider. Patient management can be guided with the help of the results of these two types of tests along with the physician's assessment of cytology history, other risk factors, and professional guidelines.

Qiagen has also developed a new generation of screening test called the careHPV test [131]. The careHPV test has promising clinical implications for cervical cancer screening. Cervical cancer incidence and mortality is higher in developing countries, where regular screening is absent and there are limited resources. The careHPV test uses a battery-operated instrument, easy-to-use reagents and a simple procedure. Therefore, medical workers in screening sites in remote areas can be easily trained to operate the system, perform tests and report results. The careHPV test may facilitate early detection of pre-malignant cervical lesions in low resource settings.

Other Markers

Other markers that monitor oncogenesis of cervical cancers, such as p16 and HPV messenger RNA (mRNA), are also available commercially and considered to have potential roles in future cervical cancer screening and clinical management [132]. Ideally, these markers should have high positive predictive value for progression of cervical cancers, such as prediction of HSIL, to be potentially clinically useful.

$P16^{INK4A}$ is a cell cycle inhibitor whose expression is increased in response to the expression of hrHPV oncogenes E6 and E7 in CIN2+ [133]. Physiologically, Rb may act as a negative regulator of $P16^{INK4A}$ expression [134]. The mechanism is lost when Rb is inactivated by hrHPV E7. Several studies have shown the clinical utility of this biomarker to improve ascertainment of difficult histological interpretations, and in triage of risk for CIN2+ in ASC-US and LSIL [135, 136]. However, $P16^{INK4A}$

was also found to be expressed in metaplastic, atrophic and endocervical cells, which represent different cell differentiation instead of preneoplastic conditions [137]. More studies are needed to verify the value of P16^{INK4A} immunocytostaining in cervical cancer screening.

HPV mRNA testing for hrHPV may be better correlated with the progression of preinvasive cervical lesions. First, HPV E6 expression is regulated at transcriptional or post-transcriptional level. HPV-16 E6/E7 has different transcripts that are either unspliced (full length-FL-E6/E7 transcripts) or spliced. Only FL E6 protein was found to bind strongly to p53, promote its degradation and be more strongly associated with tumorigenicity [138, 139]. Hence, full-length E6/E7 mRNA transcripts may serve as a better, more accurate marker than E6/E7 DNA. Second, almost all HPV DNA assays detect presence of viral DNA by detecting the L1 region, which may be deleted upon integration of the viral genome into the host cell. Since HPV mRNA testing detects E6/E7 transcripts, it may correlate well with the transforming activity of HPV in precancerous or cancerous cells [109].

PreTect HPV-Proofer (NorChip, AS, Klokkarstua, Norway) represents a new generation of assays focused on the pathogenic factors that underlie the development of HPV-associated tumors – the constitutive expression of the viral oncogenes E6 and E7 [140–142]. PreTect HPV-Proofer is a commercially available HPV RNA assay based on nucleic acid sequence-based amplification technology, detecting type-specific E6/E7 mRNA expression from carcinogenic HPV types 16, 18, 31, 33 and 45. A second mRNA-based assay is the Aptima HPV Assay (GenProbe, Inc, San Diego, CA), a 14-type E6/E7 mRNA test approved by Conformité Européenne (CE). A recent study compared APTIMA HPV assay and Digene HC2 test and showed 91% clinical sensitivity and >55% specificity for detection of CIN2+ in APTIMA assay, with 95% and 47% in the Digene HC2 test [143]. The introduction of mRNA testing has great potential in increasing the diagnostic accuracy of Pap smear and DNA test through utilizing the understanding of E6 and E7 deregulation in HPV-associated tumors. By identifying type-specific E6 and E7 mRNA, HPV mRNA testing can enable better identification of infections that are transient and infections that are more likely to persist and induce HSIL+ lesions in the future.

Clinical Management of Pre-malignant Cervical Lesions

Screening and detection of pre-malignant cervical lesions require concomitant therapies in order to be effective in lowering cervical cancer incidence. Current conventional clinical management of abnormal (ASC-US or ASC-H) or SIL interpretation of Pap smears consists of colposcopy, cervical biopsy, endocervical sampling, cervical conization and other treatment modalities (for comprehensive guidelines, see [120, 144]). In general, women with ASC-US can: (1) undergo reflex-testing for hrHPV and colposcopy if hrHPV positive, (2) be followed by repeated Pap smears at 6 and 12 months, or (3) be referred directly for evaluation by colposcopy. Women with ASC-H or LSIL are often referred for colposcopic examination while women whose

Pap smears indicate HSIL are referred immediately for treatment such as loop electrosurgical excision procedure (LEEP) or colposcopy examination.

Colposcopy is a stereoscopic binocular magnification procedure that provides a three-dimensional visualization of the tissue surfaces examined [5]. Before colposcopic examination, a 3–5% solution of acetic acid is applied to the cervical surface to dehydrate cells and remove mucus. Colposcopic diagnosis is based on the morphologic evaluation of surface contour, color tone, border and subepithelial vascular network of cervical tissue examined. The examination is limited to the exocervix and outer third of the endocervical canal. To evaluate lesions within the endocervix, an endocervical sampling (or endocervical curettage) is usually performed during the colposcopic examination. Endocervical sampling contributes to the diagnostic accuracy of the colposcopic evaluation [145–147]. During colposcopic evaluation, if necessary, cervical biopsy is performed at the regions with the most remarkable abnormality using a punch biopsy instrument.

Cervical conization (cone biopsy) is a technique that may follow the colposcopic examination with both diagnostic and therapeutic purposes. Cervical conization is conically shaped cutting of the cervix. Indications for a cervical conization include: normal colposcopy but persistent abnormal cytology or positive endocervical sampling; abnormal cytology but squamocolumnar junction not visualized under colposcopy; lesions not visualized in its entirety under colposcopy; microinvasive carcinoma or adenocarcinoma in situ on biopsy; and lack of correlation among cytologic, colposcopic and histologic findings [5].

Treatment modalities for preinvasive lesions of the cervix include cryosurgery, carbon dioxide laser or loop electrosurgical excision procedure [5]. Cryosurgery is a cryodestructive method for ablating SIL by using a cryoprobe below −22°C applied to the cervix. In experienced hands, the failure or residual rate (5–15%) and the long-term recurrence rate (0.1%) of cryosurgery do not exceed that of therapeutic conization [148, 149]. Another method is the carbon dioxide laser, which utilizes parallel beams of uniform wavelength (10.6 μm) to create a very high energy density on targeted cervical premalignant lesions. The tissue fluids boil and expand, and the cells are evaporated and destroyed. Since less necrosis is caused, it permits more rapid healing with less vaginal discharge than cryosurgery [150]. However, the major disadvantage of carbon dioxide laser is its high cost. The loop electrosurgical excision procedure is another technique that is used with increasing frequency to treat premalignant cervical lesions. A tissue specimen is obtained by a thin wire loop electrode that simultaneously cuts and coagulates the tissue. Because a tissue specimen is obtained, the method is both diagnostic and therapeutic.

HPV Vaccination

Preventive HPV Vaccines

In order to develop preventive HPV vaccines, it is important to generate protective humoral immune responses that are capable of neutralizing the HPV virus by targeting

L1 and/or L2 HPV viral capsid proteins. In the early 1990s, investigators began the search for a way to produce HPV 16 L1 capsid proteins that could be used for the building blocks for the virus-like particles (VLPs) in the preventive HPV vaccines [151]. Early studies suggested that L1-protective epitopes were probably dependent on native conformation due to poor effectiveness of vaccination with denatured L1 [152, 153]. Subsequent efforts showed that the expression of recombinant L1 in mammalian [154, 155], insect [156, 157], yeast [158] and even bacterial cells [159] results in spontaneous assembly of VLPs that were morphologically and immunologically [156, 157, 160] similar to native virions. Vaccination of animal models with L1 VLPs protects them from subsequent exposure to the homologous virus [152]. Later, a landmark controlled trial of HPV-preventive vaccine in human subjects showed that vaccination three times with HPV-16 L1 VLPs formulated in the adjuvant alum provided 100% protection from the natural acquisition of persistent HPV-16 infection over an average of 17.4 months [161]. Impressively, all cases of incident HPV16-related CIN were confined to the placebo group, indicating that vaccination protects against HPV-related disease. L1 VLP vaccines could produce high titers of neutralizing IgG antibodies, even up to 40 times those found in natural infection with HPV-16 [162, 163].

There are currently two commercially available, FDA-approved HPV vaccines in the United States – Gardasil and Cervarix (for review, see [164]). Gardasil is a quadrivalent vaccine produced by Merck containing recombinant L1 VLPs for HPV genotypes 6, 11, 16 and 18 whereas the bivalent vaccine Cervarix produced by GlaxoSmithKline contains L1 VLPs for HPV-16 and 18 (Table 21.1). Cervarix and Gardasil, are produced in insect cells and yeast, respectively. Gardasil was approved in 2006 and in October 2009, Cervarix was FDA-approved in the United States for use in girls and young women ages 10–25 [165]. Recently, the use of Gardasil was also FDA-approved or use in boys and men (aged 9–26) for the prevention of genital warts caused by HPV-6 and HPV-11 and to help prevent the spread of cervical cancer [166]. To date, Cervarix and Gardasil clinical trials have been very encouraging with regard to safety and efficacy in generating neutralizing antibodies [167–177]. However, the antibody response generated is type-restricted to those HPV genotypes contained within the vaccines, although there is some low-level cross-protection against other closely related genotypes (HPV-16 cross-protects HPV-31; HPV-18 cross-protects HPV-45) [178]. It is estimated that a preventive vaccine would need to contain the eight most common HPV types found in cancer to create >90% protection against cervical cancer – a costly and complex process [179]. Furthermore, due to the high prevalence of HPV in the population and slow process of cervical carcinogenesis, it is estimated that a reduction in cervical cancer rates will take at least 20 years after mass vaccination.

The main issues for future generations of preventive vaccines are making the vaccine more cost-effective in order to increase availability of the vaccine in developing countries and increasing the number of HPV types covered in order to maximize protection against HPV-associated malignancies. A potential approach to substantially reduce the cost of producing L1 vaccines is the employment of L1 capsomers produced in recombinant *Escherichia coli*. The production of the vaccine in *E. coli*

Table 21.1 Comparison of currently available preventive HPV vaccines

	Cervarix®	Gardasil®
Manufacturer	GlaxoSmithKline	Merck
Vaccine composition	HPV-16, 18 VLP	HPV-6, 11, 16, 18 VLP
Antigen (per dose)	20 μg HPV 16 L1 20 μg HPV 18 L1	40 μg HPV 6 L1 20 μg HPV 11 L1 40 μg HPV 16 L1 20 μg HPV 18 L1
Antigen source	Baculovirus expression system in *Trichoplusia ni* insect cells	Yeast expression system in *Saccharomyces cerevisiae*
Adjuvant	AS04: 500 μg aluminum hydroxide, 50 μg MPL (3-O-desacyl-4′-monophosphoryl lipid A)	Alum: 225 μg aluminum hydroxyphosphate sulfate
Recommended administration	Intramuscular injection of 0.5 mL dose at 0, 1, 6 months	Intramuscular injection of 0.5 mL dose at 0, 2, 6 months
Approx price (USD)	$100 per dose	$120 per dose
Approved for ages	Females: 10–25	Females: 9–26 Males: 9–26
Protection (HPV types)	HPV-16, 18 Cross-protection: HPV-31, 33, 45	HPV-6, 11, 16, 18 Cross-protection: HPV-31
Antibody titers of HPV-16 and HPV-18 at month 7 in a head to head trial [167]	HPV16: 31715 HPV 18: 13732	HPV 16: 8682 HPV 18: 1886
	Cevarix produced 3.7-fold higher antibody titers for HPV-16 and 7.3-fold higher antibody titers for HPV-18 than did Gardasil	

has been successful in generating protective antibodies in animal models [180–182]. Additionally, L1 capsomer vaccines are stable at room temperature, negating the need for refrigeration. Needle-free routes of administration such as transdermal application [183] and nasal inhalation [184] have also been investigated, with potential implications for future L1 capsomer vaccines.

A method to overcome the genotype restriction of L1 vaccines is through polyvalent L1 vaccines containing VLPs for several HPV types. Merck is currently recruiting for Phase II clinical trials of a nine-valent vaccine, V503 [185]. Another attractive strategy is the employment of the highly conserved and thus cross-reactive L2. L2-based vaccines can also be produced using *E. coli* to reduce costs and increase availability to the developing world. However, L2 vaccines are less immunogenic than their L1 counterparts, generating relatively lower titers of neutralizing antibodies, and consequently would most likely be boosted with the use of an adjuvant (for review, see [186, 187]).

Therapeutic HPV Vaccines

Although preventive HPV vaccines are safe and effective in preventing HPV infection, they are unlikely to impact HPV prevalence and cervical cancer rates for many years. The currently available preventive vaccines are relatively expensive and require appropriate facilities of storage, precluding their availability to developing countries. Furthermore, since HPV-infected basal epithelial cells, cervical cancer cells and its precursor cells do not express detectable levels of capsid protein (L1 and/or L2), preventive vaccines are unlikely to be effective in the elimination of pre-existing infection and HPV-related cancer [188]. Current commercial preventive vaccines have also demonstrated an inability to treat established lesions [164]. In order to further reduce the burden of HPV infections and cervical cancer worldwide, therapeutic vaccines are being developed.

Therapeutic HPV vaccines should focus on HPV viral antigens that are constitutively expressed in HPV-associated malignancies and its precursors. From our understanding of the molecular pathogenesis of cervical cancer, HPV E6 and E7 proteins represent ideal target antigens for therapeutic HPV vaccines. Since they are expressed only in tumor cells and not in normal cells, there is no issue of immune tolerance. Furthermore, they are constitutively expressed in malignant cervical cells. Currently, there are various forms of therapeutic vaccines targeting E6 and E7 that have been tested in preclinical and clinical trials, such as live vector-based vaccines, peptide or protein-based vaccines, tumor-cell based vaccines, dendritic cell-based vaccines, DNA-based vaccines and RNA-based vaccines (for a review, see [189]). Promising preclinical data has led to several ongoing or completed clinical trials.

Conclusion

There have been many significant advances in methods for the early detection and subsequent management of pre-malignant cervical lesions. The conventional Pap smear has dramatically decreased cervical cancer rates in industrialized countries. As developing countries have limited access to resources needed for screening programs, the creation of the cost-effective and simple HPV test suitable for remote areas may offer great promise in further impacting cervical cancer incidence. Additionally, the insight gained from knowledge of pathogenesis of HPV infections and its progression to cervical cancer has also been used to develop type-specific HPV DNA tests and E6/E7 mRNA-based assays. These new tests have higher specificity and positive predictive value, potentially reducing unnecessary stress and costs for women with transient infections and allowing for better identification of infections more likely to persist and become HSIL+ lesions. Furthermore, a significant milestone has been reached in the development and recent approval of Cervarix and Gardasil for the prevention of cervical cancer. It is foreseeable that the future strategy of cervical cancer prevention will shift from traditional screening by Pap smear to the primary prevention with HPV vaccination combined with secondary detection of pre-invasive cervical lesions by HPV testing. The combination of our increased understanding of HPV virology, optimization of screening and detection methods of pre-invasive cervical lesions, clinical management of these lesions and implementation of preventive vaccination programs may offer the opportunity to eradicate cervical cancer.

Acknowledgements This review is not intended to be an encyclopedic one, and the authors apologize to those not cited. This work was supported by the NCI SPORE in Cervical Cancer P50 CA098252, NCI 1RO1 CA114425-01 and 1RO1 CA118790.

References

1. Parkin DM, Bray F, Ferlay J, Pisani P (2005) Global cancer statistics, 2002. CA Cancer J Clin 55(2):74–108
2. Broders A (1932) Carcinoma in situ contrasted with benign penetrating epithelium. JAMA 99:1670–1674
3. Richart RM (1973) Cervical intraepithelial neoplasia. Pathol Annu 8:301–328
4. Richart RM (1969) A theory of cervical carcinogenesis. Obstet Gynecol Surv 24(7 Pt 2): 874–879
5. Wright TC KR, Ferenczy A (2002) Precancerous lesions of the cervix. In: Kurman R (ed) Blaustein's pathology of the female genital tract, 5th edn. Springer-Verlag, New York, pp 253–324
6. Bergeron C, Barrasso R, Beaudenon S, Flamant P, Croissant O, Orth G (1992) Human papillomaviruses associated with cervical intraepithelial neoplasia. Great diversity and distinct distribution in low- and high-grade lesions. Am J Surg Pathol 16(7):641–649
7. Kalantari M, Karlsen F, Johansson B, Sigurjonsson T, Warleby B, Hagmar B (1997) Human papillomavirus findings in relation to cervical intraepithelial neoplasia grade: a study on 476 Stockholm women, using PCR for detection and typing of HPV. Hum Pathol 28(8):899–904
8. Lorincz AT, Reid R, Jenson AB, Greenberg MD, Lancaster W, Kurman RJ (1992) Human papillomavirus infection of the cervix: relative risk associations of 15 common anogenital types. Obstet Gynecol 79(3):328–337
9. Lungu O, Sun XW, Felix J, Richart RM, Silverstein S, Wright TC Jr (1992) Relationship of human papillomavirus type to grade of cervical intraepithelial neoplasia. JAMA 267(18):2493–2496
10. Franquemont DW, Ward BE, Andersen WA, Crum CP (1989) Prediction of 'high-risk' cervical papillomavirus infection by biopsy morphology. Am J Clin Pathol 92(5):577–582
11. (1989) The 1988 Bethesda System for reporting cervical/vaginal cytological diagnoses. National Cancer Institute Workshop. JAMA 262(7):931–934
12. Luff RD (1992) The Bethesda System for reporting cervical/vaginal cytologic diagnoses: report of the 1991 Bethesda workshop. The Bethesda System Editorial Committee. Hum Pathol 23(7):719–721
13. Durst M, Gissmann L, Ikenberg H, zur Hausen H (1983) A papillomavirus DNA from a cervical carcinoma and its prevalence in cancer biopsy samples from different geographic regions. Proc Natl Acad Sci U S A 80(12):3812–3815
14. Boshart M, Gissmann L, Ikenberg H, Kleinheinz A, Scheurlen W, zur Hausen H (1984) A new type of papillomavirus DNA, its presence in genital cancer biopsies and in cell lines derived from cervical cancer. EMBO J 3(5):1151–1157
15. Hoory T, Monie A, Gravitt P, Wu TC (2008) Molecular epidemiology of human papillomavirus. J Formos Med Assoc 107:198–217
16. Roden R, Wu TC (2006) How will HPV vaccines affect cervical cancer? Nat Rev Cancer 6(10):753–763
17. Munger K, Baldwin A, Edwards KM, Hayakawa H, Nguyen CL, Owens M, Grace M, Huh K (2004) Mechanisms of human papillomavirus-induced oncogenesis. J Virol 78(21):11451–11460
18. Kurman RJ, Malkasian GD Jr, Sedlis A, Solomon D (1991) From Papanicolaou to Bethesda: the rationale for a new cervical cytologic classification. Obstet Gynecol 77(5):779–782
19. Ho GY, Bierman R, Beardsley L, Chang CJ, Burk RD (1998) Natural history of cervicovaginal papillomavirus infection in young women. N Engl J Med 338(7):423–428

20. Trimble CL, Piantadosi S, Gravitt P et al (2005) Spontaneous regression of high-grade cervical dysplasia: effects of human papillomavirus type and HLA phenotype. Clin Cancer Res 11(13):4717–4723
21. Kines RC, Thompson CD, Lowy DR, Schiller JT, Day PM (2009) The initial steps leading to papillomavirus infection occur on the basement membrane prior to cell surface binding. Proc Natl Acad Sci U S A 106(48):20458–20463
22. Patterson NA, Smith JL, Ozbun MA (2005) Human papillomavirus type 31b infection of human keratinocytes does not require heparan sulfate. J Virol 79:6838–6847
23. Day PM, Baker CC, Lowy DR, Schiller JT (2004) Establishment of papillomavirus infection is enhanced by promyelocytic leukemia protein (PML) expression. Proc Natl Acad Sci U S A 101(39):14252–14257
24. Day PM, Lowy DR, Schiller JT (2003) Papillomaviruses infect cells via a clathrin-dependent pathway. Virology 307(1):1–11
25. Conger KL, Liu J-S, Kuo S-R, Chow LT, Wang TSF (1999) Human papillomavirus DNA replication. Interactions between the viral E1 protein and two subunits of human DNA polymerase alpha/primase. J Biol Chem 274:2696–2705
26. Han Y, Loo Y-M, Militello KT, Melendy T (1999) Interactions of the papovavirus DNA replication initiator proteins, bovine papillomavirus type 1 E1 and simian virus 40 large T antigen, with human replication protein A. J Virol 73:4899–4907
27. Loo Y-M, Melendy T (2004) Recruitment of replication protein A by the papillomavirus E1 protein and modulation by single-stranded DNA. J Virol 78:1605–1615
28. Masterson PJ, Stanley MA, Lewis AP, Romanos MA (1998) A C-terminal helicase domain of the human papillomavirus E1 protein binds E2 and the DNA polymerase alpha-primase p68 subunit. J Virol 72:7407–7419
29. Demeret C, Goyat S, Yaniv M, Thierry F (1998) The human papillomavirus type 18 (HPV18) replication protein E1 is a transcriptional activator when interacting with HPV18 E2. Virology 242(2):378–386
30. Steger G, Corbach S (1997) Dose-dependent regulation of the early promoter of human papillomavirus type 18 by the viral E2 protein. J Virol 71:50–58
31. Doorbar J, Ely S, Sterling J, McLean C, Crawford L (1991) Specific interaction between HPV-16 E1-E4 and cytokeratins results in collapse of the epithelial cell intermediate filament network. Nature 352(6338):824–827
32. Hwang ES, Nottoli T, Dimaio D (1995) The HPV16 E5 protein: expression, detection, and stable complex formation with transmembrane proteins in COS cells. Virology 211(1):227–233
33. Crusius K, Rodriguez I, Alonso A (2000) The human papillomavirus type 16 E5 protein modulates ERK1/2 and p38 MAP kinase activation by an EGFR-independent process in stressed human keratinocytes. Virus genes 20(1):65–69
34. Disbrow GL, Hanover JA, Schlegel R (2005) Endoplasmic reticulum-localized human papillomavirus type 16 E5 protein alters endosomal pH but not trans-Golgi pH. J Virol 79:5839–5846
35. Straight SW, Herman B, McCance DJ (1995) The E5 oncoprotein of human papillomavirus type 16 inhibits the acidification of endosomes in human keratinocytes. J Virol 69:3185–3192
36. Oh ST, Longworth MS, Laimins LA (2004) Roles of the E6 and E7 proteins in the life cycle of low-risk human papillomavirus type 11. J Virol 78(5):2620–2626
37. Thomas JT, Hubert WG, Ruesch MN, Laimins LA (1999) Human papillomavirus type 31 oncoproteins E6 and E7 are required for the maintenance of episomes during the viral life cycle in normal human keratinocytes. Proc Natl Acad Sci U S A 96(15):8449–8454
38. Stoler MH, Rhodes CR, Whitbeck A, Wolinsky SM, Chow LT, Broker TR (1992) Human papillomavirus type 16 and 18 gene expression in cervical neoplasias. Hum Pathol 23(2):117–128
39. Durst M, Glitz D, Schneider A, zur Hausen H (1992) Human papillomavirus type 16 (HPV 16) gene expression and DNA replication in cervical neoplasia: analysis by in situ hybridization. Virology 189(1):132–140
40. Oh JM, Kim SH, Cho EA, Song YS, Kim WH, Juhnn YS (2010) Human papillomavirus type 16 E5 protein inhibits hydrogen peroxide-induced apoptosis by stimulating ubiquitin/proteasome-mediated degradation of Bax in human cervical cancer cells. Carcinogenesis 31(3):402–410

41. Oh JM, Kim SH, Lee YI, Seo M, Kim SY, Song YS, Kim WH, Juhnn YS (2009) Human papillomavirus E5 protein induces expression of the EP4 subtype of prostaglandin E2 receptor in cyclic AMP response element-dependent pathways in cervical cancer cells. Carcinogenesis 30(1):141–149
42. Kim SH, Oh JM, No JH, Bang YJ, Juhnn YS, Song YS (2009) Involvement of NF-kappaB and AP-1 in COX-2 upregulation by human papillomavirus 16 E5 oncoprotein. Carcinogenesis 30(5):753–757
43. Stoppler MC, Straight SW, Tsao G, Schlegel R, McCance DJ (1996) The E5 gene of HPV-16 enhances keratinocyte immortalization by full-length DNA. Virology 223(1):251–254
44. zur Hausen H (2002) Papillomaviruses and cancer: from basic studies to clinical application. Nat Rev Cancer 2(5):342–350
45. Duensing S, Munger K (2004) Mechanisms of genomic instability in human cancer: insights from studies with human papillomavirus oncoproteins. Int J Cancer 109(2):157–162
46. Horner SM, DeFilippis RA, Manuelidis L, DiMaio D (2004) Repression of the human papillomavirus E6 gene initiates p53-dependent, telomerase-independent senescence and apoptosis in HeLa cervical carcinoma cells. J Virol 78(8):4063–4073
47. Plug-DeMaggio AW, Sundsvold T, Wurscher MA, Koop JI, Klingelhutz AJ, McDougall JK (2004) Telomere erosion and chromosomal instability in cells expressing the HPV oncogene 16E6. Oncogene 23(20):3561–3571
48. Jackson S, Harwood C, Thomas M, Banks L, Storey A (2000) Role of Bak in UV-induced apoptosis in skin cancer and abrogation by HPV E6 proteins. Genes Dev 14(23):3065–3073
49. Oda H, Kumar S, Howley PM (1999) Regulation of the Src family tyrosine kinase Blk through E6AP-mediated ubiquitination. Proc Natl Acad Sci U S A 96(17):9557–9562
50. Li X, Coffino P (1996) High-risk human papillomavirus E6 protein has two distinct binding sites within p53, of which only one determines degradation. J Virol 70(7):4509–4516
51. Crook T, Tidy JA, Vousden KH (1991) Degradation of p53 can be targeted by HPV E6 sequences distinct from those required for p53 binding and trans-activation. Cell 67(3):547–556
52. Werness BA, Levine AJ, Howley PM (1990) Association of human papillomavirus types 16 and 18 E6 proteins with p53. Science 248(4951):76–79
53. Scheffner M, Werness BA, Huibregtse JM, Levine AJ, Howley PM (1990) The E6 oncoprotein encoded by human papillomavirus types 16 and 18 promotes the degradation of p53. Cell 63(6):1129–1136
54. Klingelhutz AJ, Foster SA, McDougall JK (1996) Telomerase activation by the E6 gene product of human papillomavirus type 16. Nature 380(6569):79–82
55. Rincon-Orozco B, Halec G, Rosenberger S et al (2009) Epigenetic silencing of interferon-kappa in human papillomavirus type 16-positive cells. Cancer Res 69(22):8718–8725
56. Cheng S, Schmidt-Grimminger DC, Murant T, Broker TR, Chow LT (1995) Differentiation-dependent up-regulation of the human papillomavirus E7 gene reactivates cellular DNA replication in suprabasal differentiated keratinocytes. Genes Dev 9(19):2335–2349
57. Heck DV, Yee CL, Howley PM, Munger K (1992) Efficiency of binding the retinoblastoma protein correlates with the transforming capacity of the E7 oncoproteins of the human papillomaviruses. Proc Natl Acad Sci U S A 89(10):4442–4446
58. Gage JR, Meyers C, Wettstein FO (1990) The E7 proteins of the nononcogenic human papillomavirus type 6b (HPV-6b) and of the oncogenic HPV-16 differ in retinoblastoma protein binding and other properties. J Virol 64(2):723–730
59. Munger K, Werness BA, Dyson N, Phelps WC, Harlow E, Howley PM (1989) Complex formation of human papillomavirus E7 proteins with the retinoblastoma tumor suppressor gene product. EMBO J 8(13):4099–4105
60. Gonzalez SL, Stremlau M, He X, Basile JR, Munger K (2001) Degradation of the retinoblastoma tumor suppressor by the human papillomavirus type 16 E7 oncoprotein is important for functional inactivation and is separable from proteasomal degradation of E7. J Virol 75(16):7583–7591
61. Munger K, Basile JR, Duensing S, Eichten A, Gonzalez SL, Grace M, Zacny VL (2001) Biological activities and molecular targets of the human papillomavirus E7 oncoprotein. Oncogene 20(54):7888–7898

62. Zerfass K, Schulze A, Spitkovsky D, Friedman V, Henglein B, Jansen-Durr P (1995) Sequential activation of cyclin E and cyclin A gene expression by human papillomavirus type 16 E7 through sequences necessary for transformation. J Virol 69(10):6389–6399
63. Jones DL, Alani RM, Munger K (1997) The human papillomavirus E7 oncoprotein can uncouple cellular differentiation and proliferation in human keratinocytes by abrogating p21Cip1-mediated inhibition of cdk2. Genes Dev 11(16):2101–2111
64. Funk JO, Waga S, Harry JB, Espling E, Stillman B, Galloway DA (1997) Inhibition of CDK activity and PCNA-dependent DNA replication by p21 is blocked by interaction with the HPV-16 E7 oncoprotein. Genes Dev 11:2090–2100
65. Zerfass-Thome K, Zwerschke W, Mannhardt B, Tindle R, Botz JW, Jansen-Durr P (1996) Inactivation of the cdk inhibitor p27KIP1 by the human papillomavirus type 16 E7 oncoprotein. Oncogene 13(11):2323–2330
66. Martin LG, Demers GW, Galloway DA (1998) Disruption of the G1/S transition in human papillomavirus type 16 E7-expressing human cells is associated with altered regulation of cyclin E. J Virol 72(2):975–985
67. Menges CW, Baglia LA, Lapoint R, McCance DJ (2006) Human papillomavirus type 16 E7 up-regulates AKT activity through the retinoblastoma protein. Cancer Res 66(11):5555–5559
68. McDougall JK (1994) Immortalization and transformation of human cells by human papillomavirus. Curr Top Microbiol Immunol 186:101–119
69. Thomas JT, Laimins LA (1998) Human papillomavirus oncoproteins E6 and E7 independently abrogate the mitotic spindle checkpoint. J Virol 72(2):1131–1137
70. Zhao W, Noya F, Chen WY, Townes TM, Chow LT, Broker TR (1999) Trichostatin A up-regulates human papillomavirus type 11 upstream regulatory region-E6 promoter activity in undifferentiated primary human keratinocytes. J Virol 73(6):5026–5033
71. Kalantari M, Calleja-Macias IE, Tewari D, Hagmar B, Lie K, Barrera-Saldana HA, Wiley DJ, Bernard HU (2004) Conserved methylation patterns of human papillomavirus type 16 DNA in asymptomatic infection and cervical neoplasia. J Virol 78(23):12762–12772
72. Turan T, Kalantari M, Calleja-Macias IE et al (2006) Methylation of the human papillomavirus-18 L1 gene: a biomarker of neoplastic progression? Virology 349(1):175–183
73. Turan T, Kalantari M, Cuschieri K, Cubie HA, Skomedal H, Bernard HU (2007) High-throughput detection of human papillomavirus-18 L1 gene methylation, a candidate biomarker for the progression of cervical neoplasia. Virology 361(1):185–193
74. Durst M, Dzarlieva-Petrusevska RT, Boukamp P, Fusenig NE, Gissmann L (1987) Molecular and cytogenetic analysis of immortalized human primary keratinocytes obtained after transfection with human papillomavirus type 16 DNA. Oncogene 1(3):251–256
75. Pirisi L, Yasumoto S, Feller M, Doniger J, DiPaolo JA (1987) Transformation of human fibroblasts and keratinocytes with human papillomavirus type 16 DNA. J Virol 61(4):1061–1066
76. Munger K, Phelps WC, Bubb V, Howley PM, Schlegel R (1989) The E6 and E7 genes of the human papillomavirus type 16 together are necessary and sufficient for transformation of primary human keratinocytes. J Virol 63(10):4417–4421
77. Hawley-Nelson P, Vousden KH, Hubbert NL, Lowy DR, Schiller JT (1989) HPV16 E6 and E7 proteins cooperate to immortalize human foreskin keratinocytes. EMBO J 8(12):3905–3910
78. Chen TM, Pecoraro G, Defendi V (1993) Genetic analysis of in vitro progression of human papillomavirus-transfected human cervical cells. Cancer Res 53(5):1167–1171
79. Seagon S, Durst M (1994) Genetic analysis of an in vitro model system for human papillomavirus type 16-associated tumorigenesis. Cancer Res 54(21):5593–5598
80. Psyrri A, DeFilippis RA, Edwards AP, Yates KE, Manuelidis L, DiMaio D (2004) Role of the retinoblastoma pathway in senescence triggered by repression of the human papillomavirus E7 protein in cervical carcinoma cells. Cancer Res 64(9):3079–3086
81. Steenbergen RD, Walboomers JM, Meijer CJ, van der Raaij-Helmer EM, Parker JN, Chow LT, Broker TR, Snijders PJ (1996) Transition of human papillomavirus type 16 and 18 transfected human foreskin keratinocytes towards immortality: activation of telomerase and allele losses at 3p, 10p, 11q and/or 18q. Oncogene 13(6):1249–1257

82. Klingelhutz AJ, Barber SA, Smith PP, Dyer K, McDougall JK (1994) Restoration of telomeres in human papillomavirus-immortalized human anogenital epithelial cells. Mol Cell Biol 14(2):961–969
83. Kim NW, Piatyszek MA, Prowse KR et al (1994) Specific association of human telomerase activity with immortal cells and cancer. Science 266(5193):2011–2015
84. Meyerson M, Counter CM, Eaton EN et al (1997) hEST2, the putative human telomerase catalytic subunit gene, is up-regulated in tumor cells and during immortalization. Cell 90(4):785–795
85. Steenbergen RD, Kramer D, Meijer CJ et al (2001) Telomerase suppression by chromosome 6 in a human papillomavirus type 16-immortalized keratinocyte cell line and in a cervical cancer cell line. J Natl Cancer Inst 93(11):865–872
86. Sprague DL, Phillips SL, Mitchell CJ, Berger KL, Lace M, Turek LP, Klingelhutz AJ (2002) Telomerase activation in cervical keratinocytes containing stably replicating human papillomavirus type 16 episomes. Virology 301(2):247–254
87. Backsch C, Wagenbach N, Nonn M, Leistritz S, Stanbridge E, Schneider A, Durst M (2001) Microcell-mediated transfer of chromosome 4 into HeLa cells suppresses telomerase activity. Genes Chromosomes Cancer 31(2):196–198
88. Backsch C, Rudolph B, Kuhne-Heid R et al (2005) A region on human chromosome 4 (q35.1→qter) induces senescence in cell hybrids and is involved in cervical carcinogenesis. Genes Chromosomes Cancer 43(3):260–272
89. Poignee M, Backsch C, Beer K et al (2001) Evidence for a putative senescence gene locus within the chromosomal region 10p14-p15. Cancer Res 61(19):7118–7121
90. Uejima H, Mitsuya K, Kugoh H, Horikawa I, Oshimura M (1995) Normal human chromosome 2 induces cellular senescence in the human cervical carcinoma cell line SiHa. Genes Chromosomes Cancer 14(2):120–127
91. Snijders PJ, van Duin M, Walboomers JM, Steenbergen RD, Risse EK, Helmerhorst TJ, Verheijen RH, Meijer CJ (1998) Telomerase activity exclusively in cervical carcinomas and a subset of cervical intraepithelial neoplasia grade III lesions: strong association with elevated messenger RNA levels of its catalytic subunit and high-risk human papillomavirus DNA. Cancer Res 58(17):3812–3818
92. van Duin M, Steenbergen RD, de Wilde J, Helmerhorst TJ, Verheijen RH, Risse EK, Meijer CJ, Snijders PJ (2003) Telomerase activity in high-grade cervical lesions is associated with allelic imbalance at 6Q14-22. Int J Cancer 105(5):577–582
93. Koi M, Morita H, Yamada H, Satoh H, Barrett JC, Oshimura M (1989) Normal human chromosome 11 suppresses tumorigenicity of human cervical tumor cell line SiHa. Mol Carcinog 2(1):12–21
94. Hampton GM, Penny LA, Baergen RN et al (1994) Loss of heterozygosity in cervical carcinoma: subchromosomal localization of a putative tumor-suppressor gene to chromosome 11q22-q24. Proc Natl Acad Sci U S A 91(15):6953–6957
95. Steenbergen RD, Kramer D, Braakhuis BJ, Stern PL, Verheijen RH, Meijer CJ, Snijders PJ (2004) TSLC1 gene silencing in cervical cancer cell lines and cervical neoplasia. J Natl Cancer Inst 96(4):294–305
96. Shingai T, Ikeda W, Kakunaga S et al (2003) Implications of nectin-like molecule-2/IGSF4/RA175/SgIGSF/TSLC1/SynCAM1 in cell-cell adhesion and transmembrane protein localization in epithelial cells. J Biol Chem 278(37):35421–35427
97. Boles KS, Barchet W, Diacovo T, Cella M, Colonna M (2005) The tumor suppressor TSLC1/NECL-2 triggers NK-cell and CD8+ T-cell responses through the cell-surface receptor CRTAM. Blood 106(3):779–786
98. Soto U, Das BC, Lengert M, Finzer P, zur Hausen H, Rosl F (1999) Conversion of HPV 18 positive non-tumorigenic HeLa-fibroblast hybrids to invasive growth involves loss of TNF-alpha mediated repression of viral transcription and modification of the AP-1 transcription complex. Oncogene 18(21):3187–3198
99. Soto U, Denk C, Finzer P, Hutter KJ, zur Hausen H, Rosl F (2000) Genetic complementation to non-tumorigenicity in cervical-carcinoma cells correlates with alterations in AP-1 composition. Int J Cancer 86(6):811–817

100. Finzer P, Soto U, Delius H, Patzelt A, Coy JF, Poustka A, zur Hausen H, Rosl F (2000) Differential transcriptional regulation of the monocyte-chemoattractant protein-1 (MCP-1) gene in tumorigenic and non-tumorigenic HPV 18 positive cells: the role of the chromatin structure and AP-1 composition. Oncogene 19(29):3235–3244
101. Cheung TH, Leung JO, Chung TK, Lam SK, To KF, Wong YF (1997) c-fos overexpression is associated with the pathoneogenesis of invasive cervical cancer. Gynecol Obstet Invest 43(3):200–203
102. Heselmeyer K, Schrock E, du Manoir S, Blegen H, Shah K, Steinbeck R, Auer G, Ried T (1996) Gain of chromosome 3q defines the transition from severe dysplasia to invasive carcinoma of the uterine cervix. Proc Natl Acad Sci U S A 93(1):479–484
103. Papanicolaou GN, Traut HF (1941) The diagnostic value of vaginal smears in carcinoma of the uterus. Am J Obstet Gynecol 42:193–206
104. Parkin DM (1991) Screening for cervix cancer in developing countries. In: Miller AB (ed) Cancer screening. Cambridge University Press, Cambridge, pp 184–198
105. Cibas ES, Alonzo TA, Austin RM et al (2008) The MonoPrep Pap test for the detection of cervical cancer and its precursors. Part I: results of a multicenter clinical trial. Am J Clin Pathol 129(2):193–201
106. ACOG (2009 Dec) ACOG Education Pamphlet AP085 – The Pap Test
107. (1989) The 1988 Bethesda System for reporting cervical/vaginal cytologic diagnoses. Developed and approved at a National Cancer Institute Workshop, Bethesda, Maryland, U.S.A., December 12–13, 1988. Anal Quant Cytol Histol 11(5):291–297
108. Solomon D, Davey D, Kurman R et al (2002) The 2001 Bethesda System: terminology for reporting results of cervical cytology. JAMA 287(16):2114–2119
109. Zappacosta R, Rosini S (2008) Cervical cancer screening: from molecular basis to diagnostic practice, going through new technologies. Technol Cancer Res Treat 7(3):161–174
110. MonoPrep Pap Test – P040052. 2006. [cited 2010 Jan 2]; Available from: http://www.fda.gov/MedicalDevices/ProductsandMedicalProcedures/DeviceApprovalsandClearances/Recently-ApprovedDevices/ucm078291.htm
111. ThinPrep Pap Test. 2009 [cited 2010 Jan 2]; Available from: http://www.thinprep.com/index.html
112. BD SurePath Liquid-based Pap Test. 2010. [cited 2010 Jan 3]; Available from: http://www.bd.com/tripath/products/surepath/index.asp
113. Bernstein SJ, Sanchez-Ramos L, Ndubisi B (2001) Liquid-based cervical cytologic smear study and conventional Papanicolaou smears: a metaanalysis of prospective studies comparing cytologic diagnosis and sample adequacy. Am J Obstet Gynecol 185(2):308–317
114. Davey E, D'Assuncao J, Irwig L, Macaskill P, Chan SF, Richards A, Farnsworth A (2007) Accuracy of reading liquid based cytology slides using the ThinPrep Imager compared with conventional cytology: prospective study. BMJ 335(7609):31
115. Nance KV (2007) Evolution of Pap testing at a community hospital: a ten year experience. Diagn Cytopathol 35(3):148–153
116. Papillo JL, St John TL, Leiman G (2008) Effectiveness of the ThinPrep Imaging System: clinical experience in a low risk screening population. Diagn Cytopathol 36(3):155–160
117. Schiffman M, Adrianza ME (2000) ASCUS-LSIL Triage Study. Design, methods and characteristics of trial participants. Acta Cytol 44(5):726–742
118. Manos MM, Kinney WK, Hurley LB et al (1999) Identifying women with cervical neoplasia: using human papillomavirus DNA testing for equivocal Papanicolaou results. JAMA 281(17):1605–1610
119. Cox JT (2009) History of the use of HPV testing in cervical screening and in the management of abnormal cervical screening results. J Clin Virol 45(Suppl 1):S3–S12
120. Wright TC Jr, Massad LS, Dunton CJ, Spitzer M, Wilkinson EJ, Solomon D (2007) 2006 consensus guidelines for the management of women with abnormal cervical screening tests. J Low Genit Tract Dis 11(4):201–222
121. Wright TC Jr, Massad LS, Dunton CJ, Spitzer M, Wilkinson EJ, Solomon D (2007) 2006 consensus guidelines for the management of women with abnormal cervical cancer screening tests. Am J Obstet Gynecol 197(4):346–355

122. Arbyn M, Buntinx F, Van Ranst M, Paraskevaidis E, Martin-Hirsch P, Dillner J (2004) Virologic versus cytologic triage of women with equivocal Pap smears: a meta-analysis of the accuracy to detect high-grade intraepithelial neoplasia. J Natl Cancer Inst 96(4):280–293
123. Wright TC Jr, Lorincz A, Ferris DG, Richart RM, Ferenczy A, Mielzynska I, Borgatta L (1998) Reflex human papillomavirus deoxyribonucleic acid testing in women with abnormal Papanicolaou smears. Am J Obstet Gynecol 178(5):962–966
124. Caussy D, Orr W, Daya AD, Roth P, Reeves W, Rawls W (1988) Evaluation of methods for detecting human papillomavirus deoxyribonucleotide sequences in clinical specimens. J Clin Microbiol 26(2):236–243
125. The digene HPV Test. 2009. [cited 2010 Jan 4]; Available from: http://www.thehpvtest.com/default.html
126. Sandri MT, Lentati P, Benini E et al (2006) Comparison of the Digene HC2 assay and the Roche AMPLICOR human papillomavirus (HPV) test for detection of high-risk HPV genotypes in cervical samples. J Clin Microbiol 44(6):2141–2146
127. Roche Molecular Diagnostics Amplicor HPV Test. 2009 [cited 2010 Jan 4]; Available from: http://molecular.roche.com/diagnostics/hpv_ctng/hpv_test_1.html
128. Day SP, Hudson A, Mast A et al (2009) Analytical performance of the Investigational Use Only Cervista HPV HR test as determined by a multi-center study. J Clin Virol 45(Suppl 1):S63–S72
129. FDA Approves Two Hologic HPV Tests. 2009 March 13 [cited 2010 Jan 4]; Available from: http://www.hologic.com/news-releases/view/173-year.2009_173-id.234881444.html
130. Cervista HPV. 2009. [cited 2010 Jan 4]; Available from: http://www.cervistahpv.com/index.html
131. Qiao YL, Sellors JW, Eder PS et al (2008) A new HPV-DNA test for cervical-cancer screening in developing regions: a cross-sectional study of clinical accuracy in rural China. Lancet Oncol 9(10):929–936
132. Cuschieri K, Wentzensen N (2008) Human papillomavirus mRNA and p16 detection as biomarkers for the improved diagnosis of cervical neoplasia. Cancer Epidemiol Biomarkers Prev 17(10):2536–2545
133. Villa LL (2008) Assessment of new technologies for cervical cancer screening. Lancet Oncol 9(10):910–911
134. Lambert AP, Anschau F, Schmitt VM (2006) p16INK4A expression in cervical premalignant and malignant lesions. Exp Mol Pathol 80(2):192–196
135. Horn LC, Reichert A, Oster A et al (2008) Immunostaining for p16INK4a used as a conjunctive tool improves interobserver agreement of the histologic diagnosis of cervical intraepithelial neoplasia. Am J Surg Pathol 32(4):502–512
136. Carozzi F, Confortini M, Dalla Palma P et al (2008) Use of p16-INK4A overexpression to increase the specificity of human papillomavirus testing: a nested substudy of the NTCC randomised controlled trial. Lancet Oncol 9(10):937–945
137. Eleuterio J Jr, Giraldo PC, Goncalves AK, Cavalcante DI, de Almeida Ferreira FV, Mesquita SM, Morais SS (2007) Prognostic markers of high-grade squamous intraepithelial lesions: the role of p16INK4a and high-risk human papillomavirus. Acta Obstet Gynecol Scand 86(1):94–98
138. Asadurian Y, Kurilin H, Lichtig H, Jackman A, Gonen P, Tommasino M, Zehbe I, Sherman L (2007) Activities of human papillomavirus 16 E6 natural variants in human keratinocytes. J Med Virol 79(11):1751–1760
139. Wise-Draper TM, Wells SI (2008) Papillomavirus E6 and E7 proteins and their cellular targets. Front Biosci 13:1003–1017
140. Dixon EP, King LM, Adams MD et al (2008) Isolation of RNA from residual BD SurePath liquid-based cytology specimens and detection of HPV E6/E7 mRNA using the PreTectt HPV-Proofer assay. J Virol Methods 154(1–2):220–222
141. Jeantet D, Schwarzmann F, Tromp J, Melchers WJ, van der Wurff AA, Oosterlaken T, Jacobs M, Troesch A (2009) NucliSENS EasyQ HPV v1 test - Testing for oncogenic activity of human papillomaviruses. J Clin Virol 45(Suppl 1):S29–S37
142. Szarewski A, Ambroisine L, Cadman L et al (2008) Comparison of predictors for high-grade cervical intraepithelial neoplasia in women with abnormal smears. Cancer Epidemiol Biomarkers Prev 17(11):3033–3042

143. Dockter J, Schroder A, Hill C, Guzenski L, Monsonego J, Giachetti C (2009) Clinical performance of the APTIMA HPV Assay for the detection of high-risk HPV and high-grade cervical lesions. J Clin Virol 45(Suppl 1):S55–S61
144. Wright TC Jr, Massad LS, Dunton CJ, Spitzer M, Wilkinson EJ, Solomon D (2007) 2006 consensus guidelines for the management of women with cervical intraepithelial neoplasia or adenocarcinoma in situ. J Low Genit Tract Dis 11(4):223–239
145. Helmerhorst TJ (1992) Clinical significance of endocervical curettage as part of colposcopic evaluation. A review. Int J Gynecol Cancer 2(5):256–262
146. Hoffman MS, Sterghos S Jr, Gordy LW, Gunasekaran S, Cavanagh D (1993) Evaluation of the cervical canal with the endocervical brush. Obstet Gynecol 82(4 Pt 1):573–577
147. Klam S, Arseneau J, Mansour N, Franco E, Ferenczy A (2000) Comparison of endocervical curettage and endocervical brushing. Obstet Gynecol 96(1):90–94
148. Mitchell MF, Tortolero-Luna G, Cook E, Whittaker L, Rhodes-Morris H, Silva E (1998) A randomized clinical trial of cryotherapy, laser vaporization, and loop electrosurgical excision for treatment of squamous intraepithelial lesions of the cervix. Obstet Gynecol 92(5):737–744
149. Townsend DE, Richart RM (1983) Cryotherapy and carbon dioxide laser management of cervical intraepithelial neoplasia: a controlled comparison. Obstet Gynecol 61(1):75–78
150. Stafl A, Wilkinson EJ, Mattingly RF (1977) Laser treatment of cervical and vaginal neoplasia. Am J Obstet Gynecol 128(2):128–136
151. Zhou J, Sun XY, Davies H, Crawford L, Park D, Frazer IH (1992) Definition of linear antigenic regions of the HPV16 L1 capsid protein using synthetic virion-like particles. Virology 189(2):592–599
152. Breitburd F, Kirnbauer R, Hubbert NL, Nonnenmacher B, Trin-Dinh-Desmarquet C, Orth G, Schiller JT, Lowy DR (1995) Immunization with viruslike particles from cottontail rabbit papillomavirus (CRPV) can protect against experimental CRPV infection. J Virol 69(6):3959–3963
153. Lin YL, Borenstein LA, Ahmed R, Wettstein FO (1993) Cottontail rabbit papillomavirus L1 protein-based vaccines: protection is achieved only with a full-length, nondenatured product. J Virol 67(7):4154–4162
154. Hagensee ME, Yaegashi N, Galloway DA (1993) Self-assembly of human papillomavirus type 1 capsids by expression of the L1 protein alone or by coexpression of the L1 and L2 capsid proteins. J Virol 67(1):315–322
155. Heino P, Dillner J, Schwartz S (1995) Human papillomavirus type 16 capsid proteins produced from recombinant Semliki Forest virus assemble into virus-like particles. Virology 214(2):349–359
156. Kirnbauer R, Booy F, Cheng N, Lowy DR, Schiller JT (1992) Papillomavirus L1 major capsid protein self-assembles into virus-like particles that are highly immunogenic. Proc Natl Acad Sci U S A 89(24):12180–12184
157. Rose RC, Reichman RC, Bonnez W (1994) Human papillomavirus (HPV) type 11 recombinant virus-like particles induce the formation of neutralizing antibodies and detect HPV-specific antibodies in human sera. J Gen Virol 75(Pt 8):2075–2079
158. Sasagawa T, Pushko P, Steers G, Gschmeissner SE, Hajibagheri MA, Finch J, Crawford L, Tommasino M (1995) Synthesis and assembly of virus-like particles of human papillomaviruses type 6 and type 16 in fission yeast *Schizosaccharomyces pombe*. Virology 206(1):126–135
159. Nardelli-Haefliger D, Roden RB, Benyacoub J et al (1997) Human papillomavirus type 16 virus-like particles expressed in attenuated Salmonella typhimurium elicit mucosal and systemic neutralizing antibodies in mice. Infect Immun 65(8):3328–3336
160. Ghim SJ, Jenson AB, Schlegel R (1992) HPV-1 L1 protein expressed in cos cells displays conformational epitopes found on intact virions. Virology 190(1):548–552
161. Koutsky LA, Ault KA, Wheeler CM, Brown DR, Barr E, Alvarez FB, Chiacchierini LM, Jansen KU (2002) A controlled trial of a human papillomavirus type 16 vaccine. N Engl J Med 347(21):1645–1651

162. Evans TG, Bonnez W, Rose RC et al (2001) A Phase 1 study of a recombinant viruslike particle vaccine against human papillomavirus type 11 in healthy adult volunteers. J Infect Dis 183(10):1485–1493
163. Harro CD, Pang YY, Roden RB et al (2001) Safety and immunogenicity trial in adult volunteers of a human papillomavirus 16 L1 virus-like particle vaccine. J Natl Cancer Inst 93(4):284–292
164. Harper DM (2009) Currently approved prophylactic HPV vaccines. Expert Rev Vaccines 8(12):1663–1679
165. FDA Approves New Vaccine for Prevention of Cervical Cancer. 2009 Oct 16 [cited 2009 Dec 29]; Available from: http://www.fda.gov/NewsEvents/Newsroom/PressAnnouncements/ucm187048.htm
166. FDA Approves New Indication for Gardasil to Prevent Genital Warts in Men and Boys. 2009 Oct 16 Dec 29 2009 [cited 2009 Dec 29]; Available from: http://www.fda.gov/NewsEvents/Newsroom/PressAnnouncements/ucm187003.htm
167. Einstein MH, Baron M, Levin MJ et al (2009) Comparison of the immunogenicity and safety of Cervarix() and Gardasil((R)) human papillomavirus (HPV) cervical cancer vaccines in healthy women aged 18-45 years. Hum Vaccin 5(10):705–719
168. Munoz N, Manalastas R Jr, Pitisuttithum P et al (2009) Safety, immunogenicity, and efficacy of quadrivalent human papillomavirus (types 6, 11, 16, 18) recombinant vaccine in women aged 24-45 years: a randomised, double-blind trial. Lancet 373(9679):1949–1957
169. Kjaer SK, Sigurdsson K, Iversen OE et al (2009) A pooled analysis of continued prophylactic efficacy of quadrivalent human papillomavirus (Types 6/11/16/18) vaccine against high-grade cervical and external genital lesions. Cancer Prev Res (Phila Pa) 2(10):868–878
170. Paavonen J, Naud P, Salmeron J et al (2009) Efficacy of human papillomavirus (HPV)-16/18 AS04-adjuvanted vaccine against cervical infection and precancer caused by oncogenic HPV types (PATRICIA): final analysis of a double-blind, randomised study in young women. Lancet 374(9686):301–314
171. David MP, Van Herck K, Hardt K, Tibaldi F, Dubin G, Descamps D, Van Damme P (2009) Long-term persistence of anti-HPV-16 and -18 antibodies induced by vaccination with the AS04-adjuvanted cervical cancer vaccine: modeling of sustained antibody responses. Gynecol Oncol 2009 Dec; 115 (3 Suppl):51–56
172. Rowhani-Rahbar A, Mao C, Hughes JP, Alvarez FB, Bryan JT, Hawes SE, Weiss NS, Koutsky LA (2009) Longer term efficacy of a prophylactic monovalent human papillomavirus type 16 vaccine. Vaccine 27(41):5612–5619
173. Garland SM, Hernandez-Avila M, Wheeler CM et al (2007) Quadrivalent vaccine against human papillomavirus to prevent anogenital diseases. N Engl J Med 356(19):1928–1943
174. Paavonen J, Jenkins D, Bosch FX et al (2007) Efficacy of a prophylactic adjuvanted bivalent L1 virus-like-particle vaccine against infection with human papillomavirus types 16 and 18 in young women: an interim analysis of a phase III double-blind, randomised controlled trial. Lancet 369(9580):2161–2170
175. Reisinger KS, Block SL, Lazcano-Ponce E et al (2007) Safety and persistent immunogenicity of a quadrivalent human papillomavirus types 6, 11, 16, 18 L1 virus-like particle vaccine in preadolescents and adolescents: a randomized controlled trial. Pediatr Infect Dis J 26(3):201–209
176. Mao C, Koutsky LA, Ault KA et al (2006) Efficacy of human papillomavirus-16 vaccine to prevent cervical intraepithelial neoplasia: a randomized controlled trial. Obstet Gynecol 107(1):18–27
177. Block SL, Nolan T, Sattler C et al (2006) Comparison of the immunogenicity and reactogenicity of a prophylactic quadrivalent human papillomavirus (types 6, 11, 16, and 18) L1 virus-like particle vaccine in male and female adolescents and young adult women. Pediatrics 118(5):2135–2145
178. Harper DM, Franco EL, Wheeler CM et al (2006) Sustained efficacy up to 4.5 years of a bivalent L1 virus-like particle vaccine against human papillomavirus types 16 and 18: follow-up from a randomised control trial. Lancet 367(9518):1247–1255

179. Munoz N, Bosch FX, Castellsague X, Diaz M, de Sanjose S, Hammouda D, Shah KV, Meijer CJ (2004) Against which human papillomavirus types shall we vaccinate and screen? The international perspective. Int J Cancer 111(2):278–285
180. Chen XS, Garcea RL, Goldberg I, Casini G, Harrison SC (2000) Structure of small virus-like particles assembled from the L1 protein of human papillomavirus 16. Mol Cell 5(3):557–567
181. Rose RC, White WI, Li M, Suzich JA, Lane C, Garcea RL (1998) Human papillomavirus type 11 recombinant L1 capsomeres induce virus-neutralizing antibodies. J Virol 72(7):6151–6154
182. Li M, Cripe TP, Estes PA, Lyon MK, Rose RC, Garcea RL (1997) Expression of the human papillomavirus type 11 L1 capsid protein in Escherichia coli: characterization of protein domains involved in DNA binding and capsid assembly. J Virol 71(4):2988–2995
183. Rechtsteiner G, Warger T, Osterloh P, Schild H, Radsak MP (2005) Cutting edge: priming of CTL by transcutaneous peptide immunization with imiquimod. J Immunol 174(5):2476–2480
184. Nardelli-Haefliger D, Lurati F, Wirthner D, Spertini F, Schiller JT, Lowy DR, Ponci F, De Grandi P (2005) Immune responses induced by lower airway mucosal immunisation with a human papillomavirus type 16 virus-like particle vaccine. Vaccine 23(28):3634–3641
185. Merck. A study of V503 in Preadolescents and Adolescents. 2009 [cited 2009 Dec 20]; Available from: http://clinicaltrials.gov/ct2/show/NCT00943722
186. Roden RB, Gravitt P, Wu TC (2008) Towards global prevention of human papillomavirus-induced cancer. Eur J Immunol 38(2):323–326
187. Roden R, Monie A, Wu TC (2006) The impact of preventive HPV vaccination. Discov Med 6(35):175–181
188. Schiller JT, Castellsague X, Villa LL, Hildesheim A (2008) An update of prophylactic human papillomavirus L1 virus-like particle vaccine clinical trial results. Vaccine 26(Suppl 10):K53–K61
189. Hung CF, Ma B, Monie A, Tsen SW, Wu TC (2008) Therapeutic human papillomavirus vaccines: current clinical trials and future directions. Expert Opin Biol Ther 8(4):421–439

Chapter 22
Pre-malignant Disease in the Prostate

Alastair D. Lamb, Anne Y. Warren, and David E. Neal

Abstract Carcinoma of the prostate (CaP) is the most common non-cutaneous cancer in men and the second most common cause of cancer related death. Mortality remains high despite improvements in diagnosis in the developed world. A better understanding of the mechanisms involved in the development of prostate cancer should allow targeted diagnosis, prevention and treatment, and may improve mortality. In this chapter, we outline the two principal pre-malignant histological types, prostate intraepithelial neoplasia (PIN) and atypical small acinar proliferation (ASAP) and the likelihood of progression to CaP if these diagnoses are made. We then assess current understanding of factors contributing to the initiation of pre-malignant disease and progression to CaP as they relate to stem cells, inflammation, diet and specific genetic mutations or aberrant pathways. Finally, we discuss the translational potential of these factors in early detection and prevention of CaP.

Introduction

Carcinoma of the prostate (CaP) is the most common non-cutaneous cancer in men and the second most common cause of cancer related death, killing approximately 10,000 men annually in the UK [1]. The majority of prostate cancer deaths occur in men aged 65 and over (Fig. 22.1); however, the disease is also found amongst younger men, with prevalence rates of up to 30% in 30–50 year olds reported on post-mortem analysis [2]. There is a 15-fold variation in prostate cancer mortality rates worldwide, and although North America ranks first in terms of incidence, mainly owing to high levels of PSA testing, it is eighth for mortality, with the highest mortality rates being recorded in the Caribbean (Fig. 22.2). Countries with higher levels of PSA testing detect a greater proportion of early stage disease, the consequent lead-time bias

A.D. Lamb (✉)
CRUK Cambridge Research Institute, Addenbrooke's Hospital, University Department of Uro-Oncology, Cambridge CB2 0QQ, UK
e-mail: alastair.lamb@cancer.org.uk

R.C. Fitzgerald (ed.), *Pre-Invasive Disease: Pathogenesis and Clinical Management*,
DOI 10.1007/978-1-4419-6694-0_22,

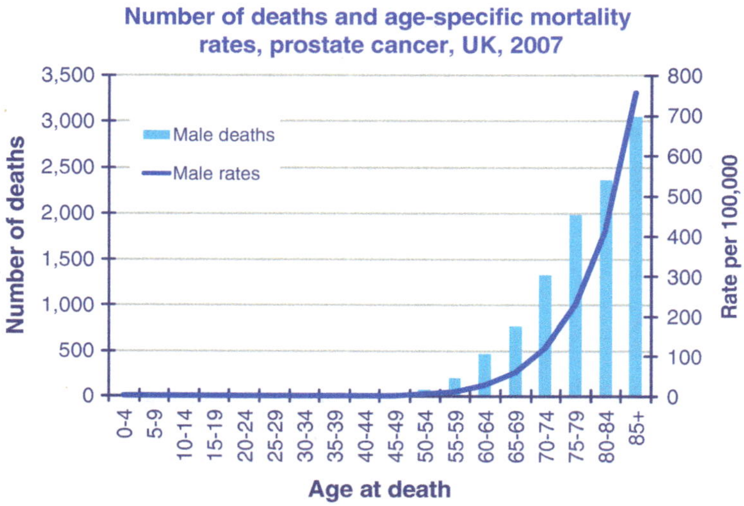

Fig. 22.1 UK age-specific mortality rates in 2007

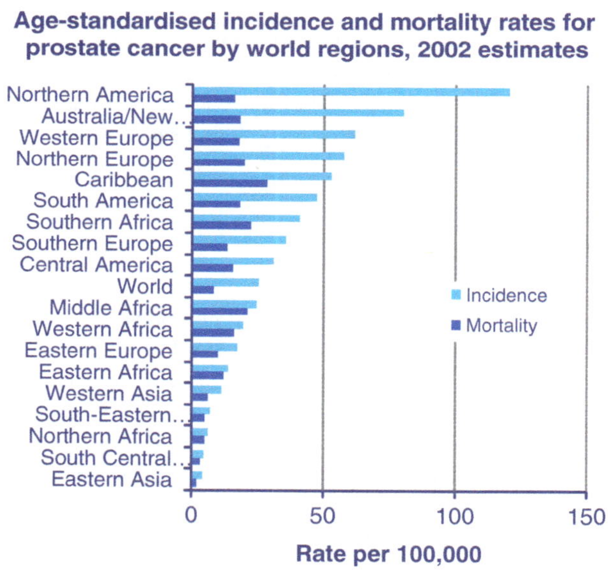

Fig. 22.2 World age-standardised incidence and mortality in 2002

giving higher survival rates compared to incidence [3]. Overall in the United Kingdom, prostate cancer mortality was fairly stable, but began to increase in the early 1980s. Mortality peaked in the early 1990s when the age-standardised death rate reached 30 per 100,000 in 1992. Since then there has been a slight fall in rates and in 2007, the age standardised rate was 25 per 100,000 (Fig. 22.3) [4]. Prostate cancer mortality remains high despite improvements in diagnosis in the developed world.

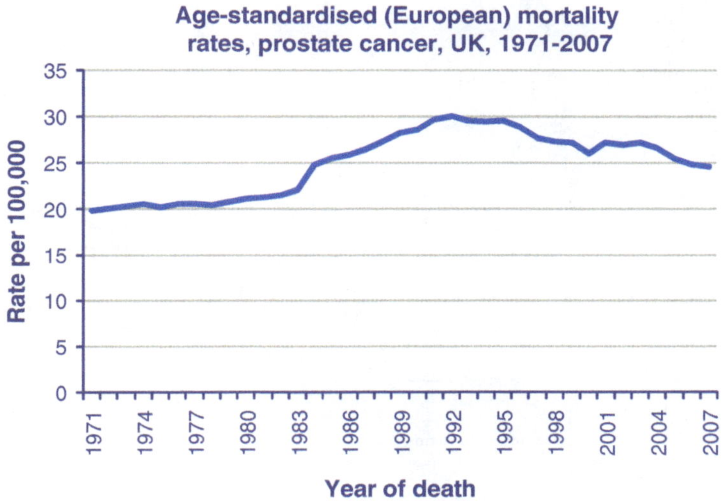

Fig. 22.3 UK mortality rates for three decades with age standardised to European averages

A better understanding of the mechanisms involved in the development of prostate cancer would allow targeted diagnosis, prevention and treatment, and may improve mortality.

Prostate cancer is a heterogeneous, often multifocal disease with numerous factors contributing to its initiation and progression. In this chapter, the two principal pre-malignant histological types will be outlined and current understanding of factors contributing to development of CaP will be assessed as they relate to stem cells, inflammation, diet and specific genetic mutations or aberrant pathways. Finally, the translational potential of these factors in early detection and prevention of CaP will be discussed.

Normal Prostate

The prostate is an accessory sexual organ with *exocrine* and *endocrine* functions, responsible for production and storage of 25–30% of constituents of the seminal fluid. Prostatic fluid is alkaline, which protects spermatozoa in the acidic environment of the vagina. The protein content of prostatic secretions is less than 1% and includes proteolytic enzymes, prostate acid phosphatase and prostate specific antigen as well as minerals such as zinc (free and protein bound) which has antimicrobial and semen coagulant effects [5, 6].

The prostate develops as part of the urogenital sinus (endodermal in origin) with contributions from the *Wolffian ducts* and from the surrounding mesenchyme. The prostate consists of branching ducts and *acini* which are often referred to as prostate glands collectively. The cells lining ducts and acini are identical with the exception of the larger peri-urethral ducts that have a urothelial lining. There are four main

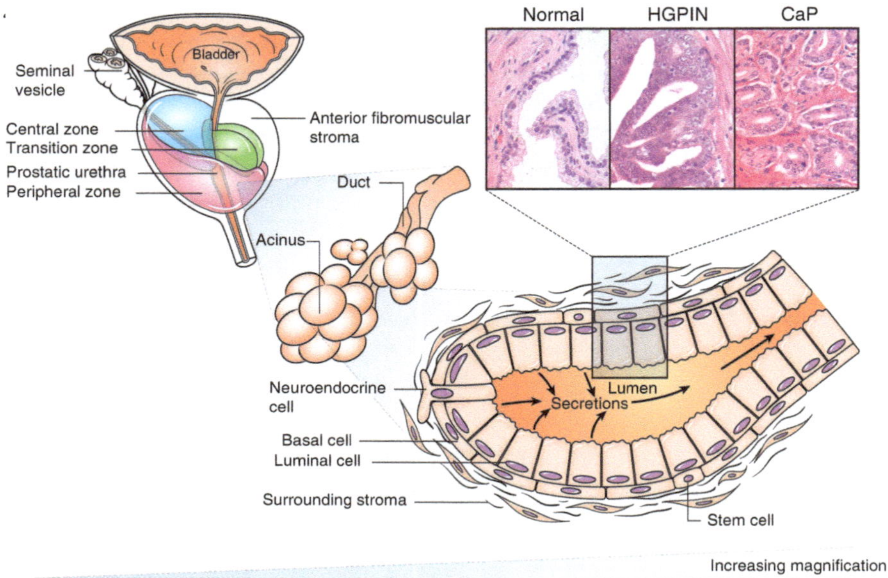

Fig. 22.4 Schematic of the prostate from organ to glands (ducts and acini). Different cell-types shown. Haematoxylin and Eosin sections show normal prostate, prostatic intraepithelial neoplasia (PIN) and Gleason score 6 carcinoma

anatomically distinct cell types (Fig. 22.4). First, prostate basal cells form a largely structural basal layer encircling each prostatic duct or acinus. Second, luminal (or glandular) cells form a columnar layer that make up the functional secretory surface of the glandular lumen. Third, rare neuroendocrine cells are interspersed between the basal and luminal cells. These are endocrine and sensory cells thought to share structural, functional and metabolic properties with neuronal cells found in the prostate. They secrete neuroendocrine peptides that support epithelial growth and viability [7]. Fourth, stromal cells surround the prostate glandular structures to guide and support growth and differentiation of the epithelium. Stromal cells include fibroblasts, myofibroblasts and smooth muscle cells and are derived from mesenchyme. Stem cells are generally thought to reside in the basal layer of the prostate contributing to all epithelial cell types of the prostate. The significance of prostate stem cells in development of prostate cancer will be discussed.

Prostatic Intraepithelial Neoplasia

Prostatic intra-epithelial neoplasia (PIN) is defined as the presence of cytologically atypical cells within a generally normal ductal or acinar outline in the presence of a basal layer of cells. PIN is conventionally divided into low grade (LG) and high grade (HG). Morphologically, HGPIN is identified by enlarged, crowded, often multilayered nuclei with irregular spacing, prominent nucleoli and amphophilic cytoplasm, features also found in high *Gleason* grade carcinoma (Fig. 22.4) [8]. The essential distinguishing feature between HGPIN and carcinoma is the presence of basal cells, which, though often patchy in HGPIN are always present [9]. LGPIN, by contrast, shows a lesser degree of atypia and lacks prominent nucleoli. Clinically, LGPIN is not reported as such because of poor reproducibility and uncertain diagnostic significance, instead being classified as benign prostatic tissue [10]. Genetic and molecular factors contributing towards the development of PIN will be discussed in subsequent sections.

There is strong histological evidence implicating HGPIN as a pre-neoplastic lesion. Morphologically, HGPIN is primarily found in the peripheral zone, in proximity to invasive CaP [11], is multifocal and similar in cytological appearance to CaP [6], and it generally precedes CaP by at least 10 years, consistent with a linear progression [2, 12]. At a cellular level, HGPIN displays similar chromosomal abnormalities to early invasive CaP [13] as well as similar markers of differentiation [14]. However, the question remains open as to whether PIN is truly a precursor lesion of CaP or whether the two conditions are simply commonly associated.

A diagnosis of PIN has important clinical implications. There is general consensus regarding the diagnosis of HGPIN and also regarding the general relationship of HGPIN to CaP [8, 15, 16]. The reported incidence of HGPIN on transrectal ultrasound (TRUS) biopsy varies considerably at 0.6–24% (mean 7.7%), largely dependent on variation in the population under study, with HGPIN incidence increasing with age [17]. There is less consensus regarding the actual risk of diagnosing CaP on repeat biopsy with figures ranging from 50% from studies in the 1990s compared to 20% in recent studies, which is little different from the risk after a "normal" biopsy [17, 18]. The explanation lies in the extent of HGPIN and timing of biopsy. HGPIN that is multifocal and present throughout the gland, as determined by involvement of multiple (two or more cores) biopsies, is associated with a 39–80% risk of CaP depending on the study [19, 20]. Similarly, delaying biopsy has been reported to increase the detection rate of CaP from 25% at 6 months to 44.6% at 1 year [21]. This has led to the advice that patients with HGPIN in more than one core should have repeat biopsies after a 1 year interval [22].

Atypical Small Acinar Proliferation

Atypical small acinar proliferation (ASAP) describes a group of small, often closely packed, acini that are regarded by the pathologist as being atypical, but lacking in sufficient morphological abnormalities to be regarded as unequivocally diagnostic of carcinoma. Although generally used to indicate a suspicion of malignancy, this term encompasses a range of pathological conditions including benign mimics of CaP such as atypical adenomatous hyperplasia (AAH) in the transition zone, reactive atypia and atrophy, high grade PIN and acini that are cytologically suspicious, but too few in number to allow a confident diagnosis of malignancy [8, 23]. ASAP is detectable in a mean of 5% of biopsies and is accepted as being highly predictive for CaP on subsequent biopsies, with a 34–60% second biopsy detection rate [17, 24]. Advice at the time of writing is for repeat biopsy in the presence of ASAP within 3–6 months [22].

The Role of Stem Cells in the Initiation of Prostate Cancer

Stem cells or early progenitors in the prostate are thought to reside in the basal layer of the prostate. This is based on the observation that there is preferential survival of the basal layer of the prostate during androgen ablation with apoptosis of androgen receptor (AR)-expressing differentiated luminal cells [25]. It is supported by findings that mice null for the basal cell marker p63 are born without prostates (or mammary glands) [26, 27]. The existence and site of prostate stem cells has been most recently elucidated following studies incorporating murine renal-subcapsular grafting of a single adult mouse prostate stem cell defined by *Lin⁻Sca-1⁺CD133⁺CD44⁺CD117⁺* and located in the periurethral prostate. These cells are able to generate functioning secreting prostate tissue with long term self renewal capacity as demonstrated by serial transplantation in vivo [28]. This prostate tissue contains all three epithelial cell-types including neuroendocrine cells, dispelling previous notions that this rarer prostate cell may have a distinct cell of origin, common with surrounding neuroectodermal or stromal cells (Fig. 22.5) [7]. The peri-urethral region in the mouse prostate is rich in basal cells and characterized by a morphologically distinct band of smooth muscle rich in TGF-β, known to promote stem cell quiescence, consistent with this site being a prostate stem cell niche [29]. However, the site of prostate stem cells remains controversial, with another recent paper identifying cells in the luminal epithelium with full regenerative potential, defined by NKX3-1⁺CK18⁺AR⁺ [30], and these studies are yet to be replicated with human tissue. This debate has important implications for the cell of origin in prostate cancer.

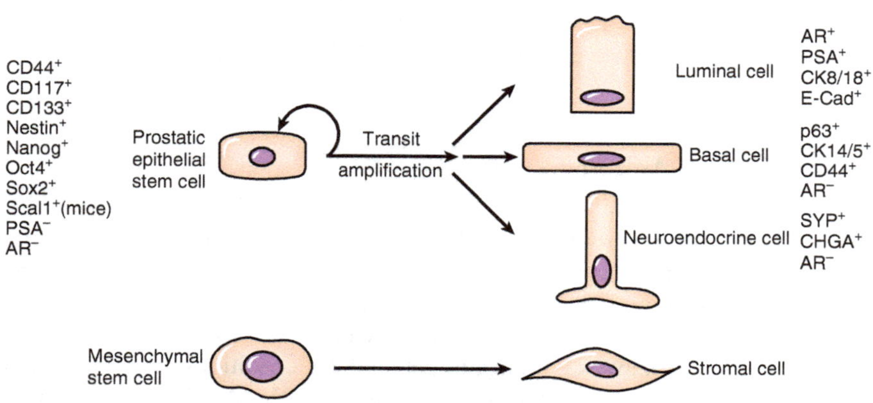

Fig. 22.5 Cell lineages of the prostate. The three epithelial cell types of the prostate are derived from a single epithelial stem cell. Stromal constituents are independently derived. Surface markers for different cell types as shown

The current dogma of stem cells as quiescent, slow-cycling cells, able to self-renew and pluripotent provides a strong case for these cells being the cell of origin in cancer. This was originally proposed in acute myeloid leukaemia [31], and subsequently many epithelial cancers including prostate [32–34]. Pathways that normally govern self-renewal or proliferation – such as PI3K [35], Wnt [36], SHh [37] and Notch [36] in haematopoietic, neural and epithelial systems – if dysregulated can contribute to tumorigenesis, for example in colon and mammary cancer, medulloblastoma, leukaemia and CaP. There are two main reasons for this. First, because stem cells have activated machinery for self-renewal, maintaining this activation may be easier than turning it on de novo. Second, if a number of mutations are required for neoplastic transformation to take place, then cells with longer lifespans have greater potential to accumulate these mutations and drive cancer [38]. The specific mutations involved in prostate cancer will be discussed later in this chapter.

Several properties of human prostate cancer suggest the disease may arise from a stem-like cancer initiating cell. The progression to androgen independent castrate resistant prostate cancer (CRPC) during androgen ablation therapy is consistent with prostate tumours containing populations of androgen-independent cells that survive and can expand in the absence of androgen. Given their androgen independent nature, prostate stem cells are a possible candidate. If the population of cells with such tumour regenerative potential is small this would fit with conventional wisdom regarding a precursor stem cell. However, it is also possible that a larger proportion of cells in a prostate tumour retains stem-like potential (a tumour is, after all, by definition, not fully differentiated), and when stressed by androgen ablation these cells alter their phenotype in a manner that is advantageous to their survival. One example of this is the propensity for castrate resistant prostate cancer to display a luminal to neuroendocrine shift [39].

Sub-populations of cells within prostate cancer cell lines with increased proliferative capacity in vitro and increased tumour initiating and metastatic capacity in vivo have been shown to possess a $CD44^{+}CD133^{+}CD117^{+}$ profile similar to prostate stem cells [34, 40, 41], as well as expressing $\alpha 2\beta 1$integrin consistent with membrane adhesional properties encouraging metastasis [34], and demonstrate higher levels of Oct4, Sox2, Nanog, Nestin [41–43], all markers of "stemness" or pluripotency. They are predominantly AR^{-}. However, they are also $p63^{-}$ [24, 41], suggesting that cancer stem cells are probably an intermediate cell type; not luminal, but not truly basal either.

In summary, prostate cancers are heterogeneous and contain subpopulations of cells that have increased tumorigenic potential compared to surrounding cells. These cells are characterised by markers that are similar, if not identical to those thought to define prostate stem cells. These "cancer stem cells" are thought by some to be the sites of initiation and maintenance of prostate cancer.

There are several questions that still need to be answered. First, most work on prostate cancer stem cells has been performed on cells that are already malignant – if prostate cancer stem cells really are transformed normal prostate stem cells then what is or are the initiating event/s? Which factors dysregulate the self-renewal pathways in normal prostate cancer stem cells? Second, can it be assumed that prostate cancer stem cells really are dysregulated normal prostate stem cells? Or, are they committed progenitors/transit amplifying cells which retain some self-renewal and multipotent properties? Or are they de-differentiated terminally differentiated (luminal) cells that re-acquire stem-like properties and phenotypic versatility when stressed (e.g. by androgen deprivation)? Third, if prostate cancer stem cells are the initiating event in prostate cancer, and the source of repopulation in recurrent tumours, is there a unifying pathway that can be targeted therapeutically either to destroy the stem cells with malignant potential, or to prevent expansion of their malignant progeny? There is no clear answer to any of these three questions at the time of writing.

The Role of Inflammation in the Initiation of Prostate Cancer

Chronic inflammation is implicated in the development of a diverse range of human cancers, with evidence causally linking it to several cancers of the gastrointestinal tract, bladder and lung [44]. In these cancers, inflammation often collaborates with environmental exposures such as dietary toxins to increase the risk further [45]. The molecular mechanisms that underlie the pathogenesis of inflammation-associated cancer are complex and involve both the adaptive and innate immune system [46–48]. The release of highly reactive compounds such as hydrogen peroxide, nitric oxide and superoxide by activated phagocytic cells of the innate immune system damages DNA in epithelial cells, leading to increased cell division to replace these damaged cells, these dividing cells then being further exposed to mutagenic agents. The release of cytokines by inflammatory cells promotes cell proliferation and stimulates angiogenesis further enhancing tumorigenesis. In addition, during chronic inflammation, T and B cell-mediated antibody activity of the adaptive immune response can cause excessive and prolonged activation of innate immune cells [47].

The prostate has been shown to harbour focal areas of epithelial atrophy, sometimes associated with inflammatory infiltrates. These are common in the ageing prostate and often encompass a large fraction of the peripheral zone [49]. Despite the atrophic architectural appearance, there is an increased fraction of epithelial cells in such lesions. One term that has been used to describe those which are also associated with an inflammatory infiltrate is proliferative inflammatory atrophy (PIA) [50]. These areas of PIA have been observed to transition to HGPIN and adenocarcinoma in morphological studies [51–54], although some debate persists regarding this continuum and the validity of the separation of PIA from other forms of atrophy [55, 56].

In most cases, the precise cause of prostatic inflammation is unclear. However, potential sources include (Fig. 22.6):

- Infectious agents (viral or bacterial)
- Reflux of urine into the prostatic ducts
- Hormonal agents (e.g. oestrogen)
- Dietary factors [57]

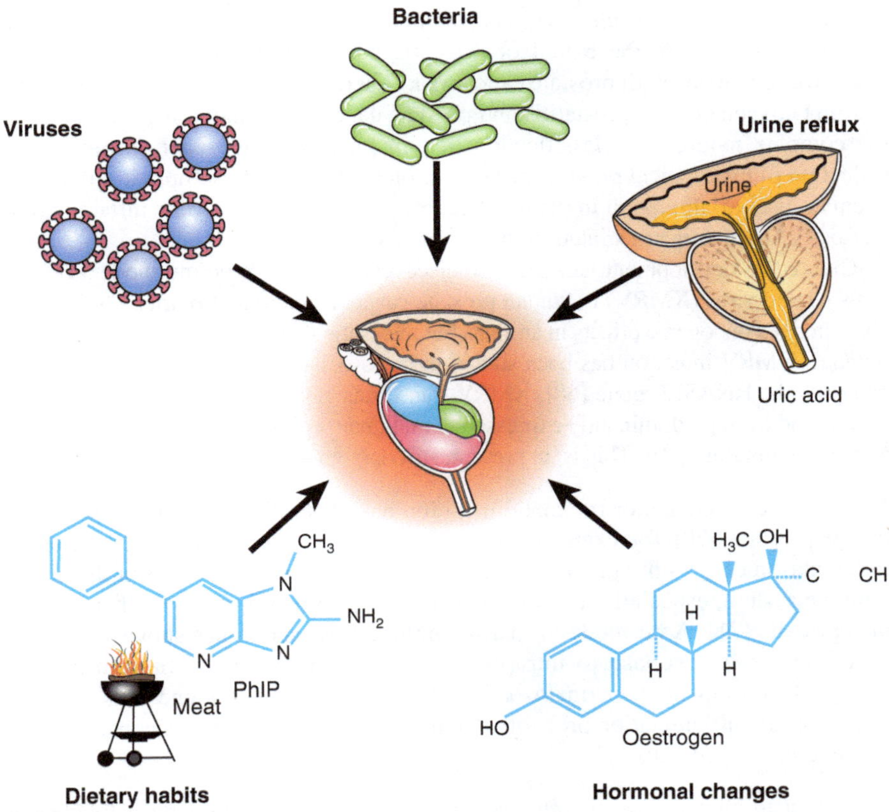

Fig. 22.6 Causes of inflammation in the prostate

Infectious agents. Sexually transmitted organisms that are known to infect the prostate include *Gonorrhoea* [58], *Chlamydia* [59], and *Trichomonas vaginalis* [60], while non-sexually transmitted bacteria include Gram-negative organisms such as *Escherichia coli* [61]. These can cause acute or chronic prostatitis, however severe acute inflammation and formation of prostatic abscesses is rare with antibiotic treatment, although TRUS biopsy of the prostate does increase this risk [62]. Nonetheless, asymptomatic infection and inflammation can still occur [58]. Viruses such as human papillomavirus (HPV) [63], cytomegalovirus (CMV) [64] and human herpes simplex virus (HSV) [65] have been detected in the prostate, although the extent to which they elicit an inflammatory response is largely unknown. It is possible that, in analogy to H. pylori in gastritis, there is a previously unidentified causative organism for PIA [57]. There is limited evidence linking specific infectious organisms with prostate cancer risk. This amounts to a lack of data rather than negative data per se, most likely due to the difficulties in assaying colonisation of the prostate. With prostatic massage being the only means of accurately obtaining prostatic fluid cultures directly from the prostate it is difficult to accurately identify and quantify the extent of prostatic colonisation [66] and to correlate causative organisms with prostate cancer risk. There is also no evidence of an association between clinical prostatitis and prostate cancer, although this may be due to the complex nature and classification of clinical prostatitis which is not a true reflection of histological prostate inflammation [67]. The link is implicit. Infectious agents cause inflammation in the prostate, often chronic, and chronic inflammation causes PIA which is associated with prostate cancer risk.

One recent development has been the discovery of Xenotropic murine leukaemia-virus related virus (XMRV) in human prostate cancers. Gammaretroviruses have well-characterised oncogenic effects in animals but this is the first such virus known to infect humans. XMRV infection has been shown to be associated with a common polymorphism of the RNASEL gene [68]. XMRV transcripts and protein, when present, have been found to be predominantly expressed in malignant epithelial cells, especially more aggressive tumours [69]. This is, at present, still only an associative link.

Urine reflux. Chemical or traumatic irritation have been linked with inflammation in the prostate [70] for example, uric acid has been shown to directly engage inflammasomes, pro-inflammatory intracytoplasmic complexes in cells of the innate immune system, especially macrophages, resulting in recruitment of other inflammatory cells [71]. A rat model of partial urethral obstruction has shown increased Cox-2 levels in response to intraprostatic urinary reflux [72]. In addition the retrograde movement of spermatozoa into the prostate has been found in association with prostatic inflammation probably due to the adaptive immune response to these immune privileged cells [73].

Hormonal influence – oestrogen. Increased levels of oestrogens have long been seen to affect the growth and development of the prostate, which is known to express oestrogen receptor-α (ERα) primarily in the stroma and oestrogen receptor-β (ERβ) in the epithelium [74, 75]. Administration of oestrogens to neonatal rodents induces developmental defects, but also results in inflammation as well as hyperplasia, dysplasia or PIN [51]. It is therefore reasonable to associate oestrogens with chronic inflammation and prostate cancer risk in the adult prostate, although further work needs to be done.

In summary many mechanisms might lead to prostate epithelial inflammation. Continuous exposure to the stimulating agent can set up a sustained or chronic inflammatory response leading to PIA and potentially to cancer. Questions that still need to be answered include: first, does the breakdown of prostate epithelial cells (e.g. in response to chemical injury) release antigens that either initiate an autoimmune response or reduce tolerance to future injuries? Indeed, a T-cell immune response to PSA in patients with chronic prostatitis has already been reported [76]. Second, do the endogenous inflammatory cells present in normal prostate, such as T-lymphocytes contribute to PIA and carcinogenesis? Methods such as automated quantitative image analysis are crucial to answer this [77]. Third, are there specific polymorphisms or mutations in inflammation-related genes that predispose an area of PIA to initiation of prostate cancer? Aspects of this last question will be answered later in this chapter.

The Role of Diet in the Initiation of Prostate Cancer

Epidemiological studies have revealed a link between prostate cancer incidence and mortality and the consumption of red meat and animal fats [78]. North-east Asian and Northern Atlantic populations have the lowest international prevalence of prostate cancer and yet they assume western risk profiles within two generations on migration [79]. This is generally thought to be due to dietary factors. Saturated and monounsaturated animal fat as well as linoleic acid have been associated in a number of case control and cohort studies with a higher risk of prostate cancer [80, 81]. By contrast, Japanese studies have demonstrated a negative association with soybean products, isoflavones, and long-chain polyunsaturated fatty acids such as eicosapentaenic acid (EPA) and docosahexanoic acid (DHA) [82]. In addition trace metals such as zinc supplements in the VITamins And Lifestyle (VITAL) cohort have been associated with a decreased risk of advanced prostate cancer [83].

Studies of the Mediterranean diet (Greece in particular) have revealed a protective effect for lycopenes, selenium, vitamin E, pulses and high plasma 1,25-dihydroxyvitamin D levels. Foods high in calcium such as milk, which is also rich in insulin-like growth factor-1 (*IGF-1*), increase the risk of prostate cancer [84].

Mechanisms by which dietary fat could affect CaP development include effects on insulin IGF-1 [85], steroid hormone metabolism, free radical damage and fatty acid metabolism pathways. Transgenic mice fed with low versus high fat diets have shown a significant delay in progression from mouse PIN to CaP and a reduction in AKT activation consistent with an IGF-mediated role (see explanatory box) [86]. This study used the *probasin* directed Hi-Myc model of mouse CaP; as yet, it has not been replicated in other models.

One mechanism by which meats might stimulate cancer development is through the formation of heterocyclic amines (HCAs), molecules produced by cooking red meat at high temperatures, and which can be metabolised to DNA damaging agents. Rat exposure to the most abundant HCA, 2-amino-1-methyl-6-phenylimidazo[4,5-b] pyridine (PhIP), results in intestinal carcinomas, mammary tumours and CaP [87, 88]. PhIP has also been shown to recruit epithelial macrophages and stromal mast cells and induce PIA before inducing PIN and CaP [89].

Recently, it has been shown that genistein, the major isoflavone of soy, and resveratrol, a polyphenolic phytoalexin found in red wine and grape-derived products, suppress the development of CaP in transgenic rat models when administered either alone or in combination. These nutritional polyphenols reduce cell proliferation and induce apoptosis by reducing levels of growth factors such as IGF-1 and steroid signalling proteins such as SRC-3 [90].

In summary, although conclusive evidence is limited, it is possible that a diet high in soybean products, fish, fruit and vegetables, and low in red meat, dairy products and calcium, similar to the Japanese or Greek diets may reduce the risk of prostate cancer [91]. However, well-designed epidemiological studies such as nested case-control studies with nutritional analyses of blood samples are needed to confirm these associations. In addition further laboratory studies in vivo models of prostate cancer are required to elucidate the mechanisms.

The Role of Specific Genetic Mutations and Pathways in the Initiation of Prostate Cancer (Table 22.1)

NKX3-1/8p. The NKX3-1 homeobox gene regulates prostate epithelial differentiation. One of the commonest events in prostate carcinogenesis (in ~80% of CaP) is loss of specific regions of chromosome 8p which encodes NKX3-1 [92]. Fluorescence in situ hybridisation (FISH) and allelic imbalance analysis studies concur that loss of 8p12-21 is an early event, while 8p22 is more common in advanced CaP [93]. Chromosome 8p deletions are also present in lung and colorectal tumours, but NKX3-1 expression is restricted to the prostate in adult tissues. NKX3-1 homozygous mutant mice develop PIN by 1 year of age [94]. In the intact adult mouse prostate, all luminal cells and 10% of basal cells express Nkx3-1. Expression is virtually abolished on castration and quickly restored after androgen re-administration. The small number of residual Nkx3-1 expressing cells has been further characterised with serial single cell transplantation and with lineage-marked Nkx3-1 knock-in mice to show that HGPIN and CaP develops from these cells in an inducible PTEN deletion mouse model of CaP. Nkx3-1 is therefore proposed as a marker of a cell of origin for CaP. As discussed earlier in this chapter, these cells also express the androgen receptor (AR) and keratin 18 (CK18) consistent with a luminal origin [30].

PTEN. Mutations involving phosphatase and tensin homolog deleted on chromosome 10 (PTEN) are common with loss of function mutations being reported in ~30% of primary cancers and ~60% of metastatic lesions [95]. PTEN dephosphorylates phophatidylinositol 3,4,5-triphosphate (PIP3) which is a product of phosphoinositide 3-kinase (Pi3K) activity. Increased levels of PIP3 in PTEN-deficient conditions alter the rate of protein translation, susceptibility to apoptosis and *anoikis*, entry in the cell cycle, differentiation and motility [35]. Key downstream effectors of PIP3 are PDK1, AKT and mTOR1&2, which play a fundamental role in supporting cancer cell metabolism, growth and survival [96]. Deletion of PTEN in the developing murine prostate leads to early onset and rapidly progressive neoplasia [97]. Cre-recombinase mediated PTEN excision in the murine prostate gland after puberty instead leads to a gradual onset of pre-malignant conditions within 16–20 weeks, following by progression to CaP at 1 year [98]. The delayed latency occurred despite evidence of prominent AKT/mTOR activation from the time of PTEN deletion. This indolent evolution of the disease after PTEN deletion in the mature mouse is reflective of disease initiation and progression in humans and is

Table 22.1 Common genetic and somatic changes in initiation of CaP

Gene	Location	Notes
Nkx3-1 [30, 117, 118]	8p12-22	Homeodomain transcription factor. Prostate specific – suppresses growth of epithelial cells/maintains prostate stem cells. One allele frequently deleted in primary tumours. Possible marker of CaP cell of origin
PTEN [98, 119]	10q23.31	Lipid phosphatase that suppresses cell proliferation and increases apoptosis. One allele lost in ~30% of primary tumours. Mutations in 60% of metastatic lesions. Constitutive PTEN deletion in mouse prostates leads to rapid CaP. Post-pubescent deletion leads to PIN and slow development of CaP at 1 year
AKT [99]	14q32.32	Pi3K pathway. Inhibited by PTEN. Activation of murine AKT induces uniform highly penetrant PIN. Only progresses to CaP if there is a secondary hit (e.g. p27)
Myc [107, 108, 120]	8q24	Transcription factor with multiple regulatory roles in epithelial proliferation, senescence, apoptosis and metabolism. Overexpression can directly transform cells. Amplified in ~70% of castrate resistant tumours
ERG ETV 1-4 [101, 103, 104] (ETS)	21q22.3 7p21.2 19q13.12 1q21-q23 17q21.31	Encode ETS transcription factors. Fusion transcripts with androgen-regulated TMPRSS2 present in ~50% of CaP at all disease stages. Particularly implicated in progression of PIN to CaP
p27 [99, 121] (CDKN1B)	12p12.3	Cell cycle regulator – regulates cyclin-CDK to inhibit cell cycle progression. Reduced levels observed in CaP progression. Ablation of p27 in mouse PIN induces CaP
Rb [122]	13q	Cell cycle regulator. Infrequently mutated in humans but homozygous mutant mice develop hyperplasia, dysplasia and CaP
Telomerase [123]	Chromosome termini	Maintains chromosomal stability. Shortened telomeres found in >90% of PIN and CaP
E-cadherin [124]	16q22.1	Cell adhesion. Prevents migration of epithelial cells. Reduced expression in PIN and CaP
c-Met [125, 126]	7q31	Tyrosine-kinase receptor. Overexpressed in PIN, CaP and metastasis. Levels repressed by normal AR signalling
FGFs [127, 128]	7:15q15-21.1 8:10q24 10:5p12-13	Growth factors. Regulators of prostate growth. FGF7 & 10 associated with progression in TRAMP mice. FGF8 enhances cell migration
p53 [118, 129]	17p13.1	Regulates apoptosis/senescence in response to DNA damage or telomere dysfunction. Mutations less common in primary CaP but occur in 50% of castrate resistant cancers
AR [130]	Xq11-12	Expressed in most primary CaP. Amplified or mutated in ~30% of castrate resistant tumours

consistent with PTEN deletion being one of the key genetic modifications accumulated in the development of prostate cancer. Inactivation of PTEN leads to deregulated PI3K signalling and subsequent AKT activation. Transgenic overexpression of AKT1 in luminal cells of the ventral murine prostate has been shown to induce PIN with increased expression of senescence markers which are proposed to limit progression to CaP. Only on genetic ablation of $p27^{Kip1}$ does progression occur. Similarly, in humans, senescence markers such as p27 are seen to be elevated in PIN that does not progress to CaP as opposed to cancer-associated PIN and CaP [99]. This is consistent with the need for a double hit: lesions initiated by PTEN deletion and upregulation of AKT also need inactivation of cell cycle limiters such as p27 in order for progression to CaP to take place.

TMPRSS2-ETS. Gene fusions involving members of the ETS family of transcription factors occur frequently in human CaP. The TMPRSS2-ERG fusion gene is generated by an interstitial deletion on chromosome 21 or by reciprocal translocation and is the most common rearrangement in CaP, being found in ~50% of localised tumours [100]. Cell line experiments suggest that the androgen-responsive promoter elements of TMPRSS2 mediate overexpression of ERG (or other ETS family members) [101]. Microdissection and fluorescence in situ hybridisation (FISH) studies have shown that, when present, the fusion is detected in essentially all the malignant cells within a focus of tumour, as well as in adjacent PIN. However, it is less commonly found in premalignant PIN when there is no tumour present [102]. Mice with probasin driven overexpression of ERG alone do not develop premalignant changes [103]. However, when TMPRSS2-ERG fusion mice are crossed with PTEN deletion/AKT activation, all mice develop PIN at 6 months, and CaP by 10–12 months [104]. This suggests that PI3K pathway changes are necessary for disease initiation and development of PIN, while ETS fusion rearrangements play a role in disease progression from PIN to CaP.

Myc/8q24. Chromosome 8q24 is an established risk locus for many common epithelial cancers, including prostate, colon, breast and bladder. It was originally discovered by fine mapping of a prostate cancer linkage peak from a family based study [105]. Most of the *single nucleotide polymorphisms* (SNPs) at 8q24 are contained within an approximately 500 kb sequence devoid of well-characterised genes. However, c-Myc, a well known oncogene in these cancers is nearby [106]. Copy number gain and amplification of 8q24 and increased c-Myc activity has been shown as an early event in some prostate cancers and in a high proportion of resistant tumours [107,108]. c-Myc has been shown to have varying oncogenic/tumour suppressor effects, from direct malignant transformation of benign cells in culture and induction of a pro-resistance phenotype [109] to increases in cell proliferation rates and recruitment of quiescent stem cells into rapidly dividing intermediate progenitors [91], to induction of apoptosis and senescence via effects on p53 and p21 [110, 111]. Overexpression of c-Myc in mouse prostates under the control of probasin (Lo-Myc) and probasin/AR promoters (Hi-Myc) leads to development of murine PIN and rapid development of invasive CaP within 6–12 months. These mice were also found to have a distinct loss of Nkx3-1 expression at the transition from PIN to CaP but Nkx3-1 is not directly regulated by c-Myc [108]. With c-Myc having such varied effects it remains crucial to delineate its direct targets in prostate carcinogenesis and to clarify its interaction with the other pathways mentioned here. Cooperativity between c-Myc and PTEN deletion has been recently shown in development of HGPIN and CaP. PTEN deletion alone in mouse prostates was shown to activate p53, thought to have a "protective" senescent effect to limit the extent of malignant transformation. However, concomitant c-Myc activation suppressed the protective effect, probably by regulation of p21, to magnify the proliferative and tumorigenic effect [109].

SNPs/GWAS. Genome-wide association studies (GWAS) have emerged as a powerful approach to identify common disease alleles without prior knowledge of position or function. Genotype frequencies are compared between cases and controls at large numbers of single nucleotide polymorphisms (SNPs), chosen to report on most known common variants in the genome [112]. This technique has identified several interesting loci associated with CaP. Most recently, analysis of around 500,000 SNPs in 2,000 cases and controls, followed up with analysis of smaller numbers of SNPs in greater numbers of cases (4,000 cases in the second stage; 16,000 in the third) have revealed prostate cancer susceptibility loci in 14 separate chromosomal regions [112, 113], as well as eight loci in the 8q24 region [114] (Table 22.2) and it is expected that more will soon follow. These studies confirm that CaP is genetically complex and

Table 22.2 Single nucleotide polymorphisms (SNPs) associated with prostate cancer

Chromosome	SNP Marker	Potentially causative genes
3 [111]	rs2660753	*CHMP2B, POU1F1*
6 [111]	rs9364554	*SLC22A3, SLC22A2, LPAL2, LPA*
7 [111]	rs6465657	*LMTK2, BHLHB8*
10 [111]	rs7920517, rs10993994	*MSMB*
11 [111]	rs7931342	
19 [111]	rs2659056, rs266849, rs2735839	*KLK2, KLK3(PSA)*
X [111]	rs594561	*X NUDT10, NUDT11, GSPT2, MAGED1/4B/4, CTD-2267G17.3, XAGE2/1C/1D/5/3, SSX8/7/2/2B, SPANXN5, TMEM29B/29*
8q24 [113]	rs12543663, rs10086908, rs1016343, rs13252298, rs6983561, rs620861, rs6983267, rs10090154	*c-Myc*
2p21 [112]	rs1465618	*THADA*
2q31 [112]	rs12621278	*ITGA6*
4q32 [112]	rs17021918	*PDLIM5*
4q24 [112]	rs7679673	*TET2*
8p21 [112]	rs2928679, rs1512268	*NKX3-1*
11p15 [112]	rs7127900	*IGF2, IGF2AS, INS, TH*
22q13 [112]	rs5759167	*TTLL1, BIK, MCAT, PACIN2*

Potentially causative genes coded by or regions of regulation associated with these SNPs as shown

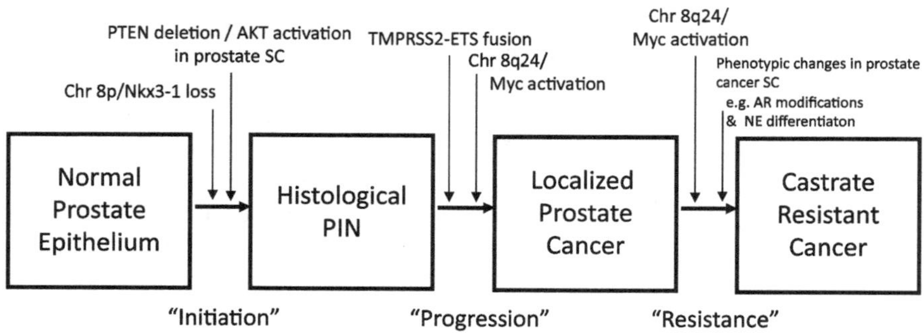

Fig. 22.7 Summary of current knowledge of the key steps involved in the initiation and progression of prostate cancer, as well as in development of resistant disease (not covered in this chapter). *SC* stem cell; *AR* androgen receptor; *NE* neuroendocrine

help to clarify the genetic architecture of CaP. Few of these loci are located directly within exon coding sequences (with the exception of MSMB and LMTK2) suggesting that diverse regulatory pathways are likely to be involved.

In summary, there are multiple specific genetic and regulatory pathway changes that occur in the development of CaP, some of which have been outlined here (Fig. 22.7). There is no doubt that there is parallel and chronological heterogeneity with a variety of factors interacting alongside each other in initiation of PIN and at subsequent progression to CaP and also to more resistant disease. A more complete understanding of these changes and their interactions will provide biomarkers for disease risk and deliver targets for therapeutic manipulation.

Implications for Early Detection and Prevention of Prostate Cancer

Specificity in therapeutic targeting of cancer stem cells will always be difficult. We are in a unique position with prostate cancer in that the patient population who develop the disease are rarely in need of their prostate. Therefore, a treatment targeted specifically to prostate stem cells, even if not specific to prostate cancer stem cells, is a viable option. However, few of the markers for prostate cancer stem cells discussed in this chapter is specific to the prostate. There is one exception: NKX3-1 is specific to the prostate after puberty and is a putative marker for the cell of origin for prostate cancer. If the cells that accumulate the genetic changes responsible for initiation and progression of prostate cancer could be destroyed then prostate cancer would not develop/progress. No compounds capable of this have yet been developed.

By contrast, treatment of inflammation is well established. The results of multicentre randomised controlled trials are awaited, for example studying the effect of non-steroidal anti-inflammatories (NSAIDS) in prevention of CaP.

However, a recent study of neoadjuvant celecoxib in clinically localised prostate cancer reported no difference in primary or secondary outcomes [115]. The search continues for an effective way to manipulate CaP risk by anti-inflammatory treatment: a randomised trial assessing the effect of treatment at the pre-malignant stage is needed. The discovery of viruses associated with CaP such as XMRV also raises the possibility of using vaccines or anti-retroviral drugs to treat CaP-associated infections and lower the risk the disease. Given its association with higher risk disease, XMRV might also serve as a useful marker to identify patients that would most benefit from early treatment [69].

Biomarkers of disease risk and likelihood of recurrence and progression will be an important means of targeting appropriate treatment. Biomarker information can be readily obtained from serum or urine samples, attractive to patients because of their non-invasive nature. In addition, more detailed analysis of prostate biopsy material with particular attention to field tumourigensis of 'near normal' tissue [115], will allow more information to be obtained from currently available material. Functional understanding is not a prerequisite for a biomarker to be useful in providing diagnostic and prognostic information when candidates have been rigorously validated by correlation of tissue expression and clinical outcome. For example, microseminomaprotein-beta (MSMB) expression is consistently high in normal prostate tissue and PIN, but lost in CaP [116]. This could be useful in assisting TRUS biopsy diagnostics and in directing the need for repeat biopsy. However, given the heterogeneity of prostate cancer development, a more complete knowledge of the key genetic players and their functional interactions will be required and this will most likely lead to a validated panel of diagnostic and prognostic markers for use in the clinical setting.

The identification of prostate cancer susceptibility genes by GWAS has a variety of clinical implications. The location of SNPs within regions that directly code for MSMB and LMTK2 suggest that these proteins might have a role in prostate cancer screening or provide potential therapeutic targets [111]. There are also implications for risk counselling although the relative risks conferred by each loci is modest (odds ratio of 2 at best) suggesting that "at-risk" SNP identification will be most useful at a population rather than individual level.

Conclusion

Prostate cancer is a heterogeneous disease with multiple factors contributing to the development of pre-malignant lesions and progression to adenocarcinoma. The role of cancer stem cells, inflammation, diet and certain specific genetic changes have been discussed in this chapter. With the identification of specific dietary factors contributing to the development of CaP the outlook is positive for lifestyle modification making a significant difference to the impact felt by this disease. It may be that targeting particular high risk populations identified through SNP profiling could lead to early preventative interventions. Prostate cancer research is a rapidly developing field with a healthy commitment of personnel and resources and new genetic players are being identified all the time. The jigsaw of heterogeneity is beginning to be pieced together and, it is hoped, will soon provide us with exciting new additions to the currently available diagnostic and therapeutic options.

Comment Boxes

Exocrine: Exocrine glands secrete their products (excluding hormones and other chemical messengers) into ducts (duct glands) which lead directly into the external environment. They are the counterparts to endocrine glands, which secrete their products (hormones) directly into the bloodstream (ductless glands) or paracrine glands that release hormones that affect only target cells nearby the release site. Examples include the sweat and salivary glands (exocrine), stomach, liver, pancreas, and prostate (mixed).

Wolffian duct: The Wolffian duct is a paired organ found in mammals during embryogenesis. It was named by Caspar Friedrich Wolff in 1759. It connects the primitive kidney to the cloaca and serves as a clustering site for embryonic cells of the reproductive tracts. The Wolffian duct goes on to form the epididymis, vas deferens and seminal vesicles.

Acinus: Acinus refers to the cluster of cells that make up the termination of an exocrine gland such as the prostate. Acinus is Latin for berry.

Gleason: The Gleason staging system is based upon the microscopic architectural appearance (size, spacing and irregularity) of the prostate glands. The pathologist assigns a grade (from 1 to 5) to the most common tumour pattern and a second grade to the next most common. The combined score is the Gleason score. In practice the lowest score commonly allocated is 6 and the highest score is 10.

$Lin^{-}Sca\text{-}1^{+}CD133^{+}CD44^{+}CD117^{+}$: Cells can be sorted according to the presence of cell surface proteins which act as specific markers for different groups of cells. These particular cell surface markers have been proposed as the unique signature of stem cells in the mouse prostate.

IGF-1: Insulin-like growth factor (IGF-1) is a protein hormone similar to insulin in molecular structure. It has an important role in child growth and continues to have anabolic effects in adulthood. It is stimulated by growth hormone. 98% is protein bound by one of 6 binding proteins (IGF-BP). It binds to IGF-1 receptor (IGF1R), a tyrosine kinase receptor, to initiate intracellular signalling and is one of the most potent activators of Pi3K/AKT signalling and has been implicated in carcinogenesis.

Probasin (PB): Probasin (PB) is a prostate-specific nuclear and secreted protein found in differentiated luminal epithelial cells. The probasin promoter is used in mouse and rat models to direct transgene expression specifically to prostate epithelial cells. This commonly-used technology may not allow for tumour initiating events that occur in undifferentiated prostate stem cells.

Anoikis: Apoptosis triggered by detachment of anchorage-dependent cells from surrounding extracellular matrix. Metastatic tumour cells resist anoikis to allow survival and attachment at distant sites. Anoikis is a Greek derivative meaning "the state of being without a home".

SNPs: A single-nucleotide polymorphism (SNP, pronounced *snip*) is a DNA sequence variation occurring when a single nucleotide in the genome (or other shared sequence) differs between members of a species (or between paired chromosomes in an individual). For example, two sequenced DNA fragments from different individuals, AAGCCTA to AAGCTTA, contain a difference in a single nucleotide.

References

1. Office for National Statistics (UK) (2007) Mortality statistics: cause, 2005 Newport: Office for National Statistics
2. Sakr WA, Haas GP, Cassin BF, Pontes JE, Crissman JD (1993) The frequency of carcinoma and intraepithelial neoplasia of the prostate in young male patients. J Urol 150(2 Pt 1):379–385
3. Hsing AW, Tsao L, Devesa SS (2000) International trends and patterns of prostate cancer incidence and mortality. Int J Cancer 85(1):60–67
4. Cancer Research UK cancerstats (2009) http://info.cancerresearchuk.org/cancerstats/types/prostate/mortality/index.htm
5. Patel M, Chhasatia M, Parmar P (2010) Antibacterial and DNA interaction studies of zinc(II) complexes with quinolone family member, ciprofloxacin. Eur J Med Chem 45(2):439–446
6. Yoshida K, Kawano N, Yoshiike M, Yoshida M, Iwamoto T, Morisawa M (2008) Physiological roles of semenogelin I and zinc in sperm motility and semen coagulation on ejaculation in humans. Mol Hum Reprod 14(3):151–156
7. Shariff AH, Ather MH (2006) Neuroendocrine differentiation in prostate cancer. Urology 68(1):2–8
8. Parkinson MC (1995) Pre-neoplastic lesions of the prostate. Histopathology 27(4):301–311
9. Hedrick L, Epstein JI (1989) Use of keratin 903 as an adjunct in the diagnosis of prostate carcinoma. Am J Surg Pathol 13(5):389–396
10. Epstein JI, Grignon DJ, Humphrey PA, McNeal JE, Sesterhenn IA, Troncoso P et al (1995) Interobserver reproducibility in the diagnosis of prostatic intraepithelial neoplasia. Am J Surg Pathol 19(8):873–886
11. Bostwick DG, Brawer MK (1987) Prostatic intra-epithelial neoplasia and early invasion in prostate cancer. Cancer 59(4):788–794
12. Bostwick DG, Amin MB, Dundore P, Marsh W, Schultz DS (1993) Architectural patterns of high-grade prostatic intraepithelial neoplasia. Hum Pathol 24(3):298–310
13. Sakr WA, Macoska JA, Benson P, Grignon DJ, Wolman SR, Pontes JE et al (1994) Allelic loss in locally metastatic, multisampled prostate cancer. Cancer Res 54(12):3273–3277
14. Nagle RB, Brawer MK, Kittelson J, Clark V (1991) Phenotypic relationships of prostatic intraepithelial neoplasia to invasive prostatic carcinoma. Am J Pathol 138(1):119–128
15. Bostwick DG, Montironi R, Sesterhenn IA (2000) Diagnosis of prostatic intraepithelial neoplasia: prostate working group/consensus report. Scand J Urol Nephrol Suppl (205):3-10
16. Bostwick DG, Qian J (2004) High-grade prostatic intraepithelial neoplasia. Mod Pathol 17(3):360–379

17. Epstein JI, Herawi M (2006) Prostate needle biopsies containing prostatic intraepithelial neoplasia or atypical foci suspicious for carcinoma: implications for patient care. J Urol 175(3 Pt 1):820–834
18. Gallo F, Chiono L, Gastaldi E, Venturino E, Giberti C (2008) Prognostic significance of high-grade prostatic intraepithelial neoplasia (HGPIN): risk of prostatic cancer on repeat biopsies. Urology 72(3):628–632
19. Netto GJ, Epstein JI (2006) Widespread high-grade prostatic intraepithelial neoplasia on prostatic needle biopsy: a significant likelihood of subsequently diagnosed adenocarcinoma. Am J Surg Pathol 30(9):1184–1188
20. Schoenfield L, Jones JS, Zippe CD, Reuther AM, Klein E, Zhou M et al (2007) The incidence of high-grade prostatic intraepithelial neoplasia and atypical glands suspicious for carcinoma on first-time saturation needle biopsy, and the subsequent risk of cancer. BJU Int 99(4):770–774
21. Roscigno M, Scattoni V, Freschi M, Raber M, Colombo R, Bertini R et al (2004) Monofocal and plurifocal high-grade prostatic intraepithelial neoplasia on extended prostate biopsies: factors predicting cancer detection on extended repeat biopsy. Urology 63(6):1105–1110
22. Oderda M, Gontero P (2009) High-grade prostatic intraepithelial neoplasia and atypical small acinar proliferation: is repeat biopsy still necessary? BJU Int 104(11):1554–1556
23. Bostwick DG, Srigley J, Grignon D, Maksem J, Humphrey P, van der Kwast TH et al (1993) Atypical adenomatous hyperplasia of the prostate: morphologic criteria for its distinction from well-differentiated carcinoma. Hum Pathol 24(8):819–832
24. Scattoni V, Roscigno M, Freschi M, Briganti A, Fantini GV, Bertini R et al (2005) Predictors of prostate cancer after initial diagnosis of atypical small acinar proliferation at 10 to 12 core biopsies. Urology 66(5):1043–1047
25. English HF, Santen RJ, Isaacs JT (1987) Response of glandular versus basal rat ventral prostatic epithelial cells to androgen withdrawal and replacement. Prostate 11(3):229–242
26. Yang A, Schweitzer R, Sun D, Kaghad M, Walker N, Bronson RT et al (1999) p63 is essential for regenerative proliferation in limb, craniofacial and epithelial development. Nature 398(6729):714–718
27. Signoretti S, Waltregny D, Dilks J, Isaac B, Lin D, Garraway L et al (2000) p63 is a prostate basal cell marker and is required for prostate development. Am J Pathol 157(6):1769–1775
28. Leong KG, Wang BE, Johnson L, Gao WQ (2008) Generation of a prostate from a single adult stem cell. Nature 456(7223):804–808
29. Salm SN, Burger PE, Coetzee S, Goto K, Moscatelli D, Wilson EL (2005) TGF-{beta} maintains dormancy of prostatic stem cells in the proximal region of ducts. J Cell Biol 170(1):81–90
30. Wang X, Kruithof-de Julio M, Economides KD, Walker D, Yu H, Halili MV et al (2009) A luminal epithelial stem cell that is a cell of origin for prostate cancer. Nature 461(7263):495–500
31. Bonnet D, Dick JE (1997) Human acute myeloid leukemia is organized as a hierarchy that originates from a primitive hematopoietic cell. Nat Med 3(7):730–737
32. Watkins DN, Berman DM, Burkholder SG, Wang B, Beachy PA, Baylin SB (2003) Hedgehog signalling within airway epithelial progenitors and in small-cell lung cancer. Nature 422(6929):313–317
33. Stingl J, Eirew P, Ricketson I, Shackleton M, Vaillant F, Choi D et al (2006) Purification and unique properties of mammary epithelial stem cells. Nature 439(7079):993–997
34. Collins AT, Berry PA, Hyde C, Stower MJ, Maitland NJ (2005) Prospective identification of tumorigenic prostate cancer stem cells. Cancer Res 65(23):10946–10951
35. Hawkins PT, Anderson KE, Davidson K, Stephens LR (2006) Signalling through Class I PI3Ks in mammalian cells. Biochem Soc Trans 34(Pt 5):647–662
36. Yardy GW, Bicknell DC, Wilding JL, Bartlett S, Liu Y, Winney B et al (2009) Mutations in the AXIN1 gene in advanced prostate cancer. Eur Urol 56(3):486–494
37. Karhadkar SS, Bova GS, Abdallah N, Dhara S, Gardner D, Maitra A et al (2004) Hedgehog signalling in prostate regeneration, neoplasia and metastasis. Nature 431(7009):707–712
38. Reya T, Morrison SJ, Clarke MF, Weissman IL (2001) Stem cells, cancer, and cancer stem cells. Nature 414(6859):105–111
39. Vias M, Ramos-Montoya A, Mills IG (2008) Terminal and progenitor lineage-survival oncogenes as cancer markers. Trends Mol Med 14(11):486–494

40. Richardson GD, Robson CN, Lang SH, Neal DE, Maitland NJ, Collins AT (2004) CD133, a novel marker for human prostatic epithelial stem cells. J Cell Sci 117(Pt 16):3539–3545
41. Gu G, Yuan J, Wills M, Kasper S (2007) Prostate cancer cells with stem cell characteristics reconstitute the original human tumor in vivo. Cancer Res 67(10):4807–4815
42. Patrawala L, Calhoun T, Schneider-Broussard R, Li H, Bhatia B, Tang S et al (2006) Highly purified CD44+ prostate cancer cells from xenograft human tumors are enriched in tumorigenic and metastatic progenitor cells. Oncogene 25(12):1696–1708
43. Sotomayor P, Godoy A, Smith GJ, Huss WJ (2009) Oct4A is expressed by a subpopulation of prostate neuroendocrine cells. Prostate 69(4):401–410
44. Coussens LM, Werb Z (2002) Inflammation and cancer. Nature 420(6917):860–867
45. Groopman JD, Kensler TW (2005) Role of metabolism and viruses in aflatoxin-induced liver cancer. Toxicol Appl Pharmacol 206(2):131–137
46. Condeelis J, Pollard JW (2006) Macrophages: obligate partners for tumor cell migration, invasion, and metastasis. Cell 124(2):263–266
47. de Visser KE, Eichten A, Coussens LM (2006) Paradoxical roles of the immune system during cancer development. Nat Rev Cancer 6(1):24–37
48. Kim S, Takahashi H, Lin WW, Descargues P, Grivennikov S, Kim Y et al (2009) Carcinoma-produced factors activate myeloid cells through TLR2 to stimulate metastasis. Nature 457(7225):102–106
49. McNeal JE (1988) Normal histology of the prostate. Am J Surg Pathol 12(8):619–633
50. De Marzo AM, Marchi VL, Epstein JI, Nelson WG (1999) Proliferative inflammatory atrophy of the prostate: implications for prostatic carcinogenesis. Am J Pathol 155(6):1985–1992
51. Putzi MJ, De Marzo AM (2000) Morphologic transitions between proliferative inflammatory atrophy and high-grade prostatic intraepithelial neoplasia. Urology 56(5):828–832
52. Wang W, Bergh A, Damber JE (2009) Morphological transition of proliferative inflammatory atrophy to high-grade intraepithelial neoplasia and cancer in human prostate. Prostate 69(13):1378–1386
53. Elkahwaji JE, Hauke RJ, Brawner CM (2009) Chronic bacterial inflammation induces prostatic intraepithelial neoplasia in mouse prostate. Br J Cancer 101(10):1740–1748
54. Tomas D, Kruslin B, Rogatsch H, Schafer G, Belicza M, Mikuz G (2007) Different types of atrophy in the prostate with and without adenocarcinoma. Eur Urol 51(1):98–103; discussion 03–04
55. Billis A (1998) Prostatic atrophy: an autopsy study of a histologic mimic of adenocarcinoma. Mod Pathol 11(1):47–54
56. Bostwick DC, Cheng L (eds) (2008) Urologic surgical pathology. Chapter 8: Non-neoplastic diseases of the prostate, 2nd ed. Mosby Elsevier, Philadelphia, PA
57. De Marzo AM, Platz EA, Sutcliffe S, Xu J, Gronberg H, Drake CG et al (2007) Inflammation in prostate carcinogenesis. Nat Rev Cancer 7(4):256–269
58. Handsfield HH, Lipman TO, Harnisch JP, Tronca E, Holmes KK (1974) Asymptomatic gonorrhea in men. Diagnosis, natural course, prevalence and significance. N Engl J Med 290(3):117–123
59. Poletti F, Medici MC, Alinovi A, Menozzi MG, Sacchini P, Stagni G et al (1985) Isolation of *Chlamydia trachomatis* from the prostatic cells in patients affected by nonacute abacterial prostatitis. J Urol 134(4):691–693
60. Stark JR, Judson G, Alderete JF, Mundodi V, Kucknoor AS, Giovannucci EL et al (2009) Prospective study of *Trichomonas vaginalis* infection and prostate cancer incidence and mortality: Physicians' Health Study. J Natl Cancer Inst 101(20):1406–1411
61. Drach GW (1975) Prostatitis: man's hidden infection. Urol Clin North Am 2(3):499–520
62. Ozden E, Bostanci Y, Yakupoglu KY, Akdeniz E, Yilmaz AF, Tulek N et al (2009) Incidence of acute prostatitis caused by extended-spectrum beta-lactamase-producing *Escherichia coli* after transrectal prostate biopsy. Urology 74(1):119–123
63. Zambrano A, Kalantari M, Simoneau A, Jensen JL, Villarreal LP (2002) Detection of human polyomaviruses and papillomaviruses in prostatic tissue reveals the prostate as a habitat for multiple viral infections. Prostate 53(4):263–276
64. Samanta M, Harkins L, Klemm K, Britt WJ, Cobbs CS (2003) High prevalence of human cytomegalovirus in prostatic intraepithelial neoplasia and prostatic carcinoma. J Urol 170(3):998–1002

65. Doble A, Harris JR, Taylor-Robinson D (1991) Prostatodynia and herpes simplex virus infection. Urology 38(3):247–248
66. Batstone GR, Doble A (2003) Chronic prostatitis. Curr Opin Urol 13(1):23–29
67. Sutcliffe S, Giovannucci E, De Marzo AM, Leitzmann MF, Willett WC, Platz EA (2006) Gonorrhea, syphilis, clinical prostatitis, and the risk of prostate cancer. Cancer Epidemiol Biomarkers Prev 15(11):2160–2166
68. Urisman A, Molinaro RJ, Fischer N, Plummer SJ, Casey G, Klein EA et al (2006) Identification of a novel Gammaretrovirus in prostate tumors of patients homozygous for R462Q RNASEL variant. PLoS Pathog 2(3):e25
69. Schlaberg R, Choe DJ, Brown KR, Thaker HM, Singh IR (2009) XMRV is present in malignant prostatic epithelium and is associated with prostate cancer, especially high-grade tumors. Proc Natl Acad Sci U S A 106(38):16351–16356
70. Kirby RS, Lowe D, Bultitude MI, Shuttleworth KE (1982) Intra-prostatic urinary reflux: an aetiological factor in abacterial prostatitis. Br J Urol 54(6):729–731
71. Martinon F, Petrilli V, Mayor A, Tardivel A, Tschopp J (2006) Gout-associated uric acid crystals activate the NALP3 inflammasome. Nature 440(7081):237–241
72. Liu W, Li SW, Zheng XM, Hu LQ, Luo Y (2008) Intraprostatic urinary reflux associated prostatitis caused by partial urethral obstruction in the rat model. Zhonghua Nan Ke Xue 14(1):11–14
73. Chen X, Zhao J, Salim S, Garcia FU (2006) Intraprostatic spermatozoa: zonal distribution and association with atrophy. Hum Pathol 37(3):345–351
74. Huang L, Pu Y, Alam S, Birch L, Prins GS (2004) Estrogenic regulation of signaling pathways and homeobox genes during rat prostate development. J Androl 25(3):330–337
75. Huang L, Pu Y, Alam S, Birch L, Prins GS (2005) The role of Fgf10 signaling in branching morphogenesis and gene expression of the rat prostate gland: lobe-specific suppression by neonatal estrogens. Dev Biol 278(2):396–414
76. Ponniah S, Arah I, Alexander RB (2000) PSA is a candidate self-antigen in autoimmune chronic prostatitis/chronic pelvic pain syndrome. Prostate 44(1):49–54
77. Lamb AD, Qadan M, Roberts S, Timlin H, Campbell FM, Gregor K, et al (2009) CD4+ and CD8+ T-lymphocyte scores cannot reliably predict progression in patients with benign prostatic hyperplasia (BPH). BJU Int *in print–DOI awaited*
78. Michaud DS, Augustsson K, Rimm EB, Stampfer MJ, Willet WC, Giovannucci E (2001) A prospective study on intake of animal products and risk of prostate cancer. Cancer Causes Control 12(6):557–567
79. Shimizu H, Ross RK, Bernstein L, Yatani R, Henderson BE, Mack TM (1991) Cancers of the prostate and breast among Japanese and white immigrants in Los Angeles County. Br J Cancer 63(6):963–966
80. Whittemore AS, Kolonel LN, Wu AH, John EM, Gallagher RP, Howe GR et al (1995) Prostate cancer in relation to diet, physical activity, and body size in blacks, whites, and Asians in the United States and Canada. J Natl Cancer Inst 87(9):652–661
81. Giovannucci E, Ascherio A, Rimm EB, Colditz GA, Stampfer MJ, Willett WC (1993) A prospective cohort study of vasectomy and prostate cancer in US men. JAMA 269(7):873–877
82. Mori M, Masumori N, Fukuta F, Nagata Y, Sonoda T, Sakauchi F et al (2009) Traditional Japanese diet and prostate cancer. Mol Nutr Food Res 53(2):191–200
83. Gonzalez A, Peters U, Lampe JW, White E (2009) Zinc intake from supplements and diet and prostate cancer. Nutr Cancer 61(2):206–215
84. Itsiopoulos C, Hodge A, Kaimakamis M (2009) Can the Mediterranean diet prevent prostate cancer? Mol Nutr Food Res 53(2):227–239
85. Yu H, Rohan T (2000) Role of the insulin-like growth factor family in cancer development and progression. J Natl Cancer Inst 92(18):1472–1489
86. Kobayashi N, Barnard RJ, Said J, Hong-Gonzalez J, Corman DM, Ku M et al (2008) Effect of low-fat diet on development of prostate cancer and Akt phosphorylation in the Hi-Myc transgenic mouse model. Cancer Res 68(8):3066–3073

87. Knize MG, Felton JS (2005) Formation and human risk of carcinogenic heterocyclic amines formed from natural precursors in meat. Nutr Rev 63(5):158–165
88. Sugimura T, Wakabayashi K, Nakagama H, Nagao M (2004) Heterocyclic amines: mutagens/carcinogens produced during cooking of meat and fish. Cancer Sci 95(4):290–299
89. Nakai Y, Nelson WG, De Marzo AM (2007) The dietary charred meat carcinogen 2-amino-1-methyl-6-phenylimidazo[4, 5-b]pyridine acts as both a tumor initiator and promoter in the rat ventral prostate. Cancer Res 67(3):1378–1384
90. Harper CE, Cook LM, Patel BB, Wang J, Eltoum IA, Arabshahi A et al (2009) Genistein and resveratrol, alone and in combination, suppress prostate cancer in SV-40 tag rats. Prostate 69(15):1668–1682
91. Ma RW, Chapman K (2009) A systematic review of the effect of diet in prostate cancer prevention and treatment. J Hum Nutr Diet 22(3):187–199; quiz 200–202
92. Chang M, Tsuchiya K, Batchelor RH, Rabinovitch PS, Kulander BG, Haggitt RC et al (1994) Deletion mapping of chromosome 8p in colorectal carcinoma and dysplasia arising in ulcerative colitis, prostatic carcinoma, and malignant fibrous histiocytomas. Am J Pathol 144(1):1–6
93. Abate-Shen C, Shen MM (2000) Molecular genetics of prostate cancer. Genes Dev 14(19):2410–2434
94. Kim MJ, Bhatia-Gaur R, Banach-Petrosky WA, Desai N, Wang Y, Hayward SW et al (2002) Nkx3.1 mutant mice recapitulate early stages of prostate carcinogenesis. Cancer Res 62(11):2999–3004
95. Tomlins SA, Rubin MA, Chinnaiyan AM (2006) Integrative biology of prostate cancer progression. Annu Rev Pathol 1:243–271
96. Faivre S, Kroemer G, Raymond E (2006) Current development of mTOR inhibitors as anticancer agents. Nat Rev Drug Discov 5(8):671–688
97. Wang S, Gao J, Lei Q, Rozengurt N, Pritchard C, Jiao J et al (2003) Prostate-specific deletion of the murine Pten tumor suppressor gene leads to metastatic prostate cancer. Cancer Cell 4(3):209–221
98. Luchman HA, Benediktsson H, Villemaire ML, Peterson AC, Jirik FR (2008) The pace of prostatic intraepithelial neoplasia development is determined by the timing of Pten tumor suppressor gene excision. PLoS One 3(12):e3940
99. Majumder PK, Grisanzio C, O'Connell F, Barry M, Brito JM, Xu Q et al (2008) A prostatic intraepithelial neoplasia-dependent p27 Kip1 checkpoint induces senescence and inhibits cell proliferation and cancer progression. Cancer Cell 14(2):146–155
100. Kumar-Sinha C, Tomlins SA, Chinnaiyan AM (2008) Recurrent gene fusions in prostate cancer. Nat Rev Cancer 8(7):497–511
101. Tomlins SA, Rhodes DR, Perner S, Dhanasekaran SM, Mehra R, Sun XW et al (2005) Recurrent fusion of TMPRSS2 and ETS transcription factor genes in prostate cancer. Science 310(5748):644–648
102. Perner S, Mosquera JM, Demichelis F, Hofer MD, Paris PL, Simko J et al (2007) TMPRSS2-ERG fusion prostate cancer: an early molecular event associated with invasion. Am J Surg Pathol 31(6):882–888
103. Carver BS, Tran J, Chen Z, Carracedo-Perez A, Alimonti A, Nardella C et al (2009) ETS rearrangements and prostate cancer initiation. Nature 457(7231):E1; discussion E2–E3
104. King JC, Xu J, Wongvipat J, Hieronymus H, Carver BS, Leung DH et al (2009) Cooperativity of TMPRSS2-ERG with PI3-kinase pathway activation in prostate oncogenesis. Nat Genet 41(5):524–526
105. Amundadottir LT, Sulem P, Gudmundsson J, Helgason A, Baker A, Agnarsson BA et al (2006) A common variant associated with prostate cancer in European and African populations. Nat Genet 38(6):652–658
106. Jia L, Landan G, Pomerantz M, Jaschek R, Herman P, Reich D et al (2009) Functional enhancers at the gene-poor 8q24 cancer-linked locus. PLoS Genet 5(8):e1000597
107. Taylor BS, Schultz N, Hieronymus H, Gopalan A, Xiao X, Carver BS et al (2010) Integrative genomic profiling of human prostate cancer. Cancer Cell 18(1):11–22

108. Ellwood-Yen K, Graeber TG, Wongvipat J, Iruela-Arispe ML, Zhang J, Matusik R et al (2003) Myc-driven murine prostate cancer shares molecular features with human prostate tumors. Cancer Cell 4(3):223–238
109. Bernard D, Pourtier-Manzanedo A, Gil J, Beach DH (2003) Myc confers androgen-independent prostate cancer cell growth. J Clin Invest 112(11):1724–1731
110. Kim J, Eltoum IE, Roh M, Wang J, Abdulkadir SA (2009) Interactions between cells with distinct mutations in c-MYC and Pten in prostate cancer. PLoS Genet 5(7):e1000542
111. Watt FM, Frye M, Benitah SA (2008) MYC in mammalian epidermis: how can an oncogene stimulate differentiation? Nat Rev Cancer 8(3):234–242
112. Eeles RA, Kote-Jarai Z, Giles GG, Olama AA, Guy M, Jugurnauth SK et al (2008) Multiple newly identified loci associated with prostate cancer susceptibility. Nat Genet 40(3):316–321
113. Eeles RA, Kote-Jarai Z, Al Olama AA, Giles GG, Guy M, Severi G et al (2009) Identification of seven new prostate cancer susceptibility loci through a genome-wide association study. Nat Genet 41(10):1116–1121
114. Al Olama AA, Kote-Jarai Z, Giles GG, Guy M, Morrison J, Severi G et al (2009) Multiple loci on 8q24 associated with prostate cancer susceptibility. Nat Genet 41(10):1058–1060
115. Antonarakis ES, Heath EI, Walczak JR, Nelson WG, Fedor H, De Marzo AM et al (2009) Phase II, randomized, placebo-controlled trial of neoadjuvant celecoxib in men with clinically localized prostate cancer: evaluation of drug-specific biomarkers. J Clin Oncol 27(30):4986–4993
116. Nonn L, Ananthanarayanan V, Gann PH (2009) Evidence for field cancerization of the prostate. Prostate 69(13):1470–1479
117. Whitaker HC, Warren AY, Eeles R, Kote-Jarai Z, Neal DE (2010) The potential value of microseminoprotein-beta as a prostate cancer biomarker and therapeutic target. Prostate 70(3):333–340
118. Bhatia-Gaur R, Donjacour AA, Sciavolino PJ, Kim M, Desai N, Young P et al (1999) Roles for Nkx3.1 in prostate development and cancer. Genes Dev 13(8):966–977
119. Lei Q, Jiao J, Xin L, Chang CJ, Wang S, Gao J et al (2006) NKX3.1 stabilizes p53, inhibits AKT activation, and blocks prostate cancer initiation caused by PTEN loss. Cancer Cell 9(5):367–378
120. Li J, Yen C, Liaw D, Podsypanina K, Bose S, Wang SI et al (1997) PTEN, a putative protein tyrosine phosphatase gene mutated in human brain, breast, and prostate cancer. Science 275(5308):1943–1947
121. Gil J, Kerai P, Lleonart M, Bernard D, Cigudosa JC, Peters G et al (2005) Immortalization of primary human prostate epithelial cells by c-Myc. Cancer Res 65(6):2179–2185
122. Yang RM, Naitoh J, Murphy M, Wang HJ, Phillipson J, deKernion JB et al (1998) Low p27 expression predicts poor disease-free survival in patients with prostate cancer. J Urol 159(3):941–945
123. Li C, Larsson C, Futreal A, Lancaster J, Phelan C, Aspenblad U et al (1998) Identification of two distinct deleted regions on chromosome 13 in prostate cancer. Oncogene 16(4):481–487
124. Zhang W, Kapusta LR, Slingerland JM, Klotz LH (1998) Telomerase activity in prostate cancer, prostatic intraepithelial neoplasia, and benign prostatic epithelium. Cancer Res 58(4):619–621
125. Umbas R, Isaacs WB, Bringuier PP, Schaafsma HE, Karthaus HF, Oosterhof GO et al (1994) Decreased E-cadherin expression is associated with poor prognosis in patients with prostate cancer. Cancer Res 54(14):3929–3933
126. Pisters LL, Troncoso P, Zhau HE, Li W, von Eschenbach AC, Chung LW (1995) c-met proto-oncogene expression in benign and malignant human prostate tissues. J Urol 154(1):293–298

127. Verras M, Lee J, Xue H, Li TH, Wang Y, Sun Z (2007) The androgen receptor negatively regulates the expression of c-Met: implications for a novel mechanism of prostate cancer progression. Cancer Res 67(3):967–975
128. Djakiew D (2000) Dysregulated expression of growth factors and their receptors in the development of prostate cancer. Prostate 42(2):150–160
129. Darby S, Sahadevan K, Khan MM, Robson CN, Leung HY, Gnanapragasam VJ (2006) Loss of Sef (similar expression to FGF) expression is associated with high grade and metastatic prostate cancer. Oncogene 25(29):4122–4127
130. Bookstein R, MacGrogan D, Hilsenbeck SG, Sharkey F, Allred DC (1993) p53 is mutated in a subset of advanced-stage prostate cancers. Cancer Res 53(14):3369–3373
131. Visakorpi T, Hyytinen E, Koivisto P, Tanner M, Keinanen R, Palmberg C et al (1995) In vivo amplification of the androgen receptor gene and progression of human prostate cancer. Nat Genet 9(4):401–406

Part IV
Common Threads

Chapter 23
Early Disease, Early Detection, Early Treatment: Some Common Threads and Some Important Problems

John D. Potter

Abstract This chapter attempts to summarise and comment on the preceding chapters. It begins with some thoughts on differences between prevention and treatment. It notes that we have achieved a great deal in the accumulation of empirical data on cancer but still lack a coherent overall theory. The chapter then discusses, in the light of the rest of the book, the classification of cancers into five groups, based on the likely effectiveness of screening, early detection, and subsequent treatment and prevention strategies. It then notes, again referring to the earlier chapters, the next steps that might better inform our detection of early lesions. A section on the development, testing, and use of new screening markers follows, with an emphasis, as elsewhere in the chapter, on the problem of studies that are too small. The final section is concerned with the repeated failure of chemoprevention to deliver on its promise. It notes, in particular, the very primitive approach that we take in using single agents, a practice that we abandoned decades ago in chemotherapy, because clonal selection and progression are known to result. We do not yet seem to have noticed that the same is frequently true with chemoprevention.

Much of human medical history can be characterized, at its best, as the healer providing comfort and support to the patient while both waited for the condition to improve or to worsen and perhaps kill. This picture can be decorated with the use of some more-effective, but often less-effective, sometimes bizarre, remedies but time has almost always been a key element in therapy. Some medical systems have been better than others at prevention (e.g. Ayurveda, Chinese medicine) but, until the twentieth century, there was little difference in the effectiveness of treatment. The development in the nineteenth century of the germ theory of infectious disease

[1]It is ironic that antibiotic therapy has become less and less rational and now, itself, is producing subclasses of previously treatable infectious disease that are rapidly lethal and spreading.

J.D. Potter (✉)
Division of Public Health Sciences, Fred Hutchinson Cancer Research Center,
1100 Fairview Avenue North, PO Box 19024. Seattle, WA, 98109-1024 USA
e-mail: jpotter@fhcrc.org

R.C. Fitzgerald (ed.), *Pre-Invasive Disease: Pathogenesis and Clinical Management*,
DOI 10.1007/978-1-4419-6694-0_23,

led eventually to a rational approach to diagnosis and treatment.[1] Antibiotics joined a handful of existing empirically effective therapeutic agents (e.g., digitalis) but did so perhaps as the first agents used to directly combat what were known to be causal agents of disease. Indeed, the development of germ theory eventually not only led to effective therapeutic approaches to infection but also provided a theoretical underpinning for already existing empirical approaches to prevention: improved living conditions; clean water; hygiene; quarantine.

The discovery of the natural history and aetiology of deficiency diseases (exogenous like vitamin deficiencies; endogenous like Type I diabetes mellitus) again led to rational approaches to therapy and prevention. The twentieth century also saw the emergence of an understanding of the natural history of cardiovascular disease, to the point where precursor states (for example, the hyperlipidaemias, hypertension) have themselves become the focus of therapy and provide targets for the prevention of both coronary heart disease and stroke.

Cancer has proved to be more elusive, partly because it is a multiplicity of different diseases (even within the same organ), partly because many of the organs are not readily accessible (consider, for example, pancreas, brain, ovary, lung), and partly because we still do not have a very complete theoretical understanding of the cause and progression of cancer. If this last is not so, why do we seek to explain the international variation of cancer (which, for some cancers, measures more than 2 orders of magnitude) among a spectrum of specific allelic variants that carry a 10–20% excess risk?

Nonetheless, despite this failure of theory, our empirical understanding of cancer has improved greatly due to: large-scale epidemiologic studies, which have provided evidence for most of the known environmental and host factors (for example, smoking, radiation, microbiologic agents, asbestos, solvents, hormones, obesity, lack of physical activity); markedly improved imaging modalities; similarly improved direct-visualization capacity (endoscopic access to most hollow organs); and histologic, and subsequently molecular, characterization of normal and pathologic tissues. Even if these developments have not resulted in a complete and coherent theory of cancer, they have allowed a much better description of its natural history, such that much earlier manifestations of the disease can be identified, examined, and treated. This, in turn, has allowed improved screening, earlier diagnosis, treatment at earlier stages, and improved survival.

It is this empirical success that has driven the search for a better understanding of early disease and for better ways to detect and treat these early lesions.

Early Detection: Some Classes of Cancers

If early lesions are useful in the detection and possible interruption of the course of a fatal cancer, the first important question that arises is whether cancers detected early and treated successfully are just a random subset of all cancers. If the answer to that is "Yes", then the more lesions that are detected early, the greater will be the improvement in cancer survival across the population. If, however, early-detected lesions are biologically distinct (if they are slower growing, more benign, for instance, this would facilitate early detection), then increasing the detection rate of such lesions, which may have more favorable outcomes irrespective of when they are detected, will have a more modest impact on survival patterns.

The second important question is how often are early lesions of no clinical significance for the individual concerned, even if they are clearly both on the pathobiologic pathway to cancer and have predictive power for clinical cancer at the population level. There is evidence for several cancers that, indeed, surveillance results in the detection of lesions that would never present clinically. This is true not only of PSA-detected prostate cancer [1] but also of mammography-detected breast cancer [2]. This is important because there is good evidence that mammographic-screening programs reduce breast cancer mortality; therefore, at least some early-detection approaches not only over-diagnose and over-treat some individuals but also result in overall population benefit. This complex balance among individual benefit and harm and population benefit (and perhaps population harm in some circumstances) will only become more difficult to achieve as possible new modalities detect other cancers at yet earlier stages and, therefore, detect even more precancers. The data in Chap. 22 on early prostate lesions (PIN and ASAP) and their possible causes and progression may eventually provide a basis for more rational early intervention but, at present, we cannot distinguish aggressive lesions that kill from those that will cause no clinical problem within the lifetime of the patient; this, for prostate (and other) cancers, is the key screening issue. Indeed, what needs to be established for *each* cancer for which there is enough understanding of early lesions and the technologic capacity to detect such lesions, is whether the detection and treatment of such early disease actually results in benefit. The field has moved very slowly towards the acceptance of this need, despite the fact that we laid out the blueprint almost a decade ago [3]. This paper is much cited, but its philosophic underpinnings do not drive the whole research programme. We need much better powered studies and considerably improved integration across biologic, clinical, and population research.

There is a second group of cancers in which screening, early detection, and treatment work very well. This group includes mouth, skin, colorectal, and cervix cancers. These organs allow direct visualization of the relevant epithelium (see Chap. 12) and, for colon and skin (and sometimes for cervix), both diagnosis and curative treatment can be accomplished at the same time. This results in extensive saving in time and effort for both patient and therapist [4]. It seems appropriate to ask whether we can improve on such direct visualization by molecular or other screens. For instance, colonoscopy is very expensive, so a first-stage test that uses additional data to identify those who will most probably benefit from such screening would be very valuable, not only in populations that can afford widespread colonoscopic screening, but especially in those that cannot. There are some possible directions (see Chap. 18) but no strong candidates have emerged to replace insensitive, non-specific FOBT as a first-stage screen. For both colon and skin, because we detect non-malignant/pre-malignant lesions, there is a reduction of incidence (screening for most cancers increases incidence even if it reduces case fatality), which is the probable explanation of the declining incidence of colorectal cancer in whites in United States. Again, there are more lesions detected and removed than would ever present as clinical disease – and, perversely, still a very high incidence of both skin and colorectal cancer.

It is unclear whether direct visualization modalities can be applied more widely to routinely screen other hollow organs but the possibility of imaging other organs in ways that could parallel mammography in impact, does not seem far-fetched. What we learn from modalities that screen, diagnose, and treat in one sitting is that these have a considerable impact on mortality, despite considerable over-diagnosis and over-treatment. They might be regarded as the closest we currently have to a gold standard for early detection. For multicentric, more diffuse lesions, such as Barrett's oesophagus (see Chap. 16), even when they are accessible to endoscopy, there is no equivalent simple strategy to the excision of polyps or skin BCCs. Nonetheless, in Chap. 12, Vikneswaran and Wang describe a variety of endoscopic ablation techniques, particularly of mucosa. However, if the underlying problem is not epithelial but more derived from tissue architecture, including stroma [5, 6], (see Chap. 2) or especially if there is a systemic disorder, then ablation may only be a temporary solution or even, eventually, a source of selective pressure (see Chap. 7) that facilitates, rather than impairs, progression. It is noteworthy in this context that endoscopic removal of adenomatous colorectal polyps almost always ablates the relevant stroma as well.

A third group of cancers includes those where causal agents are detectable and either preventable by immunization in high-risk populations (for example, hepatitis B), treatable (for example, hepatitis C), or both (HPV). Stomach cancer could fall into the detectable-and-treatable-agent group (*Helicobacter pylori*) or even be immunizable against, but there are few appropriate research or implementation programmes in the relevant populations. Much is known about *H. pylori* infection and about the emergence and progression of premalignant lesions (see Chap. 17); there would appear to be many steps in the process that could be expected to improve the currently poor survival, from immunization to the detection of metaplasia and dysplasia, but, to date, effective immunization in support of the intrinsic immune response has been elusive and the disease often remains clinically silent until very late. Stomach is still the second most common cancer in the world, only recently bumped from the top spot by lung cancer, which is itself one of the most preventable but least detectable cancers.

A fourth group of cancers includes those where we have some capacity to detect disease before it presents clinically, but no evidence that this is effective in reducing mortality. Some of these cancers are accessible to direct visualization, for example oesophagus and stomach, but these are thought to occur too infrequently in many general populations (though not in Japan, where stomach cancer remains high) to be applied without preliminary screening to enrich for a truly high-risk group. Nonetheless, colon cancer occurs much less frequently than stomach cancer worldwide, so the choice that we make regarding population screening depends, in part, on cost to the individual patient as well as cost to the society per screen-detected cancer. Other screening approaches include the use of specific blood markers (for example ovary [7]) or imaging (see Chap. 14) but large questions remain for these, not least because of the very large studies that are needed to establish the efficacy of screening and, in addition, because of the way in which the waters have been muddied by studies done less well than is appropriate [8].

The final group includes those cancers where we lack most of the necessary understanding to detect early disease. The most prominent of this group is pancreas cancer. In Chap. 19, Matthaei and Maitra identify two at-risk groups that they regard as proper targets of screening: firstly, those from known pancreas-cancer families (whether the germline lesion is known or not); and secondly, those diagnosed with asymptomatic pancreatic cysts, which frequently include mucinous precursors of pancreas cancer. These are important groups clinically but account for a very small proportion of the pancreas-cancer burden in the population. This cancer exemplifies above all others (but see also Chap. 8) the value of animal models. The disease in humans remains occult clinically, even as it is beginning to yield some molecular secrets. Animal models that are specifically constructed to mimic the human disease present the best opportunity we have to explore early markers for screening and diagnosis, molecular and histologic progression, response to therapy, and prevention [9–11]. At present, many would argue that lung also falls into this final category; indeed, Bach argues that all relevant studies show that early-stage histologically confirmed lung cancers that have been identified by screening are not themselves precursors of advanced disease and, thus, do not provide a useful route to early detection [12].

Next Steps

What does current research hold for understanding early disease sufficiently well to improve the detectability, treatment, and survival of human cancers? The chapters in this book have provided us with some excellent directions, but we are not close to cost-effective population screening modalities that are based on molecular-level understanding.

As already noted, we lack a coherent global theory of cancer, even though we have a rich understanding of many aspects of the biology of cancer. Part 1 exemplifies both of these features of our understanding: as the individual chapters show, several aspects of cancer biology can be laid out in detail:

1. There may be a role for cancer stem cells (analogues of stem cells in developing embryonic tissues). In Chap. 1, Wright, using Barrett oesophagus and other metaplasias as models, notes the way in which whole epithelial fields become genetically unstable, leading to widespread mutations. He argues that, in stomach cancer, the data show that the process involves monoclonal conversion from gastric stem cells and that, subsequently, crypt fission leads to clonal spread. He further notes that, in Barrett oesophagus, aberrant stem cells arise in a multifocal way. He says, in his final sentence, “We need to find out much more about how

mutant clones become dominant and spread, and how competition between clones promotes the development of cancer in humans." However, it seems to me that the most important question to ask is why the metaplasias arise in the first place. What makes an epithelial field unstable? How much are we missing because we lack a comprehensive theory [6]?

2. There is very consistent evidence that inflammation acts as an important stimulus to neoplastic growth (see Chap 2). For instance, there are a variety of chronic inflammatory conditions (without causal agents, at least to date), for example, chronic ulcerative colitis, Barrett esophagus, as well as some known infectious conditions, for example, chronic viral hepatitis and chronic *H pylori* infection, that markedly elevate cancer risk. In addition, many tumors over-express the pro-inflammatory COX2. Further, epidemiologic data, animal studies, and human intervention trials have established that aspirin and other non-steroidal anti-inflammatory drugs inhibit carcinogenesis in rats and humans (see also Chap. 11). Finally, genetic variation in both metabolic and signalling parts of the inflammation network modify cancer and pre-cancer risk.
3. The ways in which the readability of DNA can be ordered and disordered by normal and abnormal DNA de/methylation and histone de/acetylation provide yet another set of tools for screening that, nonetheless, remain to establish their worth (see Chap. 4).
4. In Chap. 3, Pharoah takes the position that genetic predisposition is not only important in aetiology, but also can be used in the screening of individuals for cancer risk. This is clearly a useful tool in the clinical screening of individuals who are members of rare high-risk families, allowing management decisions to be made on the basis of carrier state. Pharoah focuses most of his discussion on breast cancer but other familial cancers are similar, even pancreas (see Chap. 19). He reaches a little further in making the proposal that polygenic profiles, combined with known "lifestyle risk factors" (which, we should note again, explain international variation considerably better on their own than does genetic variation), could be used as a basis for population-based screening. He then takes a final step, arguing: "It would be possible to offer every woman a personalized screening program in which age of starting screening would vary, based on her breast-cancer risk profile. A test using the thirteen known loci would identify 10% of women with a relative risk of 1.55 or greater, which corresponds to a 10 year risk of 2.3% at age 40." Appropriately, he then notes that there "are, of course, many issues and questions that need to be addressed before such an approach became standard practice." For the foreseeable future, genetic screening will be a management tool most appropriate in the clinic, rather than the population and not really a useful way to undertake widespread screening.
5. Chapter 7 moves towards a more comprehensive theoretical basis for further thinking about cancer, arguing that progression can be usefully characterized as somatic evolution. Therefore, Maley et al. argue further, prevention (perhaps even therapy?) becomes an exercise in purposefully changing the selection pressures on clones of pre-cancer cells to prevent or delay progression. They note

(as have others – see the section on chemoprevention below), that some attempts at chemoprevention have been diametrically counterproductive. They describe a well thought-out approach both to better characterizing the nature of somatic evolution and to developing strategies and agents to push selection in a different direction or deny any selective advantage to the pre-cancer cells: they propose, among other steps, identifying (epi)genetic causes of resistance and testing for them prior to intervention; developing markers for the forms of (epi)genetic instability that tend to generate resistance to the intervention; and intervening prior to genomic instability. They promote the idea of using multiple agents as a proper approach to the problem of malignant clonal selection by agents designed to be beneficial. To date, there are few empirical data to support the utility of this approach, but it has the advantage of being consistent with much wider aspects of biology and of explaining data that many others are ignoring. It needs testing thoroughly. The authors note: "Finally, we should develop cancer prevention interventions with the goal of preventing, channeling or managing somatic evolution. Because somatic evolution is at the heart of neoplastic progression, it must be at the heart of how we manage the disease."

6. Finally, "-omics" approaches to the biology of cancer have been employed to understand progression, to classify tumours to predict response to therapy, and to develop markers of risk, progression, prognosis, and recurrence. In Chap. 6, Busuttil and Boussioutas describe this field as involving large-scale network analysis of biologic processes (for example, genetic variants, gene expression, proteins, signalling pathways, metabolic processes). In pursuit of early detection markers, studies of cancer are increasingly giving way to studies of pre-cancer. Success to date has been, at best, modest. The chapter is particularly important because it captures at least 2 issues, one technical, one design, that plague the studies in this area. The authors note that sample preparation is often poorly carried out – and, one might add, often differentially carried out, so that cases and controls are almost certain to show differences [13]. They note: "Improper tissue collection and storage may compromise RNA and/or DNA integrity and may result in poor quality data." The design issue is one which is discussed above, but their succinct summary of it is worth repeating: "A major criticism that we have, of several publications reviewed during the process of preparing this chapter, is the number of studies involving small numbers of samples." They briefly spoil this key insight by then confusing observations and experiments [14] but they are right that study size is a central problem (perhaps *the* central problem) across the whole field of early detection.

There is no chapter on the role of stroma and tissue organization per se (although some authors address it in passing (for example, see Chaps. 5, 7 and 16) but that area too, has added greatly to what we know [15]. Nonetheless, at present, these various aspects of cancer biology (stem cells, inflammation, epigenetics, genetics, clonal selection, "-omics", stroma) remain to be integrated into a unified theory and this, in turn, hampers our capacity to identify, visualize, treat, and prevent the early lesions that give rise to clinical cancer.

How will we Develop, Test, and Use New Screening Tests?

Some new techniques that show promise were discussed in Parts 1 and 2. Tissue, blood, and body fluids can provide the material to explore an extensive range of biomarkers using expression, proteins, metabolites etc (see Chap. 9). Because all indications are that a global screen for cancer is unlikely in the near future, our primary concern is what is happening in the tissue of interest (of interest for reasons other than symptoms, in the case of population screening). However, many tissues, as we have already noted, are not readily accessible. Hence the interest in surrogate tissues; for example, is a buccal swab in smokers useful for describing what is happening at cell and tissue level in the lung or larynx? The value of blood and urine is that they are, respectively a fluid that has been everywhere and its ultrafiltrate. They are thus, jointly, a resource that carries discarded cells and cell products, a vast range of metabolites, nutrients, etc., as well as immune and blood cells. We are, nonetheless, currently poorly equipped to fully exploit these resources: for cell-focussed assays, we remain ignorant about how large many tumours have to be before there are detectable numbers of cells – and whether that occurs before the cancer is detectable by other means; for proteins, metabolites, etc., the comparable problem is concentration; for both, there is the question of timing and time-interval for screening to be cost-effective. As an interesting place to look, it seems worthwhile to ask whether there are multiplier phenomena such that small concentrations of an abnormal metabolite provide a readable magnified signal in the immune system or in an endocrine response.

The advantage of DNA or RNA as screening substrates (genetics, epigenetics, expression) is having four bases in essentially equal proportions in the setting of rather uniform structures. Proteins, in contrast, show extensive structural variation and a dynamic range across about 12 orders of magnitude. Given the pathophysiologic variation within and between humans and within and between stages of disease, an ensemble of markers looks most attractive as a concept (e.g., a positive first-stage test is one where three out of five markers of interest are positive – this works as a diagnostic classifier e.g., in colorectal cancer to define micro-satellite instability) but remains elusive in practice for screening, not least because there are very few single markers with appropriate characteristics that could be concatenated into an ensemble for any cancer. And for every marker, we need a defined series of increasingly large studies to establish its utility in practice [3], (see also Chap. 9).

Another approach that attempts to encompass the whole organ (like direct visualization and less indirectly than using biomarkers) is the use of imaging (see Chap. 10). At its simplest, this is an X-ray technique, such as mammography but there are an increasing number of ways to enhance metabolic, chemical, and physical signals in order to detect static or dynamic pathophysiologic changes in tissue that may be the hallmarks of an early lesion. In this regard, it is worth considering an important lesson from mammography: mammographic density is itself a (heritable) marker of breast cancer risk [16], but this is an empirical observation without any substantial theoretical explanation for its capacity to predict disease. In the absence of a comprehensive theory on what exactly we should look for, in order to image, say, an early pancreas, lung, or ovary lesion, we are likely to make slow progress. Again, some empirical findings will get us started (tissue anoxia, the Warburg effect, tissue density) but a more complete theory would be better.

All such tests must eventually prove to be sensitive (a high capacity to identify those with disease), specific (a high capacity to exclude those without disease). Screening tests always identify some individuals who are, in fact, without disease (false positives) and, in the case of cancer screening, these people suffer distress as they go through further diagnostic procedures. The most important issue, however, is to minimize the number of those who, in fact, have disease but are screen-negative (false negatives). These are always the most poorly served in a screening programme. In practice, there is always a trade-off between sensitivity and specificity and, with an effective screening tool, the cut point will be driven by considerations of cost. If we are to have an extensive capacity to detect many cancers early, there will have to be further technical developments across a variety of screening modalities.

Chemoprevention

Imagine for a moment that we can solve the problem of how to identify true precursors of clinical cancer, the eradication of which would have important consequences for both the quality and duration of a patient's life; that is, imagine that we can detect an early cancer or pre-cancer not only with high sensitivity, but also with high specificity. From that position, we could then treat those with real disease and be sure that the vast majority of those who are negative on a screening test are truly disease-free.

How can we manage these true early lesions that we identify with sensitivity, specificity, and precision? For some lesions, the choice is easy: we are already able to remove many early colorectal, breast, skin, and cervical lesions surgically or with topical treatment. And, with many of these interventions, even the risks of over-treatment are modest. However multiple, diffuse disease (oral leukoplakia, Barrett's oesophagus, ulcerative colitis, diffuse multifocal pre-neoplastic disease of breast, even of pancreas) are much more difficult to treat definitively and require regular surveillance and intermittent surgical or topical therapy, at least until we learn how to reverse the underlying process.

Chemoprevention, a clinical analogue of public-health prevention strategies, is often proposed (see Chap. 11) as a method of reducing cancer incidence and mortality but has a wider context in possibly lowering risk of other chronic diseases. Chemoprevention has had some successes but a number of highly visible failures; failures, in this context, encompass not only null results but, more crucially, a finding of harm when the agent was specifically hypothesized to protect or reduce risk.

Maley et al., in Chap. 7, allude to this and provide some data but, in a recent invited AACR presentation [17], I detailed a more comprehensive catalogue of deleterious consequences and the differences from study settings in which chemoprevention was successful, specifically:

1. The β-carotene trials showed that not only does supplemental high-dose β-carotene not reduce cancer incidence, it increases risk in high-risk groups (ATBC [18, 19]). As I noted when the results were published [20], "A null answer to the chemoprevention question can mean: good hypothesis, good science, but wrong agent. An increase in risk, however, strongly suggests that the [theory], not the agent, is wrong." Subsequently, it has been shown that β-carotene supplementation is not only deleterious, but it actually attenuates the protective effects of vegetables and fruits on lung cancer risk in the very population in which one of the trials was carried out [21].
2. Classic NSAIDs provide chemopreventive benefit against metachronous adenomatous polyps [22, 23] but colorectal cancer reduction is not consistently seen and shows sex differences, with effectiveness against CRC in men perhaps [24] but not in women [25]. Although aspirin is beneficial in heart disease, GI bleeding remains a concern in relation to widespread use as a cancer preventive. Finally, specific COX-2 inhibitors are not appropriate in low-risk individuals or the general population because of their serious cardiovascular consequences [26–28].
3. Folate prevents neural-tube defects and almost certainly prevents early-stage or early-life colon lesions as the epidemiology consistently shows. However, folate promotes even early-stage lesions in polyp formers as the clinical-trial data show [29]. In this regard, there are relevant animal experiments and, of course, it has been long established that anti-folates are excellent chemotherapeutic agents [30]. Further, this same trial showed an excess of prostate cancer in the active (folate) arm compared with placebo [31]. In all three of these cases — β-carotene, NSAIDs, folate — there are deleterious consequences as a result of agents that were thought to be generally benign and hypothesized to be specifically effective against cancer; and in all three cases, deleterious consequences arose in the setting of attempts at single-agent chemoprevention.
4. Vitamins C and E, for instance, generally show neither beneficial nor deleterious consequences for cancer in populations where nutrition levels are adequate. However, in a deficient population, use of specific supplements has been shown to have clear benefits, including cancer prevention [32], when used in combinations not as single agents, and in doses designed to overcome known deficiency not at supra-physiologic levels, as has been the case in many of the other trials of chemoprevention.
5. There is an extensive body of literature – epidemiologic, animal experimental, small-scale human mechanistic trials, and large-scale clinical trials – pointing towards a protective role for calcium (particularly in the presence of adequate vitamin D) in colorectal neoplasia [33, 34]. However, there is some concern that it may not be beneficial for prostate cancer [35].

6. Sex steroid hormones were hypothesized in 1980 to reduce risk of colon cancer [36]. In 1983, we showed that oral contraceptives were associated with lower risk of colon cancer [37] and subsequently that post-menopausal hormones (PMH) were associated with reduced risk of colorectal adenomas [38]. In 2004, almost a quarter century after the original hypothesis, it was shown in a well conducted clinical trial, that PMH prevents CRC [39]. However, in the interim, it had been shown, in the same clinical trial, that PMH was deleterious for breast cancer [40] and even for coronary heart disease [41]. Naturally occurring soy estrogens may be effective against breast cancer when consumed in low doses in food and from an early age, at least as early as adolescence, but not later in life [42].
7. The problem of chemoprevention is not confined to cancer: there have also been deleterious outcomes from the use of single agents against heart disease and this casts light on the problem of primitive thinking about chemoprevention generally. Rosiglitazone is a PPAR-γ agonist that has been used to control diabetes but the pseudo-physiologic reasoning that reducing high levels of glycated hemoglobin will improve health outcomes was proved false as patients treated in this way had substantial increases in myocardial infarction and death from cardiovascular causes [43]. These findings that were late in the life of the drug and elicited strong condemnation [44].
8. Nonetheless, some single agents have beneficial effects, e.g., statins lower risk of both heart disease [45] and prostate cancer [46] and tamoxifen is clearly beneficial in preventing ER+ breast cancer, particularly in women with a prior history but may increase ER- contralateral cancers [47]. It seems likely that these agents may work as a result of having pleiotropic effects, interdicting more than one pathway and thus acting like a multi-agent intervention. As noted above, multi-agent interventions work against cancer, particularly in deficient populations. Furthermore, diet (low-dose and multi-agent by necessity) and exercise interventions reduce the risk of several cancers – again consistent with the notion that multiple strategies, and multiple agents in physiologic doses, can be effective.

As often as possible, chemotherapy in the treatment of cancer involves multiple agents in order to prevent clonal selection. We need to ask what light this long and successful experience (especially in the treatment of childhood cancer) sheds on the theory and practice of chemoprevention. Do we even have a theory that underpins chemoprevention? Do we need to reconsider the whole enterprise? For early detection to be effective, we need a strategy to prevent, not enhance, progression. As a research and practice community, there is much for us to do.

References

1. Etzioni R, Penson DF, Legler JM, di Tommaso D, Boer R et al (2002) Overdiagnosis due to prostate-specific antigen screening: lessons from U.S. prostate cancer incidence trends. J Natl Cancer Inst 94(13):981–990
2. Zahl PH, Strand BH, Maehlen J (2004) Incidence of breast cancer in Norway and Sweden during introduction of nationwide screening: prospective cohort study. BMJ 328(7445): 921–924

3. Pepe MS, Etzioni R, Feng Z, Potter JD, Thornquist MD et al (2001) Phases of biomarker development for early detection of cancer. J Natl Cancer Inst 93:1054–1061
4. Subramanian S, Bobashev G, Morris RJ (2009) Modeling the cost-effectiveness of colorectal cancer screening: policy guidance based on patient preferences and compliance. Cancer Epidemiology Biomarkers Prev 18(7):1971–1978
5. Bissell MJ, Labarge MA (2005) Context, tissue plasticity, and cancer: are tumor stem cells also regulated by the microenvironment? Cancer Cell 7(1):17–23
6. Potter JD (2007) Morphogens, morphostats, microarchitecture and malignancy. Nat Rev Cancer 7(6):464–474
7. Palmer C, Duan X, Hawley S, Scholler N, Thorpe JD et al (2008) Systematic evaluation of candidate blood markers for detecting ovarian cancer. PLoS One 3(7):e2633
8. Henschke CI, Yankelevitz DF, Libby DM, Pasmantier MW, Smith JP et al (2006) Survival of patients with stage I lung cancer detected on CT screening. N Engl J Med 355(17):1763–1771
9. Hingorani SR, Petricoin EF, Maitra A, Rajapakse V, King C et al (2003) Preinvasive and invasive ductal pancreatic cancer and its early detection in the mouse. Cancer Cell 4(6):437–450
10. Hingorani SR, Wang L, Multani AS, Combs C, Deramaudt TB et al (2005) Trp53R172H and KrasG12D cooperate to promote chromosomal instability and widely metastatic pancreatic ductal adenocarcinoma in mice. Cancer Cell 7(5):469–483
11. Izeradjene K, Combs C, Best M, Gopinathan A, Wagner A et al (2007) Kras(G12D) and Smad4/Dpc4 haploinsufficiency cooperate to induce mucinous cystic neoplasms and invasive adenocarcinoma of the pancreas. Cancer Cell 11(3):229–243
12. Bach PB (2008) Is our natural-history model of lung cancer wrong? Lancet Oncol 9(7):693–697
13. Petricoin EF, Ardekani AM, Hitt BA, Levine PJ, Fusaro VA et al (2002) Use of proteomic patterns in serum to identify ovarian cancer. Lancet 359(9306):572–577
14. Potter JD (2001) At the interfaces of epidemiology, genetics, and genomics. Nat Rev Genet 2:142–147
15. Bissell MJ, Radisky D (2001) Putting tumours in context. Nat Rev Cancer 1:46–54
16. Vachon CM, Sellers TA, Carlson EE, Cunningham JM, Hilker CA et al (2007) Strong evidence of a genetic determinant for mammographic density, a major risk factor for breast cancer. Cancer Res 67(17):8412–8418
17. Potter J (2009) Chemoprevention: why do we keep getting it wrong? Presentation for 2009 AACR-American Cancer Society Award for Research Excellence in Cancer Epidemiology and Prevention, 100th AACR Meeting, Denver CO
18. Cancer Prevention Study Group ATBC (1994) The effect of vitamin E and beta carotene on the incidence of lung cancer and other cancers in male smokers. N Engl J Med 330:1029–1035
19. Omenn G, Goodman G, Thornquist M, Balmes J, Cullen M et al (1996) Effects of a combination of beta carotene and vitamin A on lung cancer and cardiovascular disease. N Engl J Med 334:1150–1155
20. Potter JD (1996) Chemoprevention: pharmacology or biology? Oncology 10:1487–1488
21. Neuhouser ML, Patterson RE, Thornquist MD, Omenn GS, King IB et al (2003) Fruits and vegetables are associated with lower lung cancer risk only in the placebo arm of the beta-carotene and retinol efficacy trial (CARET). Cancer Epidemiol Biomarkers Prev 12(4):350–358
22. Baron JA, Cole BF, Sandler RS, Haile RW, Ahnen D et al (2003) A randomized trial of aspirin to prevent colorectal adenomas. N Engl J Med 348(10):891–899
23. Sandler RS, Halabi S, Baron JA, Budinger S, Paskett E et al (2003) A randomized trial of aspirin to prevent colorectal adenomas in patients with previous colorectal cancer. N Engl J Med 348(10):883–890
24. Flossmann E, Rothwell PM (2007) Effect of aspirin on long-term risk of colorectal cancer: consistent evidence from randomised and observational studies. Lancet 369(9573):1603–1613

25. Cook NR, Lee IM, Gaziano JM, Gordon D, Ridker PM et al (2005) Low-dose aspirin in the primary prevention of cancer: the Women's Health Study: a randomized controlled trial. JAMA 294(1):47–55
26. Arber N, Eagle CJ, Spicak J, Racz I, Dite P et al (2006) Celecoxib for the prevention of colorectal adenomatous polyps. N Engl J Med 355(9):885–895
27. Bertagnolli MM, Eagle CJ, Zauber AG, Redston M, Solomon SD et al (2006) Celecoxib for the prevention of sporadic colorectal adenomas. N Engl J Med 355(9):873–884
28. Psaty BM, Potter JD (2006) Risks and benefits of celecoxib to prevent recurrent adenomas. New Engl J Med 355(9):950–952
29. Cole BF, Baron JA, Sandler RS, Haile RW, Ahnen DJ et al (2007) Folic acid for the prevention of colorectal adenomas: a randomized clinical trial. JAMA 297(21):2351–2359
30. Ulrich CM, Potter JD (2007) Folate and cancer – timing is everything. JAMA 297(21):2408–2409
31. Figueiredo JC, Grau MV, Haile RW, Sandler RS, Summers RW et al (2009) Folic acid and risk of prostate cancer: results from a randomized clinical trial. J Natl Cancer Inst 101(6):432–435
32. Qiao Y-L, Dawsey SM, Kamangar F, Fan J-H, Abnet CC et al (2009) Total and cancer mortality after supplementation with vitamins and minerals: follow-up of the Linxian general population nutrition intervention trial. J Natl Cancer Inst 101(7):507–518
33. Baron JA, Beach M, Mandel JS, van Stolk RU, Haile RW et al (1999) Calcium supplements for the prevention of colorectal adenomas. N Engl J Med 340:101–107
34. Grau MV, Baron JA, Sandler RS, Haile RW, Beach ML et al (2003) Vitamin D, calcium supplementation, and colorectal adenomas: results of a randomized trial. J Natl Cancer Inst 95(23):1765–1771
35. Kristal AR, Cohen JH, Qu P, Stanford JL (2002) Associations of energy, fat, calcium, and vitamin D with prostate cancer risk. Cancer Epidemiology Biomarkers Prev 11(8):719–725
36. McMichael AJ, Potter JD (1980) Reproduction, endogenous and exogenous sex hormones, and colon cancer: a review and hypothesis. J Natl Cancer Inst 65(6):1201–1207
37. Potter J, McMichael A (1983) Large bowel cancer in women in relation to reproductive and hormonal factors: a case-control study. J Natl Cancer Inst 4:703–709
38. Potter JD, Bostick RM, Grandits GA, Fosdick L, Elmer P et al (1996) Hormone replacement therapy is associated with lower risk of adenomatous polyps of the large bowel: the Minnesota Cancer Prevention Research Unit Case-Control Study. Cancer Epidemiol Biomarkers Prev 5(10):779–784
39. Chlebowski RT, Wactawski-Wende J, Ritenbaugh C, Hubbell FA, Ascensao J et al (2004) Estrogen plus progestin and colorectal cancer in postmenopausal women. N Engl J Med 350(10):991–1004
40. Chlebowski RT, Hendrix SL, Langer RD, Stefanick ML, Gass M et al (2003) Influence of estrogen plus progestin on breast cancer and mammography in healthy postmenopausal women: the Women's Health Initiative Randomized Trial. JAMA 289(24):3243–3253
41. Manson JE, Hsia J, Johnson KC, Rossouw JE, Assaf AR et al (2003) Estrogen plus progestin and the risk of coronary heart disease. N Engl J Med 349(6):523–534
42. Shu XO, Jin F, Dai Q, Wen W, Potter JD et al (2001) Soyfood Intake during adolescence and subsequent risk of breast cancer among Chinese women. Cancer Epidemiology Biomarkers Prev 10(5):483–488
43. Nissen SE, Wolski K (2007) Effect of rosiglitazone on the risk of myocardial infarction and death from cardiovascular causes. N Engl J Med 356(24):2457–2471
44. Psaty BM, Furberg CD (2007) Rosiglitazone and cardiovascular risk. N Engl J Med 356(24):2522–2524
45. Ridker PM, Danielson E, Fonseca FAH, Genest J, Gotto AM Jr et al (2008) Rosuvastatin to prevent vascular events in men and women with elevated C-reactive protein. N Engl J Med 359(21):2195–2207
46. Platz EA (2007) Epidemiologic musing on statin drugs in the prevention of advanced prostate cancer. Cancer Epidemiology Biomarkers Prev 16(11):2175–2180
47. Li CI, Malone KE, Weiss NS, Daling JR (2001) Tamoxifen therapy for primary breast cancer and risk of contralateral breast cancer. J Natl Cancer Inst 93(13):1008–1113

Index

H

I

Kolibri 360 GmbH
Ferdinand-Jühlke-Straße 7
99095 Erfurt, Deutschland
produktsicherheit@kolibri360.de